FOURTH EDITION

HEARING IN CHILDREN

FOURTH EDITION

Hearing in Children

Jerry L. Northern, Ph.D.

Professor
Department of Otolaryngology/Pediatrics
University of Colorado
School of Medicine
Denver, Colorado

Head
Audiology Services
University Hospital
Denver, Colorado

Marion P. Downs, Dr.H.S.

Professor Emerita
Department of Otolaryngology
University of Colorado
School of Medicine
Denver, Colorado

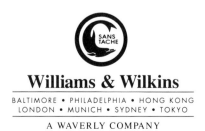

Williams & Wilkins

BALTIMORE • PHILADELPHIA • HONG KONG
LONDON • MUNICH • SYDNEY • TOKYO

A WAVERLY COMPANY

Editor: John P. Butler
Associate Editor: Linda Napora
Copy Editor: Dana Knighten
Designer: Norman Och
Illustration Planner: Lorraine Wrzosek
Production Coordinator: Raymond E. Reter

Copyright © 1991
Williams & Wilkins
428 East Preston Street
Baltimore, MD 21202, U.S.A.

Accurate indications, adverse reactions, and dosage schedules for drugs are provided in this book, but it is possible that they may change. The reader is urged to review the package information data of the manufacturers of the medications mentioned.

Printed in the United States of America

First Edition 1974
Second Edition 1978
Third Edition 1984

Library of Congress Cataloging-in-Publication Data

Northern, Jerry L.
    Hearing in children / Jerry L. Northern, Marion P. Downs. — 4th ed.
      p. cm.
    Includes bibliographical references and index.
    ISBN 0-683-06574-2
    1. Hearing disorders in children. I. Title.
    [DNLM: 1. Hearing Disorders—in infancy & childhood. 2. Hearing
Tests—in infancy & childhood. WV 271 N874h]
RF291.5.C45N67   1991
618.92′0978—dc20
DNLM/DLC
for Library of Congress   90-13107
                                           CIP

94 95
5 6 7 8 9 10

Preface
to the Fourth Edition

The 6-year period since publication of the Third Edition of *Hearing in Children* has been absolutely explosive in terms of new technological developments in the diagnosis and management of hearing-impaired children. The new publications and articles on hearing in children have been prolific. It is a testimony to this progress that little of the original material in the earliest editions of *Hearing in Children* is present in this new edition.

With each new edition of *Hearing in Children*, we have deleted dated material as we added current information, thereby maintaining the reasonable size of this textbook. For example, we dropped nearly 300 references from the bibliography (primarily those works written before 1972) while adding more than 280 new references in this Fourth Edition. Every chapter has been reviewed and rewritten or revised.

The reader will find new material on the controversial relationship of otitis media to hearing, speech and language development, new medical findings related to cytomegalovirus, meningitis, perilymph fistula, and persistent fetal circulation disorder. Our introductory chapter has been revised completely for readers who are new to the field of pediatric audiology. The hearing aid chapter, also reorganized and greatly updated, now includes discussions of real-ear measurements in pediatric hearing aid fittings, as well as details about the growing use of cochlear implants in deaf children. The chapter on hearing screening includes the newest hearing screening protocols for all age groups of children; the 1990 Joint Committee Position Statement for Infant and Newborn Hearing Screening is also included.

Of major significance since the publication of the last edition of *Hearing in Children* has been the change in status of my good friend and coauthor, Marion P. Downs. Dr. Downs is now Professor Emerita, having reached that pinnacle known as "retirement." As those of you who know her can attest, "retirement" has little relation to the activity level demonstrated by this grand lady as she pursues an only slightly diminished professional life, with somewhat more time and emphasis on tennis, travel, skiing, her great-grandchildren, and continuation of her own projects. Her influence on this new edition is clear; however, for better or worse, the actual responsibility for this fourth edition of *Hearing in Children* is now in my hands.

J.L.N.

Acknowledgments

First Edition. A book of this magnitude cannot be assembled and written without the help of many other people. We would like to pay special tribute and thanks to five of our colleagues and good friends who gave graciously of their valuable time and personal material for our benefit—LaVonne Bergstrom, M.D.; Isamu Sando, M.D.; Janet M. Stewart, M.D.; Marlin Weaver, M.D.; and Winfield McChord, Jr., M.S.

Many others responded to our needs, willingly and unselfishly, to provide requested information at a moment's notice: Carol Amon, M.A.; Owen Black, M.D.; Carol Cox, M.A.; Kathleen O. Foust, M.A.; William K. Frankenberg, M.D.; W. G. Hemenway, M.D.; Brian Hersch, M.D.; Aram Glorig, M.D.; Mrs. Page T. Jenkins; Darrel Teter, Ph.D.; Pat Tesauro, M.A.; and Harold Weber, M.A. Connie H. Knight, M.A., Audiologist at the Georgia Retardation Center, Atlanta, was our Research Associate and gathered much of the material presented in the "Index of Selected Birth Defect Syndromes," Sharon Mraz was out Editorial Assistant. Patricia Jenkins Thompson, M.A., diligently proofread and critiqued our efforts.

Y. Oishi, M.D., served as our primary photographer, Miriam Eliachar illustrated the chapter pictures and embryology figures; and Anita McGuire typed the entire manuscript. We would also like to acknowledge the cooperation of the publishing staff at Williams & Wilkins, especially William R. Hensyl who encouraged us to write this textbook.

And finally, we would like to extend our appreciation and thanks to our spouses, families, children, and friends, who will long remember (as will we!) this period of time during which we were too busy, too preoccupied, or too tired—our Year of the Book, 1973.

Second Edition. Once again numerous colleagues came to our aid to provide advice, share materials, and labor in the libraries to help prepare this Second Edition of *Hearing in Children.* We would like to express our warmest thanks to Jeff Adams, Marlin Cohrs, Roni Halpern, Donna Lutz, Winfield McChord, Deborah Smith, Steven Staller, Darrel Teter, Harold Weber, and Janet Zarnoch. We are particularly grateful for the contributions of Mrs. Kathleen Bryant, Speech Pathologist at the University of Colorado Medical Center. Patsy Tormey, our helpful secretary, typed the manuscript and quietly tolerated our many revisions. Ruby Richardson at Williams & Wilkins nudged us gently, but firmly, throughout this revision. And finally, we appreciate the helpful comments and critique provided by our professional friends who took time to respond to a lengthy questionnaire regarding the first edition. Their guidance and suggestions have greatly influenced this second edition of *Hearing in Children.*

Third Edition. We are again grateful to a new cadre of friends, students, and associates who have responded to our requests for help with this third edition. We would like to thank David Asher, James R. Curran, Sandra Abbott Gabbard, Marianne Geisler, Christine Gerhardt, Kathryn Grose, Katherine Pike Gerkin, Deanie

Johnson, Deborah Kinder, Sharon A. Mitchell, Patrick Sullivan, M.D., and Ann Wilson. Patsy Tormey-Meredith typed the new manuscripts again, but this time during maternity leave. We were delighted to work again with William R. Hensyl, of Williams & Wilkins, who was the original perpetrator of *Hearing in Children*.

Fourth Edition. We are indebted to many of our colleagues for their supportive efforts. Especially helpful through their review, critical commentary, and useful suggestions were: Julia M. Davis, Judith S. Gravel, Sandy Friel-Patti, M. Suzanne Hasenstab, Deborah Hayes, John and Claire Jacobson, Susan Jerger, Robert W. Keith, and Laszlo Stein. We thank them for their time and effort. And, once again, we are most thankful to our ever-dependable secretary/friend Patsy Tormey-Meredith, for bearing with us again in typing (and retyping) the manuscript. A special thanks is extended to the University Hospital audiology staff for their patience, understanding and support during the many months spent preparing this new Edition.

Contents

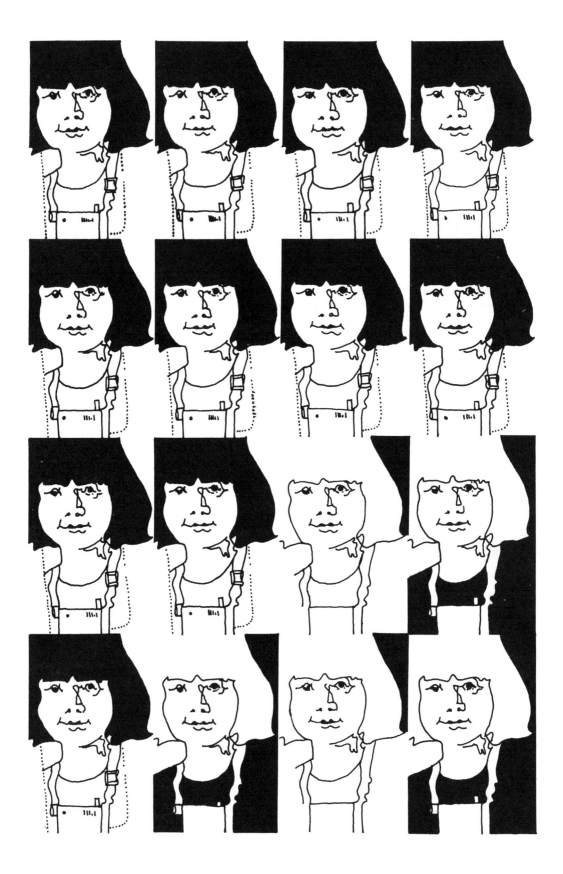

CHAPTER 1

Hearing and Hearing Loss in Children

Long ago the function of hearing became the building stone upon which our intricate human communication system was constructed. If predawn man had not inherited an ear, he might have resorted instead to signing with his fingers or scratching marks upon the sand to share his thoughts with others. The result would have been an awkward method of communication that could have slowed, for millennia, our so-called progress. For good or bad, we have developed the ear and the vocal mechanism as the media through which language is customarily learned and communicated. An illustration of the interdependence of the ear and speech is found in the direct relationship between the frequencies that make speech intelligible and the differential sensitivity of the human ear. The human ear is most sensitive precisely at the frequencies of speech. The question of which of these factors came first is an ontogenic mystery no one has yet solved.

The structure of language is unique to *Homo sapiens*, although experimenters have demonstrated that signed symbols and other visual language forms can be taught to chimpanzees and believe that the beginnings of true language are evidenced in these primates (Gardner and Garner, 1969; Premack and Premack, 1972; Savage-Rumbaugh et al., 1980). Other investigators insist that the conceptual system learned by these primates is not linguistic; i.e., they (the primates) do not "think in words"; instead they use a signalization system that is far removed from the higher symbolization and syntax of human language (Terrace et al., 1979).

But neither group would question that between the laboriously learned signal response of the chimpanzee and the first voluntary sentence of the 18 month old baby lies "a whole day of creation" (Langer, 1957).

The human baby appears to be born with "preexistent knowledge" of language—specialized neural structures in the brain that await auditory experience with language to trigger them into functioning. These structures are dependent on auditory stimulation for their emergence, providing of course that other developmental factors are normal.

The auditory-linked acquisition of language is further unique to human beings because it is a time-locked function related to early maturational periods in the infant's life. The longer auditory language stimulation is delayed, the less efficient will be the language facility. The reason is that critical periods exist for the development of biologic functions, and language is one of the biologic functions of humans (Chomsky, 1966; Lenneberg, 1967). A baby who is deprived of appropriate language stimulation during this first 2 or 3 years of life will never fully attain his or her best potential language function, whether the deprivation is from lack of hearing or from lack of high-quality language experience.

It is for these reasons that it is urgent to attack the hearing problems of children with all the skill, knowledge and insights of which we are capable. The prevention of hearing loss in children protects the right of children to their essential humanity, which lies in optimal language function.

EARLY IDENTIFICATION OF HEARING PROBLEMS IN CHILDREN

Hearing loss in children is a silent, hidden handicap: it is hidden because children, especially infants and toddlers, cannot tell us that they are not hearing well; it is a handicap because, if undetected and untreated, hearing loss in children can lead to delayed speech and language development, social and emotional problems, and academic failure. It is unnecessary for a child to suffer these consequences. By detecting hearing loss as early as possible, even as young as the newborn period, effective treatment, which significantly reduces the handicap of hearing loss, can be applied. All too often, however, identification of a child's hearing loss is delayed because parents are unaware that any child, even a newborn infant, can receive an accurate hearing test. Unfortunately, routine medical care seldom includes the simple hearing evaluation that could identify those children with hearing loss (American Academy of Audiology, 1989).

The problem of hearing loss in children is significant if we consider the following facts:

- One child in 1000 is born with profound deafness.

- An additional 2 children in 1000 will acquire deafness in early childhood.

- Infants who need intensive medical care during the newborn period are at special risk for hearing loss, resulting in 1 child in 50 from intensive care nurseries being hearing impaired.

- Ear infection, the most common infectious disease of childhood, is associated with hearing loss.

- Nearly 100% of all children will develop some period of hearing loss related to ear infections during the period from birth through 11 years of age.

- Ten percent to 15% of children who receive hearing screening at school fail because they cannot hear within normal limits.

During 1989, the United States federal government accepted a new commitment aimed at reducing the harmful effects of childhood hearing loss. In a statement released by the United States Public Health Service, the former Surgeon General C. Everett Koop, M.D., observed that Helen Keller, who was born without sight or hearing, often said that she regretted her deafness more than her blindness. A portion of Dr. Koop's statement regarding his belief that early identification of hearing problems in children is essential is presented below:

Deafness in infants is a serious concern because it interferes with the development of language—that which sets humans apart from all other living things. The longer a child's deafness goes undiscovered, the worse the outcome is likely to be. Language remediation, which is what specialists call the process of teaching hearing-impaired children to communicate, must begin as early as possible, because language develops so rapidly in the first few months of life. For example, by 6 weeks, a normally hearing infant is more attracted to human speech than to any other sound. A 6-month-old baby already has an ability to analyze language—to break it down into its parts—to put those parts back together again and to store language in its brain and retrieve it. By 18 months, most children are producing simple sentences.

Fortunately, many of the negative results of deafness in babies can be prevented or substantially lessened. Many research studies have demonstrated that early intervention with hearing-impaired children results in improved language development, increased academic success and increased lifetime earnings. Early intervention actually saves money, since hearing-impaired children who receive early help require less costly special education services later.

If it is to be effective, early intervention with deaf children should begin before the child's first birthday. Unfortunately, we are not doing a very good job of detecting infant deafness in the United States. A recent report to Congress and the President by the Commission on Education of the Deaf pointed out that the average age at which profoundly deaf children in this country are identified is 2½ years. In contrast, the average age at which such children are identified in Israel and Great Britain is 7 to 9 months.

Clearly, we must do a much better job of early identification if we are to reduce the unnecessary suffering, poor educational performance and lack of productivity that so often accompany deafness. Three groups of people must work together.

Parents are in the best position to identify their child's hearing difficulties. We need to do a better job of making parents aware of the danger signals and of the sources of help that are available to them.

Physicians need to become more responsive to parents' concerns about their child's hearing. Too often, those concerns are brushed aside or ignored. Yet, a recent study found that parents of hearing-impaired children knew about their baby's hearing loss an average of 7 months before it was diagnosed and that almost half of them were given poor advice, such as "don't worry about it" or "wait until the child starts school," when they told their doctors about their concerns.

State agencies can help by initiating high-risk screening programs, such as those currently in operation in Utah, Colorado, Oklahoma, Tennessee and several other states. Research indicates that such programs are able to identify up to 75% of infants who are born deaf or with hearing impairments.

Many others can help too, of course, from older brothers and sisters to grandparents and babysitters. We in the federal government are committed to doing our part. The 1986 Education of the Deaf Act, which authorized the creation of the Commission on the Education of the Deaf, was a first step. At the National Institutes of Health, a new research institute, the National Institute of Deafness and Communication Disorders, has been authorized and is now in formation.

I am optimistic. I foresee a time in this country, in the near future, in fact, when no child reaches his or her first birthday with an undetected hearing impairment. It's a tall order, yes, but if we all work together, I believe we can fill it [C. Everett Koop, M.D., Surgeon General of the United States Public Health Service, Department of Health and Human Services, 1989].

According to the American Academy of Audiology (1989), more than 7000 professionally trained audiologists are available with appropriate skills and equipment to evaluate the hearing of any child at any age with a high degree of accuracy. The hearing of newborn infants can be tested by a sophisticated evoked potential technique, the auditory brainstem response, that accurately identifies even mild degrees of hearing loss; for children with a developmental age of 6 months or older hearing can be assessed by traditional behavioral procedures that permit identification of any degree of hearing loss. Once hearing loss is identified, medical or audiologic intervention can be initiated immediately. At the first sign of hearing loss, children, even newborn infants, should receive a formal audiologic evaluation by a properly accredited audiologist.

WHAT IS A HANDICAPPING HEARING LOSS?

It is first necessary to ask if there is a definition for hearing loss in children. At what point does hearing in children cease to be normal and become abnormal? This question has never been satisfactorily researched or resolved. The problem is that no one has adequately defined the parameters of a hearing handicap or described the best method of securing the necessary data for such definition. Thus it has been extremely difficult to estimate the prevalence of hearing handicaps, for unless there are agreed upon criteria, there is no way to determine the rate of occurrence. A review of governmental attempts to resolve this dilemma reveals the complexity of the problem.

The Health Examination Survey of the Department of Health, Education and Welfare undertook, in 1963–1970, to collect hearing data on a representative sample of children 6–11 years of age (Leske, 1981). Ear, nose, and throat examinations, audiologic tests, and a parental health questionnaire were given to a sample of the United States child population. The estimate of the prevalence of "hearing handicaps" was obtained from a parents' questionnaire, which inquired if their child had "trouble hearing?" An equivalent of 1 million children 6–11 years old (4%) was judged to be hearing handicapped on the basis of this question. Yet the audiometric hearing tests collected by the survey revealed fewer than 1% of the children to be handicapped, using a criterion of average loss (500–2000 Hz) of 26 dB hearing level (HL) as a beginning hear-

Table 1.1.
Distribution of Hearing Test Results in Children Ages 4–11 Years by Age: Community Sample, Selected Areas in Washington, D.C., 1971[a]

Hearing Test Result	Age of Child (% Distribution)				
	4–5 yr	6–7 yr	8–9 yr	10–11 yr	Total All Ages
Bilateral normal	76.2	78.8	84.8	84.8	81.1
Bilateral speech loss	4.1	1.7	1.1	1.9	2.2
Unilateral speech loss	5.1	4.6	3.7	4.5	4.5
Bilateral nonspeech loss	4.8	4.5	4.1	5.2	4.6
Unilateral nonspeech loss	9.7	10.4	6.2	3.7	7.6
Total	99.9	100.0	99.9	100.1	100.0
Total number	402	443	406	388	1639[b]

[a]From D.M. Kessner, C.K. Snow, and J. Singer: Assessment of medical care in children, Washington, D.C.: In: *Contrasts in Health Status*. National Academy of Sciences, 1974.
[b]Excludes 31 who could not be tested.

ing loss. The National Speech and Hearing Survey of 1968–1969 used the same criterion on a sample of children tested in grades 1–12 and found a prevalence of 0.73% (Hull et al., 1971).

On the ear examinations of the Health Examination Survey, the children found to have abnormalities of the eardrum were significantly more likely to have had trouble hearing as reported by their parents. Yet the hearing test findings showed small differences between those with normal and those with abnormal eardrum findings.

Evidently a credibility gap existed in the survey between what parents thought and what the government team decreed as hearing handicap. Either the parents misjudged their children's ability to hear, or the scientific criterion of adequacy was in error. Which was the case? Resolving this question is critical to the activities of schools, government agencies, and health facilities whose task it is to identify hearing loss in children.

A classic survey reported by Jordan and Eagles (1961) obtained otoscopic examinations and auditory thresholds on 4067 5–10 year old school children. They found that 6% of the children who could be examined otoscopically had bilateral, abnormal findings and 12% had unilateral abnormalities. Some 13% of the children could not be given otoscopic examination because of cerumen in the ear canal. When the individual

pathologies were compared with the threshold audiometry, it was found that 50% of the children with serous otitis media had hearing better than 15 dB HL. In other words, even a 15 dB HL screening criterion would have missed more than half of the children with serous otitis media. Another comparison revealed that of 30 children with dry perforations of the eardrum, 12 (40%) would have been missed by a 15 dB HL screening criterion.

These authors pointed out that audiometric screening—and even threshold audiometry—may not identify the majority of children with significant ear pathology. Does this mean that there is no relationship between ear disease and hearing loss? Most certainly not. It merely means that one of them has been incorrectly defined. Inasmuch as ear disease is an observable fact, while "hearing loss" is only a concept, the concept needs to be altered to fit the fact.

Kessner et al. (1974) for the National Academy of Sciences examined a sample numbering 1639 of the children in health agencies in the Washington, D.C. area, conducting audiometric studies on the 4–11 year old group. They chose as their criterion for a significant hearing loss the level of 15 dB or greater (500–2000 Hz). Their results are summarized in Table 1.1. This chart shows that 2.2% of the children had bilateral losses in the speech range (500–2000 Hz) of 15 dB or greater and 4.5% had

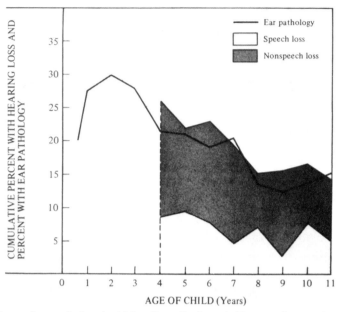

Figure 1.1. Prevalence of ear pathology in children 6 months through 11 years of age and prevalence of hearing loss by type of loss in children 4–11 years of age. (Reprinted with permission from D. M. Kessner, C. K. Snow, and F. Singer: Assessment of medical care in children. In: *Contrasts in Health Status*. Washington, D.C., National Academy of Sciences, 1974.)

unilateral losses in the speech range of 15 dB or greater, for a total of 6.7% with significant hearing losses in one ear or both ears. Most interesting is the fact that in a group of 4–5 year olds, 4.1% had significant hearing losses in both ears—a figure almost identical with that of the Health Examination Survey derived from the parents' questionnaire. In the Kessner study the mean threshold difference between those with the normal ears and those diagnosed as having serous otitis media were only 7.4 dB in the speech range. Children with normal ears had mean thresholds of 7.8 dB, while children with otitis media had mean thresholds of 15.2 dB.

The occurrence of both ear pathology and hearing loss is age-related in all studies of prevalence. Kessner's report demonstrated the relationship of both factors to age (Fig. 1.1). The rate of ear pathology peaks at age 2 with 30% abnormal ears and declines by age 11 to 15% abnormal ears. It can be seen that the age trend for hearing loss parallels that for ear pathology. Although no hearing data were obtained for children under age

4, the strong correlation between hearing loss and ear pathology in the 4–11 year olds led the authors to assume the same trend in the under 4 year old group. If one extrapolates from the data for the 4–11 year olds, it appears that 15% of the 2 year olds will have losses in the speech range greater than 15 dB in at least one ear. Further extrapolation from the Table 1.1 shows that one third of the total speech-range losses (4–11 years) are bilateral. Applying this rate to the children 2 years and under leaves 5% of these children with significant bilateral hearing loss.

This is not to say that unilateral hearing losses are innocuous. On the contrary, most clinical observers believe that unilateral losses are a great deal more handicapping than any available measure can show. A study by Boyd (1974) did demonstrate that 30% of a group of children with unilateral deafness but normal hearing in the other ear had a mean academic achievement lag of 1.12 years. Bess and Tharpe (1984) also found a significant effect of unilateral hearing loss on the educational, linguistic, and

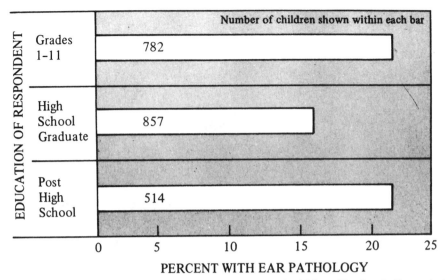

Figure 1.2. Education level of parents and prevalence of hearing loss in children. (Reprinted with permission from D. M. Kessner, C. K. Snow, and F. Singer: Assessment of medical care in children. In: *Contrasts in Health Status*. Washington, D.C., National Academy of Sciences, 1974.)

auditory perceptual development of children.

Other variables, besides ear disease and laterality, should be mentioned when looking at prevalence rates. One of the most interesting demographic findings in these large sample studies was that there were not the expected hearing loss differences between the various races. In fact, the Kessner study found the prevalence rates of both ear pathology and hearing loss to be almost twice as high in white children as in black children—a condition that may be unique to the Washington, D.C. area. The most consistent demographic association was the education level of parents: the higher the educational attainment, the lower the prevalence of hearing loss (Fig. 1.2). There is a lesser but significant association with family income: the higher the income, the lower the rate of hearing loss (Fig. 1.3).

Another demographic association was found in the National Health Survey between regions of the United States and hearing loss. Children living in the South had less sensitive hearing in the middle frequencies (for frequencies below 6000 Hz), with children living in the West having the most sensitive hearing in those frequencies (frequencies lower than 4000 Hz).

Minimal Criteria for Hearing Loss. The 1979 American Academy of Otolaryngology and American Council of Otolaryngology *Guide for the evaluation of hearing handicap* gives directions to compensation agencies for rating the percentage of hearing loss in industrial compensation and concerns adults only. Handicap is rated in terms of the ability to hear everyday speech in quiet and noise, but it is measured in terms of pure tone threshold. The average of the thresholds at 500, 1000, 2000, and 3000 Hz was thought to reflect a realistic degree of the understanding of speech in both quiet and noise. Although 3000 Hz was a new addition to the previous criteria, it was selected because of its importance to hearing speech in noise or when speech is distorted.

In the 1979 *Guide*, only hearing loss averages greater than 25 dB are considered handicapping for compensation rating. This "low-fence" value of 25 dB has been used for many years to evaluate the hearing of adults, with the inherent assumption, apparently, that adults do not experience

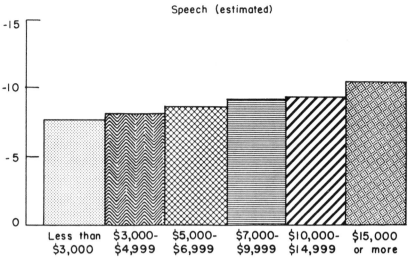

Speech (estimated)

Figure 1.3. Income level of parents and hearing levels of children. (Reprinted with permission from *Hearing Levels of Children by Demographic and Socioeconomic Characteristics*. Washington, D.C., United States, Department of Health, Education and Welfare, 1972.)

communication difficulties until their hearing impairment exceeds this value (average of thresholds from 500 to 3000 Hz). But how realistic is it to apply this low-fence value to children's hearing needs? It is our contention that children have a more critical need for hearing during their developmental and school years than adults require for the understanding of everyday speech. We believe strongly that 15 dB HL should be considered the lower limit of normal hearing for children and impairment begins with each decibel of hearing loss greater than 15 dB HL (Figs. 1.4 and 1.5).

For the adult, all the contextual strategies of interpreting speech have been firmly implanted. Indeed, an adult does not have to hear all of the speech sounds in order to put together the concept of what is said. Speech can be badly distorted or interrupted and still be intelligible to an adult. But a child who is just learning to interpret speech and language needs to hear acutely in order to develop the strategies necessary for his or her adult skills. Even infants must hear well if they are to lay the groundwork for later language skills.

Many people may question why a 15 dB loss may result in language delays. The reasons lie in the nature of speech sounds, with

the major amount of speech energy residing in the voiced vowels and consonants. The unvoiced consonants /s, p, t, k, th, f, sh/ contain so little speech energy that they often fall below even normal hearing thresh-

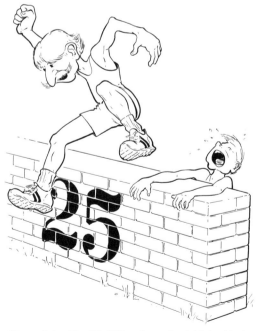

Figure 1.4. The 25 dB "low fence," established to define the beginning of hearing loss in adults, may be too severe to serve as the "low-fence" figure for children's hearing loss.

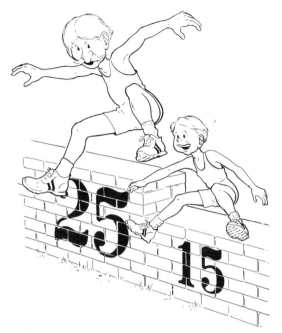

Figure 1.5. Normal hearing "low fence" for the beginning of hearing loss in children may be more appropriate at 15 dB HL because of their more critical need for hearing all the intricacies of speech.

olds in average rapid conversation as shown in Figure 1.6. Those of us who have learned speech and language know so well all the strategies for understanding speech in context that our brains can fill in automatically for the missing sounds. But the child or infant just learning speech relationships has a need to hear all sounds clearly in order to implant the perceptions solidly.

Skinner (1978) listed a number of liabilities to a child's language learning when a mild hearing loss exists:

- **Lack of Constancy of Auditory Clues When Acoustic Information Fluctuates.** When a child does not hear speech sounds in the same way from one time to another, there is a confusion in abstracting the meanings of words due to inconsistent categorization of speech sounds.

- **Confusion of Acoustic Parameters in Rapid Speech.** Even the normal hearing child suffers from variations of speech occurring between speakers and even in the same speaker. Frequency, duration, and intensity vary as a result of differences between speakers of age, sex, and personality. The child with mild hearing loss will be confused in language learning as a result.

- **Confusion in Segmentation and Prosody.** The child with a mild loss may miss linguistic boundaries such as plurals, tenses, intonation, and stress patterns. These factors are requisite to meaningful interpretation of speech.

- **Masking of Ambient Noise.** According to French and Steinberg (1947), the normal child required a signal-to-noise ratio of +30 dB at 200–6000 Hz in order for speech learning to take place. It is rare in our modern culture for such a ratio to be present. Public school classes have no better signal-to-noise ratio than +12 dB. A child with even mild loss is handicapped in such situations.

- **Breakdown of Early Ability to Perceive Speech Sounds.** Almost at birth the infant begins to learn to discriminate speech sounds. Studies have shown that at 1–4 months the infant can discriminate between most of the English speech sound pairs. By 6 months the infant recognizes many of the speech sounds of language and is making ongoing cataloging of speech sounds as discussed in Chapter 4. If these sounds are not perceived early, due to a hearing loss, learning can be impeded.

- **Breakdown in Early Perceptions of Meanings.** Often, during ordinary speech, the normal listener misses some unstressed or elided words or sounds that he or she is able to fill in by context. But when an infant's hearing loss results in missing many of these soft or inaudible sounds, there is confusion in word naming, difficulty in developing classes of objects, and misunderstanding of multiple meanings.

- **Faulty Abstraction of Grammatical Rules.** When short words are soft or elided as they often are, it becomes more

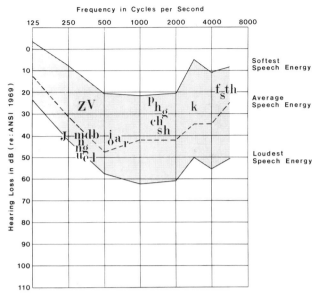

Figure 1.6. Average range of speech energy in dB HL is shown in audiogram form, with average range of softest and loudest speech energy in conversation. (Adapted from Skinner (1978) and Dudich et al. (1975).)

difficult for a slightly hearing impaired child to identify the relationships between words and to understand word order.

- **Subtle Stress Patterns Missing.** The mild conductive hearing loss is worse in the low frequencies than in the high frequencies. The emotional content of speech, its rhythm, and its intonation are communicated through the low frequencies. When these are lost, the emotional content of speech is confused—a condition that would impair learning of the speech milieu.

Contrary to conventional wisdom, mild conductive losses may even be more handicapping than mild sensorineural losses. A conductive loss muffles the sound that is heard, whereas in a sensorineural loss the full loudness sensation of the sound is heard (Fig. 1.6). In a conductive loss of 30 dB, speech of 50 dB will be heard at 20 dB loudness sensation, whereas in a sensorineural loss of 30 dB, 50 dB speech will be heard at almost 50 dB loudness sensation.

The diagnosis of a handicapping hearing loss in any given case, then, lies in an entire diagnostic process that includes not only ear examinations and hearing tests but also measures of a child's receptive and expressive language, vocalization or speech levels, and behavioral functioning. Such diagnostic evaluations can be made by enlisting other disciplines that will determine if the child is language-delayed sufficiently to warrant educational intervention. The identification of these children, of course, lies in the hands of the family practice physician and the pediatrician, for they are the source of primary care. Therefore, they will require directives as to when to apply measures of language competence to determine whether a handicapping hearing loss is present.

The foregoing concepts can be used in proposing a realistic definition of hearing loss in children, namely: "A handicapping hearing loss in a child is any degree of hearing that reduces the intelligibility of a speech message to a degree inadequate for accurate interpretation or learning." Such a definition recognizes that it may not be possible to place specific measure on what handicaps a child's ability to learn. Too many variables are present in the learning process of children: amount of parental stimulation, quality

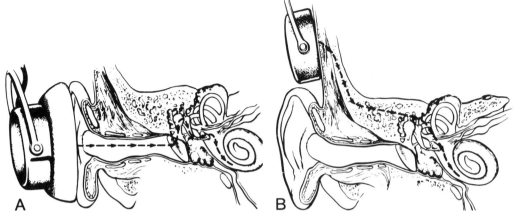

Figure 1.7.   The two pathways of sound resulting in "hearing." *Broken arrow lines* show routes of air conduction hearing pathway (**A**) and bone conduction hearing pathway (**B**). (Reprinted with permission from Zenatron Corporation, Chicago, Illinois.)

of parental stimulation, innate intelligence, age of onset of hearing loss, personality factors, health conditions, and socioeconomic status. These variables may so affect the learning abilities of children that a 10 dB loss will be a handicap to one child, whereas a 25 dB loss will not handicap another.

NATURE OF HEARING LOSS

In the simplest of descriptions, we hear everyday sounds through two physiologic pathways. The traditionally known route of sound is the air conduction pathway in which sound waves enter the external ear canal and cause the tympanic membrane to vibrate and transmit the sound energy across the three small bones of the middle ear. As the footplate of the third small bone (the stapes) vibrates, the vibrations cause eddies of otic fluid to move within the cochlear portion of the inner ear. Vibration of the inner ear fluid bends minute sensory cell hairs, which starts the neural phenomenon we recognize as "hearing." A second route for sound also exists, known as the bone conduction pathway. Since the cochlear is actually encased in the bones of the skull, any vibration to the skull will create the same eddies of fluid motion in the cochlear, causing the hair cells to bend, again resulting in the neural phenomenon we recognize as "hearing."

Under most circumstances, air-conducted sounds and bone-conducted sounds are perceived by us as exactly the same sound. By comparing the sound transmission of air-conducted sound versus bone-conducted sound during a hearing test session, we can determine the basic etiology of hearing loss (Fig. 1.7). See Chapter 2 for a more thorough discussion of the physiology of hearing and the auditory pathways.

Hearing losses are generally categorized as conductive or sensorineural. When a combination of both types of hearing loss occurs, we speak of a mixed-type hearing loss. When auditory dysfunction can be shown to exist, yet peripheral hearing mechanisms are within normal limits, the loss is categorized as a central auditory problem.

Conductive Hearing Loss.   Interference of any sort in the transmission of sound from the external auditory canal to the inner ear causes conductive hearing loss. The inner ear, in such cases, is capable of normal function, but the sound vibration is able to stimulate the cochlea only with increased stimulus intensity via the normal air conduction pathway (Fig. 1.8).

The conductive-type loss is characterized by a hearing loss for air-conducted sounds, while sounds conducted to the inner ear directly by bone via the skull and temporal

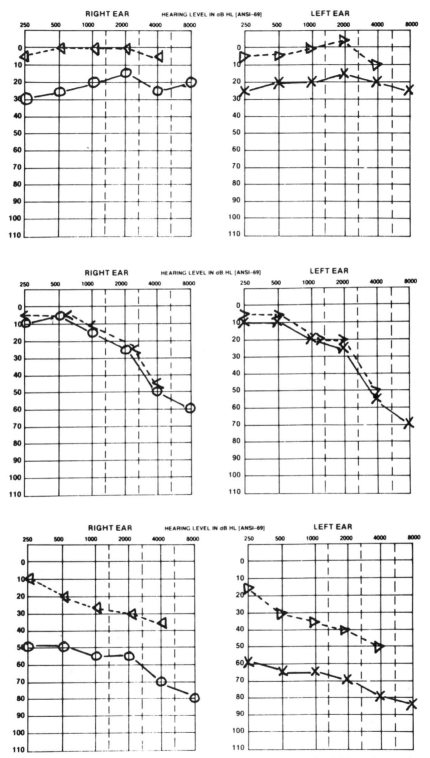

Figure 1.8. Example audiograms showing bilateral conductive hearing loss (*top*), bilateral sensorineural hearing loss (*center*), and bilateral mixed-type hearing loss (*bottom*).

bone are heard normally. When the air-conductive pathway is totally blocked as in atresia, stenosis, complete stapes fixation, or ossicular discontinuity, a maximal 60-dB air conduction hearing loss will exist. Although some conductive hearing losses may resolve spontaneously, frequently some residual of middle ear effusion (MEE) may remain for long periods of time. Conductive-type hearing loss is often associated with craniofacial malformations. Most conductive hearing losses can be corrected through medical treatment or surgery.

Sensorineural Hearing Loss. Hearing impairment occurs when damage has been sustained by the sensory end organ or cochlear hair cells, or the dysfunction may be the fault of the auditory nerve. Traditionally, damage to the sensory end organ is not easily differentiated from neuronal damage, so the resultant hearing loss is lumped under the category "sensorineural." Testing techniques such as electrocochleography and auditory evoked potentials offer promise as objective means of differentiating between sensory and neural hearing impairment (see Chapter 6).

In sensorineural hearing losses the air and bone conduction thresholds are nearly the same. Sensorineural hearing losses may easily be overlooked during physical examination, since the external auditory canal and tympanic membrane will appear normal. Progressive sensorineural hearing loss may be related to bony disease causing encroachment on the auditory nerve or membraneous labyrinth, metabolic disease, serious bacterial and viral infections as well as familial inheritance. This type of hearing loss is nearly always irreversible.

Mixed Hearing Loss. When both a sensorineural loss and a conductive hearing loss are present, the result is a mixed hearing loss. The audiogram shows less-than-normal bone conduction thresholds closer to normal levels than the air conduction thresholds. A significant air conduction-to-bone conduction gap between threshold

levels may exist, which should disappear when the conductive portion of the hearing loss is ameliorated. The mixed hearing loss, however, improved only as much as the degree of air conduction-to-bone conduction gap, and hearing levels are not likely to return to normal limits.

Central Auditory Dysfunction. This type of impairment is not necessarily accompanied by a decrease in auditory sensitivity but tends to manifest itself in varying degrees as a decrease in auditory comprehension. For example, the child may have a normal audiogram but be unable to recognize or interpret speech. Central auditory dysfunction is a complex topic and is discussed more fully in Chapter 4.

Degree and Severity of Hearing Loss. An important consideration of any hearing loss is its degree of impairment. Common terms used to identify degree of loss include mild hearing loss, moderate hearing loss, severe hearing loss, profound hearing loss, and anacusis or total hearing loss. Sometimes, borderline categories of hearing impairment are described with a combination of terms such as "moderately severe" hearing loss.

Additional consideration regarding the severity of the hearing loss must be given to its unilateral or bilateral presence. The child with a totally dead ear on one side but with a normal ear on the other side may function adequately in many situations. The child will fail the school screening test, however, and presents special problems to the audiologist who tests his or her hearing. This youngster's auditory abilities will be lacking in circumstances where sound localization is needed or in instances when noise exists to compete with the signal of interest. Refer to the section in this textbook on management of the child with unilateral deafness (Chapter 5) for more information.

A complete description of a youngster's hearing loss should include its presence as unilateral or bilateral, in addition to a term that identifies its degree of auditory impairment as well as a statement regarding the type of loss as conductive, sensorineural, or mixed. From the physician's diagnosis a description of the cause of the hearing loss can be made. Samples of hearing loss descriptions might include unilateral, severe sensorineural hearing loss due to mumps or a bilateral, moderate conductive hearing loss due to MEE.

EFFECT OF HEARING LOSS ON SPEECH AND LANGUAGE

Reduced or defective hearing sensitivity does not cause one specific kind of communication problem. The effects of a hearing loss depend primarily on its degree, configuration, and stability and on the age of onset. In the hearing-impaired child, language development is also influenced by the extent and type of early training; the type and timing of amplification; visual, emotional, and intellectual factors; and family attitude. Age of onset of the hearing loss is an especially important factor in language development. A child who sustains significant hearing loss after he or she has acquired language (3 or 4 years of age) will have a less severe linguistic deficit than the child whose hearing loss is present at birth or develops within the first few months of life.

The major effect of a hearing impairment is the loss of audibility for some or all of the important acoustic speech cues. Elderly persons with hearing loss typically complain of their inability to understand speech. Conversation may be loud enough for them, but they cannot understand the words because they miss part of the acoustic information cues.

Traditionally, there has been disagreement as to how different degrees of hearing loss should be categorized. The term *hearing-impaired* generally includes a broad range of hearing ability from mildly hearing-impaired to profoundly deaf. *Deaf* is defined as having a hearing loss greater than 70 dB HL, which precludes the understanding of speech through audition. *Hearing-impaired* is defined as having a loss of at least 15 dB HL, which makes the understanding of speech through audition more difficult as the degree of hearing loss increases. An individual with a loss greater than 70 dB HL is likely to have speech and language production and expression problems associated with deafness (see Table 1.2).

Mild Hearing Loss (15–30 dB HL). A 15–30 dB loss will have mild impact on communication and language learning. Vowel sounds are heard clearly, but voiceless consonants may be missed. In children with a 15–30 dB HL loss, auditory learning dysfunction after the first year results in inattention, mild language delay, and mild speech problems. This hearing-impaired child hears only the louder, voiced speech sounds. The short unstressed words and less intense speech sounds (such as voiceless stops and fricatives) are inaudible. The acoustic cues of speech that are audible may be perceived differently by someone with a conductive loss than by someone with a sensorineural hearing loss.

Moderate Hearing Loss (30–50 dB HL). These children miss almost all of the speech sounds at conversational level, but they understand language with the help of hearing aid amplification. Children with such losses may show inattention, language retardation, speech problems, and learning problems. Children with moderate hearing loss will have difficulty learning abstraction in the meaning of words and the grammatical rules of language, because they cannot hear some of the speech sounds and they hear others inaccurately. With this degree of hearing loss, vowels are heard better than consonants. Short, unstressed words such as prepositions and relational words, as well as word endings (-s, -ed), are particularly difficult to hear. This reduction of information can lead to confusion among speech sounds and word meanings, limited vocabulary, difficulty with multiple meanings of words, difficulty in developing object classes, confusion of grammatical rules, errors in word placement in sentences, and omission of articles, conjunctions, and prep-

Table 1.2.
Handicapping Effects of Hearing Loss in Children

Average Hearing Level 500–2000 Hz	Description	Possible Condition	What Can Be Heard without Amplification	Handicapping Effects (If Not Treated in First Year of Life)	Probable Needs
0–15 dB	Normal range	Conductive hearing losses	All speech sounds	None	None
15–25 dB	Slight hearing loss	Conductive hearing losses, some sensorineural hearing losses	Vowel sounds heard clearly; may miss unvoiced consonants sounds	Mild auditory dysfunction in language learning	Consideration of need for hearing aid; speechreading, auditory training, speech therapy, preferential seating
25–30 dB	Mild hearing loss	Conductive or sensorineural hearing loss	Only some of speech sounds, the louder voiced sounds	Auditory learning dysfunction, mild language retardation, mild speech problems, inattention	Hearing aid, speechreading, auditory training, speech therapy
30–50 dB	Moderate hearing loss	Conductive hearing loss from chronic middle ear disorders; sensorineural hearing losses	Almost no speech sounds at normal conversational level	Speech problems, language retardation, learning, dysfunction, inattention	All of the above, plus consideration of special classroom situation
50–70 dB	Severe hearing loss	Sensorineural or mixed losses due to a combination of middle ear disease and sensorineural involvement	No speech sounds at normal conversational level	Severe speech problems, language retardation, learning dysfunction, inattention	All of the above, probable assignment to special classes
70+ dB	Profound hearing loss	Sensorineural or mixed losses due to a combination of middle ear disease and sensorineural involvement	No speech or other sounds	Severe speech problems, language retardation, learning dysfunction, inattention	All of the above, probable assignment to special classes

ositions. The speech articulation of the individual with moderate hearing loss includes omitted and distorted consonants. Strangers may have some difficulty understanding the speech of the individual with moderate hearing loss.

Severe Hearing Loss (50–70 dB HL). Language and speech will not develop spontaneously in children with severe hearing loss, but with early special education and amplification with hearing aids, these children may eventually function as well as hard-of-hearing persons. Without amplification, children with severe hearing loss

cannot hear sounds or normal conversation. They can hear their own vocalizations, loud environmental sounds, and only the most intense speech when spoken loudly at close range. With the use of hearing aids, they can discern vowel sounds and differences in manner of consonant articulation. This degree of hearing loss generally results in severe language problems, speech problems, and learning dysfunction.

Profound Hearing Loss (70 dB HL or Greater). Children with this degree of loss can only learn language and speech with intensive special education. Without amplification through hearing aids, individuals with profound hearing loss are generally unable to hear sound. With amplification, they may hear the rhythm patterns of speech, their own vocalizations, and loud environmental sounds. Profound hearing loss results in severe language retardation, speech problems, and learning dysfunction in children and adults.

Deaf children commonly have voice, articulation, resonance, and prosody problems. Their vocal pitch is frequently higher than that of normal-hearing people, and the prosodic features of intonation and stress are lost, giving their voices a monotonous quality. The speech of deaf children is characterized by (*a*) slow temporal patterning, (*b*) inefficient use of the breath stream, (*c*) prolongation of vowels, (*d*) distortion of vowels, (*e*) abnormal rhythm, (*f*) excessive nasality, and (*g*) addition of an undifferentiated neutral vowel between abutting consonants. The articulation of the severely-to-profoundly hearing-impaired has been observed to have excessive mandibular movement, lack of tongue movement, posterior tongue positioning, voiced-voiceless confusions for consonants, problems with coarticulation, substitution of visible sounds for those difficult to see, better articulation for initial speech sounds than for medial or final speech sounds, stop/plosive confusion, and the intrusion of an undifferentiated neutral vowel between abutting consonants. Studies of speech intelligibility indicate that, at best, naive listeners understand 20–25% of deaf speech. Deaf children use concrete rather than abstract words and poor syntactic constructions.

The categorization of hearing impairment into terms such as mild and moderate is particularly misleading and, perhaps, an unfortunate practice. To have a mild or moderate hearing loss certainly implies minimal dysfunction. Wohlner (as cited by Matkin, 1986) found that young children categorized with "mild" bilateral sensorineural hearing loss showed delay in development of at least 2 years in expressive oral language by the age of 7 years. Children in the study with "moderate" hearing impairment at age 7 scored below the norms for normal-hearing 4 year olds!

ACOUSTIC CHARACTERISTICS OF SPEECH SOUNDS

General American English speech sounds are often described in terms of the way they are produced (Northern and Lemme, 1986). In traditional articulatory phonetics, the main divisions are (*a*) voicing, related to vocal fold vibration, e.g., voiced or voiceless; (*b*) place, related to articulators used to constrict the vocal tract, e.g., tongue or lips; and (*c*) manner, related to degree of nasal, oral, or pharyngeal cavity construction, e.g., plosives, fricatives, nasals. Thus /b/ in the word *be* is a voiced bilabial plosive. In contrast, acoustic phonetics identifies speech sounds in terms of acoustic parameters-frequency composition, relative intensities, and durational changes.

Vowels are characterized by periodicity produced by vocal fold vibration. Vowel quality is determined by energy in several frequency regions, called *formants*, whose center frequency depends on the shape of the vocal tract. The first three formants are the most important for correct recognition of English vowels. Vowels are usually more intense and relatively longer than consonants. As we have seen, the glides /w,j/ and semivowels /r,l/ resemble vowels.

Fricative consonants are characterized by aperiodic noise and may be voiced or voiceless. They are frequently classified in voiced-unvoiced cognate pairs. Each member of the pair is articulated in the same way and has similar acoustic characteristics except for the presence or absence of voicing. The frequency regions differentiate consonant pairs; for example, the /ʒ,ʃ/ pair has energy between 2500 and 4500 Hz, while the /z,s/ pair has energy in the frequency region of 3500 through 8000 Hz. The /h/, /f/, and /ə/ have less energy than the rest of the fricatives.

Plosive consonants or stop consonants are produced when air pressure is built up to the point of complete closure in the vocal tract and is then released abruptly, causing a burst of air. A silent period followed by a burst of air is distinctive in plosives and identifies them as different from other consonants. The unvoiced plosives are characterized by an aspiration period prior to the onset of the succeeding voiced vowel; the voiced plosives are characterized by the burst of air immediately preceding the onset of the succeeding vowel. Acoustic cues for differentiation among the various plosives are the frequency of the released burst and the second formant transitions; i.e., changes in the center frequency of energy in the burst of /b/ and /p/ are relatively low frequency, those of /d/ and /t/ are relatively high frequency, and those of /k/ vary with the adjacent vowel. The frequency and intensity of general English sounds during conversational speech are compared with common environmental sounds in Figure 1.9.

Variation in Acoustic Parameters of Speech Sounds. Skinner (1978) suggested that infants would recognize speech sounds with relative ease if they were not spoken in rapid succession and if their acoustic features were constant. However, speech-sound acoustic cues vary (*a*) each time an individual speaker produces a speech sound, (*b*) from speaker to speaker, and (*c*) with changes in phonetic context as they are modified by adjacent speech sounds and stress patterns.

Most children and adults recognize the ambiguous, sometimes even distorted, acoustic cues provided in everyday conversation with remarkable ease. While there are multiple acoustic cues for recognizing speech sounds, other cues include the general speech situation or context, our previous experience and expectations and, most importantly, our knowledge of the language. Speech recognition depends partially on the acoustic signal and partially on the listener's language experience. Through extensive listening experiences, the infant learns where the boundaries of speech sounds and words occur in connected speech. The process is called *segmentation* (see Chapter 4).

In different listening environments over a period of time, the average intensity of speech varies between 50 and 70 dB sound pressure level (SPL) with an average of about 65 dB SPL. Ordinary background noise varies between approximately 35 and 68 dB SPL. For normal-hearing adults, the situation where noise is 10–15 dB below the level of speech does not create difficulty in listening, since they can fill in missing acoustic cues. In contrast, the linguistically unsophisticated infant cannot fill in the missing acoustic details, and speech energy needs to be 30 dB louder than the background masking noise.

Connected speech carries suprasegmental information, which depends on the rhythm of speech and consists of stress and intonation patterns as well as durational characteristics. Stressed speech sounds or words are longer in duration, more intense, and higher in fundamental frequency than unstressed speech sounds. Change in the fundamental frequency of voiced sounds contributes to intonation, which helps us identify sentence type. There is little definitive information about the specific role of suprasegmental parameters, but within broad limits they can be specified for various grammatical configurations.

An ingenious scheme to show what happens with a mild 20 dB loss was devised by Dobie and Berlin (1979). They undertook to find out what kind of speech perception problems such a child would have in language learning situations. They treated recorded speech sample utterances, first by recording them through correcting filters, which shaped the signal as if it were processed through an ear at about the 40-phon level. They then displayed these utterances oscillographically and attenuated them by 20 dB, to simulate how a person with a 20 dB conductive hearing loss would perceive the material. The readings of these treated utterances revealed the following two observations: (*1*) there was

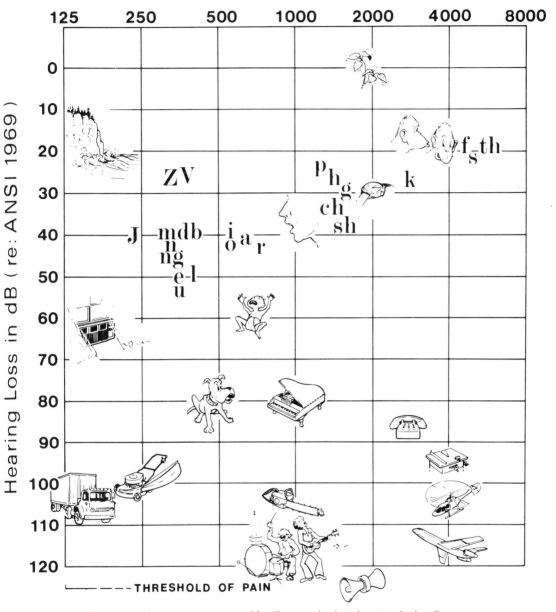

Figure 1.9. Frequency spectrum of familiar sounds plotted on standard audiogram.

a potential loss of transitional information, especially plural endings and related final-position fricatives; and (2) very brief utterances or high-frequency information could conceivably either be distorted or degraded if signal-to-noise conditions were less than satisfactory. Dobie and

Berlin reasoned that on the basis of their findings, a child with a 20 dB hearing loss might be handicapped acoustically in the following ways:

- Morphologic markers might be lost or sporadically misunderstood; for example,

"Where are Jack's gloves to be placed?" might be perceived as "Where Jack glove be place?"

- Very short words that are often elided in connected speech (see "are" and "to" above) will lose considerable loudness because of the critical relationship between intensity, duration, and loudness.

- Inflections or markers, carrying subtle nuances such as questioning and related intonation contouring, can at the very best be expected to come through inconsistently.

OTITIS MEDIA AND COMMUNICATIVE DISORDERS

Otitis media is the most common of childhood diseases and one of the most frequent reasons for a child to need medical attention. By definition, otitis media is inflammation of the middle ear, which is nearly always the result of poor eustachian tube function. Often, otitis media is evidenced by the presence of fluid in the middle ear space, which compromises the traditional sound pathway to the cochlea and creates some degree of conductive hearing loss. A more thorough discussion of the medical aspects and treatment for otitis media is presented in Chapter 3.

Nearly every aspect of otitis media raises controversial debate. While recurrent otitis media is a well-recognized medical problem in children, the treatment and the management of children with this disorder have been the focus of numerous international conferences and comprehensive national research efforts in various countries around the world. The short- and long-term effects of otitis media and the accompanying mild-to-moderate conductive hearing loss on child development are even less well understood. It is surprising that so little substantive data and information are known about the natural course of this problem and that so much controversy surrounds the relative efficacity and risks of medical and surgical treatments, as well as the outcome results for management of the speech and language

delays considered by many to be the direct result of the transient and recurrent mild conductive hearing loss. Excellent summaries of multidisciplinary workshops concerned with otitis media identification and management have been published by Bluestone et al. (1983, 1986).

The hearing acuity of children with otitis media with effusion (fluid) in the middle ear has been well-documented by Fria et al. (1985). Average air conduction thresholds based on careful audiometric examination of 762 children with documented MEE was 27 dB HL at 500, 1000, and 4000 Hz, with a somewhat better average hearing threshold of 20 dB HL at 2000 Hz. Bone conduction thresholds in this study sample were not affected by the presence of MEE. Hearing acuity was approximately 10 dB worse in children with bilateral disease than in children with unilateral effusion. Otoscopic observation of an air-fluid level or air bubbles within the middle ear fluid was generally associated with less hearing impairment.

The economic considerations of otitis media as a medical disorder affect our national health expenditures in an overwhelming fashion. Otitis media represents huge financial considerations, which affects the income of numerous professionals, pharmaceutical companies, hospital admissions, and surgical billings as described in the statements below taken from an excellent book prepared for parents, *Ear Infections in Your Child*, authored by K. Grundfast and C. J. Carney (1987):

- The total yearly costs related to management of otitis media in the United States is estimated to be as high as $2 billion. These costs include medical costs of physician fees and surgery, prescribed medications, and speech-language audiology examinations;

- Thirty million visits per year to physicians are estimated to take place for the diagnosis and treatment of otitis media. This includes emergency visits, follow-up visits, consultations with ENT [ear, nose, and throat] specialists, hearing tests, and evaluation of speech and language;

• It is estimated that on any one day in the United States, up to 30% of children are suffering an ear infection or have an abnormal middle ear condition. This means that up to 900,000 children a day may suffer an ear-related condition;

• Before the age of 6, 90% of children in the U.S. will have had at least one ear infection. Half of the children who have one ear infection before the age of 1 will have six or more episodes in the next 2 years. Nearly 20% of children who suffer ear infections will require, at some time, surgery to correct the problem.

The role of otitis media relative to the development in children of cognitive and linguistic function has divided the involved professionals into two opposing points of view. Menyuk (1986) described these two opposing positions concerning the relationship of persistent otitis media and speech and language disorders. One viewpoint is that otitis media has no effect on speech and language development in children because the hearing loss is only slight and short-term and the child's hearing returns to normal between the recurring episodes of MEE. The other viewpoint is that persistent otitis media does have a detrimental effect on speech and language development because of the fluctuating hearing loss during the early years of life and that this inconsistent auditory-receptive status creates problems for some children with mild-to-moderate hearing loss. A mountain of research studies has been conducted over the past decade to substantiate one or the other of the viewpoints. Unfortunately, as pointed out by Paradise (1981) and Ventry (1983), the research design in a large number of these projects has been less than adequate to reach significant conclusions, and thus we are left with a confusing array of statistics that both viewpoint camps use to support their polar positions.

A complete review of the literature pertaining to the developmental sequelae thought to be associated with otitis media is beyond the scope of this textbook. In recent years, a number of excellent publications have summarized the overwhelming accumulation of such studies, and interested readers are referred to Kavanagh (1986), Hasenstab (1987), Haggard and Hughes (1988), and Chalmers et al. (1989). Brief descriptions of seminal research publications of otitis media and developmental sequelae are presented below to provide the reader with a sense of the history of this research body and an overview of various efforts to study this perplexing problem. In spite of the acknowledged shortcomings of these research studies, the overall picture is that linguistic, cognitive, and behavioral effects can be documented as real sequelae of otitis media. The important factors seem to be the onset of the recurrent problem in the first few months of life and the duration of time the child has MEE (and thus conductive hearing loss) during the initial 2 years.

One of the first reports on the developmental effect of early ear disease was made by a psychologist working with language learning problems (Eisen, 1962). He identified a child with auditory learning difficulties who had had a history of otitis media in early childhood, starting in infancy. Although this child now had normal hearing, Eisen blamed the early otitis media for causing irreversible auditory language learning problems. He believed that a new syndrome had been identified and called it the "quondam hard-of-hearing" ("at one-time hard-of-hearing") syndrome.

In a classic study by Holm and Kunze (1969) an experimental group of children 5½–9 years old was identified who had had no other medical problems except middle ear disease that had had its onset before the age of 2. Hearing levels had fluctuated from normal to greater than 25 dB. A well-matched control group of children with no history of ear disease was used for comparison. Each group was given a battery of

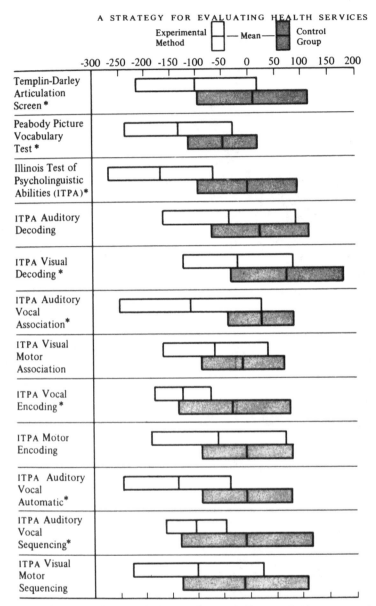

Figure 1.10. Holme and Kunze study of matched groups (see text). (Reprinted with permission from D. M. Kessner and C. E. Kalk: A Strategy for evaluating health services. In: *Contrasts in Health Status*. Washington, D.C., National Academy of Sciences, 1973.)

tests, including the Illinois Test of Psycholinguistic Abilities (ITPA), the Peabody Picture Vocabulary Test, the Templin-Darley Tests of Articulation, and the Mecham Verbal Language Development Scale. As shown in Figure 1.10, the otitis media group showed significant lowered scores in all tests requiring the receiving or processing of auditory stimuli or the pro-

duction of a verbal response. But essentially no differences were found in tests requiring visual skills. All language skills were lower in the experimental groups.

Virgil Howie, a pediatrician with a long-time interest in problems presented by young children with otitis media, studied the whole of his private practice caseload and noted that one group of children could be identified as "otitis-prone" (Howie et al., 1975). These children had had six or more recurrent bouts of otitis media before the age of 6 years. With additional analysis of the children who fell into this "otitis-prone" category, Howie et al. noted that the majority had had their first episode of otitis media during the first 18 months of life. This finding has been replicated in numerous other subsequent studies that verify that if a child has an initial bout of otitis media very early in life, the chances of recurrent episodes of MEE are great. On the other hand, the research shows that if a child's first bout of otitis media occurs later than the age of 18 months, the child is likely to have only a singular, or a few isolated, occasions of MEE during childhood.

Howie (1975) also identified two matched groups of paired children from his private practice: one group having had no otitis media during the first year (12 months) of life, and the other group having had at least three documented episodes of otitis media during this time period. He applied the Wechsler Adult Intelligence Scale (WISC) IQ test to the two groups of matched children at the age of 7 years to determine that the mean IQ scores of the otitis media group were significantly lower than the mean IQ scores obtained by the nonotitis group. A similar finding was reported by Paradise (1976b) who compared the IQs of a group of 32 cleft palate children, two thirds of whom had aggressive otologic management of their otitis media with repeated myringotomy and ventilation tube placement, and the other third of whom received "poor" otologic management of their otitis media. The mean IQ of the children in the aggressive care group was 110 compared with 98 in the poor-care group.

An important research effort was conducted by Teele et al. (1984) on some 2500 Boston children, all of whom were evaluated in a prospective manner. The children were examined before 3 months of age and routinely thereafter for presence of middle ear disease. The children had generally normal developmental history and were strati-

fied for study purposes by the estimated daily presence of MEE, gender, type of health care, and socioeconomic status. The project, known as the Boston Cohort Study, found a significant correlation between estimated time spent with MEE (unilateral or bilateral) and low test scores on vocabulary, comprehension and verbal ability. The Boston Cohort Study data showed that it is the history of otitis media in the first 6 months of life that accounts for the significant differences in cognitive abilities.

Needleman (1977) identified 20 children ages 3–8 years with recurrent serous otitis media that had begun between birth and 18 months and continued for at least 2 years. She compared this group with a matched group of otitis-free children, studying the comprehension and production of aspects of the phonologic system as measured by various tests. She found the otitis media group to score significantly lower than the nonotitis group in production of phonemes and words, in production of phonemes in connected speech, in the use of combinations of phonemes and word endings, and in varying morphologic contexts. She pointed out that the phonologic skills that were deficient were necessary for reading skills and that this fact may account for the educational retardation of the children who have had early otitis media.

A group of middle-class children with early and recurrent otitis media were followed by Sak and Ruben (1982). A control group of the unaffected siblings of these children were also followed. The two groups were given an extensive battery of language tests. The scores of the siblings with early MEE were consistently lower than those of their matched siblings with statistical significance in four areas of auditory learning.

Eight hundred and seventy children were seen by pediatricians at ages 6 weeks, 6 months, and 1, 1½, 2, 3, and 4½ years (Bax, 1981). A highly significant relationship was found between language delay at 2 years and the reported incidence of MEE in the previous 6 months. At age 3 years, the percentage of MEE was twice as high among children showing delay as among children with normal language development. Although parental report was the source of information, the large numbers involved suggests a causal relationship.

Early language scales (Receptive, Expressive Emergent Language Scale, REEL; Sequenced Inventory of Communication Development, SICD) were given to a group of infants who had been in intensive care and developed documented MEE and to a parallel group with normal ear history (Friel-Patti et al., 1982). The results at 12, 18, and 24 months show marked and significant language delays in the effusion group compared with the controls. The significant fact is that 43% of the MEE group had language delay greater than 6 months, compared with only 7% in the MEE-free children. Language delay occurred in 22% of children who had been in intensive care and did not develop MEE but in 72% of these who developed MEE.

An extremely well designed, prospective study known as the Dallas Cooperative Project has been following a cohort of more than 450 middle-class, normally developing children with concurrent and repeated measures of hearing, MEE, and language development (Friel-Patti et al., 1986; Roland et al., 1989; Friel-Patti and Finitzo, 1990). Measurements on the cohort children have been collected in a variety of settings, including a pediatrician's office, a community hearing-speech-language center, and home/day care settings. Among other findings, the Dallas Cooperative Project reported significant correlations for hearing over time and days with effusion over the same time period. These measures were then related to emerging language patterns at 12, 18, and 24 months of age and found to show significant negative correlations beginning with receptive language at 12 months, and by 18 and 24 months, both expressive and receptive scores were significantly related to hearing thresholds. Receptive language scores were significantly

higher for children who had hearing better than 20 dB HL as early as 12 months of age. By 2 years of age, both receptive and expressive language performance were higher for children who had better hearing between 6 and 18 months of age. Thus, these findings confirm that there is a definite causal relationship between otitis media and language performance based on hearing levels (Fig. 1.11).

In summary, it appears that the relationship between communicative disorders and otitis media with MEE creates opportunities and new challenges for audiologists and educators. Although one can be critical of the small-sample retrospective studies so often published in this area, the more recent, well-planned, large-sample prospective studies such as the Boston Cohort Study and the Dallas Cooperative Project confirm the suspected association between frequency occurrence of otitis media during early childhood and impaired speech and delayed language development. Many will claim it is still too early to reach such conclusions, but to wait for a definitive answer while the suspicion remains is an untenable position for those of us who are advocates for optimal child development conditions.

EAR DISEASE IN INDIAN AND ESKIMO CHILDREN

Otitis media has been one of the most serious health problems among the native American Indian and Eskimo populations of North America. Much effort and money have been expended over the past years to gain control over the widespread problems of alcoholism and tuberculosis among American Indians. The success in these health problems, however, brought to light a new health problem—otologic disease and hearing impairment.

Health problems are readily evident among native American populations because of their poor home conditions, harsh physical and psychologic environment, inadequate water facilities, crowded living conditions, unsanitary waste disposal, inad-

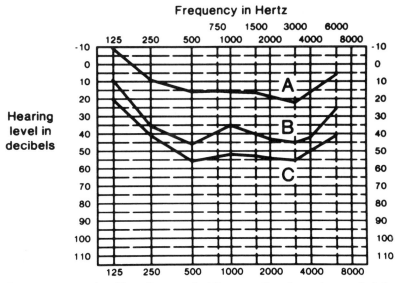

Figure 1.11. *Curves* represented on this audiogram reflect the perception of speech presented at normal conversational levels. Conversational speech exceeds *curve A* 90% of the time, *curve B* 50% of the time, and *curve C* only 10% of the time. (From W. Olsen: Speech spectrum, audiograms and functional gain. *The Hearing Journal* 37(8):25, 1984.)

equate refrigeration, nonexistent insect control, and poor nutrition. With federal financial support during the late 1960s, great strides in the health care for American Indians and Eskimos were made. Cultural barriers, poverty, poor transportation, and lack of education about issues continue to make solutions to health problems more difficult.

Hearing Impairment in Eskimos. As early as 1957 it was reported that the prevalence of active otitis media in Eskimo children was as high as 17% (Hayman and Kester). In fact, ear disease in these children was such a common occurrence that Eskimo parents did not consider otorrhea to be a disease. Brody (1964, 1965) reported a study in which 31% of an Eskimo village population had at least one episode of draining ears within the evaluation year, with two thirds of the ear disease group indicating more than one episode of otorrhea. He indicated that ear pathology in Eskimos is established by the age of 2 years, and those children who by age 2 did not have draining ears were unlikely to develop ear pathology.

Several additional studies on Eskimo populations have been published confirming the extraordinarily high incidence of middle ear disease. D. Reed et al. (1967) followed 378 Eskimo children during their first 4 years after birth. They reported that the *frequency* of episodes had more influence on the degree of hearing impairment than did the age of onset of the initial otorrhea episode. Reed and Dunn (1970) found that 43% of 641 Eskimo children experienced 532 episodes of otitis media, with the highest incidence occurring in children less than 2 years of age. Kaplan et al. (1973) reported that 38% of a group of Eskimo children had one or more bouts of otorrhea prior to age 1 and 76% of these children commonly experienced otorrhea when they were subsequently evaluated at 7–10 years of age.

Ear Disease in American Indians. Review of publications dealing with the incidence of ear disease in various American Indian populations also shows a high percentage of middle ear disorders. Johnson in 1967 reported the incidence of chronic otitis media in the Navajo population to be 12–15 times higher than that found in Caucasian Americans.

Jaffe (1968b) studied the incidence of ear diseases of all types in the Navajo. Aural atresia was found in 58 of 60,000 persons. Chronic suppurative otitis media was the most common Navajo otologic disease with 4.2% central perforations in 2,000 patients. Jaffe cites inbreeding among the Navajos as a major cause of frequently seen bifid uvula and aural atresias. One hundred years ago there were only 5,000 Navajos, while current Navajo population is estimated to be at least 150,000.

Other reports have been published on various American Indian tribes (Zonis, 1968; Gregg et al., 1970; Axelsson and Lewis, 1974; McCandless, 1975; Johnson and Watrous, 1978; Fischler et al., 1985). Nelson and Berry (1984) confirmed the high levels of chronic otitis media in the Navajos and cited concern over the current era of financial cutbacks in health care for native Americans.

MANAGEMENT OF THE CHILD WITH OTITIS MEDIA

When a child presents with otitis media and there is an indication that it may be a recurrent problem, a speech and language evaluation screening test must be recommended. Whether or not the child turns out to be otitis-prone, the evaluation will serve as a baseline for future references. It is particularly urgent to be zealous about applying these evaluations in the first 2 years of life, for during this period of critical language learning 3 months of poor hearing is an eternity in the development of language skills. The sequence of management of these children follows.

Medical Intervention. Medical treatment is the first line of defense in otitis media. The choice of treatment depends on the specialty training of the responsible physician, and the treatment regimen may vary considerably among physicians (see Chapter 3). The American Academy of Pediat-

rics published a policy statement in 1984 concerning the medical management of otitis media with a special caution regarding the relationship between middle ear disease and language development:

There is growing evidence demonstrating a correlation between middle ear disease with hearing impairment and delays in the development of speech, language and cognitive skills. A parent or other caretaker may be the first person to detect such early symptoms as irritability, decreased responsiveness and disturbed sleep. Middle ear disease may be so subtle that a full evaluation for this condition should combine pneumatic otoscopy, and possibly tympanometry, with a direct view of the tympanic membrane. This statement is not meant to be a recommendation for specific treatment methods. *When a child has frequently recurring acute otitis media and/or middle ear effusion persisting for longer than 3 months, hearing should be assessed and the development of communicative skills must be monitored.*

The Committee feels it is important that the physician inform the parent that a child with middle ear disease may not hear normally. Although the child may withdraw socially and diminish experimentation with verbal communication, the parent should be encouraged to continue communicating by touching and seeking eye contact with the child when loudly and clearly speaking. Such measures, along with prompt restoration of hearing whenever possible, may help to diminish the likelihood that a child with middle ear disease will develop a communicative disorder. Middle ear disease can occur in the presence of sensory neural hearing loss. *Any child whose parent expresses concern about whether the child hears should be considered for referral for behavioral audiometry without delay* [italics ours].

Ruben (1986) points out that treatment for otitis media is directed at the return to "normal," and he outlines two forms of medical intervention. The initial choice of treatment is the administration of antibiotics for chronic and/or recurrent otitis media. This medical treatment appears to be efficacious for about half of the patients, with the other half harboring MEE with accompanying hearing loss.

Those patients who do not respond by returning to "normal" are candidates for the second treatment approach, which consists of surgical placement of a tympanostomy tube (also known as ventilation tubes) through the tympanic membrane to permit aeration of the middle ear space and, hopefully, improved hearing. Ruben points out that the insertion of a tympanostomy tube does not ensure that the threshold of hearing will return to "normal." Further, the drawback to this treatment is that as a surgical procedure, certain risks and complications may be expected in a small percentage of cases.

Language and Speech Screening. Delayed early language milestones are often the keystone for identifying possible developmental delay in children and may indicate slow cognitive development or the presence of hearing loss. Further, many studies have noted that children who are experiencing otitis media with effusion may score poorer on tests of articulation than those children who are otitis-free. From a retrospective point of view, speech-language pathologists often comment that children with significant history of otitis media are noted to have phonologic or articulation deficiencies. Children who are identified with significant communication deficiencies should be referred for diagnostic language evaluation and possible remediation through speech therapy (Paden et al., 1987, 1989).

Our suggested guideline is that if MEE exists for 3 months despite vigorous medical or surgical treatment or if the hearing impairment persists after 3 months, a language screening test should be applied. Coplan et al. (1982) developed a useful screening test for language development known as the Early Language Milestone (ELM) Scale with which we have had good success in young children between 12 and 26 months of age (Walker et al., 1989). Coplan's ELM Scale has been well-normed for the presence of 41 language milestones during the first 36 months of life in normal children. The ELM Scale is a brief language assessment tool with both receptive and expressive items that are specifically age-related, and it reportedly yields 97% sensitivity and 93% specificity as a detector of developmentally delayed children.

Since language delay can be a significant factor in the identification of young children with mild-to-moderate hearing impairment or history of otitis media with effusion, it behooves the audiologist to develop competency in the observation of normal speech-language milestones as well as skill in administering language screening tests. Naturally, when a child is noted to be functioning at a level significantly less than normal for his or her age, referral should be made for a comprehensive language evaluation and a thorough hearing evaluation.

Educational Intervention. If the child fails the language screening test at age level, an initial program that encourages home language stimulation may be recommended. During the past decade, the areas of early development, education and, especially, infant intervention have become ever-expanding fields for study and research. Since the 1960s there has been an increase in awareness for the value of early intervention for young children in general, particularly for infants and toddlers who have handicaps or who are at risk for developing handicaps. Research suggests that early intervention with infants, in which problems are identified and treated as early as possible, can make a significant difference later in their physical, cognitive, and social abilities and can minimize the effects of present or potential handicaps (Weiner and Koppelman, 1987).

The impact of these research findings has resulted in a new federal law, passed in 1986, known as Public Law 99-457, which requires that early intervention and special education services be provided to children (ages birth through 5 years) who have handicaps or who are at risk for developing handicaps. Public Law 99-457 should increase parents' access to early intervention programs where audiology is one of the twelve special services identified by name. Through these programs, parents can understand more about their baby's abilities, make decisions about the goals they have for their baby, and discover ways to stimulate their baby's growth and development. In many cases, parents can get support in adjusting to and meeting the needs of an infant with handicaps or delays. But certainly one of the most important functions of such programs is to help parents develop a close and satisfying relationship with their child. When parents find ways to enjoy their baby and are able to give the needed support, they very likely will increase the prospect that their child will have a happier and more productive life within the family and the community.

Traditionally, the approach to delivering services to very young children has focused on identifying strengths and weaknesses, then remediating deficits and "teaching" the child the needed skills. In recent years, however, the focus in many early intervention programs offers a more positive approach for children, their families, and the professionals who work with them. This approach, often referred to as prevention-intervention, recognizes that not all problems or deficits can be "fixed" through many of the medical or educational therapies available and that parents and professionals cannot change the long-term problems that occur at birth, such as brain damage or severe hearing loss. Parents and professionals can, however, minimize or prevent impairments from causing secondary handicaps, such as emotional problems, or problems with thinking or communicating. They can work through child's strengths to help their child develop alternative or compensatory learning strategies (Campbell and Wilcox, 1986).

While many programs focus on parents being given advice and educational and therapeutic tasks to do at home, others are beginning to develop systems that recognize parents and professionals as equal partners. In such programs, professionals serve as consultants to families, helping them determine the goals and activities they want for their child. The changes in the approaches taken and attitudes adopted by professionals working with parents reflect a focus on family needs, with an emphasis on enhancing the child's growth, development, and sense of well-being, rather than a singular focus on correcting a problem. Parents need to be regarded as full partners in this effort and to be valued as prime contributors in decisions made about their child's program and progress.

We know from research studies on early childhood development that infants learn, respond, and interact from the moment they are born. Infants learn through social contact and active participation. And of course, the behavior of infants affects their parents, just as parents affect their babies. It is generally accepted that an infant's earliest interactions with its environment can significantly, although not totally, affect future language and communication development (Hanson, 1984).

We believe that the child at risk for any developmental delay, whether from auditory deprivation or neurologic condition, requires a stepped-up language enrichment program such as those offered in child developmental centers under the direction of a qualified speech-language pathologist. However, the initial step may be the instigation of a simple program designed to improve parent-infant interaction and communication. Such a program has been designed by Dr. Noel Matkin of the University of Arizona as a useful list of suggestions for parents of children with middle ear problems, which he has been kind enough to permit us to reproduce below:

- **The Importance of Talking.** Talking to your child is necessary for his or her language development. Since children usually imitate what they hear, how much you talk to your child, what you say, and how you say it will affect how much and how well your child talks.

- **Look.** Look directly at your child's face and wait until you have his or her attention before you begin talking.

- **Control Distance.** Be sure that you are close to your child when you talk (no farther than 5 feet). The younger the child, the more important it is to be close.

- **Loudness.** Talk slightly louder than you normally do. Turn off the radio, TV, dishwasher, etc. to remove background noise.

- **Be a Good Speech Model**
  —Describe to your child daily activities as they occur.
  —Expand what your child says. For example, if your child points and says "car," you say, "Oh, you want the car."
  —Add new information. You might add, "That car is little."
  —Build vocabulary. Make teaching new words and concepts a natural part of every day's activities. Use new words while shopping, taking a walk, washing dishes, etc.
  —Repeat your child's words using adult pronunciation.

- **Play and Talk.** Set aside some times throughout each day for "play time" for just you and your child. Play can be looking at books, exploring toys, singing songs, coloring, etc. Talk to your child during these activities, keeping the conversation at his or her level.

- **Read.** Begin reading to your child at a young age (under 12 months). Ask a librarian for books that are right for your child's age. Reading can be a calming-down activity that promotes closeness between you and your child. Reading provides another opportunity to teach and review words and ideas. Some children enjoy looking at pictures in magazines and catalogs.

- **Don't Wait.** Your child should have the following skills by the ages listed below:
  18 months: 3-word vocabulary
  2 years: 25–30-word vocabulary and several 2-word sentences.

2½ years: At least a 50-word vocabulary and 2-word sentences consistently.

- **If Your Child Doesn't Have These Skills, Tell Your Doctor.** A referral to an audiologist and speech pathologist may be indicated. Hearing and language testing may lead to a better understanding of your child's language development.

Hearing Aid Placement. A mild ear-level hearing aid, with appropriate limitations on maximum saturation and gain, can be considered even for a young infant. The obvious drawbacks are that it is difficult to convince parents of the necessity for such an extreme antidote, and there are problems in keeping such an instrument on an infant. Hearing aid placement is a feasible procedure only if (*a*) the parents are highly motivated, (*b*) continual guidance by an audiologist or speech therapist is obtained, (*c*) a total support system by doctor, parent, and therapist is in effect, and (*d*) a period of diagnostic therapy with a loaner hearing aid is initiated to judge the effectiveness of the aid.

MULTIDISCIPLINARY MANAGEMENT OF THE CHILD WITH OTITIS MEDIA

By the time a child with recurrent otitis media reaches age 2, his or her parents may be purchasing services from a variety of professionals: pediatrician, otologist, audiologist, and speech/language pathologist. Although decisions made by these various individuals may be in the best interest of the child, the decisions may not be consistent with each other, disrupting the continuity of the child's care and creating a financial burden for the family. Scharfenaker et al. (1987) described a multidisciplinary clinic staffing to treat and manage children with recurrent episodes of otitis media.

The otitis media clinic is similar to other multidisciplinary clinics in that at one appointment, various professionals evaluate a child's medical and developmental status relative to otitis media, share results at a staffing, and make recommendations for further care. The clinic, therefore, performs as a body of professionals who provide a consensus of recommendations for the child's primary caregivers.

The disciplines involved include otology, pediatrics, speech/language pathology, and audiology. The role of the otologist is to assess middle ear status and the health of the child as it may relate to middle ear problems. This is accomplished through use of pneumatic otoscopy and microscopic examination. Evaluation of tonsils, adenoids, allergies, constant congestion, and eustachian tube dysfunction are some additional areas of assessment. The pediatrician is responsible for overall evaluation of the child's health, including developmental concerns. In addition, the pediatrician conducts a review of the patient's medical chart prior to each clinic and identifies pertinent information relative to otitis media. Routine speech/language screenings are administered by the speech/language pathologist, who also provides information on language stimulation techniques to be used by the parents at home. The audiologist performs tympanometry and audiometry.

Consideration for entry into the otitis media clinic is determined by any one or a combination of the following factors: (a) three episodes of otitis media within 3–6 months; (b) 3 months of effusion; and (c) one or more episodes of otitis media prior to 6 months of age.

During the otitis media clinic, children and their parents rotate between four stations: otology, pediatrics, speech/language pathology, and audiology. A staffing follows the clinic, at which each of the professionals describes their findings, and suggestions for management are agreed upon and discussed with the parents.

ECONOMIC BURDEN OF CHILDHOOD DEAFNESS

A major concern that has a significant impact on parents when they learn that their child is hearing-impaired or deaf is the worry about the unknown economic burden that looms as an impending problem to be faced during the child's lifetime. Although no specific amount of money can be identified that will apply to every hearing-impaired or deaf child, we can at least give consideration to a number of possible factors that may be included to make the child's daily living optimal for communication and education purposes. This information may be used for parents' financial planning or for medical-legal purposes in establishing compensation awards for inadvertent hearing loss resulting from an accident with pecuniary obligations or as the conclusion of an iatrogenic misadventure of medical treatment that is identified as the determinant of the child's hearing impairment.

It is a thought-provoking exercise to consider the economic burden created by childhood deafness. A number of general areas should be considered, including routine medical and audiologic expenses over the lifetime of the child, special educational and vocational expenses required because of the hearing impairment that are above and beyond those expenses incurred by parents of children with normal hearing. The deaf child will require a number of special living expenses for assistive listening devices and aids to meet ordinary daily life circumstances. And finally, there is the question of loss of income born by every profoundly deaf individual, over the course of their adult working lifetime, which is due to their inability to obtain employment of full and equal status with the average, normal-hearing adult. In addition to specific expenditures that can be estimated, consideration must include a number of intangible costs of deafness that affect the deaf person in childhood and throughout their adult life. Although statistics to determine the precise economic penalty of deafness are not available, our cursory overview reveals a potential enormous financial obligation to be shared among the child's parents, state and federal social service agencies, as well as the hearing-impaired individual. The amounts shown below are our estimates of approximate costs, based on 1990 dollar values, calculated for a child of 1 year of age with severe hearing impairment with a life expectancy, according to the National Center for Health Statistics, of 71 years:

**Medical and Audiologic
Expenses** **$75,000**

- Otolaryngology consultations twice annually until 16 years of age and then annual evaluations throughout adult life
- Audiologic services twice annually until age 18 and as necessary throughout adult life
- Hearing aids, batteries, maintenance, and insurance based on binaural amplification devices used daily and replaced every 4 years throughout life

**Education and Training
Expenses** **$750,000**

- Parent-infant program training; speech, language, and auditory training therapy during preschool years; private school for the hearing-impaired, with special educational tutoring services as needed through age 18; computer-assisted learning systems; Gallaudet University, National Technical Institute for the Deaf, or regular college with interpreter services

Special Living Expenses **$100,000**

- Baby-cry amplifier, personal FM auditory system, special signaling devices to include door bells, telephone TTY system, fire alarm, alarm clock, wristwatch with necessary replacements and upgrades as needed throughout life, special interpreter fees as needed for daily living, telecaption system for television, captioned films and videos for entertainment and recreational purposes, hearing dog services including provisions for food, shelter, transportation, and medical care

Loss of Income .... **$300,000 to $500,000**

- Based on a work life expectancy of 50 years and a comparison of the average annual salary with the fact that em-

ployed deaf adults earn 30% less annually than a normal-hearing person (Schein and Delk, 1974). It can be further noted that unemployment of deaf adults is more than twice the United States national unemployment figure and more than 20% of deaf adults actually report no income (based on Internal Revenue Service statistics)

It may be seen from the above cost estimates that the economic burden of deafness can easily exceed the staggering figure of 1 million dollars over an average lifetime! These calculations do not take into account any possible future technologic advances such as a cochlear implant device with surgical implantation and follow-up rehabilitation, maintenance, and replacement. These calculations, incidentally, have formed the basis of at least two actual compensation settlements within the past year, to infants and their families, for iatrogenic incidences that resulted in profound deafness.

INTANGIBLE COSTS OF DEAFNESS

The price of deafness is not limited to economic costs. One must also take into consideration the deep wounds of emotional trauma to the parents and family of the child found to be hearing-impaired. Many have compared the parent's realization of deafness in their child to an actual death, inasmuch as the parents have "lost" the normal child they thought they would have. Many of the parents go through a denial phase (during which they may go from clinic to clinic, searching for a diagnosis and cure that will allow their child to be normal); an anger phase (during which they may lash out at clinicians and doctors and try to place blame); a mourning phase (during which they experience sadness and depression over the deafness); and, finally, an acceptance phase (which allows them to become active participants in the child's habilitation process).

Other intangible costs accrue to the families and to the individual who has the hearing loss. They comprise a never-ending recital of problems that only begin with the initial realization of the deafness.

Breakdown of Normal Family Communications. Parents are denied the pleasure of being understood easily by their child and of hearing their child speak normally. Their child does not come when they call, does not obey their verbal commands, can neither be praised nor reprimanded orally, and cannot play the kinds of games the rest of the family plays—all these things present difficulties for the parents of a child with severe hearing loss.

In addition, other children in the family are markedly deprived of the attention of their parents, who must spend a great deal of time in coping with the needs of the deaf child. The extra time required to teach that child the basic elements of living as well as communicating, is taken away from the other siblings, who may suffer from this deprivation. The deaf child suffers as well, for jealousy and anger can arise from siblings that is directed at him or her.

Problems in School. The deaf child is isolated from peers in every educational system circumstance. As the mainstreamed child in normal-hearing classes, he or she stands aside while the other children play games involving verbal commands. In the classroom he or she requires special attention and help that sets him or her apart from peers. Studies have shown that although a deaf child may learn well in a mainstreamed environment, he or she is scarred by psychologic feeling of inferiority and poor self-image (Davis et al., 1986). In a special school for the deaf he or she is among deaf peers but is only able to communicate fully with them if signing is the mode of communication.

Language learning is always impaired to some degree in the deaf child. The average language level of the young deaf adult has been shown to be often equivalent to third or fourth grade level. This fact has ac-counted for the poorer earning power of the deaf. But it also deprives them of one of the great joys of life: an appreciation of humor that relies on verbal play or on an understanding of some of our daily usages. For example, expressions such as "put your best foot forward" can only be taken literally by a deaf child without additional explanation.

Speech defects seriously diminish the social relations of the deaf with normal-hearing peers. Nothing makes a child an outcast more than "funny speech," and children are notoriously cruel to a child with any deviations from the norm. Few children with severe to profound hearing losses have speech that approaches normalcy, so they must forever be "different."

Problems in Adulthood. The lower income of the deaf necessitates a more modest lifestyle than is possible for their peers, consigning them to a lower level of living than their potential abilities would have allowed them. When it comes to marriage, the choices of the deaf are narrowed. If the deaf person has been led by his or her family and educational environment to expect to find a hearing mate, he or she may be doomed to disappointment.

One of the most devastating problems facing the deaf is dealing with the demands of the "hearing establishment." Society is organized around hearing people, and major adjustments have to be made to cope with them. How can one explain to the Internal Revenue Service the problems one is having with taxes? How can one go to court and plead a case without communicating directly? How can one explain to one's doctor what the medical problem is? How can one get out of a burning building in time without hearing the fire alarm? And what if one has lost a child in the shopping mall—how does one mobilize the facility to find the lost child? These are but a few of the problems confronting the severely hearing-impaired adult in everyday life.

Going through a college program for normal-hearing people requires a supreme effort by the deaf person. In order to profit from lectures a notetaker and/or an interpreter to sign during the lectures may be necessary. Most colleges now have these special helps available for the deaf youth, but it requires constant concern and application to keep up with the college requirements. The hearing-impaired or deaf college student may depend on elaborate augmentative communication devices in lieu of helpful colleagues.

The choice of a career is limited for the deaf individual. He or she cannot become a physician without sufficient hearing to interpret heart beats and chest sounds, and he or she cannot become a trial lawyer unless speech is adequate for understanding in a court room. Many other occupations are closed to the deaf adult if they require verbal communication with hearing people.

It is to the everlasting credit of the human spirit that deaf people are able to rise above these problems and lead the productive and happy lives that most of them have, for despite all the limitations described above, the deaf community is a cohesive, supportive group whose members are most often as contented as their normal-hearing peers.

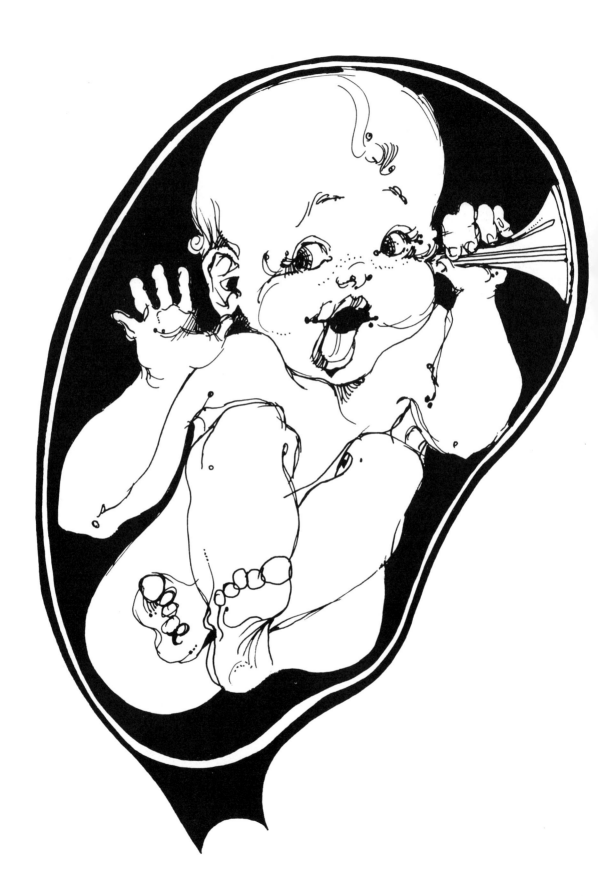

CHAPTER 2

Auditory Mechanism

The embryologic development of the ear is of more than academic interest to the clinician. An understanding of embryologic relationships helps the physician in his or her diagnosis and the audiologist in his or her plan for early identification and management of hearing loss. If one is aware of the timetable of prenatal development and the association of the various structures with each other, the suspicion of deafness and its subsequent diagnosis and treatment become easier. Although the major changes in the development of the ear take place in the mother's womb, first as an embryo and later as a fetus, the baby becomes a more progressively complex structure with time. Several mechanical processes occur concurrently to produce the final structure, including enlargements, constrictions, and foldings, which are further modified by evaginations and invaginations. However, development of the auditory structure does not cease, nor is it totally complete, at the time of birth.

Knowledge of the origins of auditory structures can be diagnostically significant to the clinician. For example, when an infant presents with a congenital skin disorder, the clinician considers the fact that the skin and the otocyst both originate from ectoderm. It may then be logical to suspect that anomalies of the cochlear structures could have occurred contiguously with the skin disorder and that a search for severe sensorineural deafness is in order.

Similarly, the timing of development of the various organ systems guides us to suspect that a hearing loss may have occurred at the same time that other systems were affected. A noxious influence on the fetus at 2 months of gestation may result in a mal-

formation of the pinna developing at that time. The pinna malformation, however, does not necessarily imply malformation of the ossicles of the middle ear. Although the ossicles of the middle ear share partially the same time clock as the pinna in embryologic development, the origins of the structures are different. On the other hand, an insult to one may well result in a related insult to the other.

Principles such as these allow us to look for the occult symptom of hearing loss whenever an overt embryologically related symptom becomes evident. The prognosis for auditory function can then be estimated from what is known of the origin and the expected pathology. A review of the embryologic development of the ear and its related structures will clarify some of these principles.

PHYLOGENY

Unfortunately, "ears" and "hearing" are often synonyms to the naive student who may be unaware that the ability to hear is actually a secondary acquired characteristic of the ear. The primary responsibility of the auditory organ is maintaining equilibrium. The study of comparative anatomy confirms that hearing is important only to higher forms of vertebrates, but the basic function of equilibrium remains essentially unchanged in the phylogenetic evolution between fish and humans.

In many fish, amphibians, and reptiles the paired internal ears are devoted primarily to functions related to equilibrium. In these creatures the membranous labyrinth of the inner ear is filled with endolymph, and two distinct saclike structures are generally present, the utricle and saccule. An endolymphatic duct extends upward from these two sacs and terminates within the brain case as the endolymphatic sac. A structure known as the lagena, which is actually the forerunner of the cochlea, is formed as a depression pocket in the floor of the saccule. Even in these lower vertebrates, branches of the auditory nerve are associated in the sensory sacs with end organs known as macula.

The macula-type of sensory cell is found in all vestibular systems and is the basic means of transforming equilibrium information into neural codes. These sensory end organs, much like the human cochlear hair cells, have hairlike projections embedded in an overlying gelatinous material, the cupula. In the utricular and saccular maculae and often in the primitive lagena, this gelatinous material becomes a thickened structure in which are deposited crystals of calcium carbonate. Technically speaking, the very small crystals in the human otolithic membrane are otoconia (Greek word meaning "ear dust"), while the somewhat larger concretions of some other vertebrates are otoliths (Greek word meaning "ear stones"). However, the two terms are often used interchangeably (Nolte, 1988)

An interesting equilibrium system utilized by the crayfish is described by Storer et al. (1979). The crayfish has a small sac known as the statocyst located at the base of each antenna. The statocyst contains a ridge of sensory hairs to which sand grains are attached by mucus to form structures called statoliths. The action of gravity on the statoliths causes the sensory hairs to bend, informing the crayfish of its present orientation. Each time the crayfish molts, it loses the statolith lining and must acquire new grains of sand to deposit in the statocyst. The crayfish shows disorientation in an aquarium with no foreign debris particles following molting. When iron filings are placed in the aquarium, the crayfish will pick some up for use in its statocyst, and then its equilibrium may be controlled with

a magnet held in various positions along the sides of the aquarium.

All vertbrates are, of course, dependent on information concerning turning movements provided by the semicircular canals. In every jawed vertebrate, three such canals arise from each utricle. The three canals are at right angles to each other and represent the three planes of space. Each canal has an enlargement at one end known as an ampulla. Within the ampulla is a sensory end organ, the crista. Displacement of the endolymph in the semicircular canal causes displacement of the cupula attached to the cristae, bending the sensory hairs and initiating neural impulses.

Some fish and amphibians have a peculiar sensory system termed the lateral line system. The receptor organ of the lateral line is the neuromast, a generalized name applied to nerve receptors that demonstrate a hairlike projection enclosed in a flexible mass of gelatinous material—the cupula. Neuromasts are generally located on the surface skin of the water-dwelling organism. Evidence of embryonic development of the sensory endings in the human cochlea—which closely resembles the externally placed neuromast organs—may indicate that the internal ear originated phylogenetically as a specialized, deeply sunk portion of the lateral line system.

As animals evolved to become landdwelling creatures, adaptations in the hearing sense organ were necessitated to process airborne sound waves. Changes were in order to transmit sounds and amplify them to the inner ear, which was usually set deeply in the skull. It is now known that a hole exists through the bird's skull connecting both ears and permitting sound localization otherwise not available because of the bird's small head size. The middle ear of amphibians and reptiles is quite similar, in the sense that the hyomandibular bone seen in the fish has changed its function to become a rodlike stapes or columella. The columella crosses the middle ear between the tympanic membrane and the oval window of the inner ear. This columellar-type middle ear ossicle is of particular interest, since human middle ear malformations may show this type of deformity. It makes one wonder if this is a throwback to our primitive evolutionary forebears (Fig. 2.1). An abnormal structure reminiscent of normal structures in "lower" animals, such as a cervical fistula or a columella ossicle, is known as a reversion structure or *atavism*.

In the mammals the external ear becomes a prominent structure known as the pinna. A more fundamental change occurs in the middle ear where, instead of a single bone, an articulated series of three ossicles between the eardrum and oval window exists. The middle ear mechanism in humans is the result of a 400 million year evolutionary process in which discarded parts from nearby structures, having lost their original function, became adapted for full use in the hearing apparatus (Himalstein, 1978). According to Romer (1977) the origin of this series of ossicles has long been debated. The question existed as to whether the three ossicles were really due to subdivisions of the columella. Careful study of paleontology and comparative anatomy, however, led to the conclusion that only the mammalian stapes is related to the lower vertebrate columella. Mammals have developed a new specialized jaw system, and the "older" jaw elements have been developed into the other two middle ear ossicles. The reptile eardrum lies close to a jaw joint known as the articular, which becomes the malleus in mammals. A second jaw bone, the quadrate, is attached to the articular in the reptile and to the hyomandibular bone (forerunner of the stapes) in the fish. The quadrate retains these primitive connections and becomes the incus in mammals. Thus, these bones, which were originally part of the gill structure in fish, developed into the jaw structure of reptiles and finally into ear structures in mammals. In Romer's words, the breathing aids of the fish developed into feeding aids in reptiles and finally into "hearing aids" in mammals!

The inner ear in birds and mammals functions from nearly identical physiologic mechanisms—auditory sensory structures vibrated by movements of a membrane located beneath them. Birds and mammals refined their hearing abilities with the advanced development of the cochlea. The number of coils present in the cochlea may vary among mammalian species. As indicated earlier in this phylogenetic discussion, the portions of the inner ear devoted to balance show little change in evolutionary development.

BASIC EMBRYOLOGY

Most audiologists have not had training or coursework in the field of embryology, so some basic background information is essential to appreciate fully the development of the ear. The reader is also referred to Zemlin (1988) for a very good discussion of the embryonic development of the facial, head, and neck regions.

All growth is the result of cell division of preexisting cells. Through a process known as mitosis, changes take place in the nucleus of a cell that produce a specific number of double structures. The cell and nucleus then subdivide into two identical "daughter" cells. At the same time, "organizers" exist in the embryo that stimulate development of associated areas and create specific differentiation of cells in the developmental process.

One of the earliest organizational developments in the embryo is the differentiation of cells into three superimposed, cellular plates called germ layers. These germ layers are known as ectoderm, mesoderm, and endoderm. Initially, the cells of each layer are virtually indistinguishable. While all the cells are descendents of the same fertilized egg, chemical changes take place. Ectoderm is generally responsible for development of the outer skin layers but also gives rise to the nervous system and the sense organs. Mesoderm is associated with skeletal, circulation structures, kidneys, and reproductive organs. Endoderm creates the digestive canal and respiratory organs. These germ layers are actually not

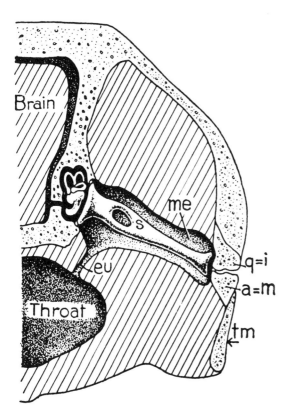

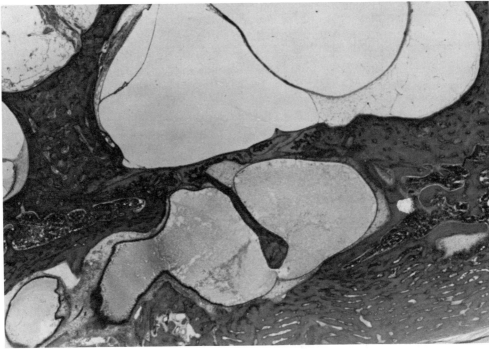

Figure 2.1. Example of an otic reversion structure. *Top*. Ventricle cross-section of the normal reptile middle ear. Abbreviations denote the following: *me* is middle ear; *s* is the columella, which is the forerunner of the stapes; *q* is the quadrate, which becomes the incus (*i*); *a* is the articular, which becomes *m*, the malleus; *tm* is to be the tympanic membrane; *eu* is the eustachian tube. (Reprinted with permission from A. S. Romer: *The Vertebrate Body,* ed. 5. Philadelphia, W. B. Saunders, 1977.) *Bottom*. Horizontal cross-section of a human middle ear from a Treacher Collins patient, showing congenital columella-type stapes with absence of malleus and incus. (Reprinted with permission from I. Sando and R. P. Wood: Congenital middle ear anomalies. *Otolaryngology Clinics of North America (Symposium)* 4:29–318, 1971.)

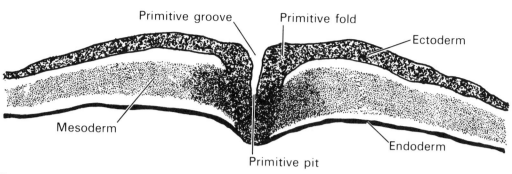

Figure 2.2. Early life of the embryo. The embryonic disc is split at about 25 hours. This drawing is made from a transverse cut through a seven-segment chick embryo. (Modified with permission from L. B. Arey: *Developmental Anatomy*. Philadelphia, W. B. Saunders, 1940.)

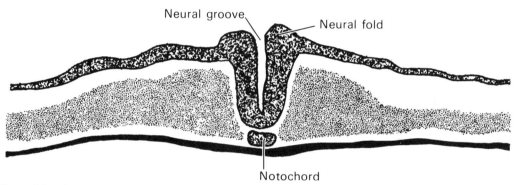

Figure 2.3. Cephalic transverse section through the fifth pair of somites in a seven-segment chick embryo. (Modified with permission from L. B. Arey: *Developmental Anatomy*. Philadelphia, W. B. Saunders, 1940.)

quite so specific in their functions as outlined above; but, as you will see, the outer and inner portions of the ear do indeed develop from ectodermal tissue, while the middle ear ossicles and the bone surrounding the inner ear originate from mesodermal tissue.

A developing baby is known as an embryo (from a Greek word meaning "to swell") during its first 8 weeks of gestation. At the end of the second week a cellular disc exists composed of the three germ layers. By the end of the first month of life, the embryo is only about a fourth of an inch long. The embryonic period terminates around the eighth week when the structure assumes a "human" appearance and is known as a fetus (from the Latin word meaning "offspring") for the remainder of the gestation period.

The ear begins its development during the early life of the embryo, so some discussion of the detailed growth of the embryo itself is worthwhile. The embryonic disc is split by a primitive streak at about 25 hours, which leads the way for development of the ectodermal-lined primitive groove and primitive fold (Fig. 2.2). The primitive groove deepens into a primitive pit, which in turn becomes the neural groove and neural fold (Fig. 2.3). An enlargement exists (the primitive knot) at the cephalic end of the primitive streak. This enlargement is destined to become the head of the organism. The ectodermal-lined neural folds come together to close off the neural groove, which is now known as the neural tube. It is during the stage of the neural tube that the earliest beginnings of the ear are seen (Snell, 1975).

DEVELOPMENT OF THE EAR

Inner Ear. Only the general essentials of the development of the ear are presented here. Readers interested in an excellent in-depth presentation on embryology of the ear are referred to Anson (1973).

The earliest demarcations of the ear in the human embryo are seen early in the third week as thickenings in the superficial ectoderm on either side of the open neural plate. These thickenings are the auditory or otic placodes and are obvious by the middle of the third week (Fig. 2.4a). About the 23rd day, the auditory placodes begin to invaginate into the surface ectoderm and are known as the auditory or otic pits. When the mouth of each auditory pit closes on or about the 30th day, it becomes the auditory vesicle or otocyst and appears as an ecto-dermal cavity lined with epithelium lateral to the now-closed neural tube as shown in Figure 2.4c.

The auditory vesicle proceeds to differentiate through a series of folds, evaginations, and elongations and takes on an elongated shape divided into a utricular-saccule area and a tubular extension known as the en-dolymphatic duct. By 4½ weeks the portion of the auditory vesicle connected to the en-dolymphatic duct can be recognized as the future vestibular portion of the labyrinth, while the more slender portion of the vesicle begins to elongate from the sacular area as the future cochlea (Fig. 2.5a.) At the end of the sixth week, three archlike outpockets are visible and destined to become the semicircular canals. At this same time the utricle and saccule become two definitive areas through a deepening construction of the vestibular portion of the auditory vesicle (Fig. 2.5b).

By the end of the seventh week, the elongated outpocketing of the saccular portion of the auditory vesicle has completed one coil of the future cochlea. During the eighth through 11th week, the two and a half coils of the cochlea are completed. The cochlear duct continues to be attached to the vestibular area by means of a narrow tube known as the ductus reuniens. The cochlear division of the eighth nerve follows the elongation and coiling of the cochlear duct, and fans its fibers out to be distributed along the duct's entire length.

During the seventh week, the complicated convolutions of the otic labyrinth continue to develop, and sensory end organs first appear as localized thickenings of epithelium in the utricle and saccule. Similar localized epithelial thickenings are found in the ampullated ends of the semicircular canals during the eighth week and in the floor of the cochlear duct at 12 weeks. These epithelial thickenings show differentiation into two types of cells including sensory cells with bristle-like hairs and supporting cells at one end. Complete maturation of the sensory and supporting cells in the cochlea does not occur until the fifth month when the entire cochlear duct has shown considerable growth and expansion.

The membranous labyrinth of the inner ear reaches its full adult configuration by the early part of the third month. At this time the otic capsule, which has been encased in cartilage, begins to ossify through a complex system of 14 different endochondral ossification centers in the petrous portion of the temporal bone. The inner ear is the only sense organ to reach full adult size and differentiation by fetal midterm. However, it should be noted that the cochlear portion of the inner ear is the last inner ear end organ to differentiate and mature. Thus, the cochlea may be subject to more possible developmental deviations, malformations, and acquired disease than the vestibular end organs.

Middle Ear. While the sensory portion of the auditory system—the inner ear—is developing, the transmission portion of the auditory mechanism is developing as the middle ear. Unlike the inner ear, which originates from ectodermal tissue, the middle ear is an endodermal structure. The middle ear cavity begins its development during the third week while the auditory pit

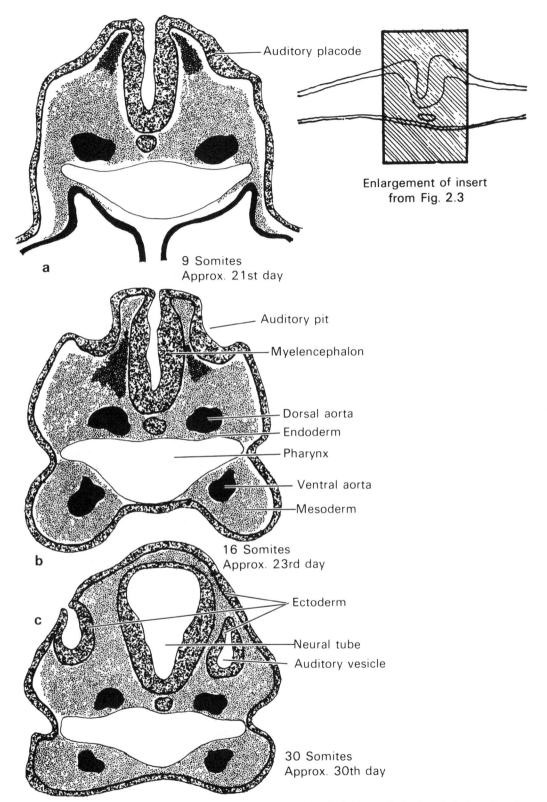

Figure 2.4. Early development of inner ear in human embryo. (Modified with permission from L. B. Arey: *Developmental Anatomy.* Philadelphia, W. B. Saunders, 1940.)

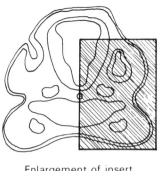

Enlargement of insert
From Fig. 2.4

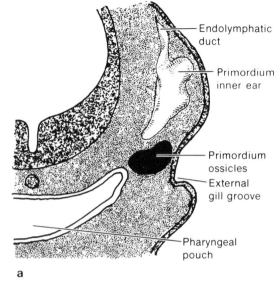

a

Approx. 4½ weeks

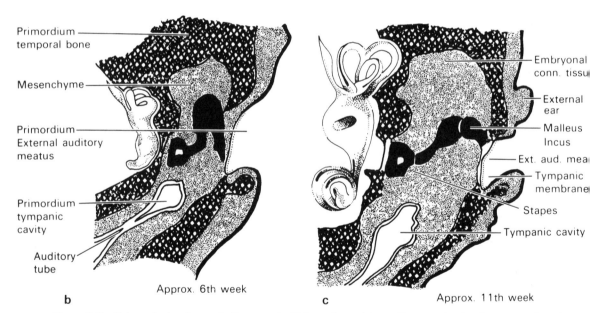

b   Approx. 6th week

c   Approx. 11th week

Figure 2.5. Schematic development of inner and middle portions of the auditory mechanism from approximately 4½ to 11 weeks. (Modified with permission from B. M. Patten: *Human Embryology*, ed. 3. New York, McGraw-Hill, 1968.)

is sinking into the neural plate to become the auditory vesicle. The tympanic cavity and the auditory tube (later known as the eustachian tube) come from an elongation of the lateral-superior edge of the endodermal-lined first pharyngeal pouch. This elongation is called the tubotympanic recess (Fig. 2.5b).

By the time the human embryo is in its fourth week, a series of five branchial grooves or "gill slits" has appeared. These grooves are in the lower head and neck region on the outside of the embryo. On the inside of the embryo a corresponding series of pharyngeal pouches develops, and the collective structures are identified as "arches." In the fish, these grooves from the outside ultimately meet the corresponding pouches on the inside to form "gills" as part of its respiratory mechanism. In humans, most of the branchial grooves do not form slits with the pharyngeal pouches; however, the embryo's passing through this developmental stage is an example of our inheritance of embryonic structure from aquatic ancestors. It is of interest that in the human embryo one of the gill pouches does actually become perforated, forming a passageway from the pharynx to the outside of the head. This passageway becomes the external ear canal and eustachian tube. The eardrum forms a barrier between these two portions of the passageway, which otherwise would directly connect the pharynx and the exterior as does the gill slit of a fish (Himalstein, 1978). Occasionally, an additional opening will occur, forming a cervical fistula or branchial cyst that is an opening on the throat between the pharynx and the surface of the neck. The exact position of the fistula depends on which of the pouches is involved.

During the second month, the tubotympanic recess approaches the embryo surface between the first and second branchial arches, known as Meckel's (or mandibular) and Reichert's (or hyoid) cartilages, respectively. By the eighth week, the tympanic cavity is present in the lower half of the future middle ear, while the upper half is filled with cellular mesenchyme (Fig. 2.5b). The classical theory of ossicle origin holds that the malleus and incus arise from Meckel's cartilage and the stapes comes from Reichert's cartilage. Pearson et al. (1970) suggests a more complex and dual origin for the ossicles. Currently, the first branchial arch is credited for most of the body structure in the malleus and incus, while the second branchial arch gives rise to the lenticular process of the incus, the handle of the malleus, and the stapes. The middle ear cavity itself also has a dual origin, with the anterior area coming from the first arch and the posterior area coming from the second arch. It is noteworthy that the mandible also arises from the first arch.

By 8½ weeks, the incus and the malleus have attained a complete cartilaginous form similar to that in an adult (Fig. 2.5c). The stapes grows as a cartilaginous structure until the 15th week. By the 15th through the 16th week, ossification begins to occur in the cartilaginous surface of the malleus and incus, which have nearly reached completion by the 32nd week. The stapes does not begin to ossify until the 18th week and continues to develop even after ossification is complete. The stapes develops further during life. Otologic surgeons recognize the stapes in a child to be more bulky and less delicate than the normal stapes seen in the adult.

As the ossicles begin to ossify, the surrounding mesenchymal tissue becomes loose and less cellular and is absorbed into the mucoperiosteal membrane of the middle ear cavity. When the ossicles are free from mesenchyma, mucous membrane connecting each ossicle to the walls of the middle ear cavity remains, eventually to become the ossicular supporting ligaments.

By the 30th week, development of the tympanum proper is almost complete. The middle ear cavity antrum is pneumatized by the 34th through 35th week, and the epitympanum is pneumatized during the last fetal month (36th to 38th week). The air cells of the temporal bone develop as outpouchings from the middle ear cavity during the 34th week. Air does not actually enter the middle ear cavity until the onset of respiration immediately after birth.

External Ear and Eardrum. The auricle develops during the third or fourth week from the first and second branchial arches (Fig. 2.6a). Actually, the auricle is derived primarily from the second branchial arch, and only the tragus seems to originate from the first branchial arch. This is about the

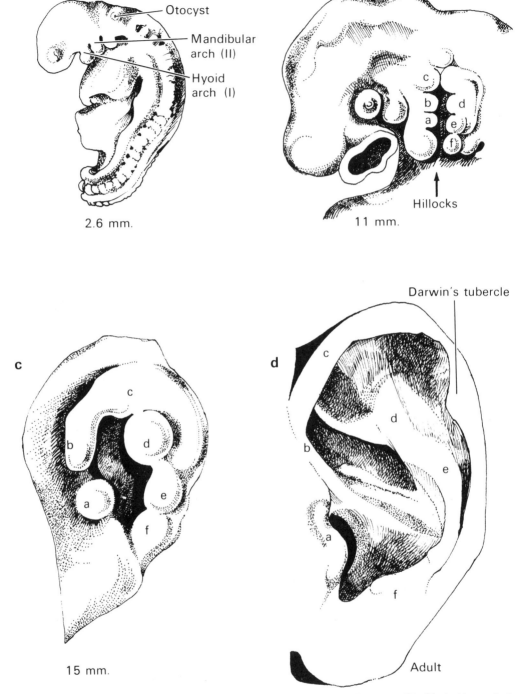

Figure 2.6. Schematic development of auricle from third to fourth week to adult stage. (Modified with permission from L. A. Arey: *Developmental Anatomy*. Philadelphia, W. B. Saunders, 1940; and from B. J. Anson: *An Atlas of Human Anatomy*, ed. 2. Philadelphia, W. B. Saunders, 1963.)

same time that the auditory vesicle is formed in the development of the inner ear.

During the sixth week, six hillocks or tissue thickenings form on both sides of the first branchial groove (Fig. 2.6*b*), arranged as three hillocks on each facing border. The ultimate shape and configuration of the adult auricle depend on the development of these six growth centers; thus many divergent forms of the auricle are within the extremely wide range of normal (Fig. 2.6*c*). Darwin's tubercle forms in some people as an irregularity in the posterior margin of the helix or outer edge of the auricle as shown in Figure 2.6*d*. At this time the mesenchymal folds of the auricle are beginning to become cartilage. From the 7th to the 20th week, the auricle continues to develop, moving from its original ventromedial position to be slowly displaced laterally by the growth of the mandible and face. At the 20th week the auricle is in the adult shape (Fig. 2.6*d*) but continues to grow in size until the individual is 9 years of age.

The external auditory meatus is derived from the first branchial groove during the fourth to fifth week. At this time, the ectodermal lining of the first branchial groove is in brief contact with the endodermal lining of the first pharyngeal pouch. Mesodermal tissue, however, soon grows between the two layers and separates the pharyngeal pouch from the branchial groove. In the eighth week, the primary auditory meatus sinks toward the middle ear cavity and becomes the outer one third of the auditory canal, surrounded ultimately by cartilage.

The ectodermal groove continues to deepen toward the tympanic cavity from the external surface until it meets a thickening of epithelial cells known as the meatal plug, which has arisen from surface ectoderm. Mesenchyme grows between the meatal plug and the epithelial cells of the tympanic cavity. These three layers of tissue, then, become the tympanic membrane composed of inner circular fibers, the fibrous middle layer of tissue, and the outer radial fiber layer, before the ninth week. The solid meatal plug, however, keeps the external auditory canal closed until the 21st week. By this time the inner and middle ear structures are well-formed and ossified. The meatal plug disintegrates and forms a canal, with the innermost layer of meatal plug epithelium becoming the squamous epithelial layer of the tympanic membrane. The external auditory canal continues to develop until the ninth year. At birth the floor of the external auditory canal has no bony portion. In the infant the external auditory canal is short and straight, while in the adult the canal is longer and curves. This suggests that the infant tympanic membrane might be easier to observe than the eardrum of the adult. That is not the case, however, because the infant tympanic membrane is in an oblique or almost a horizontal position and difficult to visualize. The bony portion of the external canal is not complete until about the seventh year. A summary of major embryologic features and their time sequence is presented in Table 2.1.

A young patient with evidence of multiple congenital anomalies related to first and second branchial arch origins is shown in Figure. 2.7. This patient has been diagnosed to have Möbius' syndrome, also termed aplasia of the sixth and seventh cranial nerves. Her cranial deformities include obvious malformations of the external ear, bilateral facial weakness producing a consistent masklike appearance, submucous cleft palate with a bifid uvula, and macrostomia or a greatly exaggerated width of the mouth resulting from failure of proper union of the maxillary and mandibular processes. She has no measurable hearing and is a student in a residential school for the deaf. Radiographic tomographic studies reveal symmetric middle ear anomalies including malleus and incus deformities, the absence of the oval window bilaterally, and mastoid dysplasia. The cochlea and semicircular canal system appear normal on the x-ray study, but the internal auditory canals are abnormally narrow, measuring only 1.5 mm in diameter instead of the normal diameter of approximately 8.0 mm.

Table 2.1.
Embryology Summary of the Ear

Fetal Week	Inner Ear	Middle Ear	External Ear
3rd	Auditory placode; auditory pit	Tubotympanic recess begins to develop	
4th	Auditory vesicle (otocyst); vestibular-cochlear division		Tissue thickenings begin to form
5th			Primary auditory meatus begins
6th	Utricle and saccule present; semicircular canals begin		Six hillocks evident; cartilage begins to form
7th	One cochlear coil present; sensory cells in utricle and saccule		Auricles move dorsolaterally
8th	Ductus reuniens present: sensory cells in semicircular canals	Incus and malleus present in cartilage; lower half of tympanic cavity formed	Outer cartilaginous third of external canal formed
9th		Three tissue layers at tympanic membrane are present	
11th	Two and one-half cochlear coils present; nerve VIII attaches to cochlear duct		
12th	Sensory cells in cochlea; membranous labyrinth complete; otic capsule begins to ossify		
15th		Cartilaginous stapes formed	
16th		Ossification of malleus and incus begins	
18th		Stapes begins to ossify	
20th	Maturation of inner ear; inner ear adult size		Auricle is adult shape but continues to grow until age 9
21st		Meatal plug disintegrates, exposing tympanic membrane	
30th		Pneumatization of tympanum	External auditory canal continues to mature until age 7
32nd		Malleus and incus complete ossification	
34th		Mastoid air cells develop	
35th		Antrum is pneumatized	
37th		Epitympanum is pneumatized; stapes continues to develop until adulthood; tympanic membrane changes relative position during first 2 years of life	

A general overview of human development is presented in Figure 2.8.

ANATOMY OF THE EAR THROUGH TEMPORAL BONE STUDY

Knowledge concerning the anatomy of the temporal bone is becoming increasingly more important to the clinician who deals with hearing loss patients. More and more journal articles and oral presentations at meetings include histologic temporal bone sections to demonstrate some aspect of deafness. Many of the significant advances in our knowledge about the etiology of deafness have come from careful study of temporal bone histologic sections. This information has influenced many areas of clinical services, including hearing aid fittings, educational recommendations and referrals, genetic counseling, and patient progress estimation.

Most speech and hearing training programs have infrequent access to normal or pathologic temporal bone sections. In fact, only a handful of nonmedical clinicians are

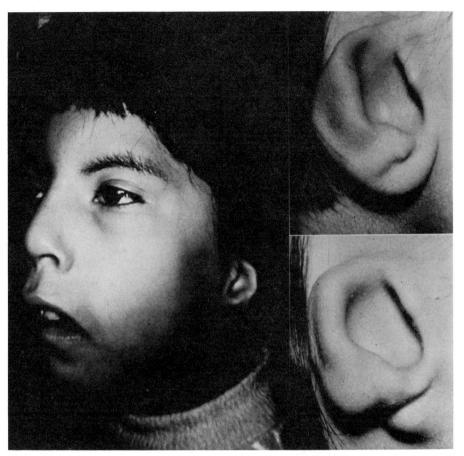

Figure 2.7.   Patient with Möbius' syndrome, with first and second branchial arch anomalies as described in the text.

experienced enough with this technical discipline to teach through the use of histologic sections. Yet this method of instruction enables the student to achieve an understanding of the anatomy of the structures of the ear and vestibular system, as well as an appreciation for the complexity of the hearing mechanism. An understanding of the anatomy of the normal temporal bone will provide the clinician with new insight into the etiology and pathology of deafness.

The paucity of temporal bone anatomic sections available for the benefit of hearing and speech students has prompted us to include this section of histologic samples from a normal temporal bone. Our own understanding of deafness has been enhanced greatly by careful study of temporal bone anatomy and pathology, and we feel that it

is important for students to examine fully the normal temporal bone sections presented in this chapter. These normal histologic samples may be used as a comparative reference for pathologic temporal bone sections shown in other chapters of this book. The clinician can extrapolate from what is known about the pathology of a given ear disease or genetic entity to other similar cases or patients. As an example, knowledge of the temporal bone pathology of meningitis deafness can suggest that when little or no hearing can be detected in a child who has had meningitis, the probability of destruction of cochlear structures is quite high. Temporal bone studies of rubella deafness often demonstrate sections of nearly normal tissues that suggest the possibility of residual hearing in a youngster

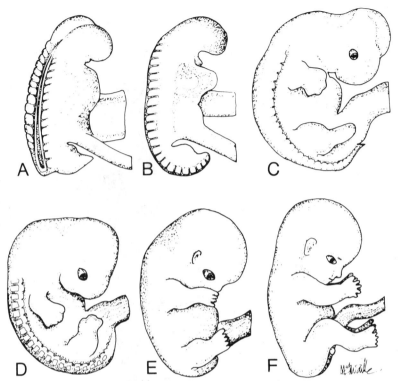

Figure 2.8. Human life and hearing develop together. **A.** The neural tube, the heart, and the brain begin to develop at 3 weeks concurrently with the auditory pit and tubotympanic recess. **B.** In the 4 week old embryo, limbs begin to appear and the otocyst develops. **C.** The embryo is only one-third inch in length at the fifth week when the auditory meatus starts to form. **D.** At 6 weeks, eyes, semicircular canals, and external ear hillocks develop. **E.** Embryonic seventh week includes initial formation of teeth, muscles, genitals, external ear, and cochlea. **F.** Now nearly 1 inch long, at 8 weeks the embryo becomes a fetus, and the middle ear ossicles and tympanic membrane begin to form.

with this disorder, despite clinical failures in obtaining measurable audiometric responses.

Temporal Bone. The temporal bone forms part of the lateral wall and base of the skull, as shown in Figure 2.9. It articulates with other bones of the skull, including the sphenoid, parietal, and occipital bones. The petrous part of the temporal bone is the most dense bone of the body and contains, among other things, most of the structures of the ear. The temporal bone is generally divided into four sections—the squamous, mastoid, petrous, and tympanic areas (Anson and Donaldson, 1967). In general terms, the squamous portion of the temporal bone is superior to the external auditory meatus; the mastoid area is posterior, while

the tympanic portion forms the anterior, inferior, and part of the posterior walls of the external auditory meatus.

The petrous portion of the temporal bone extends medially from the external auditory canal, and its middle third contains the structures of the middle and inner ear. In the petrous bone it is noteworthy that the cochlear portion of the inner ear is situated anteriorly and medially to the internal auditory meatus and the vestibular portion of the inner ear. The internal auditory meatus houses the facial nerve (seventh) which lies superior to the auditory portion of the acoustic nerve (eighth) and anterior to the superior vestibular branch of the eighth cranial nerve. The petrous bone is shown in Figure 2.10 as part of the base of the skull as seen from above.

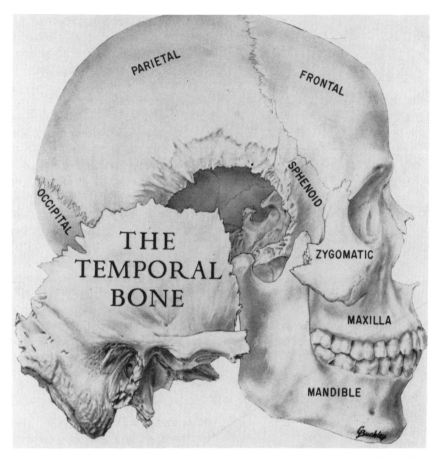

Figure 2.9. Temporal bone section of the human skull. (Reprinted with permission from B. J. Anson and J. A. Donaldson: *The Surgical Anatomy of the Temporal Bone and Ear*. Philadelphia, W. B. Saunders, 1967.)

Preparation of Temporal Bone Histologic Sections. The density of the temporal bone and the intricacy of the inner ear structures make preparation of suitable histologic slides from the gross bone specimen very difficult. The processing of a temporal bone into slides is a difficult, demanding, precise, time-consuming, and expensive procedure. Initially, the temporal bone must be removed from the skull of the donor within 24 hours of death, or the inner ear structures undergo autolysis. The bone is immediately submerged in formalin for 2 or 3 weeks for fixation of structures. An extensive decalcification process follows for some 5 weeks in an adult bone to remove the dense calcium from the temporal bone. Infant temporal bones that are hours or

days old may not show the presence of calcium after the first or second week in the decalcification solutions. Excess bone is then pared from the gross structure, the decalcification chemicals are neutralized and the bone is carefully washed.

The temporal bone is then dehydrated with ethyl alcohol solutions, infiltrated, and embedded into varying solutions of celloidin for nearly 3 months. The celloidin provides support for the bone tissues to permit sectioning with a microtome.

The temporal bone is sliced into sections 20 μm thick, forming some 400 sections from each temporal bone. Only every 10th section is initially stained with dyes, generally hematoxylin and eosin, to give the various tissues color for ease in identification.

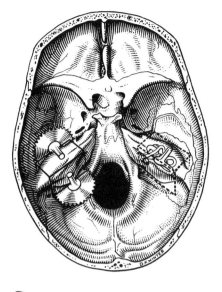

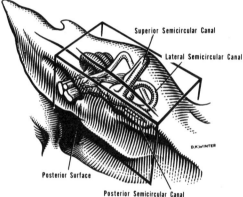

Superior Semicircular Canal

Lateral Semicircular Canal

D.K.WINTER

Posterior Surface

Posterior Semicircular Canal

Figure 2.10. Petrous portion of temporal bone shown as part of the skull viewed from above. (Reprinted with permission from J. C. Gallagher: *Histology of the Human Temporal Bone.* Washington, D. C., Armed Forces Institute of Pathology, 1967.)

The dyed sections are mounted on microscope slides, ready for reading.

Examination of the stained sections of the temporal bone under high-powered magnification takes expert skills and knowledge gained only through experience and thorough study. The entire procedure involved in preparation of a single temporal bone may involve some 5 individuals, take 9 months of time, and is estimated to cost more than $1000.

Anatomy of a Normal Temporal Bone.

An understanding of normal temporal bone

structures is necessary before one can appreciate the abnormalities found in temporal bone from patients with various kinds of deafness. Temporal bone study is usually reserved for residents in otolaryngology or physiologists interested in studying mechanisms of hearing, but there seems sufficient reason for all students of hearing disorders to have some familiarity with anatomy as demonstrated by horizontally cut, temporal bone histopathologic sections.

One must keep in mind the general level of the section under study as it was taken from the inner ear, or temporal bone block. Figure 2.11 shows the general gross structure of the inner ear. Imagine a horizontal line drawn through the most superior portion of the inner ear, and you will see that the only structure represented might be the arch of the superior semicircular canal. As the microtome cuts off horizontal sections from a temporal bone block, the superior semicircular canal will be the initial structure to be sectioned. One must then imagine how a horizontal slice of temporal bone tissue will appear when placed on a microscope slide and viewed from above. The student of temporal bone anatomy must have a draftsman's ability to imagine 3-dimensional structures from a 2-dimensional picture.

Samples sections from a horizontally sectioned petrous portion of a temporal bone are shown in the next few pages. The sections have been selected because they show specific portions of the inner ear that are of interest to audiologists. Photographs of the midmodiolar section of the cochlear and a single coil, or turn of the cochlear and a single coil, or turn of the cochlea have been included at higher magnification, so readers can appreciate these interesting structures.

Figure 2.12. Well-pneumatized mastoid can be seen in the posterior (or left) area of this section. The ampulla of the superior semicircular canal is shown as a nearly round structure enclosing the membranous labyrinth. The crista is noticeable on the anterior edge of the superior semicircular canal ampulla. The facial nerve and its genu

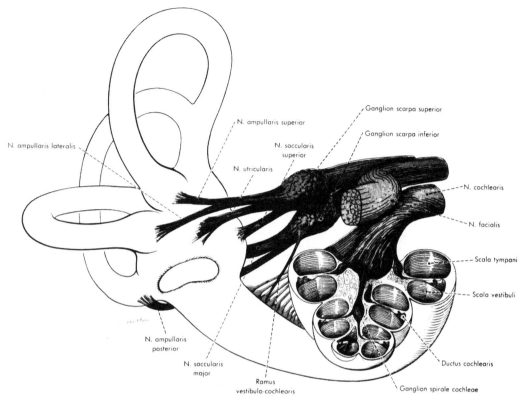

N. ampullaris superior

Ganglion scarpa superior

Ganglion scarpa inferior

N. saccularis
superior

N. ampullaris lateralis

N. utricularis

N. cochlearis

N. facialis

Scala tympani

Scala vestibuli

N. ampullaris
posterior

N. saccularis
major

Ramus
vestibulo-cochlearis

Ductus cochlearis

Ganglion spirale cochleae

Figure 2.11. Inner ear. Note the position of the facial nerve to the cochlear nerve and to the superior and inferior vestibular nerve. The cochlea is open to illustrate the midmodiolar view as observed in temporal bone sections. (Reprinted with permission from B. J. Melloni: *Some Pathological Conditions of the Eye, Ear, and Throat: An Atlas.* Chicago, Abbott Laboratories, 1957.)

are very clearly shown in this slide, which has cut across the superior portion of the internal auditory canal. Immediately anterior to the genu of the facial nerve is the dense bone of the otic capsule, which contains the cochlea. The lateral semicircular canal and its membranous labyrinth are also present at the peripheral edges of the structure.

Figure 2.13. This section is approximately 1 mm below the previous slide. The middle ear cavity is now obvious in this section and contains a cross-sectional view of the malleus and incus joined by the malleoincudal joint. The facial nerve is now encased in the facial canal. The upper portion of the basal turn of the cochlea is now present anteriorly and medially to the facial nerve. The superior branch of the vestibular nerve is visible in the internal auditory meatus and is shown passing to the macula

of the utricle. The endolymphatic duct is also present.

Figure 2.14. This section is approximately 1 mm below the section shown in the previous figure. The middle ear cavity shows the malleus and incus with its short process pointing posteriorly toward the aditus and antrum into the mastoid air spaces. The anterior mallear ligament can also be seen. The large space immediately medial to the facial nerve and canal contains the utricle. This section passes through the basal and middle turns of the cochlea that extend laterally. Reissner's membrane, the basilar membrane, and spiral ligament are obvious, even at this magnification. The modiolus is evident in the center of the basal turn of the cochlea. The inferior division of the vestibular nerve and the cochlear branch of the auditory nerve are shown in the internal auditory meatus. The endo-

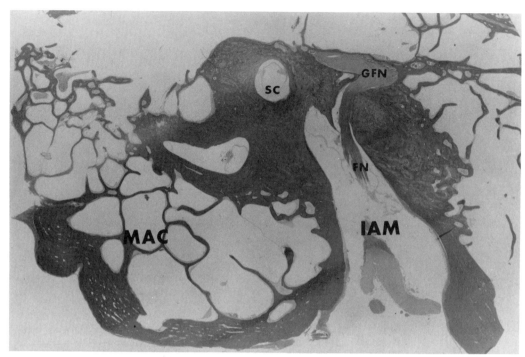

Figure 2.12. Temporal bone horizontal section showing facial nerve genu (*GFN*), facial nerve (*FN*), internal auditory meatus (*IAM*), ampulla of superior semicircular canal (*SC*), and mastoid air cells (*MAC*). (Courtesy of I. Sando, M.D.)

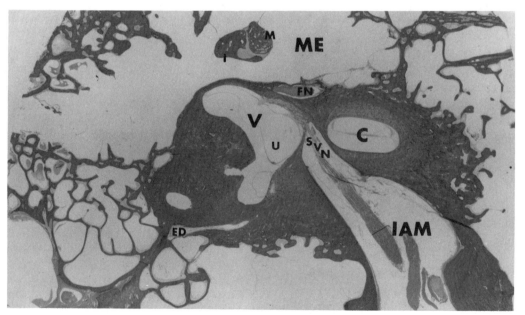

Figure 2.13. Horizontal section of normal temporal bone, showing malleus (*M*) and incus (*I*) in attic of middle ear (*ME*), utricle (*U*), basal turn of the cochlea (*C*), and superior vestibular nerve (*SVN*), feeding into vestibule (*V*) from the internal auditory meatus (*IAM*). The endolymphatic duct (*ED*) is seen at lower left corner. (Courtesy of I. Sando, M.D.)

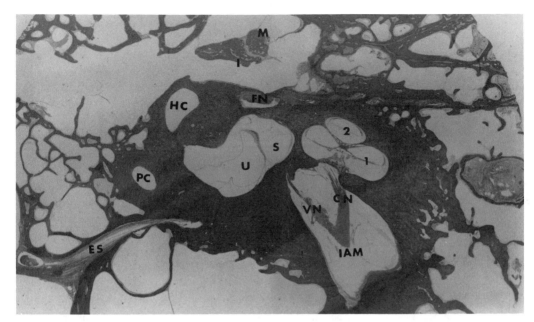

Figure 2.14. Horizontal section from normal temporal bone showing two cochlear turns, basal (*1*) and middle (*2*); vestibular (*VN*) and cochlear (*CN*) portions of the eighth nerve in the internal auditory meatus (*IAM*), the endolymphatic sac (*ES*) is shown at lower left. The utricle (*U*) and the saccule (*S*) may be seen in the vestibule. The horizontal (*HC*) and posterior (*PC*) semicircular canals are also identified. Malleus (*M*); incus (*I*); facial nerve (*FN*). (Courtesy of I. Sando, M.D.)

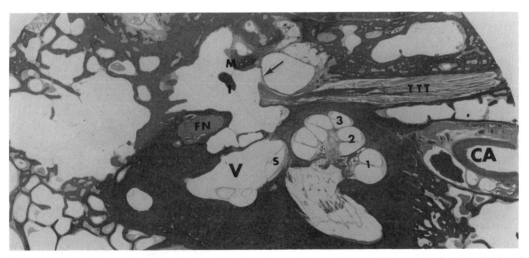

Figure 2.15. Cochlear midmodiolar horizontal section of normal temporal bone. All three coils of cochlea (*1, 2,* and *3*) are evident; the malleus (*M*) is attached to tympanic membrane; the tensor tympani muscle (*TTT*) extends through the processus cochleariformis with tensor tendon (identified by *arrow*) to malleus. *FN*, facial nerve; *V*, vestibule; *CA*, internal carotid artery; *I*, incus; *S*, saccule. (Courtesy of I. Sando, M.D.)

lymphatic sac is apparent in the posteromedial portion of the photograph.

Figure 2.15. This section is about 1 mm lower than the section shown in Figure 2.14. This section passes through the bony modiolus of the basal and middle turns of the cochlea and now includes the final cochlear turn, the apical coil. In the middle ear, the malleus and incus are no longer touching. The large tensor tympani muscle in its

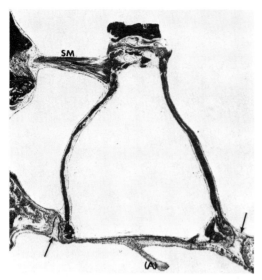

Figure 2.16. Enlargement of stapes in oval window and stapedial tendon (*SM*). Note normal attachment of stapes footplate in oval window by annular ligament (*arrows*). (Courtesy of E. L. Grandon, M.D., Cedar Rapids, Iowa.)

canal is very obvious immediately adjacent to the cochlea and running anteroposterior. This section shows the processus cochleariformis extending posteriorly into the middle ear cavity from which the small tensor tympani tendon can be seen attaching to the anterior surface of the malleus. Part of the stapedial crura can be seen with the stapes footplate in the oval window niche. (An enlargement of the stapes in the oval window with the attachment of the stapedial tendon is shown in Fig. 2.16.) The saccule and its innervation can be seen clearly in the vestibule along with the lateral semicircular canal and utricle. The large circular structure at the anterior edge of the section is the internal carotid artery. All three ossicles are difficult to demonstrate on one temporal bone section because they are not lined up equally on a single horizontal plane level.

Figure 2.17. This is an enlargement of the cochlea as viewed in Figure 2.15. It may be useful to the reader to review the gross view of the inner ear in Figure 2.11 to see how this exposure of the cochlea is obtained. This is a midmodiolar section of the cochlea showing the basal, middle, and apical turns. The nerve fibers are easily seen in the internal auditory meatus, and the ganglion cells of the spiral ganglion may be seen in Rosenthal's canal. The osseous spiral lamina extends radially from the modiolus in each turn. The basilar membrane can be seen extending from the osseous spiral lamina to the spiral ligament and stria vascularis. Reissner's membrane is seen in each coil of the cochlea, separating the scala vestibuli from the scala media. The basilar membrane supports the organ of Corti, which can just barely be seen at this magnification.

Figure 2.18. This classic view of a cochlear turn emphasizes the structures of the scala media. These structures can be observed on a human temporal bone section by increasing the magnification on a single cochlear turn. The cochlear nerve fibers are shown under the spiral osseous lamina at the left of the photograph. The limbus supports one end of the tectorial membrane, which in its natural position should extend over the outer hair cells. The tectorial membrane, however, is very often seen in distorted position as an artifact of the temporal bone preparation procedure. Reissner's membrane extends from the limbus (crista spiralis) to the edge of the spiral ligament and stria vascularis. The curve between the limbus and the organ of Corti is the internal sulcus. The lower edge of the limbus, pointing and extending toward the organ of Corti, is known as the tympanic lip, which has numerous holes termed the habenula perforata. The habenula perforata permits cochlear nerve fibers to enter the organ of Corti from below the osseous spiral lamina.

The basilar membrane supports the organ of Corti, which includes inner hair cells, outer hair cells, and the tunnel of Corti. The tunnel of Corti is formed by inner and outer pillar cells. Various supporting cells are seen next to the hair cells. Hensen's and Claudius' supporting cells are found between the outer hair cells and the external sulcus formed by the lower curve of the

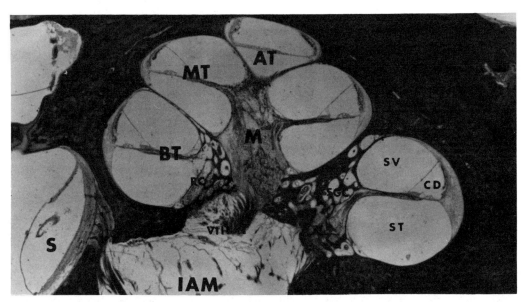

Figure 2.17. Enlargement of cochlea from horizontal temporal bone section shown in Figure 2.15. Note auditory nerve (*VIII N*) in internal auditory meatus (*IAM*) with ganglion cells (*SGC*) in Rosenthal's canal (*RC*). The cochlear basal turn (*BT*), the middle turn (*MT*), and apical turn (*AT*) are clearly shown. Three ducts are seen in each turn: the scala vestibuli (*SV*), the cochlear duct (*CD*), and the scala tympani (*ST*); the saccule (*S*) is also obvious in this view, with its innervation. *M*, modiolus. (Courtesy of I. Sando, M.D.)

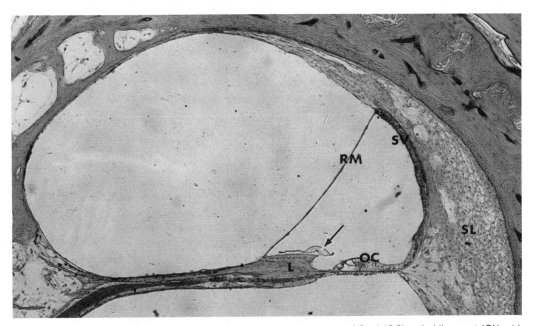

Figure 2.18. Higher magnification of one cochlear duct, showing organ of Corti (*OC*), spiral ligament (*SL*), stria vascularis (*SV*), Reissner's membrane (*RM*), tectorial membrane (*arrow*), and limbus (*L*). (Courtesy of I. Sando, M.D., and L. Bergstrom, M.D.)

stria vascularis. Nuel's space is between the outer pillar and the first row of outer hair cells. The outer hair cells are sup-ported by outer phalangeal cells (Deiter's cells). Thus, the outer hair cell rests on a Deiter's cell and extends hairs from its up-

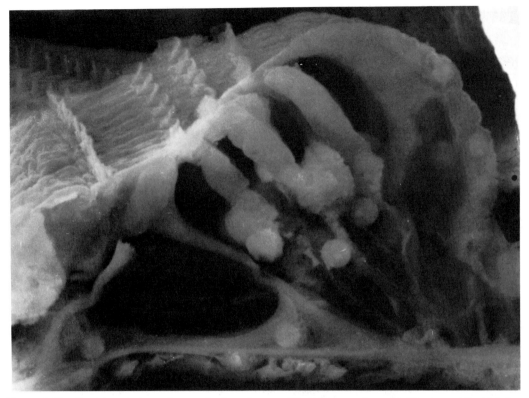

Figure 2.19. Scanning electron microscopic view of organ of Corti from a guinea pig. (Courtesy of David Asher, Ph.D., University of Colorado School of Medicine.)

per surface toward the tectorial membrane. The lower portion of the stria vascularis contains a bulge known as the spiral prominence, which contains a blood vessel, the vas prominens.

Our understanding of the anatomy and physiology of the fine structure of the inner ear has increased tremendously since utilization of the electron microscope began in 1951. The scanning electron microscope is now adding new dimension to our appreciation of inner ear structures. Unlike the conventional electron microscope, which transmits an electron beam through the specimen, the image in the scanning microscope is created by secondary electrons emitted from the excited surface of the specimen. The result is a picture similar to the image produced on a TV screen. The depth of field obtained with the scanning microscope is about 500 times that of a light microscope. An outstanding monograph has been pub-

lished by David Lim (1969) featuring 3-dimensional views of the inner ear with the scanning electron microscope. A photograph of the organ of Corti taken with a scanning electron microscope is shown in Figure 2.19.

PHYSIOLOGY OF HEARING

To appreciate fully the intricacies of hearing impairment, one must understand the normal physiology of the hearing mechanism and the nature of hearing loss. These concepts are presented lightly here only as background material so that we may develop discussion regarding the pathologies of hearing impairment in the following chapter.

The phenomenon of hearing is the result of a complex series of events. Sound energy, originating as vibration and transmitted through an elastic medium such as air, impinges on the tympanic membrane causing it to vibrate. The vibrations are transmitted to the oval window of the otic capsule by the three middle ear ossicles. In addition to serving as a conductor to the sound energy, the tympanic membrane and ossicles amplify the sound by two simple mechanical principles consisting of a slight lever action of the ossicles and the areal surface relationship between the surface area of the tympanic membrane and the funneling of sound energy onto the smaller surface area of the stapes footplate. This middle ear amplification amounts to approximately 30 dB and may be lost when defects or pathologies inhibit either or both of the amplifying mechanisms (Lipscomb, 1988).

The mechanical vibration transmitted by the stapes to the oval window induces motion in the fluids of the cochlea where the intensity and frequency of the vibrations are faithfully transmitted by traveling waves to the receptor cells for hearing. Perilymph fluid fills two ducts within the cochlea that are known as the scala vestibuli and the scala tympani. These parallel scalae communicate with each other at the helicotrema in the apical tip of the cochlear coils. When sound vibration displaces the stapes inward into the scala vestibuli, a simultaneous outward motion occurs in the scala tympani at the round window membrane; this movement is termed the round window reflex.

We also hear by bone-conducted vibrations that bypass the external and middle ear, displacing fluids of the cochlea and resulting in traveling waves that stimulate the hairs of the receptor cells within the organ of Corti.

The organ of Corti is a papillary structure resting on a basilar membrane within the scala media (cochlear duct) and is composed of sensorineural receptors and supporting elements. The organ of Corti is specifically designed to convert mechanical vibrations into electrical events transmitted to the central nervous system. According to Lippe (1986), our understanding of cochlear physiology has undergone considerable change in the past few years because of new research findings.

The vibratory fluid motion in the cochlea ultimately causes a nerve impulse, with the cochlear neural epithelium acting as a mechanical transducer. This cochlear epithelium is composed of about 16,800 hair cells in each ear. According to Dallos (1988), the hair cells are arranged in an inner row of approximately 3,500 cells, while some 14,000 hair cells are found in three parallel rows in the cochlea. The hair cells rest on supporting cells that, in turn, rest on the basilar membrane and extend into a third cochlear duct filled with endolymph fluid known as the scala media or cochlear duct. This third duct is interposed between the scala vestibuli and scala tympani throughout the entire two and a half turns of the cochlea. Hair cells have an orderly arrangement in the cochlea that is related to sound frequency. Hair cells that respond to high frequency above 2000 Hz are located in the basal turn of the cochlea, while hair cells that are tuned to stimulating frequencies below 2000 Hz are found in the middle and apical cochlear coils.

The peripheral neurons of the cochlear nerve are distributed to hair cells from beneath the basilar membrane and its supporting shelf, the osseous spiral lamina. The fluid motion of the scala tympani, due to its physical properties of width, length, thickness, mass and elasticity, displaces the basilar membrane in a traveling wave pattern, producing torsion on the hairlike processes of the cell and creating some type of mechanical-chemical change resulting in peripheral-nerve-ending stimulation (Ryan and Dallos, 1984). Thus, the vibratory energy transmitted by the tympanic membrane is transformed into neural impulse code. Interested readers are referred to Yost and Nielsen (1985) and Jahn and Santos-Sacchi (1988) for a more complete discussion of auditory physiology.

Auditory Nerve. The nerve fibers that innervate the hair cells have their cell bodies in the bipolar spiral ganglion located in Rosenthal's canal. Axons from the spiral ganglion cells join in the modiolus and collect as the auditory, or cochlear, branch of the eighth nerve. Just outside the cochlea the vestibular portion of the eighth nerve coming from the semicircular canals, utricle, and saccule joins the cochlear portion. The two portions of the eighth nerve come together like a rope and pass through the internal auditory meatus toward the medulla. The structure of the auditory nerve is orderly, with fibers from the apical quarter of the cochlea forming the core of the nerve, and around them are the fibers from the apex of the cochlea twisting one way, while the fibers from the middle turn of the cochlea twist the other way. Fifty percent of the fibers from the cochlea come from the basal coil and represent sensory elements that respond to frequencies above 2000 Hz.

Research by Spoendlin (1967, 1969) has shown that most of the afferent neurons come from the inner hair cells, whereas only some 10% of the fibers come from the outer hair cells. Each outer hair cell is, however, innervated by several different neurons, while one neuron innervates a large number of outer hair cells. The inner hair cells are innervated by a large number of different neurons, but each neuron innervates only one inner hair cell.

The eighth nerve divides again, however, before it reaches the medulla. The auditory portion divides into dorsal and ventral branches that go to corresponding nuclei in the brainstem wherein the second-order afferent auditory neuron cell bodies are located.

Experimenters have found that fibers in the eighth nerve are "tuned" to certain frequencies. That is, certain fibers are most responsive to certain stimulating frequencies. This fact is determined by inserting microelectrodes into single nerve fibers and determining the threshold for the action potential "spike" of that nerve fiber for a variety of frequencies, then plotting what is known as the response area for that particular fiber. The threshold sensitivity of a fi-

ber increases gradually and is most sensitive at its "tuned" frequency—which can then be used to name the fiber, such as "7000 Hz fiber." Most of the auditory fibers are high-frequency units, usually above 1000 Hz. More recent observations indicate that individual inner hair cells also maintain characteristic responses to "tuned" frequencies and may actually be more finely tuned than the nerve fibers (Evans, 1975). It is remarkable that only a few fibers of the eighth nerve are required to preserve good hearing. The auditory nerve must be sectioned more than halfway to have a measurable effect on auditory thresholds, and then, if indeed hearing is left, it is predominantly low-frequency hearing (Neff, 1947; Wever and Neff, 1947). To click stimuli, the individual nerve responses, tuned to different frequencies, fire in close synchrony, so that the amplitude of the action potential is representative of the number of fibers that respond (Davis, 1961).

Brainstem Pathways. Much of the brainstem auditory pathway can be seen in Figures 2.20 and 2.21 and is well-described by Nolte (1988). The higher auditory pathways are rather complex and often escape significance with students who tend only to memorize the names of the relay stations and major neuronal paths. It is important to realize that although first-order neurons from the cochlea reach the brainstem in the cochlear nuclei, most of the activity that ultimately reaches the cortex is by way of fourth-order neurons. This seemingly too complex system seldom breaks down because of alternate paths to the cerebral cortex (Lynn and Gilroy, 1984; Thompson, 1983).

Two pairs of cochlear nuclei exist, a dorsal and a ventral cochlear nucleus on each side of the medulla, but are referred to collectively as the cochlear nuclei of the medulla. Although some of the neurons of the cochlear nuclei ascend to higher nuclei on the same side of the system, most cross over to the opposite side in the trapezoid body. Auditory units in the cochlear nuclei

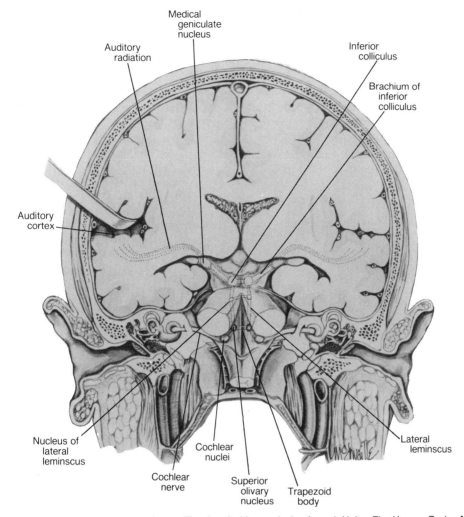

Figure 2.20. Ascending auditory pathway. (Reprinted with permission from J. Nolte: *The Human Brain: An Introduction to Its Functional Anatomy*, ed. 2. St. Louis, C. V. Mosby, 1988.)

are also sensitive to specific frequencies as we noted previously with auditory nerve fibers. Inhibitory units have also been reported in the cochlear nuclei, which under certain circumstances actually inhibit response rather than excite the unit under examination. Thus a particular frequency stimulus may excite certain neurons of the auditory system, while inhibiting other units from firing. What starts out in the cochlea as the excitation of the relatively large group of hair cells is narrowed down to a smaller group of neurons through the process of inhibition. In addition, the cochlear nuclei, like the cochlea, exhibit ton-

otopic organization, or an orderly arrangement of responsiveness to different frequencies. In fact, Rose et al. (1959) reported one unrolling of the cochlear frequency distribution in the dorsal cochlear nucleus and two separate complete frequency patterns in the ventral nuclei. The number of discharges from a single cochlear nucleus unit is apparently related to the intensity of the acoustic stimulus.

The principal terminations of second-order afferent auditory neurons are in the nuclei of the trapezoid body and superior olivary body. The superior olive is the first structure in the medulla that receives fibers

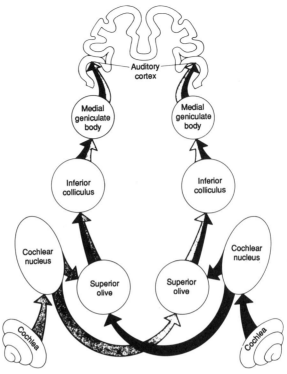

Figure 2.21. A diagrammatic scheme for the ascending auditory pathway. (Reprinted with permission from W. A. Yost and D. W. Nielsen: *Fundamentals of Hearing*. New York, Holt, Rinehart & Winston, 1977.)

from both ears, and it may play a role in the localization of sound. From here, neurons originate that course upward in the loosely compacted neurons of the lateral lemniscus to another principal relay station, the inferior colliculus. Collaterals of second- and third-order neurons are given off to the reticular formation that provides an indirect, diffuse, sensory pathway to the cerebral cortex. The reticular formation is closely related to arousal and attention during sleep and may be responsible for the fact that a crying baby may wake only the mother but no one else in the family. Or one may sleep soundly through a barrage of noise but wake suddenly upon hearing a soft familiar voice.

Most of the fibers in the lateral lemniscus pathway terminate in the inferior colliculus, but some may bypass and end in the next relay station, the medial geniculate body. So far as is known, all direct projections to the auditory cortex are relayed in the medial geniculate body. The auditory cortex is, of course, responsible for the fine discrimination necessary in the understanding of speech. The "tuning" function of the higher auditory centers including the inferior colliculus, the medial geniculate body, and the auditory cortex has been summarized by Dallos (1988): Some units at higher levels in the auditory system are frequency specific, and some are not; many units respond only to clicks with a complex spectrum and are unresponsive to pure tone signals; many units show spontaneous firing that can sometimes be inhibited by acoustic stimuli; and of the units that are frequency-specific, the response areas of the units higher up in the auditory system tend to be narrower than those units found in lower auditory centers. An estimated cell count of each of the levels in the afferent auditory pathway is presented in Table 2.2 (Schuknecht, 1974).

Attempts to map the cortical responses to auditory stimuli have identified the tem-

Table 2.2.
Afferent Auditory Pathways and Estimated Cell Count at Each Level

Cochlear nuclei	8,800
Superior olivary complex	34,000
Nuclei of lateral lemniscus	38,000
Inferior colliculus	392,000
Medial geniculate body	364,000
Auditory cortex	10,000,000

poral lobe as the responsive area, sometimes further localized as Brodmann's areas 41 and 42. The cortex has at least two tonotopic frequency projections that are the reverse of each other. Kryter and Ades (1943) established a very important fact with significant clinical implication. They showed that under appropriate conditions, cortical lesions have no appreciable effect on the absolute thresholds of pure tone stimuli. This is true even when extensive bilateral cortical lesions are made. Thus, the ability to respond to tones is not dependent upon cerebral cortex. These same investigators reported that removal of the inferior colliculi created an approximate 15 dB loss in pure tone sensitivity; destruction of the entire auditory system from the midbrain to the cortex created a pure tone loss of about 40 dB. It may be concluded that the most important aspect of auditory sensitivity to pure tones is due to intact neurons below the inferior colliculi, and a nearly normal audiogram may be obtained with a loss of 75% of the neurons of the auditory nerve.

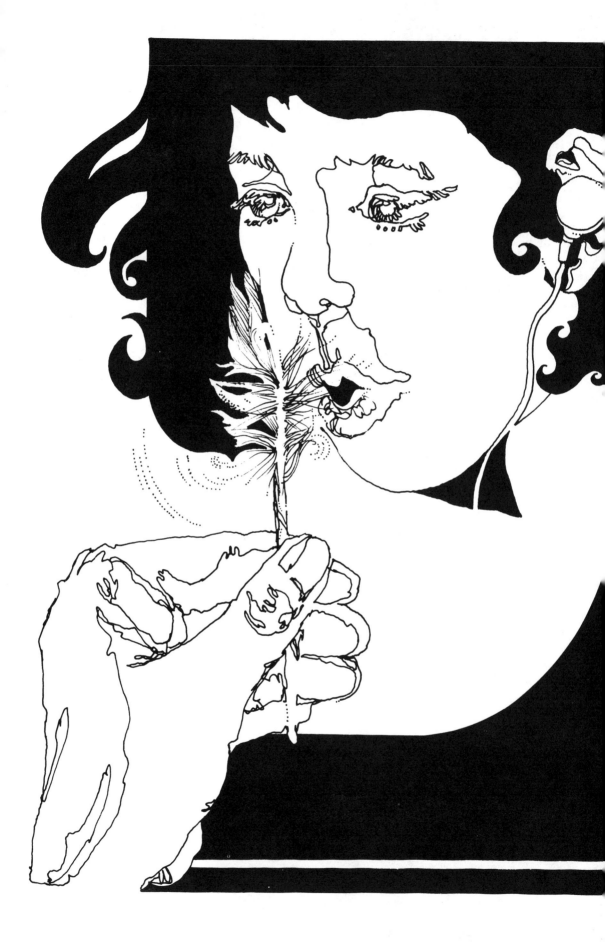

CHAPTER 3

Medical Aspects of Hearing Loss

Detailed descriptions of disorders associated with hearing loss in children are presented in most textbooks on otolaryngology, such as *Pediatric Otolaryngology* by Bluestone and Stool (1990) and *Clinical Pediatric Otolaryngology* edited by Balkany and Pashley (1986). Audiology textbooks may offer material on hearing pathology, but it is usually offered in a nonmedical manner, so that insufficient information is available to audiologists who work with medical personnel. The material presented below is not as complete as that found in otolaryngology textbooks, but it is our hope it is more pertinent to childhood disorders than that commonly found in basic audiology textbooks.

DISORDERS ASSOCIATED WITH HEARING LOSS

Conditions of the External Ear and Ear Canal.
The audiologist may have confrontation with various medical conditions involving the pinna and external auditory canal. The fitting of ear defenders for hearing conservation, the making of earmold impressions, and the insertion of immittance probe tips make it imperative for the clinician to recognize disorders of the external ear.

To recognize the presence of a diseased state, one must appreciate the normal anatomy of the pinna, the external auditory canal, and their normal variations. The pinna or auricle is an appendage attached to the side of the head, level with the middle third of the face. It is composed of a piece of elastic cartilage with numerous convolutions, covered with thin skin, and fixed in position at the lateral aspect of the external auditory canal by its direct continuity with the cartilaginous canal, auricular muscles, and auricular ligaments. Its major convolutions include the helix, anthelix, tragus, antitragus, and concha. The lobule is unique in that it contains no cartilage and, therefore, has been designated by various cultures as the appropriate place through which and on which to hang ornaments for decoration.

An opening, the external auditory meatus, in the concha leads to the external auditory canal that is cartilaginous in the lateral third and bony in the medial two thirds. The cartilage of the external auditory canal is continuous with that of the pinna except in the anterosuperior aspect. Present in the anterior cartilaginous canal wall are several fissures to permit flexibility. Hence, the curved path of the canal can be partially straightened to facilitate inspection by gently pulling posterosuperiorly on the pinna. Squamous epithelium lines the external canal and covers the tympanic membrane. This skin is thicker laterally with hair follicles, sebaceous glands, and earwax-producing glands, but it is quite thin over the more medial bony portion of the canal with fewer skin structures present. This skin is unusual because it does not flake, as does other squamous epithelium, but migrates laterally toward the external meatus, providing a self-cleaning mechanism unique to the ear canal.

At the onset of every clinical evaluation or testing procedure, one should initially note the location of the pinnae and their relationship to the remainder of the structures of the head and face. Normally, the superior border of the helix is located at the outer canthus of the eye, and the tragus is roughly level with the infraorbital rim (Fig.

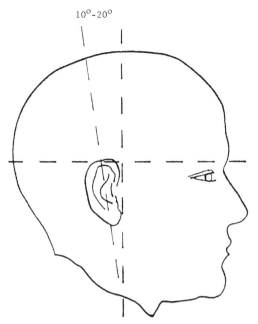

10°-20°

Figure 3.1.   Pinna in relationship to structures of face.

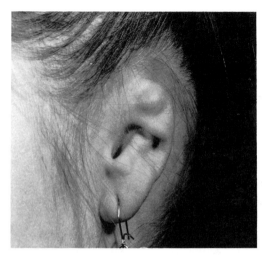

Figure 3.2.   Atretic ear canal and microtia of the pinna.

3.1). Low-set auricles are frequently associated with other anomalies of the first and second branchial cleft. Even though the pinna may have no abnormality in its location or basic shape, the alert clinician should be aware of any lump, ulcer, or lesion on the pinna.

After ascertaining that the pinna is located in the normal position, one should observe the size and shape of the auricle. The child with ears that stick out from his head in a prominent fashion may have severe social problems from the ridicule of his or her peers. Successful surgical treatment of a patient with this deformity prior to the patient's entering school may save a great deal of emotional anguish. About 90% of the time this condition is the result of an excessively deep concha and/or lack of development of the anthelical fold. Correction of these deformities is easily accomplished through an incision of the back of the pinna through which stitches are then used to hold the ear in its new position.

Atresia or Stenosis of the Canal.   Atresia is the complete closing off of the ear ca-nal, while stenosis is a narrowing of the canal. Atresia or stenosis may accompany microtia, or either may appear in conjunction with a normal auricle (Fig. 3.2). Stenosis may be congenital or acquired. The embryonic atresia plate may be solid bone or membranous; x-ray examination will help distinguish between these two possibilities. The incidence of aural atresia (with or without abnormalities of the pinnae) is estimated to be between 1 and 5 per 20,000 live births (Cooper and Jabs, 1987). Atresia is frequently observed with cranial, facial, mandibular, or acrofacial dysostoses such as Cruzon's disease or Treacher Collins' syndrome. Aural atresia may also be associated with facial, labial, and/or palatal clefts. Abnormalities of the skeletal system and visceral organs or chromosomal aberrations may also accompany atresia. Children with these defects usually suffer conductive-type hearing losses and may do well with bone conduction hearing aids if medical or surgical treatment is not in order. Jahrsdoerfer and Hall (1986) report surgical results and complications from operating on 202 patients with congenital malformations of the external ear.

Collapsed Ear Canals.   In some children the anatomy of the concha-meatal opening is such that collapse of the ear canal occurs during audiometric testing. This situation produces a conductive-type hearing loss from pressure of the earphones against the pinna, tragus and opening to the external auditory meatus. Audiometric testing will show an erroneous air-bone gap from supposed conductive hearing loss. The suspected conductive hearing loss will not be confirmed by immittance audiometry or otologic examination of the ear. Such children can be shown to have normal hearing when retested with a hollow auditory canal plug used under the earphone or when tested in sound field conditions.

Aural Discharge. The presence of fluid running from the external auditory meatus should give the clinician concern. Fluid from the external auditory canal may be divided in three categories: (*1*) clear, (*2*) cloudy, whitish, or yellow, and (*3*) bloody.

1. Clear Fluid. Clear fluid may represent cerebral spinal fluid leaking from a temporal bone fracture, which offers a ready route for access for infection into the cranial cavity. This condition requires prompt otologic consultation by physical examination, x-ray studies, and perhaps surgical exploration of the ear to confirm and repair the leakage.

2. Cloudy Fluid. Cloudy fluid usually represents inflammation of the external auditory canal, a condition known as external otitis. Less often, cloudy discharge may result from an inflamed middle ear space with existing perforation of the tympanic membrane. External otitis should be treated before performing immittance audiometry, as insertion of the probe tip may cause pain and such evaluation is unlikely to provide additional diagnostic information.

3. Blood. Blood coming from the external auditory canal frequently results from self-instrumentation of the ear canal to relieve itching or remove earwax. Blood coming from the ear canal may also be an expression of a fracture of the temporal bone and, as such, requires immediate medical consultation. Presence of these types of fluid requires immediate medical referral.

Cerumen and Foreign Bodies. Cerumen, or earwax, is a combined product of the apocrine and sebaceous glands located in the skin of the ear canal. Cerumen comes in two varieties: wet and dry. Wet earwax varies from yellowish to dark brown and, at times, even resembles blood. Dry earwax tends to be whitish scales or powdery feathery-like material. Most people's ear canals are self-cleaning of cerumen because of the migratory pattern of the epithelium toward the external auditory meatus. The cerumen may easily be wiped away with a washcloth. People with excessive production of cerumen or inadequate self-cleaning mechanism may accumulate wax in the external auditory canal, which can cause hearing loss. These individuals should have the wax removed by a physician who will frequently utilize magnification for improved visibility. The use of a Waterpic or the use of the infamous Q-tip applicator is to be condemned. Cotton tip applicators, in the hands of an aggressive parent, are a major source of lacerated ear canals, perforated eardrums, and occasional sensorineural hearing loss or deafness from displaced ossicles that are accidentally forced into the inner ear.

Children are the leading candidates to appear with a foreign object in their ear canal—objects that may include broken crayons, food, small toys, or pieces of jewelry. Hearing loss is usually not a major concern in such cases unless the foreign object has ruptured the tympanic membrane. Referral to a medical specialist for removal of the object is, of course, mandatory.

Bony Growths. Occasionally, bony outgrowths in the external auditory canal may create problems. These come in two forms: (*1*) multiple growths termed *exostoses*; and (*2*) single growths termed *osteomas*. These are the most common neoplasms of the external auditory canal and appear as smooth, hard, round nodules covered with normal skin. Exostoses do not require removal unless they cause cerumen accumulation, impair hearing, or create canal obstruction. Osteomas usually continue to grow and, hence, require surgical removal.

Inflammatory Conditions. Occasionally, just touching the pinna will cause the patient to wince or react with noticeable discomfort. Conditions most frequently responsible for this phenomenon are: (*1*) external otitis, (*2*) perichondritis, and/or (*3*) furunculosis of the external auditory canal.

1. *Otitis Externa.* Otitis externa is an inflammation of the skin of the external auditory canal, most frequently due to bacterial infection or fungal infection. The presence of water in the ear canal against the tympanic membrane provides ideal circumstances for bacterial growth. The skin of the canal on acute external otitis is usually red and quite tender, with some form of drainage present. It is of interest that external otitis is frequently found in hearing aid users. The presence of an occlusive earmold results in increased moisture in the ear canal, which seems to predispose external otitis. The otolaryngologist may suggest that the patient either switch his or her hearing aid to the opposite ear or, in certain instances, go without the aid for a while until the condition clears. The use of open-type earmolds helps prevent this possible condition (Alvord et al., 1989).

2. *Perichondritis.* Perichondritis is an inflammation of the covering of the cartilage of the ear or ear canal. It is usually secondary to trauma to the cartilage, either accidental or surgical. The pinna is usually red and tender with generalized swelling. Subperichondrial abscesses may deprive the cartilage of needed blood supply. The resultant lack of nourishment to the cartilage may cause subsequent deformities of the pinna.

3. *Furuncle.* A *furuncle* of the external canal is a boil or pimple. It is exquisitely tender because the skin of the ear canal is tightly applied to the cartilage.

Each of these conditions is usually quite painful, and the patient needs prompt medical attention.

Bullous Myringitis. Blisters occasionally form on the tympanic membrane in association with a coincident upper respiratory infection. The blisters, or bullae, represent an accumulation of fluid between the layers of the tympanic membrane and may appear to the untrained observer as acute otitis media. This disorder is extremely painful and accompanied by a feeling of pressure in the ear. Hearing levels may be within normal limits. According to Roberts (1980), bullous myringitis probably is not a separate clinical entity but is merely acute otitis media with blisters on the eardrum.

Perforations of the Tympanic Membrane. Perforations may occur from some sort of trauma, such as a blow to the side of the head, a water-skiing fall, diving, or sudden changes in air pressure, or from middle ear problems, such as acute otitis media. The tympanic membrane is about 8 mm in diameter, and perforations from acute otitis media are usually much smaller, 1–2 mm in diameter. Often these perforations will heal spontaneously.

Conductive hearing loss occurs as a consequence of poor vibration of the tympanic membrane. The degree of loss, however, is variable and dependent upon the size of the perforation and its location on the tympanic membrane. Small perforations may be obvious with hearing levels within normal limits. Immittance audiometry may be used effectively as described in Chapter 6, to identify children with perforated tympanic membranes. Complications from perforations may be very serious, and all such children should be immediately referred to a medical specialist. Parents should be advised to practice aural hygiene by keeping water out of the ear when the child is swimming or bathing, until proper medical care of the ear has been taken.

Otitis Media. Otitis media is one of the most common disorders in children. Otitis media is defined as an inflammation of the middle ear, which may or may not be infectious in origin. Middle ear effusion (MEE) is the liquid resulting from otitis media. A current hypothesis is that the different clinical types of otitis media form a continuum and are dynamically interrelated. At any specific point in the continuum, a definite clinical entity can be identified, and at another time a different clinical entity may be present in the same patient (Paparella, 1976).

The general categories of otitis media are (a) otitis media without effusion, (b) otitis media with effusion, and (c) otitis media with perforation. Each of these categories may be classified by duration into (a) acute, 0–21 days; (b) subacute, 22 days to 8 weeks; and (c) chronic, over 8 weeks. In otitis media with effusion and otitis media with perforation, the fluid or discharge may be characterized as (a) serous—thin, watery liquid; (b) purulent—pus-like liquid; or (c) mucoid—thick, viscid, mucus-like liquid (Senturia, 1976; Senturia et al., 1980).

Otitis media is most common during the first 2 years of life and decreases in incidence thereafter. The incidence of otitis media has been studied by many investigators and found to be a function of age, sex (more otitis media in boys), race (whites have a higher incidence than blacks), genetic factors, socioeconomic status, season, and climate (Teele et al., 1980b). According to Teele et al., children living in households with many members were more likely to have otitis media than were children living in households with fewer members, and children with siblings or parents who had a history of otitis media had a higher incidence of otitis media than children with parents or siblings without a history of the disease.

The incidence statistics concerning otitis media are impressive: 76–95% of all children have had at least one episode of otitis media by age 6 years (Howie et al., 1975); approximately 50% of all children have had one episode of otitis media by age 1 year; and by age 2 years, this later incidence increases to 75%. In a careful study of preschool children in Pittsburgh, Casselbrant et al. (1985) confirmed that nearly 60% of the children examined monthly for 2 years had documented otitis media with effusion that lasted approximately 2 months in duration. The prevalence of this disorder showed strong seasonal variation associated with the presence of upper respiratory tract infections (URI) and often resolved spontaneously with a high recurrance rate. According to Klein (1979), children may be divided into three general groups with regard to otitis media. Approximately one third of children have no episodes, one third may have an occasional episode, and the remaining third have frequent episodes.

Of particular importance is the "otitis-prone" child described initially by Howie et al. (1975). An otitis-prone child is the child who has the condition 6 or more times before the age of 6 years or whose initial episode of otitis media was due to *Pneumococcus* and occurred before the age of 1 year. The otitis-prone child seems destined to have continued and recurrent bouts of otitis media throughout childhood.

Recurrent tonsillitis and enlarged adenoids were once thought to be the major cause of otitis media. Bluestone (1979) reviewed several studies and concluded that no good evidence exists that tonsillectomy and adenoidectomy reduce the incidence of ear disease. The decrease in tonsillectomies and/or adenoidectomies performed each year in the United States has dropped from 981,000 in 1965, to 471,000 in 1975, to only 279,000 reported in 1983 (Grundfast and Carney, 1987). The "T & A" (short for tonsillectomy and adenoidectomy operation) is still the second most common for children, even though the true efficacy of this surgery on otitis media in children is still under study (Bluestone and Klein, 1988).

Tonsils and adenoids are part of a ring of glandular tissue encircling the back of the throat. The adenoids are located high in the throat behind the soft palate and are not visible through the mouth without special instruments. The tonsils are the two masses of tissue on either side of the back of the throat. These structures are strategically located to "sample" incoming bacteria and viruses, and they often become infected themselves. It is thought that they help form antibodies to those "germs" as part of the body's immune system to resist and fight future infections. However, chronic infections in the tonsils and adenoids can also affect nearby structures and may create blockage of the eustachian tubes. This situation creates poor eustachian tube function, leading to a lack of aeration of the middle ear spaces, thereby causing frequent or chronic ear infections and subsequent hearing loss.

Opposing points of view regarding the use of tympanostomy tubes for treatment of otitis media with effusion cite the lack of convincing evidence linking otitis media early in life to either otologic or developmental difficulties later in life. Other considerations to be weighed prior to surgical intervention include the tendency of serous otitis media to resolve spontaneously, the cost and risk of surgery, and possible sequelae of tube placement.

Eustachian tube dysfunction has long been recognized to be a significant factor in the development of otitis media. The most important function of the eustachian tube is ventilation of the middle ear space. When the eustachian tube dysfunctions from either a mechanical or a functional cause, the air trapped in the middle ear cavity is absorbed, creating negative middle ear pressure and, ultimately, transudation of fluid into the cavity. Paradise (1980) states that eustachian tube function appears less compliant in infants than in older children and adults, perhaps because the tubal wall of infants is more compliant and therefore more susceptible to collapse, creating functional obstruction.

The diagnosis of otitis media is based on clinical manifestations, physical examination of the tympanic membrane, and possibly immittance testing and routine audiom-

etry. Paradise (1980) categorizes symptoms as either specific or systemic. Specific symptoms include earache, rubbing or tugging at the ears, otorrhea (drainage), hearing impairment, and balance disturbance. Of these, only earache and otorrhea generally indicate active infection. The systemic symptoms include fever, temperament disorders and restless sleep, irritability or low-grade discomfort.

Considerable controversy and confusion exist concerning the treatment for otitis media. Tremendous benefits would be gained if recurrences of otitis media could be prevented or substantially reduced in frequency. Paradise (1980) summarizes five different approaches to the prevention of otitis media currently under evaluation: (*a*) adenoidectomy with or without tonsillectomy; (*b*) antimicrobial prophylaxis; Perrin et al. (1974) have shown a significant reduction in the number of episodes of purulent otitis media in children who were treated continuously with low-dose sulfisoxazole); (*c*) the use of tympanostomy tubes; Gebhart (1981) showed that placement of tympanostomy tubes significantly decreased the number of episodes of acute purulent otitis media); (*d*) liberal use of myringotomy as an adjunct to antimicrobials; and (*e*) the administration of polyvalent pneumococcal vaccine.

The complications associated with otitis media are not uncommon. Complications of otitis media with effusion include hearing loss, perforation of the tympanic membrane with or without suppuration, cholesteatoma, mastoiditis, petrositis, adhesive otitis media, tympanosclerosis, ossicular discontinuity, facial paralysis, and labyrinthitis. Intracranial complications include meningitis, encephalitis, brain abscess, and sinus thrombophlebitis. Finally, otitis media may impair the development of children's cognitive abilities and detrimentally influence behavior.

An extremely important finding was reported by Teele et al. (1980a) concerning persistence of MEE following medical treatment. After the first episode of otitis

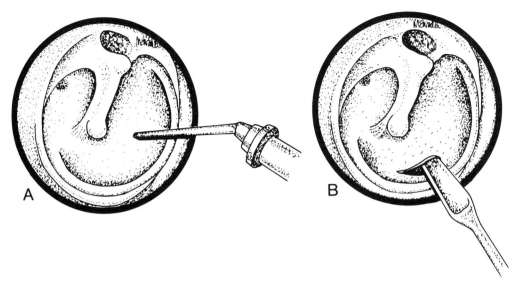

Figure 3.3. **A.** View of tympanotomy, or surgical puncture of the tympanic membrane, often used to aspirate fluid by suction for culture. **B.** Myringotomy, or surgical incision of tympanic membrane, is performed in lower half of tympanic membrane to avoid damage to middle ear ossicles. Myringotomy is conducted to provide instant relief from pain, to drain fluid from middle ear space, and thus to help initiate rapid recovery from middle ear disease.

media, 70% of the children in their study still had MEE at 2 weeks; 40%, at 1 month; 20%, at 2 months; and 10%, at 3 months. Pelton et al. (1977) also found that approximately one third of unselected children with acute otitis media had persistent fluid in the middle ear for 4 or more weeks. These statistics confirm the importance of careful and thorough medical follow-up for all children identified to have otitis media.

Acute otitis media presents suddenly with severe ear pain, redness of the tympanic membrane, and fever. Schwartz et al. (1981a) attempted to delineate a more precise definition of acute otitis media to include the bulging contour, decreased mobility and color of the tympanic membrane. In 85 infants and children diagnosed with acute otitis media, a poorly mobile, bulging, yellow, opacified tympanic membrane was most typical. The red tympanic membrane was seen in only 19% of the children, 67% had no fever, and 28% had no pain associated with their acute otitis media. In a follow-up study, Schwartz et al. (1981b) noted that approximately 10% of all cases of acute

otitis media led to persistent purulent otitis media despite adequately prescribed antibiotic treatment.

When the diagnosis of acute otitis media is in doubt or when determination of the causative agent is in question, aspiration of the middle ear fluid is performed with tympanocentesis or myringotomy as shown in Figure 3.3. In patients with an unusually severe earache, myringotomy is performed to provide immediate pain relief.

Serous otitis media is very common in infants and children and may be recalcitrant to medical treatment. If pain is present in this disorder, it is usually intermittent and rather mild (Bluestone and Shurin, 1974). Many cases of serous otitis media are unaccompanied by significant hearing loss (Cohen and Sade, 1972).

Adhesive otitis media is a thickening of the fibrous tissue of the tympanic membrane that may be accompanied by severe retraction and negative pressure in the middle ear space. When a retraction pocket forms in the superior portion of the pars tensa of the tympanic membrane, the development of cholesteatoma is probable.

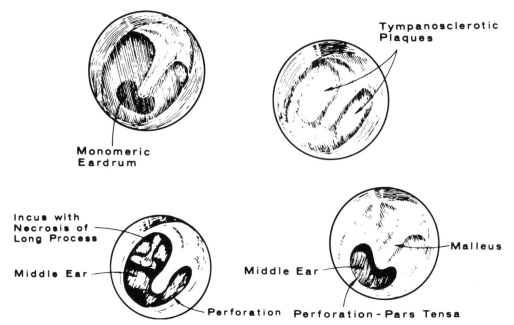

Figure 3.4.   Otoscopic views of the tympanic membrane showing some sequelae of chronic otitis media. (Courtesy of Gerald M. English, M.D., Denver, Colorado.)

Chronic otitis media most often has its onset in early childhood, between the ages of 5 and 10 years. Recurrent otitis media may halt or reverse the process of mastoid pneumatization or cause mastoid sclerosis. Severe forms of otitis media may or may not damage the middle ear ossicles, depending on the severity and duration of the disease. Severe otitis media may produce areas of osteitis in the mastoid septae, resulting in a continuous foul discharge.

During healing the middle ear and tympanic membrane may develop *tympanosclerosis*, which is hyalinized and calcified scar tissue. Tympanosclerosis deposits may cause stiffening of the tympanic membrane or fusion and fixation of the middle ear ossicles. Middle ear granulation tissue, polyps, and monomeric membrane formation are also associated with various chronic otitis media as shown in Figure 3.4.

Paparella and Brady (1970) reviewed 232 patients with chronic suppurative otitis media and mastoiditis. They found a definite increase in the incidence of sensorineural hearing loss that they suggested was due to a cochlear biochemical change created by toxic materials passed into the inner ear through the round window, resulting in gradual destruction of the organ of Corti. English et al. (1973) evaluated 404 patients with various forms of otitis media and reached conclusions in accord with the Paparella and Brady study. English et al. found that bone conduction thresholds worsened with the severity and duration of disease. Posttreatment bone conduction thresholds were unchanged from pretreatment tests, leading these authors to conclude that sensorineural hearing loss can be a natural sequela of chronic otitis media.

Middle Ear Effusions in Neonates.   A number of investigators have shown that MEE occurs commonly in neonates, both in the outpatient population and the intensive care nursery (Jaffe et al., 1970; Warren and Stool, 1971; Bland, 1972; Shurin et al., 1976). In spite of these well-documented studies, otoscopy is not routinely performed on neonates because the infant tympanic membrane is difficult to visualize (Fig. 3.5). In an infant, the external ear canal is distensible and often collapsed, and

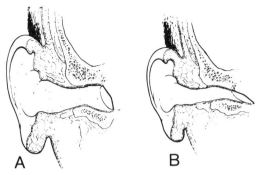

Figure 3.5. Orientation of the tympanic membrane in the adult (**A**) and in the infant (**B**). Note the horizontal plane of the infant eardrum, which makes visualization of the tympanic membrane difficult. (Reprinted with permission from T. J. Balkany, S. A. Berman, M. A. Simmons, and B. J. Jafek: Middle ear effusion in neonates. *The Laryngoscope* 88:399, 1978.)

the tympanic membrane lies in a nearly horizontal plane. Balkany et al. (1978) reported results from examining 125 consecutive infants from the neonatal intensive care unit (ICU) and found MEE to be present in some 30% of their sample. They believed that this finding was especially important and often overlooked, since unrecognized MEE may act as a focus for dissemination of bacteria into the circulation and/or central nervous system. They also found that nasotracheal intubation of longer than 7 days is highly associated with suppurative MEE.

Of special importance to audiologists is the relationship of early otitis media to subsequent language and learning difficulties. Wallace et al. (1988) conducted a prospective study of neonates from birth until 1 year of age. Their results demonstrate language deficits in otitis media children as early as 1 year of age. These researchers conclude that infants who suffer repeated episodes of bilateral otitis media during the first year of life are more likely to have reduced auditory sensitivity and to be at risk for expressive language difficulties.

Cholesteatoma. A cholesteatoma is a skin growth that occurs in the middle ear typically caused by repeated infections of this area. The repeated infections and per-

sistent negative middle ear pressure causes a retraction pocket (pouch or sac). The continuing maturation and persistent growth of the squamous epithelium (skin) into this pocket can take the form of a cyst formed by layers of old skin. Over time, the cholesteatoma can increase in size and destroy the surrounding tissues and structures of the middle ear. In otitis media with perforation, the tissues of the middle ear intermittently undergo destruction, healing and scarring during the recurrent infection process. Skin may grow from the external ear canal into the middle ear cavity or mastoid through a tympanic membrane perforation, creating a cholesteatoma.

Initially, the symptoms that are presented include drainage, sometimes accompanied by a foul odor, conductive hearing loss, fullness or pressure in or behind the ear, dizziness, and facial weakness. Usually, although not always, cholesteatoma is a unilateral problem. This is a very serious ear condition that must be examined and evaluated by an otolaryngologist. Cholesteatomas that are undiscovered or untreated can be dangerous, with resultant bone erosion leading to deafness, brain abscess, and meningitis, and rarely death can occur. Because of the seriousness of this disorder, audiologists must be extremely careful in the evaluation and referral of children with unilateral conductive hearing losses that do not respond to traditional medical treatment.

A cross-section diagram in Figure 3.6 shows an attic and a middle ear cholesteatoma. Moisture and bacteria may gain access to the cholesteatoma, creating infection and drainage. Initial treatment of the cholesteatoma may consist of careful cleaning of the debris, topical ear drops, and antibiotics to clear up the infection process. Large or complicated cholesteatomas usually require surgical removal to protect the patient from more serious complications. The purpose of the surgery is twofold: to remove the cholesteatoma and infection as well as to preserve or improve hearing. In some cases, these goals are accomplished

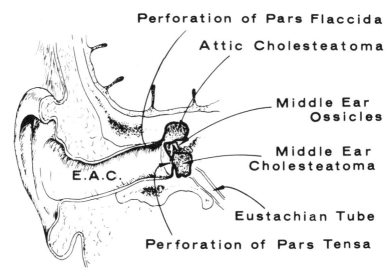

Figure 3.6. Cross-section of the external and middle ear showing an attic cholesteatoma through a perforation of the pars flaccida portion of the tympanic membrane. A perforation of the pars tensa portion of the tympanic membrane may lead to development of a middle ear cholesteatoma. (Reprinted with permission from G. M. English, J. L. Northern, and T. J. Fria: Chronic otitis media as a cause of sensorineural hearing loss. *Archives of Otolaryngology* 98:17–22, 1973.)

through two separate operations. Tos (1983) reviewed surgical results from 122 children operated on for removal of cholesteatoma. He found recurrent cholesteatoma in 12% of the patients and remarked that recurrent growth of cholesteatoma is more common in children than in adults and develops faster in young people. Follow-up visits are necessary following surgical removal of the cholesteatoma to examine the ear for possible recurrence of the skin tumor. In some patients, an open mastoid cavity is surgically created, and office visits every few months (perhaps for life) are necessary to clean out the cavity and prevent new infections.

Mastoiditis. Mastoiditis is categorized into either acute or chronic stages. The terms represent the degree of involvement of the infected mastoid air cell system. The anatomic continuity between the middle ear and the mucosal lining of the mastoid antrum allows for the coexisting inflammatory process associated with these structures. *Acute mastoiditis* is an inflammation of the ciliated mucosa of the antrum. With the onset of edema or insufficient drainage

of the mastoid mucosa, pressure is created within the air cells, causing localized discomfort. Some of the clinical manifestations of acute mastoiditis are fullness, pain, acute otitis media, tenderness, edema, and conductive hearing loss. Other clinical findings may consist of tympanic membrane destruction, depending on the status of the tympanum or epitympanum.

Chronic mastoiditis occurs with chronic inflammation of the membrane lining the mastoid antrum and ciliated cells. The bone structure is often involved in the infection. Generally, chronic mastoiditis is associated with a history of otitis media, which may be active or inactive, depending on whether or not purulent discharge is present. The symptoms of chronic mastoiditis are similar to those of acute mastoiditis, with the exception of the hearing loss, which often takes on a sensorineural component.

Acute mastoiditis was, until the 1930s and 1940s, a complication of acute otitis media in 25–50% of the cases. With the advent of antibiotics such as penicillin, the incidence of acute mastoiditis was lowered to approximately 0.4% by 1955 (Palva and Pulkinen, 1959). However, antibiotic therapy has been attributed to a "masked" presence of mastoiditis, whereby the disease is suppressed enough to reduce the symptoms but not enough to resolve the ongoing destructive process (Holt and Young, 1981).

During the preantibiotic era, some of the most life-threatening complications of mastoiditis were meningitis, brain abscess, and cerebellar abscess. Present complications still include facial nerve paralysis, labyrinthitis, meningitis, and cholesteatoma. Intracranial complications have decreased since the 1930s and 1940s along with a significant decrease in patient mortality. In cases in which antibiotics have been ineffective in treating acute mastoiditis, a simple mastoidectomy is performed with surgical drainage of the mastoid air cells. Patients with chronic mastoiditis are initially given nonsurgical treatment to dry the ear and prevent complications that would complicate surgical treatment. When medical management fails, a modified or radical mastoidectomy is performed.

Cleft Palate. Deformities of the lip and palate are among the most common major congenital malformations, occurring once in 900 newborns. A substantial number of articles have been published concerning the otologic and audiologic problems of children with overt cleft palate. The incidence of recurrent otitis media in such children is quite high and has been reported to be from 50% to 90% by various investigators.

Paradise and Bluestone (1974) reported the "universality" of otitis media findings in 50 infants with cleft palate. Paradise (1980) commented on 300 additional cleft palate infants examined during the first few months of life. Usually, sterile inflammatory effusions that vary in viscosity are found in the ears of these infants. Paradise recommends infants with cleft palate receive myringotomy and tympanostomy tube insertion at a relatively early age, within the first 6 months, if possible, especially if hearing loss seems present or discomfort or infection is present. Repeat myringotomy and

tubes may be necessary to keep the infant's ears clear and hearing normally.

Complications such as cholesteatoma and adhesive otitis may accompany MEE in cleft palate children. Hearing loss as a secondary problem to the middle ear disorder related to cleft palate is also very common and may exist in 90% of such patients (Yules 1970). The incidence and severity of middle ear problems related to the cleft palate decrease as the patient grows older.

Otologic and hearing problems associated with submucous cleft palate have been reviewed by Bergstrom and Hemenway (1971). The submucous cleft palate is an imperfect union of muscle across the soft palate that tends to "tent" when the patient phonates. The area may appear bluish, since it is covered by only nasal and oral mucosa. The dehiscence of muscle and bone may be obvious with palpation and is often accompanied by a bifid uvula. From a study of 58 patients with submucous cleft palate, Bergstrom and Hemenway reported an incidence of 39% with recurrent or chronic disease of the middle ear ranging in severity between serous otitis media to cholesteatoma. Conductive hearing loss was demonstrated by 34% of the group, while an additional 25% had either pure sensorineural or mixed-type hearing loss.

Although numerous ideas have been offered to explain the high incidence of hearing problems associated with overt and submucous cleft palate children, most clinicians agree that the deficiency of palate musculature is the probable cause of poor eustachian tube function. This results in inadequate middle ear ventilation, effusion of fluid, tympanic membrane retraction, and hearing loss. Such disease of the middle ear is most common in children between 3 and 8 years of age, which also corresponds to the increased exposure and susceptibility to URI found in this age group (Bluestone and Klein, 1988).

Clinicians should be sensitive to this increased incidence of hearing difficulty and recurrent middle ear disease in children with cleft palate. The hearing of such patients should be monitored on a regular basis with close medical follow-up. Our experiences with cleft palate children have exposed numerous youngsters with recurrent episodes of otitis media accompanied by significant hearing loss who undoubtedly miss such auditory information at school and home. Immediate medical treatment is often necessary for these children who may qualify for repeated myringotomy and ventilation tubes. Mild to moderate-power hearing aids may be in order for children who do not respond well to medical treatment, especially during the important school years.

The diagnosis of ear disease and hearing loss in the infant with cleft palate is difficult because of the small structure of the external ear and the infant's neurologic immaturity (Stool, 1971). MEE is often present in cleft palate babies when they are examined in the first days of life (Paradise and Bluestone, 1974). Too often the audiologist, however, is "only a bench-warmer" on the cleft palate team, even though the results from hearing evaluations contribute substantially to the total management of these children (Pollock, 1979).

Immittance audiometry is an especially valuable clinical procedure in children with cleft palate. The overt cleft palate is diagnosed within the first few days of life, although the submucous cleft palate may not be diagnosed until years later. Immittance audiometry may identify conductive impairments in even very young infants. (Bess et al., 1975, 1976).

Down's Syndrome (Trisomy 21). Ear abnormalities such as small pinnae, narrow external auditory canals, abnormal external ear configuration, and a strong tendency to have otitis media are commonly associated with Down's syndrome and suggest the possibility of a high incidence of conductive hearing losses in this population. In addition, it has been suggested that the Down's child may be more susceptible to URI than is the normal child, because of peculiar nasopharynx and eustachian tube development, which can adversely affect proper drainage of the sinuses and middle-ear spaces. The most complete description of hearing impairment in children with Down's syndrome, was published by M. P. Downs (1980). She noted that the Down's child may be treated medically or surgically for persistent MEE, but following treatment the conductive hearing loss may persist. She designed a comprehensive study of 107 noninstitutionalized Down's children and found 78% to have hearing loss in one or both ears. Fifty-four percent had conductive loss, 16% had sensorineural loss, and 8% had mixed-type hearing loss.

Complete otologic examinations were conducted on each of the 107 Down's children. According to Balkany et al. (1978), about 40% of the children with conductive hearing loss could not be explained by MEE or chronic otitis media. On microscopic pneumatic otoscopy the patients had normal-appearing examinations, suggesting the presence of middle ear anomalies. Seventeen operative procedures on carefully selected Down's syndrome patients revealed congenital ossicular malformations and destruction caused by inflammation due to chronic infection. Balkany (1980) recommends that children with Down's syndrome and persistent conductive hearing loss be treated aggressively to normalize hearing, to break the cycle of recurrent suppurative otitis media, and to prevent chronic ear disease.

In the audiologic evaluation of Down's syndrome children, the immittance tests (tympanometry and acoustic reflex measurement) are important to confirm hearing test results. In addition, the high incidence of conductive hearing loss in this population makes immittance audiometry an imperative part of each hearing evaluation (Northern, 1980a). Every hearing test on a Down's syndrome child should include some aspect of sound field testing (without earphones) to rule out erroneous "conductive losses" due to collapsed ear canals.

The results of this study and others (Brooks et al., 1972; Schwartz and Schwartz, 1978b) clearly show that conductive hearing loss in the Down's syndrome population is prevalent in infants and children, and often the hearing loss continues in spite of proper medical management. Down's children should not be excluded from vigorous monitoring of middle ear problems and attempts to normalize their hearing by appropriate amplification strategies. In addition, a total team approach including an ear, nose, and throat specialist, pediatrician, audiologist, and speech-language pathologist is recommended for the Down's children in order to provide optimal opportunities for advancement.

Autism. Autism is a severely debilitating disorder that has an occurrence rate of 5 in 10,000 and affects boys 3 times more often than girls (Rutter, 1965). The disorder is diagnosed by observation of a cluster of behaviors associated in some manner with central nervous system pathology (Paluszny, 1979). Rutter (1978) defines autism with the following criteria: early onset (before 30 months of age); disturbances of social relationships; disturbances of speech and language; and extremely deviant behavior characterized by preoccupation with particular objects and/or insistence on sameness. The American Psychiatric Association definition of autism (1980) adds that these patients show a pervasive lack of responsiveness to other people, gross deficits in language development and, where speech is present, often peculiarities of speech such as immediate and delayed echolalia, metaphorical language, and pronoun reversal. Autistic individuals may exhibit bizarre responses to various aspects of the environment and failure to use or comprehend verbal and nonverbal messages, with illogical and inconsistent responses to sensory, especially auditory, stimuli. For example, autistic children may be distracted, enraged, or frightened by normal background noises. This system has been termed *auditory overselectivity* by Reynolds et al. (1974).

Several auditory evaluation studies on autistic individuals have been reported in the literature. In general terms, auditory evoked brainstem response is the test of choice, and considerable effort has been conducted to identify differences in auditory brainstem response (ABR) patterns between autistic and normal children (Gillberg et al., 1983; Rosenblum et al., 1980; Tanguay et al., 1982a and b). Although minor differences in ABR patterns have been reported between normal and autistic patients, the differences are not consistent across studies, and the reports are difficult to compare, since control conditions and experimental variables are often not well-described. Some authors have attempted to use central auditory tests to speculate about the specific loci of dysfunction in autistic children (Wetherby et al., 1981). Although it is probable that the organic dysfunction is clearly implicated in autism, no precise etiologic mechanisms have been identified (Volkmar and Cohen, 1986).

Ototoxic Hearing Loss. Ototoxicity is due to the administration of certain drugs and medications that damage the cochlea and/or vestibular portion of the inner ear, causing permanent sensorineural hearing loss and often accompanied by vertigo, nausea, or gait instability. Almost any available drug, effective for treatment of certain ailments, has the potential to compromise the human system in some way. Management of illness with chemotherapy becomes a fine-line judgment, weighing the potential benefit to the patient against the risk of adverse side effects.

Antibiotics, diuretics, and antimalarial pharmaceuticals have been implicated as potentially toxic to both the auditory and vestibular systems, as well as to the kidney. Kanamycin and neomycin are the worse ototoxic drugs at this time, although other members of the aminoglycoside family, including entamycin, vancomycin, amikacin, dihydrostreptomycin, and tobramycin, have caused documented auditory problems. Streptomycin is well-known to be destructive to the vestibular system. There exists considerable individual susceptibility to these ototoxic drugs, which usually, but not always, cause bilaterally symmetrical hearing loss of varying degree, audiometric configuration, and severity. Aspirin, quinine, and diuretics are the only drugs that produce temporary hearing loss that may be reversible, fully or partially, when the patient is taken off the medication. Salamy et al. (1989) examined very low birth weight infants and found a significant association between furosemide administered for long duration with aminoglycosides and sensorineural hearing loss.

Ingestion of ototoxic drugs by pregnant women can result in a multitude of congenital abnormalities, including hearing loss, from passage of the drugs across the placenta (Siegel and McCracken, 1981). Apparently, renal failure, concomitant use of diuretics such as ethacrynic acid and furosemide, and a prolonged course of drug therapy are the most important factors in the development of fetal ototoxicity. The evaluation of aminoglycoside ototoxicity in infants is a complex problem, since these babies are receiving medical therapy for severe problems, including systemic infection, that may accompany low birthweight, jaundice, or other health disorders that are of themselves associated with deafness.

A 4 year follow-up study of 347 neonates treated with gentamicin and kanamycin was reported by Finitzo-Hieber et al. (1979). Although this was an excellent study, complete with a control group of nontreated infants, limitations in the study and failure to demonstrate ototoxicity in the experimental group of infants do not completely assure the safety of larger doses of the drugs. Suspect infants require extensive audiologic follow-up, and sometimes the mild-to-moderate hearing loss is difficult to verify. Finitzo-Hieber (1981b) has advocated the auditory brainstem response as a noninvasive procedure that can be used for measurement of auditory sensitivity in high-risk infants.

The area of vestibular testing in infants and children exposed to ototoxic drugs is even more difficult. The problem is to establish a simple, reliable, and noninvasive method of assessing vestibular function that will be tolerated by children. Eviatar and Eviatar (1983) describe a combined evaluation of postural control, developmental reflexes, and electronystagmographic data that provides useful information about the vestibular function in children.

According to Bergstrom and Thompson (1984), epithelial structures in the cochlea and vestibule show the primary damage from ototoxicity. In the cochlea, atrophy of stria vascularis, spiral ligament, sensory hair cells, and supporting cells may be seen. The basal and middle coils of the cochlea are more commonly affected than the apical coil, correlating clinically with the high-frequency hearing loss typically seen in cases of ototoxic etiology. With increased severity, the apical turn—and accordingly, the low-mid frequencies—can be involved. The outer hair cells in the cochlear duct are more vulnerable than the inner hair cells. In the vestibular system, histopathologic studies show damage to the cristae of the ampullae in the semicircular canals.

The incidence of ototoxicity in general figures or for specific drugs has not been accurately established. Thompson and Northern (1981) identify a number of risk factors that may enhance the potential risk of ototoxicity, including increased drug serum level, decreased renal function, the use of more than one ototoxic drug simultaneously or in increased daily doses or for an extended period of time, age, health, heredity, concurrent noise exposure or in the presence of preexisting problems including severe visual impairment or blindness, or drugs administered in the presence of ear symptoms such as tinnitus, hearing loss and/or dizziness.

Perilymph Fistula. A perilymph fistula (PLF) is a leak of inner ear fluid through a hole in either the round window membrane or the oval window annular ligament; this hole permits an open communication between the middle ear and the inner ear. The perilymph leak has also been found in certain cases of stapes footplate defect or may occur through the otic capsule bone from trauma or cholesteatoma erosion. The perilymph leak can occur spontaneously but more typically is the result of head trauma. The diagnosis of PLF is often difficult to make, particularly in children, and may be a diagnosis of last resort when other possible etiologies are systematically eliminated (Balkany and Pashley, 1986).

Sensorineural hearing loss is commonly associated with PLF, and many otologic surgeons perform exploratory operations to seek evidence of PLF (which can be repaired by patching) in otherwise unexplained sensorineural hearing loss. Petroff et al. (1986) summarize several facts including (*1*) the relationship between fistulas and hearing loss is not completely understood and, in PLF, may occur in normal-hearing ears; and (*2*) surgical repair of a PLF does not usually restore or improve hearing, although a successful repair may stabilize progressive sensorineural hearing loss. Some believe that the majority of PLFs may self-heal with bedrest.

PLF is a condition with a wide variety of signs and symptoms. No clear pattern of diagnostic signs may be anticipated, but "typical" symptoms may be as subtle as fluctuation in speech recognition scores, aural fullness, dysequilibrium, positive fistula test, or fluctuating severe hearing loss, which may be unilateral or bilateral (McCabe, 1989). Caution must be exercised to separate fluctuating hearing loss from fluctuations in audiologic testing in children (Myer et al., 1989). PLFs should be considered in any child with a progressive sensorineural hearing loss and intermittent dizziness that can, if left untreated, result in total hearing loss (Parnes and McCabe, 1987).

Cochlear Trauma. Skull fracture involving the occipital or squamous portion of the temporal bone may extend into the petrous portion of the temporal bone and involve the otic capsule. Should the fracture line cross the external auditory canal, laceration of the skin and bleeding of the external nal canal may occur with little permanent loss of hearing. More medial fractures may produce bleeding in the middle ear or disruption of the ossicular chain, which would create a maximal 60 dB conductive-type hearing loss. Hearing loss due to concussion may be totally or partially reversible, while hearing loss due to fracture of the cochlea is irreversible (Barber, 1969).

Relatively moderate trauma to the occiput of the skull can cause a permanent sensorineural hearing loss. Numerous animal studies have been conducted with traumatic blows to the head that produce temporary and permanent sensorineural high-frequency hearing loss. Schuknecht (1974) states that a blow to the head creates a pressure wave in the skull that is transmitted through bone to the cochlea just as a pressure wave in air is carried by the conducting mechanism, and the injury must be attributed to intense acoustic stimulation. Meningitis may occur as a late complication of temporal bone fracture.

Noise-Induced or Noise-Trauma Hearing Loss. A sound of sufficient intensity and duration can cause injury to the inner ear, producing a temporary or permanent hearing loss. The extent of noise-induced or traumatic noise-inflicted hearing loss in children is difficult to ascertain, but its presence is relatively common. A most thorough review of the literature concerning noise and children was published by Mills (1975).

A number of devices used by children produce sound levels capable of producing acoustic injury (Axelsson and Jerson, 1985). Devices with sufficiently high sound levels include firecrackers, model airplane engines, toy firearms, and fireworks (Marshall and Brandt, 1974). It has been speculated that thousands of children have permanent hearing losses that were caused by the acoustic impulses of toy caps. There appears to be no acceptable reasons for toys to produce dangerously loud sounds, but there is little doubt that even a single exposure to an impulsive noise toy can yield immediate and permanent acoustic trauma.

The issue of susceptibility of children to temporary threshold shift is still open. This question is critical in the determination of hearing hazard produced by incubators and hearing aids. Fior (1972) presented temporary threshold shift data from children between 3 and 13 years that are similar to data generally reported for adults. It is understandable that data are sparse with regard to experimental evaluation of temporary threshold shift in children because of concern to eliminate any risk of permanent auditory damage.

The hearing loss due to noise exposure typically consists of sensorineural impairment at 4000 Hz in the affected ear, regardless of the type of noise exposure. Often the traumatic noise-induced hearing loss can be related to a single identifiable noise exposure, such as the explosion of a firecracker.

Weber et al. (1967) evaluated 1000 children from Colorado with hearing loss and found 249 boys and 51 girls with noise exposure characteristic audiograms. These authors suggest that noise-induced losses are first identified in junior-senior high school boys who have a history of experience with firearms and farm machinery. Litke (1971) evaluated higher frequency hearing among 1516 South Dakota school children. He found high-frequency hearing loss in 6% of the population, with an average loss of 58 dB occurring at the highest incidence at grades 3 and 12. Litke found 5 times more boys than girls suffered high-frequency hearing loss with two thirds of the subjects showing 6000 Hz as the most involved frequency.

We are often asked by concerned parents if listening or playing loud rock-and-roll music can damage the hearing of their children. Although research in the issue of hearing loss and hard rock music is somewhat conflicting, there is little doubt that exposure to loud music can produce temporary threshold shift. Rintlemann and Borus (1968) studied rock musicians and found that only 5% of them incurred noise-induced hearing losses. Jerger and Jerger (1970) reported that eight of nine rock-and-roll musicians, aged 14–23 years, showed temporary threshold shift in excess of 15 dB on at least one frequency between 2000 and 8000 Hz, one of whom had a 38 dB shift in threshold at 3000 Hz! A study by Danenberg et al. (1987) showed that hearing threshold shift can be measured in persons attending a typical school dance with loud, live rock music.

The degree of noise young people are exposed to in daily life was measured by Siervogel et al. (1982). They placed dosimeters on 127 subjects 7–20 years old. The average daily 24 hour log equivalent sound levels ranged from 77 to 84 dBA. The noise exposures of the children were the same whether or not school was in session.

Thorough history questioning may identify unrecognized situations of excessive noise exposure. These youngsters must be carefully counseled regarding the potential hazards of additional noise exposure and fitted with ear defenders as soon as possible.

Noise Levels in Infant Incubators and the Intensive Care Unit. A visitor to the newborn ICU within a hospital is immediately aware of the high noise level. Originally, hospital nurseries were small rooms with four to eight infants in incubators or cribs with virtually no life-support equipment. However, modern technology has created a much noisier nursery environment with the use of machines for life support, diagnosis, and monitoring of baby activity. In fact, one of the greatest problems in the ICU is the multitude of sound sources, respirators, and monitors that generate both background sound and alarm signals (Kellman, 1982).

Noise levels in the ICU may be 20 dB higher than in the well-baby nursery, day and night, causing staff aggravation, fatigue, and stress, leading to potential patient care errors. Ambient noise levels in ICU have been reported to range from 56 to 77 dBA (Peltzman et al., 1970; Falk and Woods, 1973; Redding et al., 1977). This noise is generally low frequency in nature (most energy lower than 250 Hz), persistent, and continuous all hours of the day and night.

Although prolonged exposure to the noise levels characteristic of intensive care equipment and infant incubators may be harmful to the developing neonate, direct evidence for such insult has not been reported. In 1974, the American Academy of Pediatrics Committee on Environmental Hazards recommended that manufacturers of incubators reduce noise below 58 dBA.

Abramovich et al. (1979) examined the hearing of 111 perinatal intensive care survivors of birthweights 1500 g or less at a mean age of 6 years and found no evidence that ambient incubator noise of 65 dBA had affected their hearing thresholds. However, these researchers warned that with the increasing use of noise signals as auditory monitors, attention should be given to ambient noise levels to ensure that potentially damaging levels are not exceeded. Long et al. (1980) recorded 2-hour polygraphic tracings from infants' heart rate, respiratory rate, transcutaneous oxygen tension, and intracranial pressure during the routine ICU schedule. They found that sudden loud noises usually caused agitation and crying in the infants, which led to decreases in transcutaneous oxygen tension and an increase in intracranial pressure, as well as increases in heart and respiratory rate.

A number of concerned investigators have measured the ambient sound level generated within infant incubators. In general, the SPLs of incubators have been reported to be greater than 60 dBA (League et al., 1972; Falk and Farmer, 1973; Blennow et al., 1974; Douek et al., 1976). While these sound levels are not in excess of acceptable damage risk criteria, it must be remembered that infants in such incubators are usually in poor health and may be under treatment with potentially ototoxic drugs, and their noise exposure is continuous, 24 hours per day, 1440 minutes per day, from several weeks to months (Falk, 1972).

An excellent study was conducted by Bess et al. (1979) of incubator noise with different types of life-support equipment and when impulse noise was created by striking the side of the incubator or by opening and closing the doors of the storage unit. The life-support equipment increased the overall noise levels of the incubators by as much as 15–20 dBA with a predominance of high-frequency energy. The impulse signals created by striking the side of the incubator (a common practice of physicians and nurses to forcefully stimulate breathing in apneic infants) ranged from 130 to 140 dBA SPL. Opening and closing the storage unit doors created peak amplitudes of 114 dBA SPL.

Bacterial and Viral Diseases. Bacterial and viral diseases have long been recognized as causes of deafness. Both prenatal and postnatal infections have been identified as a cause of hearing loss. Maternal rubella has largely been eradicated by widespread vaccine programs, but occasionally new cases do occur. The sequelae of maternal rubella are discussed further in the "Appendix of Hearing Disorders." Congenital deafness has also been attributed to meningoencephalitis, chickenpox, and other viruses. Bacterial postnatal infections known to result in deafness due to meningogenic spread include streptococcus, pneumococcus, and staphylococcus. Acute otitis media and URI are commonly associated with bacterial meningitis.

Common viruses of the later postnatal period known to or suspected to cause deafness and/or vestibular symptoms include mumps, measles, chickenpox, influenza, and viruses of the common cold. Deafness results from damage to the inner ear as a result of direct infiltration via the internal meatus. Disease may be limited to the endolymphatic system with the inflammatory process beginning in the vascular beds (Lindsay, 1967a).

The viral diseases may cause mild to profound sensorineural hearing loss. Histopathologic effects of viral infections reported have included extensive destruction of organ of Corti, degeneration of saccule, damage or complete destruction of stria vascularis and tectorial membrane, damage or obliteration of vestibular system, and atrophy or destruction of neural pathways (Lindsay, 1976b).

Maternal infections have been demonstrated as the cause of a host of other congenital malformations and abnormalities. However, congenital infections often cause fetal death and miscarriage. Damage to the fetus attributed to congenital viral infections has included congenital malformations such as clubfoot; intrauterine growth; retardation; damage to the nervous system, including anencephaly, encephalocele, and spina bifida; congenital heart disease; and disease of other organs, such as the liver, pancreas, and adrenals.

Residuals of postnatal viral infections include nerve atrophy, notably the optic nerve, cerebral palsy, mental retardation, disturbances of respiration, muscular atrophy or paralysis, convulsions, disturbances of autonomic system, and disturbances of metabolism.

Meningitis.   Sensorineural hearing impairment is the most common complication of bacterial meningitis in infants and young children. The microorganisms associated with hearing loss include *Haemophilus influenzae*, *Neisseria meningitidis*, and *Streptococcus pneumoniae*. Infectious meningitis causes deafness as the result of bacterial labyrinthitis due to an extension of the infection from meninges. The infecting virus has been traced from the meninges to the inner ear through the cochlear aqueduct and along vessels and nerves of the internal auditory meatus (Paparella and Suguira, 1967). Serous or purulent labyrinthitis may follow with partial or complete destruction of sensory receptors in the cochlea and eighth nerve elements. Subsequent replacement of the membranous labyrinth in the cochlea and vestibular divisions of the inner ear with fibrous tissue

and bone ossification is common (Keane et al., 1979).

Although the severity of the sensorineural configuration may range between mild and profound hearing loss, the audiometric pattern is typically bilateral, symmetrical, and irreversible. Conductive hearing loss components are often noted as acute otitis media and URI are commonly associated with bacterial meningitis. Estimates of the frequency of hearing loss following bacterial meningitis, based almost entirely on retrospective studies, have been reported to be 2.4–29% of children who survive this illness (Kaplan et al., 1984). Despite the significant reduction in overall mortality due to the use of antibiotics, nearly 50% of children with bacterial meningitis still have significant handicaps.

In earlier years, clinicians anticipated partial hearing recovery in some patients following bacterial meningitis. Current research based on prospective auditory evaluations of meningitic infants with ABR techniques confirm that documented hearing improvement occurs in only isolated cases. Previous "improved" hearing levels followed meningitis may have been related to inaccurate behavioral hearing tests obtained during the acute illness stage of the disease or to resolution of the conductive element of the hearing loss. On the other hand, certain sequelae of meningitis, such as elevated intercranial pressure or neuritis of the eighth nerve, may explain temporarily reduced hearing that improves with time and treatment. When improvement in hearing is noted, the increase is more common at frequencies lower than 3000 Hz and is associated with moderate-to-severe hearing losses. A number of reports have documented cases of hearing improvement following meningitis (Roeser et al., 1975; Ozdamar et al., 1982; Guiscafre et al., 1984; Vienny et al., 1984).

Vienny et al. (1984) of Switzerland examined 51 children with bacterial meningitis hearing loss with serial ABR recordings beginning with the earliest phase of the disease. They found that 35 children (68%) always showed normal ABR recordings, 11 children (21%) had transient ABR tracing abnormalities, and 5 children (9.8%) had persistent pathologic ABR tracings and permanent sensorineural hearing impairment. This study showed the early occurrence of deafness in the course of the meningitis disease, with a crucial phase of possible recovery (or worsening) happening during the initial 2 weeks. In this cohort of patients there were no incidences of "late" deafness or "late" hearing recovery, based on thorough audiometric follow-up studies 3 months after discharge from the hospital. In one report of hearing recovery following bacterial meningitis, Guiscafre et al. (1984) of Mexico City used ABR testing to follow 32 children with early postmeningitic hearing loss and found that 22 of these patients recovered normal hearing.

In a prospective evaluation of acute bacterial meningitis in children, Dodge et al. (1984) tested the hearing of 185 infants and young children older than 1 month of age. Of this population, 19 children (10.3%) showed permanent sensorineural hearing loss. Transient conductive hearing loss was identified in 16% of the sample of patients, but in no case was there improvement of the sensorineural hearing loss with time. Based on their analyses of their data, the authors concluded that the presence of hearing impairment in postmeningitic children does not correlate with the number of days of illness (symptoms) before hospitalization or with the number of days before the initiation of antibacterial treatment. The number of children who suffer hearing loss due to meningitis is expected to decrease sharply with the recent development of a protective vaccine. The vaccine is recommended to be administered to all children at 2 years of age or, for those children who have increased risk of meningitis, such as those in day care, or for those children with other underlying disease, at 18 months of age.

Although the ABR technique has significant prognostic value in estimating hearing levels in meningitic infants, clinicians are cautioned that the ABR tests only the higher frequencies and is therefore insufficient as a singular hearing test. Clinical audiologic surveillance with behavioral testing is the only means by which to determine hearing levels with certainty at all frequencies in postmeningitic infants and young children (MacDonald and Feinstein, 1984; Cohen et al., 1988). To be sure, because hearing deficits are so common in patients with bacterial meningitis, a hearing evaluation by ABR is recommended as a routine practice as close as possible in time to hospital discharge. Follow-up audiometric evaluation must be conducted when initial findings suggest the presence of hearing loss.

Congenital Syphilis. Congenital syphilis is still one of the most important contributors to perinatal mortality and morbidity in many parts of the world. In Western countries, the disease is now relatively rare, but the recent increase in venereal disease may well mean that congenital syphilis will again become a threat to neonates (Bryan and Nicholson, 1981).

Early manifestations include nasal discharge (snuffles), rash, anemia, jaundice, and osteochondritis. Later manifestations include saddle nose, saber skin, Hutchinson teeth, mulberry molars, and other dental anomalies. Congenital syphilis may demonstrate a multitude of central nervous system abnormalities including vestibular dysfunction, sensorineural hearing loss and, occasionally, aortic valvulitis. Possible accompanying mental retardation depends on severity of neurologic damage.

Auditory impairment may not be present at birth. Onset of hearing loss is generally in early childhood, usually sudden bilaterally symmetrical hearing loss causing severe to profound impairment. The hearing loss is usually not accompanied by marked vestibular manifestations. Poor hearing function and limited use of the hearing aid can be expected as a result of neural atrophy. The general treatment of congenital syphilis consists of prompt treatment of the infant with penicillin. Treatment may be done in utero prior to delivery when an infected mother is identified (Karmody and Schuknecht, 1966).

Cytomegalic Inclusion Disease. The cytomegalovirus (CMV) is a common virus that is harmless to most people who may have actually passed through a CMV infection with no symptomatology. Although antibodies are then established, the virus itself remains in cells of the body in an inactive state, possible for the remainder of the person's life. But this inactive virus can be reactivated under certain circumstances, including pregnancy, during which time the reactivated virus is excreted in body fluids such as urine, saliva, feces, blood, semen, and cervical secretions (Ho, 1982). CMV subclinical congenital infection is the most common viral agent causing sensorineural hearing loss among neonates. CMV accounts for at least 2000 cases annually of sensorineural hearing loss (Strauss, 1985).

The CMV causes cytomegalic inclusion disease that is a generalized "herpes-like" viral infection of infants caused by intrauterine or postnatal contraction from the mother. The infection may be contracted during the perinatal period with passage down the birth canal (Peterson, 1977). It appears microscopically as large eosinophilic bodies seen within cells as "inclusions" in certain body fluids (Ward et al., 1965). The viral infection shows little pathogenicity in the mother who may be totally asymptomatic. An infant may acquire the infection during the postnatal period from breast milk, blood transfusions, or older children and adults.

One in 100 infants born in the United States has active CMV infection but appears normal at birth. Of these infants, 10–15% will develop central nervous system disabilities including hearing loss, developmental delay, psychomotor retardation, and intellectual problems. About 1 infant in 1000 live births in the United States will show severe forms of the cytomegalic inclusion disease (Stagno et al., 1982). Most infants with mild infections of CMV remain asymptomatic with no permanent sequelae and will develop within normal limits. In its most severe form, however, infants usually die during the newborn period. Pappas (1983) concludes that the majority of congenital asymptomatic CMV infections of the inner ear among pediatric patients are undetected 6 months after birth and subsequently are incorrectly attributed to unknown and/or genetic etiologies.

If the CMV disease is clinically detectable at birth, some 80% of infants have sequelae related to the central nervous system. CMV, when transmitted in utero, may be associated with a spectrum of problems including varying degrees of mental retardation, spasticity, hyperactivity, microcephaly, optic atrophy, and convulsive seizures. Associated complications may include facial weakness, cleft of the hard or soft palate, and a fairly high incidence of sensorineural hearing loss (Shinefield, 1973; Strauss and Davis, 1973). Strauss (1985) states that 20–65% of infants with symptomatic CMV infection have sensorineural hearing loss severe enough to be handicapping in 10–25%. Infants identified with subclinical CMV-caused hearing losses show nonspecific sensorineural audiometric configurations. Pappas (1983) reports data from vestibular evaluation of CMV children that indicate that selective involvement of the peripheral end organs of the vestibular system is highly probable.

Harris et al. (1984) reported data from a large-scale prospective study conducted in Sweden. Some 10,328 infants were followed for a 5-year period in which 50 (0.5%) turned out to have a congenital CMV infection. Of this group, 5 children were found to have sensorineural hearing loss—4 with total deafness and 1 with mild hearing loss.

Persistent Fetal Circulation. Infants with persistent fetal circulation (PFC), also known now as primary pulmonary hypertension (PPHN), present with severe hypoxemia, often following birth asphyxia. This cardiac abnormality, previously known as patent ductus arteriosus, is actually fairly common in children and is often associated with maternal rubella syndrome. The defect occurs as an isolated abnormality as the persistence of the normal fetal vessel that joins the pulmonary artery to the aorta. Surgical correction is usually the treatment of choice performed between the ages of 2 and 5 years.

Naulty et al. (1986) followed 11 patients with PPHN for 36 months with behavioral audiometry and auditory brainstem evaluations conducted on at least two occasions. Three of the 11 (27%) babies had bilateral, progressive hearing loss with language delays 4–12 months below age level. Sell et al. (1985) pointed out that PFC babies are potentially at risk for long-term neurologic problems because of their history of severe hypoxemia due to mechanical ventilation. Hendricks-Munoz and Walton (1988) reported sensorineural hearing loss in 21 of 40 PFC infants, 14 of whom required hearing aids. In their study, the authors report a high association of delayed onset and progressive sensorineural hearing loss. Nield et al. (1989) routinely refer, for audiologic evaluation, all infants who have been mechanically ventilated, because of PFC, for 20 days or more. PFC babies are definitely at higher risk for sensorineural hearing loss than others in the ICU, and therefore, hearing screenings and routine follow-up hearing evaluations are recommended.

Rh Incompatibility. This condition involves the destruction of Rh positive blood cells of the fetus by maternal antibodies. Complications of Rh incompatibility account for about 3% of profound hearing loss among school-age deaf children. Owing to improved technology in perinatal care, fewer cases of Rh incompatibility lead to hearing loss, even in patients with complete blood transfusions at birth. Clinical symptoms, when they occur, develop during the immediate neonatal period and include elevated bilirubin, jaundice, and possible brain damage.

Kernicterus is a condition with severe neural symptoms, associated with high levels of bilirubin in the blood (sometimes called bilirubin encephalopathy). Most infants having kernicterus die during the first week, with 80% of those surviving having complete or partial deafness. Other common residuals reported included cerebral palsy, mental retardation, epilepsy, aphasia, and behavioral disorders. Audiometric findings may show mild-to-profound sensorineural hearing loss characterized by a "cookie-bite" or "saucer-shaped" curve. Hearing loss is usually sensorineural and may be bilaterally symmetrical.

Diabetes Mellitus. Diabetes mellitus is a chronic hormonal disorder of carbohydrate metabolism that is believed to result from insulin deficiency. The exact cause of this problem is unknown, but there appears to be a strong genetic predisposition (Lowenstein and Preger, 1976). There are two types of diabetes mellitus; juvenile onset and maturity onset. Juvenile onset is the more severe of the two and usually appears suddenly in childhood or in the teens. Daily insulin injections are required to compensate for a lack of native insulin. The young untreated diabetic is often quite thin and experiences excessive hunger, thirst, need to urinate, weakness, and weight loss. Diabetics are more susceptible to infection. Long-term complications of this disorder include blindness, kidney dysfunction, and gangrene of extremities. Deafness is not an invariable accompaniment, but when it occurs it is usually a mild-to-moderate, progressive, bilaterally symmetrical sensorineural hearing loss.

In the normal body system, insulin is produced in the pancreas and is secreted directly into the bloodstream. Insulin's function is to enable glucose in the blood to enter the cells. Insulin also serves to facilitate and expedite the metabolism and storage of glucose in the cells. Fuel for metabolism, heat, and motion is provided by glucose. Any excess is stored by the cells as glycogen, fat, or both. Glucose is also stored in the liver as glycogen and, when needed, is converted back to glucose and released into the bloodstream. Normally, insulin lowers blood sugar level, while glycogen serves to raise it. In diabetics there is insufficient insulin for normal absorption of the glucose by the cells or the liver. The body senses a deficiency of glucose and sends hormonal messages to increase the delivery of glucose. The liver converts glycogen back to glucose, but the glucose still cannot be absorbed by cells without insulin so it accumulates in the blood. The liver also begins breaking down fats and amino acids for metabolism, which may give rise to acids that accumulate in blood and ultimately become poisonous to the system. Over many years, vascular changes occur and involve the small blood vessels of the body, including the capillaries, arterioles, and venules. The diameter of these vessels decreases, resulting in less blood flow (microangiopathy).

Morphologic and histologic studies of the ear generally agree that the etiology of hearing loss in diabetics is damage to the cochlear structures due to microangiopathic disturbance. Cranial nerve VIII and spiral ganglion may also be affected, but most auditory tests indicate cochlear disorder. This confusion surrounding etiology of the hearing loss leaves few clues as to the otologic and audiologic symptoms of early diabetes. However, the incidence of hearing loss is higher in diabetics than in nondiabetics of the same age (Axelssen and Fagerberg, 1968; Friedman et al., 1975).

The "typical" sensorineural hearing loss in patients with diabetes is characterized by fullness, roaring tinnitus, and fluctuations in the hearing level. Vertigo is usually not associated with diabetes. Although Carmen et al. (1988) suggest that a rising, progressively improving auditory threshold pattern correlates with diabetes, historically no specific configuration has been identified.

Acoustic Nerve Tumors. Tumors arising from the eighth nerve and ex-

tending into the cerebellar-pontine angle have been reported in children. Tumors in this area are usually neuromas originating from the vestibular portion of the eighth nerve. The hearing loss is usually a unilateral, progressive sensorineural type and may be difficult to identify, especially in children. The acoustic tumor diagnosis is generally made from ABR wave morphology abnormalities as well as specialized radiographic techniques. Acoustic tumors should be expected in all children with von Recklinghausen's neurofibromatosis (see Appendix of Hearing Disorders). Audiometric tests and vestibular procedures may contribute information to the ultimate diagnosis. Cases of acoustic tumors in children are rare.

MEDICAL REFERRAL OR TREATMENT

It is the audiologist's responsibility to insist that regular medical examinations be obtained for the hearing-impaired child. Until the child is 8 or 10 years of age, an otolaryngologic examination should be insisted upon every 6 months.

An erroneous assumption is that after a child has sustained a hearing loss, nothing more can happen to his or her ears. Not only is this belief incorrect, but there is some evidence suggesting that sensorineural hearing impairment may be accompanied by increased susceptibility to other ear disease, to noise-induced loss, or to ototoxicity (Falk, 1972). Therefore it is imperative that the hearing-impaired child be monitored more regularly than the normal-hearing child. The importance of every dB of residual hearing that the child possesses may be in exponential ratio to each dB of hearing loss.

Routine audiologic monitoring of the degree of loss pays dividends in information on changes in hearing that are pertinent for the habilitation program. A more extensive otologic and physical examination may be suggested when deterioration of the auditory threshold or the speech discrimination is found.

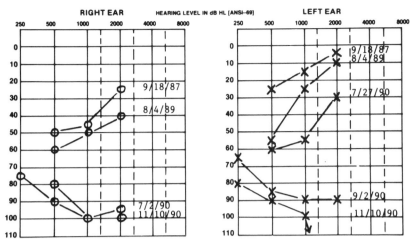

Figure 3.7. Audiogram of a patient with documented progressive bilateral sensorineural hearing loss. This child had normal hearing by observation of responses from birth to age 2½ years.

A number of important pieces of information may be noted at routine audiologic reevaluations. For example, progression of sensorineural hearing loss may occur in either a gradual or rapid manner as shown in Figure 3.7. The hearing initially deteriorated slowly over a 4 year period and then rapidly for 2 months until stabilizing.

Obviously, monitoring a temporary conductive loss superimposed on a sensorineural loss has important medical and educational implications. As hearing levels change in hearing-impaired children, hearing aid adjustments may be necessary. For this reason, tympanometry should be performed at every routine audiologic reevaluation. Attention must be given to new complaints from the child including reports of the onset of tinnitus, dizziness, or changes in the quality of sound. When change is noted during the reevaluation examination, the audiologist must be overly sensitive to the possible need for medical referral.

GENETICS

Humans take great pride in identifying distinguishing traits from one generation to the next. We enjoy speculating on the resemblance of children to their parents and question which child has, for example, the father's eyebrows or the mother's chin. With such observations begins the study of genetics and the submicroscopic structures known as genes.

Genes are found in the nuclei of the many cells that compose the body. Genes are concerned with the determination of what a person's characteristics shall be, and they form the hereditary link between one generation and the next. The characteristics of an offspring are, to a large degree, determined by the genes he or she receives from parents—from the mother through the ovum or egg and from the father through the sperm cell that fertilized that ovum at the time of conception. Genetic factors present at conception are largely unaltered throughout life. The genes are contained in chromosomes that occur in pairs. One member of each chromosome pair is inherited from the father, the other chromosome member is inherited from the mother.

The clinician concerned with hearing disorders should have some basic knowledge of genetics in hereditary inheritance. There is probably some genetic component in almost all disease processes, but the extent of this component varies. Some diseases are almost entirely determined by a person's genetic constitution, such as Down's syndrome, achondroplasia, or other individually rare conditions.

Nearly 3000 genetic disorders have been identified. Of the 3,000,000 babies born in the United States each year, 2–3% have a major genetic or congenital disease. The average person has 4–8 potentially harmful genes—out of a total of 50,000–100,000 genes that determine his or her neonatal and physical traits. A number of important technologic advances will help reduce these statistics. *Amniocentesis* (and a related procedure known as *chorionic villus sampling*) is a procedure in which physicians withdraw amniotic fluid from the mother's uterus for laboratory examination to search for abnormal cells that indicate the condition of the fetus. *Ultrasound* techniques bounce sound waves off the fetus to produce pictures. *Fetoscopy* permits the physician to examine the fetus directly with a lighted lens inserted into the uterus.

Of course, the problem of identifying an abnormal fetus may be simpler than the decision regarding abortion. The problem of deciding whether to abort a fetus is complicated by the fact that many genetic disorders present with a wide spectrum of severity. For example, some children born with cystic fibrosis have only minor symptoms throughout their life, while others die a slow death from respiratory failure. Some mildly involved Down's children may lead useful, productive lives, while others with the same chromosome picture but more severe retardation will necessarily be institutionalized for life.

The following presentation will include basic information concerning chromosomes and chromosome defects, patterns of inheritance, the genetics of deafness, and genetic counseling. Our goal is to acquaint the clinician who has had little or no formal course work in genetics with the fundamentals of this important aspect of life that contributes to many of the cases of deafness we see commonly in the patient population. We are greatly indebted to Janet Stewart, M.D., of the University of Colorado Health Sciences Center Birth Defects Clinic and Pediatrics Department, for use of her materials on genetic counseling as the basis of the following discussion.

Chromosomes and Chromosomal Defects. All hereditary material, in the form of deoxyribonucleic acid (DNA), is carried as genes on the chromosomes. All human body cells contain 23 pairs of chromosomes or 46 total chromosomes. Twenty-two of these pairs are known as autosomes; the remaining two chromosomes are called the sex chromosomes, two X chromosomes constituting a female (written as 46,XX in genetic nomenclature), and one X and Y constituting a male (46,XY). The reproduction process of the body (or somite) cells is known as mitosis, while the reproduction of the germ (or sex) cells is called meiosis.

During the process of mitosis, each chromosome becomes shortened and thickened, and splits longitudinally into two chromatids joined at the point called the centromere. This is the form in which most chromosomes are pictured. They are then aligned and split longitudinally through the centromere, separating the two chromatids that then migrate to opposite ends of the cell. Cleavage then occurs in the cell to produce two genetically similar cells. Mitosis is an elegant, yet simple, mechanism for the replication of body cells (Fig. 3.8).

Humans, like all forms of life, must reproduce if the species is to continue. An essential factor in the reproductive process is the formation of additional sperm and eggs by a special type of cell division (meiosis) that involves only the germ cells, as shown in Figure 3.9.

In this process, the chromosomes again shorten and thicken and split into two chromatids joined at the centromere as described in mitosis. Matching pairs are arranged together and at this time material may be exchanged between paired chromosomes. The paired chromosomes then separate (known as dysjunction) and move to opposite poles of the cell, forming two cells now with 23 chromosomes each (known as

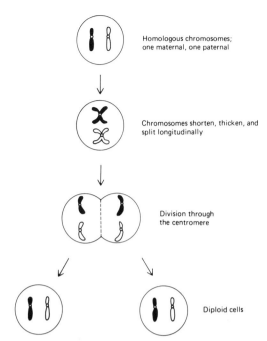

Homologous chromosomes; one maternal, one paternal

Chromosomes shorten, thicken, and split longitudinally

Division through the centromere

Diploid cells

Figure 3.8. Process of mitotic cell division. (Reprinted with permission from J. M. Stewart: Genetic counseling. In J. Clausen et al. (eds.): *Maternity Nursing Today*. New York, McGraw-Hill, 1973.)

the haploid number). Each cell contains two chromosomes—either X chromosomes, or Y chromosomes, or a combination of each. The next step in the process is simple mitotic division in which there is a longitudinal split at the centromere and migration of the chromatids to opposite poles. In this manner new ova and new sperm are formed, each with 23 chromosomes. At some future time of fertilization, one ovum and one sperm will unite to form a cell, known as the zygote, with a full 46 chromosome constitution.

Abnormalities may occur during meiotic or mitotic division, producing an individual with a chromosomal defect. These abnormalities may involve one of the autosomes or one of the sex chromosomes and consist of either too much or too little total chromosome material. In certain types of tissue and under certain conditions, chromosomes are readily visible under high magnification. A photographic record of chromosomal constitution of a cell is called a karyotype (Figs. 3.10 and 3.11). The human kary-

otype is often described in terms of "Denver system," so-called because it was formulated at the meeting of cytologists in Denver, Colorado. In the human karyotype the pairs of somatic chromosomes (autosomes) are identified by number (1–22) as nearly as possible in descending order of length and are divided into seven groups (usually designated as group A through group G). Each group is composed of chromosome pairs with similar morphologic features. The sex chromosomes are identified by the symbols X and Y.

The most common autosomal defect is known as Down's syndrome, or mongolism. The affected individual has an extra number 21 chromosome (trisomy 21) for a total of 47 chromosomes. The clinical feature of Down's syndrome are described in "Appendix of Hearing Disorders." Down's syndrome can also occur in another form. An occasional child with Down's syndrome will have only 46 chromosomes, including one large abnormal chromosome that consists of the translocation of the extra 21 to another chromosome. Clinically, the child with the translocation type of Down's syndrome is indistinguishable from the child with the more common form, trisomy 21.

Hearing loss may also occur with trisomy 13 and trisomy 18, as described more fully in the Appendix. These children usually have many severe abnormalities and rarely live beyond a few months of age. The total absence of an autosome is believed to be incompatible with life, although a few exceptions have been reported. For example, a deletion of the short arm of chromosome 5 results in severe mental retardation and a catlike cry in infancy, comprising the cri-du-chat syndrome.

Unlike the loss of autosomal material, an individual may lose one of the sex chromosomes with surprisingly little defect. Sex chromosome defects do cause disorders usually less severe than autosomal defects, such as Turner's syndrome and Klinefelter's syndrome. About 1% of residents of institutions for the retarded have sex chromosome anomalies (Robinson, 1972).

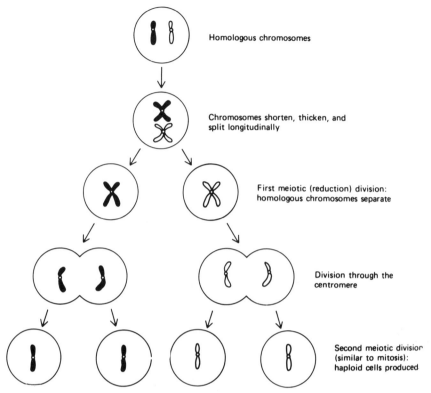

Homologous chromosomes

Chromosomes shorten, thicken, and split longitudinally

First meiotic (reduction) division: homologous chromosomes separate

Division through the centromere

Second meiotic division (similar to mitosis): haploid cells produced

Figure 3.9. Germ cell division or meiosis. (Reprinted with permission from J. M. Stewart: Genetic counseling. In J. Clausen et al. (eds.): *Maternity Nursing Today*. New York, McGraw-Hill, 1973.)

PATTERNS OF INHERITANCE

The chromosomal defects that have been described above are all grossly obvious in a standard karyotype. Defects involving single genes, however, are much more discrete and invisible by any currently used technique. The determination of the hereditary nature of an abnormality is done primarily by the careful study of an individual's family.

Genes occur in pairs and are located on homologous chromosomes. One gene is maternal in origin, and the other paternal. If the two genes have the same effect, the person is said to be "homozygous" for the gene. If the effect is different, the person is said to be "heterozygous" for the gene. The expression of each gene factor depends on its interaction with other genes and the environment. Genetic defects can be inherited in three well-known ways and in a fourth less well understood, but commonly occurring, manner.

Autosomal Dominant. A condition or trait is said to be dominantly inherited if it is manifest in the heterozygous state. This is a type of inheritance with an affected person having a 50% chance of passing the gene on to each of his or her offspring. Every afflicted person will have a similarly afflicted parent. An unaffected person in most cases does not carry the abnormal gene, and all of his or her offspring will be normal. Dominantly inherited traits have several distinguishing characteristics. They are usually milder, since the gene is passed on by the affected individual who is capable of reproduction. There is much variation in the clinical manifestations of a dominant gene, which is known as "variation in expressivity." In other words, a few persons are so very severely affected, while those at the

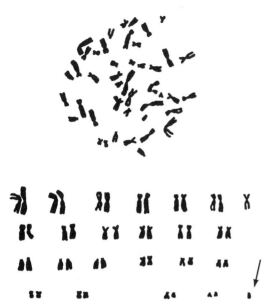

Figure 3.10. Human male karyotype with normal chromosomes. (Courtesy of A. Robinson, M.D., Cytogenetics Laboratory, University of Colorado Medical Center.)

other end of the spectrum may be so mildly affected, that they have no obvious clinical manifestation of the gene problem. If this occurs, a gene is said to have "decreased penetrance." On occasion, a dominant trait

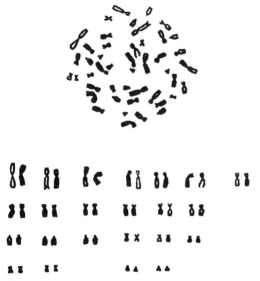

Figure 3.11. Human female karyotype with normal chromosomes. (Courtesy of A. Robinson, M.D., Cytogenetics Laboratory, University of Colorado Medical Center.)

will seem to appear as a spontaneous gene mutation. The parents of such a child are not at an increased risk for future pregnancies, although the affected person would have a 50% chance of passing the trait on to his or her offspring.

Autosomal Recessive. A condition is said to be recessively inherited if it is manifest only when the person is homozygous for the defective gene. This is a type of inheritance in which the carrier parents may often be asymptomatic with a 25% chance of producing an affected child. One half of their children will be carriers, like themselves, and 25% will be genetically normal. In many cases, recessive conditions are more severe than dominant conditions, as the abnormality is passed on by the asymptomatic carrier and the affected person need not reproduce. If a particularly recessive condition is rare, there is an increased incidence of consanguinity in the parents. Consanguinity, which refers to a marriage of parents with recent common ancestors, such as cousin to cousin or uncle to niece, has genetic significance in that there is a greatly increased chance that two parents who have a recent common ancestor may each have the same recessive gene inherited from that common ancestor. Each partner, then, could give a child this gene, so that the child would possess two such genes and be homozygous for the abnormal gene. The pattern of this type of inheritance shows a cluster of affected persons among brothers and sisters, with normal parents. It is not possible to identify such families in the general population until they have produced affected children. An example of an autosomal recessive disorder is Pendred's syndrome, a condition characterized by hearing loss and a goiter, which appears in adolescence. Both parents in some circumstances might have normal hearing with no other family history of deafness.

Sex-linked. If the gene for a particular trait or abnormality is located on the X chromosome, the condition is said to be inherited in an X-linked or sex-linked manner. The condition then is X-linked recessive if it is manifest only in the male who is homozygous; i.e., the abnormal gene on the single X chromosome is genetically unopposed. The female who has a normal gene on one X chromosome and an abnormal gene on the other is a carrier and usually asymptomatic. The carrier female passes the gene on to 50% of her sons, who then manifest the abnormality, and to 50% of her daughters, who are also carriers but who will not manifest the abnormality. The cardinal feature of an X-linked trait is the lack of male-to-male transmission, since the male may pass on his Y chromosome only to his sons. The pattern of father-daughter alternation is characteristic because affected fathers have only one X chromosome, so they must pass the gene to their daughters, and none of their sons, who get the father's Y chromosome and the mother's X chromosome. Sex-linked inheritance patterns have been familiar since biblical times when it was noted that hemophilia, as well as color blindness, seemed to be passed from unaffected females to males.

Polygenic.   Many of the more common congenital abnormalities, such as cleft lip, cleft palate, and spina bifida, are not inherited in one of the manners described above, and yet it is well-known that these defects cluster in families. It has been postulated that multiple genes contribute to these defects and that each individual has a threshold above which the abnormality will be manifest. This condition is known as polygenic inheritance. The more severe the defect, the more the predisposing genes must present. Unlike single-gene defects, the recurrence risk varies with the number of affected persons in the family.

Genetic Counseling.   Genetic counseling is often given to parents who have had one abnormal child and who are interested in knowing the potential for having additional children with the same defect. Genetic counseling may also be offered to siblings of an abnormal person and to the affected person as he or she approaches marriage age and possible parenthood. Genetic evaluation and counseling may be done in any of some 400 genetic counseling centers in the United States today.

The steps of the genetic counseling vary with the complexity of the problem but include a careful family, pregnancy, birth, and infancy history to find factors that might explain the abnormality, careful physical examination of the affected individual and other family members, and necessary laboratory work as required. When the evaluation has been completed and the diagnosis reached, the parents return for the actual counseling sessions. Both parents are generally required to attend, and the counseling is done in an unhurried and relaxed atmosphere. They are given the final diagnosis and the risk figures for future pregnancies. When possible an attempt is made by the genetic counselors to minimize guilt; however, in situations in which one parent is obviously the carrier of the gene causing the defect, it may be better to acknowledge the guilt and help the parent deal with it. In many instances more than one counseling session is necessary. There is good evidence that parents who seek genetic advice will usually make appropriate and expected decisions about future children.

The field of genetics is old yet it is filled with new discoveries. Only in 1956 were human chromosomes accurately counted, and in 1959 the first chromosomal abnormality—the trisomy 21 associated with Down's syndrome—was accurately described. Progress has been rapid, however, in the past 30 years, and many of the new techniques are of practical significance in terms of genetic counseling.

The diagrammatic construction of a family pedigree, which is a representation of the family medical history used to determine if the etiology of a disease is indeed familial, it is helpful to indicate modes of inheritance. The pedigree may provide evidence to establish whether a trait carried

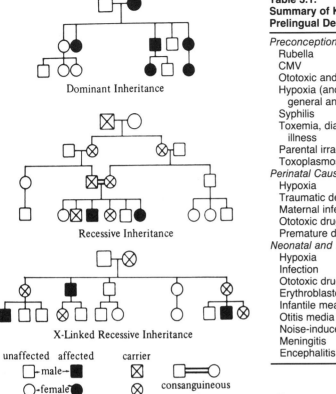

Dominant Inheritance

Recessive Inheritance

X-Linked Recessive Inheritance

unaffected	affected		carrier
□ –male–■		⊠	□══○
○ –female–●		⊗	consanguineous marriage

Figure 3.12. Family pedigrees showing simple inheritance patterns of single-gene factors. (Reprinted with permission from A. Robinson: Genetic and chromosomal disorders. In C. H. Kempe et al. (eds.): *Current Pediatric Diagnosis and Treatment.* Los Altos, California, Lange Medical Publications, 1972.)

Table 3.1.
Summary of Known Exogenous Causes of Prelingual Deafness

Preconception and Prenatal Causes
  Rubella
  CMV
  Ototoxic and other drugs, maternal alcoholism
  Hypoxia (and its possible causes: high altitude, general anesthetic, severe hemorrhage)
  Syphilis
  Toxemia, diabetes, other severe systemic maternal illness
  Parental irradiation
  Toxoplasmosis
Perinatal Causes
  Hypoxia
  Traumatic delivery
  Maternal infection
  Ototoxic drugs
  Premature delivery
Neonatal and Postnatal Causes
  Hypoxia
  Infection
  Ototoxic drugs
  Erythroblastosis fetalis
  Infantile measles or mumps
  Otitis media (acute, chronic, serous)
  Noise-induced
  Meningitis
  Encephalitis

by a single gene is dominant, recessive, or sex-linked. Simple pedigrees showing classic types of single-gene inheritance are presented in Figure 3.12.

HEREDITARY DEAFNESS

Hereditary deafness is a fairly common disease entity, occurring between 1 in 2000 and 1 in 6000 live births. We use the term "hereditary deafness" rather than "congenital deafness" in this section because we are referring to children with profound, irreversible, bilateral sensorineural hearing loss of early onset. Congenital deafness would include those children with conductive hearing loss due to osseous malformation in the middle ear. Such a condition usu-

ally creates a moderate hearing loss, often amenable to surgical intervention, and thus quite a different group of children from those we describe with hereditary childhood deafness. Everberg (1960) researched nearly 200,000 school children in Copenhagen to conclude that hereditary factors were of importance in only 10%, or 12 of 122 patients, with unilateral deafness. In studying a child with apparent congenital severe deafness, the clinician must be aware of possible exogenous, or outside, factors that can cause childhood deafness, as summarized in Table 3.1. A major contribution to the study of etiologic factors in deafness has been published by Fraser, *The Causes of Profound Deafness in Childhood* (1976).

A high percentage of congenital deafness is hereditary, according to Konigsmark (1972) and Fraser (1976). About 40% of profound childhood deafness is autosomal recessive in origin; 10%, dominant transmission; and some 3%, due to a sex-linked gene. Since deaf persons tend to marry

Table 3.2.
**Etiology of Hearing Loss as Expressed by
Manually Communicating Deaf Adults**

Etiology	Percentage	
	Northern et al. (1971c)	Schein (1965)
Unknown	35.8	32.2
Congenital	25.5	10.5
Meningitis	13.1	12.7
Scarlet fever	9.5	4.6
Result of a fall	8.1	7.7
Whooping cough	3.6	2.3
Measles	2.2	3.4
Pneumonia		2.3
Mastoiditis		1.9
Other	2.2	16.7
N =	137	1132

other deaf persons (Schein, 1965; Northern et al., 1971, 1971c), statistics regarding their potential for producing deaf offspring are of interest. The marriage of two deaf persons gives only a slightly increased risk of deafness in their children because there is small chance that two such persons would be affected by the same exact genetic deafness. Should the same recessive gene be carried by two normal-hearing parents, theoretically one fourth of their offspring would be affected and one half of their children would be carriers. However, if both parents are overtly affected by the same recessive type of hereditary deafness, they are homozygous for the trait and therefore *all* their children will be not only affected but also capable of passing the trait on to some of their offspring.

A means of identifying the causes of deafness has been accomplished by interviewing large samples of adult deaf persons. The adult deaf, however, are unfortunately poorly informed regarding the cause of their hearing problems. Such analyses are usually obtained through a written questionnaire or personal interview, but in this type of population in which language and communication are problems, such information-gathering techniques suggest caution in data interpretation. We are reminded of the deaf father who told us that he lost his hearing between the ages of 1 and 2. His parents told him that he had cut his finger badly, and the doctor had stitched up the cut without use of anesthesia. The pain was apparently so severe that his loud crying damaged his hearing. This story was from a totally deaf man married to a deaf woman, the parents of three deaf children! A summary of results from two studies of deaf adults who were asked the cause of their hearing loss (Schein, 1965; Northern et al., 1971c) is shown in Table 3.2.

Despite the large number of syndromes associated with dominant deafness, most human inherited deafness (about 90%) is of a recessive rather than dominant type. In the case of recessively inherited deafness, both parents must be the carriers of the particular gene, in which event the chance of offspring being affected is only 25%. Most of these patients have no family history of deafness, thereby making the case for hereditary etiology difficult to prove.

CLASSIFICATION OF HEREDITARY DEAFNESS

Childhood deafness associated with other defects has been observed for hundreds of years and cited in journal articles too numerous to count. Konigsmark (1969) indicates that about 70 types of hereditary deafness have been identified in humans. Only since the mid-1960s have data been available regarding the relative frequency of various syndrome complexes that include deafness.

The alert clinician is soon aware that malformations and anomalies often "run together." Congenital defects are often caused by prenatal misfortunes that may influence the development of specific body systems or create generalized malformations of all the structures undergoing growth at that time. On the other hand, when multiple congenital malformations appear together frequently, the patient can be described in terms of a "syndrome." The term syndrome is often overused and misapplied. The difficulties of syndrome classification lie in terminology problems, broad spectra of signs and symptoms, and differences in the basis of diagnosis, depending on whether the diagnosis is anatomic, histologic, or hematologic. Often, experts disagree on the diagnosis of a syndrome, or the youngster may present such a variety of symptomatic signs that clear-cut diagnosis is not possible. The definition of a syndrome depends on the level of acuity of observation and becomes easier the more pronounced the accompanying features are demonstrated.

Many children may likely be candidates for ultimate syndrome diagnosis, but hearing loss will not always be present. In addition, some disorders may manifest progressive-type hearing loss, so that although normal hearing is noted on the initial visit, these children deserve regular reevaluation. The verification of hearing loss is the realm of the audiologist who can substantiate accurately hearing levels in such children with appropriate testing techniques. A summary of communication disorders found in various syndromes was published by Siegel-Sadewitz and Shprintzen (1982). A concise system of classifying deafness was prepared by Bergstrom et al. (1971), ordered around types of hearing loss and body systems as shown in Table 3.3.

CONGENITAL MALFORMATIONS

Congenital Malformations of the Inner Ear. Although wide variety exists in anatomic abnormalities of the inner ear, four classic types exist. These include (*a*) Michel, complete failure of development of the inner ear; (*b*) Mondini, incomplete development and malformation of the inner ear; (*c*) the Scheibe membranous cochleosaccular degeneration of the inner ear; and (*d*) the Alexander malformation of the cochlear membranous system.

Knowledge of these inner ear anomalies is important for accurate diagnosis, proper treatment of the patient, and genetic counseling for the parents of the handicapped child, as well as for the patient when he (or she) is old enough to become a parent. Therefore, differentiation of the above in-

ner ear problems is crucial in the determination of whether the hearing loss in question is of a genetic or an acquired origin.

The degree of abnormal development that is actually involved in any specific patient may vary considerably from other patients with similar inner ear malformations. Diagnostic considerations must include petrous pyramid polytomography of the inner ear, as well as a complete evaluation of the hearing impairment. Malformations in the bone of the otic capsule can be detected by careful x-ray, and differential diagnosis of the Michel and Mondini aplasias are possible.

Aplasia of the inner ear implies failure of the ear to reach full development. Accordingly, inner ear aplasia is always a congenital malformation. The embryonic time of developmental failure, of course, determines the ultimate structure and appearance of the deformity. According to Schuknecht (1967), an individual may possess different degrees of aplasia in the two ears. Aplasia of the inner ear is a relatively uncommon aberration.

Michel-Type of Aplasia of the Inner Ear. The macroscopic description of this temporal bone anomaly was first described by Michel in 1863. This type of anomaly is represented by a complete absence of the inner ear and auditory nerve. The outer ear may be completely normal with a narrow middle ear cavity. The malleus and incus may be present, but the staples and stapedius muscle may be absent or abnormal. Maternal thalidomide during pregnancy has been associated with this anomaly, and it has been observed in at least one case of Klippel-Feil deformity (McLay and Maran, 1969).

Mondini Aplasia of the Inner Ear. Mondini described a temporal bone in 1791 that showed incomplete development of a flattened cochlea that consisted of only a single basal coil. In 1904, Alexander added more detail to this type of anomaly indicating involvement of the auditory nerve and the vestibular canals. Characteristic of this

Table 3.3.
Classification of Hereditary Deafness

I. CONGENITAL SENSORINEURAL HEARING LOSS DISORDERS	II. CONGENITAL CONDUCTIVE HEARING LOSS DISORDERS	IV. PROGRESSIVE HEARING LOSS DISORDERS
Craniofacial and Skeletal Disorders	**Craniofacial and Skeletal Disorders**	**Sensorineural Progressive Hearing Loss of Later Onset**
Absence of tibia	Apert's syndrome	*Craniofacial and Skeletal Disorders*
Cleidocranial dysostosis	Fanconi's anemia syndrome	Roaf's syndrome
Diastrophic dwarfism	Goldenhar's syndrome	Van Buchem's syndrome
Hand-hearing syndrome	Madelung's deformity	*Eye Disorders*
Klippel-Feil	Malformed, low-set ears	Alström's syndrome
Saddle nose and myopia	Mohr's syndrome	Cockayne's syndrome
Split-hand and foot	Otopalatodigital	Fehr's corneal dystrophy
Integumentary and Pigmentary Disorders	Preauricular appendages	Flynn-Aird
Albinism with blue irides	Proximal symphalangism	Norrie's syndrome
Congenital atopic dermatitis	Thickened ears	Optic atrophy and
Ectodermal dysplasia	Treacher Collins	diabetes mellitus
Keratopachyderma	**Integumentary and Pigmentary Disorders**	Refsum's syndrome
Lentigines	Forney's syndrome	*Nervous System Disorders*
Onychodystrophy	**Eye Disorders**	Acoustic neuromas
Partial albinism	Cryptophthalmos	Friedreich's ataxia
Piebaldness	Duane's syndrome	Herrmann's syndrome
Pili torti	**Renal Disorders**	Myoclonic seizures
Waardenburg's syndrome	Nephrosis, urinary tract	Sensory radicular
Eye Disorders	malformations	neuropathy
Hallgren's	Renal-genital syndrome	Severe infantile muscular
Laurence-Moon-Biedl-Bardet	Taylor's syndrome	dystrophy
Nervous System Disorders	III. DISORDERS OF CONGENITAL SENSORINEURAL AND/OR CONDUCTIVE HEARING LOSS	*Endocrine and Metabolic Disorders*
Cerebral palsy		Alport's syndrome
Muscular dystrophy		Amyloidosis, nephritis, and
Myoclonic epilepsy		urticaria
Opticocochleodentate	**Craniofacial and Skeletal Disorders**	Hyperprolinemia II
degeneration	Achondroplasia	Hyperuricemia
Richards-Rundel	Crouzon's syndrome	Primary testicular
Cardiovascular System Disorders	Marfan's syndrome	insufficiency
Jervell and Lange-Nielsen	Pierre Robin	**Sensorineural or Conductive Progressive Hearing Loss**
Endocrine and Metabolic Disorders	Pyle's disease	*Craniofacial and Skeletal Disorders*
Goiter	**Integumentary and Pigmentary Disorders**	Albers-Schönberg disease
Hyperprolinemia I	Knuckle pads and	Engelmann's syndrome
Iminoglycinuria	leukonychia	Osteogenesis imperfecta
Pendred's	**Eye Disorders**	Paget's disease
Miscellaneous Somatic Disorders	Möbius' syndrome	*Endocrine and Metabolic Disorders*
Trisomy 13–15	**Miscellaneous Somatic Disorders**	Hunter's syndrome
Trisomy 18	Turner's syndrome	Hurler's syndrome
		Progressive Conductive or Mixed Hearing Loss
		Otosclerosis

anomaly is that it involves both the bony capsule and the membranous labyrinth. This anomaly, which often bears both investigators' names, has been associated with Klippel-Feil and Wildervanck syndromes. It has also been found in cases of mental retardation, hydrocephalus, and hydronephrosis. Middle ear anomalies may be present in these cases, and atresia of the external canal has also been reported.

Many temporal bone studies have described this deformity, which varies considerably from one case to another and may be unilateral or bilateral (Fig. 3.13). Altmann (1950) suggested that labyrinthine hydrops may be present in Mondini dysplasia, and a

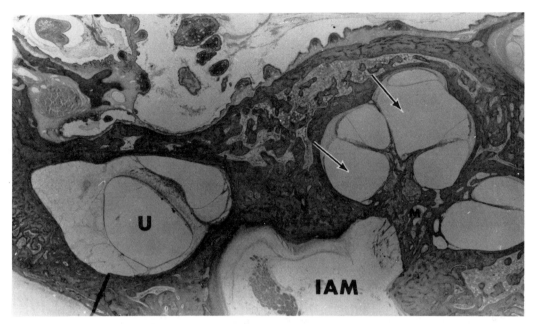

Figure 3.13. Mondini type of incomplete development with malformation of the inner ear from a patient with trisomy 13–15 syndrome. Note incompletely developed cochlea with absence of the interscalar osseous septum (*arrows*) and poorly developed modiolus (*M*). *U*, utricle; *IAM*, internal auditory meatus. (Reprinted with permission from I. Sando, B. Baker, F. O. Black, and W. G. Hemenway: Persistence of stapedial artery in trisomy 13–15 syndrome. *Archives of Otolaryngology* 96:441–447, 1972.)

new theory of management has emerged on this basis, utilizing the endolymphatic shunt operation in an effort to relieve the hydrops believed to be causing progressive hearing loss in these cases.

It has been possible recently to diagnose dysplasia through temporal bone polytomography, leading to more frequent diagnoses of this problem. Many patients report fluctuant hearing loss that tends to become progressively worse, and questioning the parents may reveal that the child has difficulty walking at that time. Electrocochleography (ECoG) may contribute to the diagnosis, as Brackmann (1977) described a type of wave form that is a multipeaked or disynchronized acoustic nerve action potential wave form that he considered characteristic of Ménière's disease. Mangabeira-Albernaz et al. (1981) found the same characteristic peak wave forms in 12 cases of Mondini dysplasia. These authors also found a suspicion of dysplasia in cases with clearly asymmetrical ECoG thresholds and in those with diphasic action potential re-

sponses. It was proposed by House (1964) that an endolymphatic subarachnoid shunt would help to prevent the fluctuation of hearing in Mondini ears and would stop the progression of the hearing loss. The theory is that the progressive loss of hair cells may result from membrane ruptures resulting from endolymphatic hydrops, as the temporal bones that have been studied do show enlarged endolymphatic sacs and ducts. According to Mangabeira-Albernaz et al. (1981), children with a complete absence of the osseous spiral lamina usually lose their hearing completely about 4 years of age, but in many cases the dysplasia is less severe and the patient continues to have hearing for many years.

As the endolymphatic shunt operations have been done only for a short period of time on Mondini cases, it is impossible to predict long-term results. Mangabeira-Albernaz et al. (1981) indicated that in 22 ears surgery did indeed stop the progression of the hearing loss, at least in the 1-year term of their report.

Scheibe Aplasia of the Inner Ear. The Scheibe abnormality of the inner ear, originally described in 1892, is characterized by involvement of only the membranous portion of the cochlea and saccule. This type of dysplasia is the most common of the inner ear aplasias. Histopathology of these inner ears shows atrophy of the stria vascularis, degeneration of the organ of Corti, and rolling up of the tectorial membrane, especially in the basal turn of the cochlea. This anomaly has been identified in cases of Waardenburg's syndrome, the cardioauditory syndrome of Jervell and Lange-Nielsen, Usher's syndrome, Refsum's syndrome, and maternal rubella.

Knowledge regarding the residual hearing in children with inner ear anomalies may be of great value in the habilitation of the child so deafened. According to Black et al. (1971a), audiometric patterns in the Michel ear should show no hearing, since no true inner ear exists. True hearing is impossible, and a hearing aid for such a patient can be of limited value. It is possible for the Mondini malformed inner ear to have some hearing, since the basal coil of the cochlea may be present with intact higher auditory pathways. The Scheibe ear may show residual hearing in the low frequencies, since in this ear the major damage is in the basal coil of the cochlea. The Scheibe and Mondini malformations may be unilateral. Black et al. (1971a) state that asymmetry of malformation is not uncommon and the patient may demonstrate one type of inner ear anomaly on one side and another type of inner ear anomaly on the other side. In such cases, x-ray findings and the degree or pattern of the hearing loss may be quite unlike each other.

More information is needed regarding the presence of these inner ear malformations. As of now, the risk of occurrence and the ratio of male-female incidence has not yet been securely determined. The bony inner ear dysplasias may be diagnosed soon after birth by x-ray, but the membranous labyrinth malformations must be inferred.

Congenital Middle Ear Malformations. Interest in middle ear anomalies has increased with the advent of microscopic surgical techniques and improved diagnostic capabilities of clinicians. Many patients with abnormal middle ears can have the deformity corrected by surgery. Since the middle ear is largely formed during the first trimester of fetal life, gross developmental anomalies of the middle ear are often related to factors that influence the fetus during that time.

Malformation of the middle ear may be due to hereditary factors or to disturbances during embryonic development. Failure in the proper development of the first and second branchial arches may result in the absence of the ossicles or a fusion of the ossicles. A malformation of the stapes footplate, however, is related to the development of the otic capsule. A disturbance in the fetal growth of the first branchial pouch may affect the eustachian tube, middle ear cavity, and the ultimate pneumatization of the mastoid air spaces.

Isolated anomalies of the middle ear ossicles are not particularly rare. Malleus anomalies include fixation or deformation of the malleus head and bony fusion of the incudomalleolar joint or absence of the malleus. Incus deficiencies may exist in isolation or in conjunction with other middle ear ossicular problems and range from total absence to a deficiency of the lenticular process. The incus may have only a fibrous connection to the malleus or be fused to the lateral semicircular canal wall. Stapes anomalies may involve fusion of the stapes head to the promontory, absence of the head and/or crura, the absence of the entire stapes itself, or the presence of a columellar ossicle. Congenital absence of the oval window or the round window may also exist as a unilateral or bilateral defect.

Middle ear anomalies should be suspected whenever other branchial arch anomalies are observed and are often noted as part of congenital syndromes. Branchial arch disorders include atresia of the external auditory canal, cleft palate, micrognathia, Pierre Robin syndrome, Treacher Collins syndrome, and low-set auricles. Disorders that feature other skeletal defects may also include middle ear anomalies such as Apert's syndrome, Klippel-Feil syndrome, and Crouzon's, Paget's, and van der Hoeve's diseases. Middle ear anomalies have been reported in disorders of connective tissue such as gargolism or Hunter-Hurler syndromes, Möbius' syndrome, and dwarfism.

Malformations of the External Ear and Canal. The auricle develops around the first branchial groove as six knoblike protrusions early in embryonic life. These six hillocks soon lose their identity as they coalesce to form the pinna. With six separate growth centers developing at differing rates, it is not surprising that a wide variation exists in final ear configurations that are within normal limits. The shape of the auricle is so different among individuals that European police forces utilize the configuration of the ear much like American police use fingerprints.

Supernumerary hillocks, known as "tags" or preauricular appendages, may remain with an otherwise normal-appearing pinna. However, the presence of tags may suggest anomalies of the external and middle ear systems. An interesting study reported from Sweden established an incidence figure for preauricular tags of 5.4 in 1000 live births. Kankkunen (1987) studied 188 Swedish babies with preauricular tags and noted that when the tag was the only facial defect, mild-to-moderate sensorineural hearing loss was found in 23% of the patients. However, in 10 patients with preauricular tags and associated facial anomalies (facial paralysis, mandibular anomalies, etc.), 8 patients had conductive hearing loss, 1 patient had a mixed-type hearing loss, and 1 patient showed sensorineural hearing loss.

Defects of the external ear and canal may be apparent without damage to the middle or inner ear structures. However, severe middle ear anomalies or aplasia of the middle ear may be associated. External ear and canal anomalies may be visible at birth, but they are often overlooked, and the defect is not noted until hearing loss is suspected or discovered. Sometimes the auricle and the opening to the external auditory meatus appear normal, but the meatus may funnel down to complete closure lateral to the tympanic membrane. If the atresia is bilateral, the child should be fitted with a bone conduction hearing aid as soon as possible. If the atresia is unilateral and normal hearing can be established in the opposite ear, treatment or habilitation is generally deferred. Aural atresias may accompany other defects of the cranium, face, skeleton, or mandible. The etiology of the aural atresia may be a chromosomal aberration, heredity, maternal thalidomide, or maternal rubella. In cases of the atretic ear canal, occasionally, thick soft tissue is found at surgery where the tympanic membrane should be, or more often a bony atresia plate of varying degrees of thickness is present.

Microtic Ear. The microtic ear has always been a problem to professionals as well as to the unfortunate possessor. Fortunately, it occurs only once in 20,000 births (Holmes, 1949), but this is often enough that we see a number of such cases each year in our clinic. The congenitally microtic ear varies from the mildly deformed ear to total absence of pinna with no external auditory meatus or to complete atresia of the canal. Unilateral microtia is about 6 times more frequent than bilateral occurrence (Dupertius and Musgrave, 1959), is more common in males than females, and is found predominantly on the right side (Brown et al., 1969).

When a patient has one normal-hearing ear, obviously the problem of unilateral microtia is not so bad. When hair styles are long, the deformity of the auricle is easily covered. Patients, however, who wish to do something about the microtia have a choice between attempted surgical improvement or the use of a prosthetic-type pinna that is attached to the side of the head by special adhesive material. According to Holmes (1949) and supported by our observations, regardless of what surgical techniques are employed, the reconstructed ear can never take the place of a normally developed pinna, and the result will never be inconspicuous. For improved hearing benefit, however, as in the patient who has bilaterally stenosed ear canals, surgical intervention may be successful. Schuchman (1971) reported the fitting of a special ear level, bone conduction hearing aid for a patient with bilateral atresia.

TEAM MANAGEMENT OF CHILDREN WITH HEARING IMPAIRMENT

The nature of modern-day hearing losses makes it increasingly imperative that a team of professional people work together to diagnose a hearing loss and chart the management of the child with a loss (Fig. 3.14). The hearing function is not an isolated phenomenon.

We have called such a group of experts the children's hearing team. Our emphasis on the team approach to diagnosis in no way minimizes the audiologist's art. The role of the audiologist in decisions concerning diagnosis and management is a vital one, to not only contribute essential information on the degree of loss, the auditory behavior and development, and the auditory functioning of the child but also to provide familiarity with training methods largely in decisions on the placement of the hearing-impaired child. Precise audiologic measurements provide the necessary objective data, but the art of audiology weighs strongly in the evaluation. The clinical insight and intuition of the experienced audiologist contribute a much needed element to the decisions that will be made. How does the child relate to the clinician? Is eye contact good? Is the behavior even minimally distractible? Does there seem to be perseveration of auditory behavior? What is the vocal quality and how does the child use his or her voice? How do parent and child relate to each other? These are the questions that can be answered more through intuition than through measurements. They are an integral part of the audiologist's art.

A summary of recommended medical workup for the child with hereditary deafness is shown in Table 3.4. Pappas and Schaibly (1984) evaluated 143 children with sensorineural hearing loss in their otolaryngology practice. They described a systematic approach to determine the specific etiology of the hearing loss and were able to confirm diagnosis in nearly 65% of this population. They concluded that a complete family and medical history and a thorough physical examination consisting of tests appropriate to the child's age level are the most important means available to the physician. Polytomography was also deemed important, as well as neonatal studies for CMV (urine viral culture) and rubella (throat viral culture).

Once the audiologist has specified that a certain degree of hearing loss exists and has delineated the status of the auditory development of the child, a standard protocol of examinations is indicated. Any of these studies, if made in isolation, will furnish only a fragment of the total picture of the child and his or her needs, but when these fragments are brought together in a team conference, the picture becomes a whole. The team together makes a diagnosis of the etiology, extent, and degree of the problem and decides on the proper management for the child.

After the initial thorough evaluation, it is customary to follow the young child every 6 months to observe his or her progress and to pick up any loose ends of diagnosis. Not until all facets are put together and the child has stabilized satisfactorily in his or her program will the child be seen only once a year. Such stabilization does not occur until the child is 5 or 6, even if he or she has been identified in infancy. From then on until adolescence the child will be seen once a year and, after that, whenever indicated.

Management of the Child. *Diagnosis.* Diagnosis is a cooperative effort of

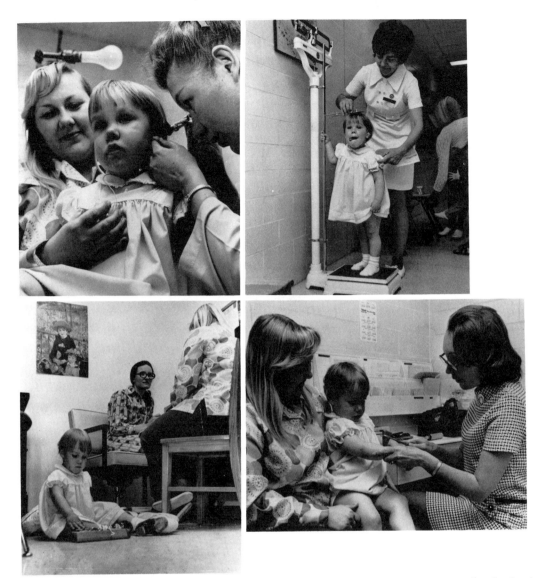

Figure 3.14. The nature of modern-day hearing losses makes it increasingly imperative that a team of professional people work together for the management of the child with hearing loss. In addition to the audiologist's services, the regularly scheduled checkup should include otologic examination (*top left*), physical examination (*top right*), social work interview (*bottom left*), and pediatric evaluation (*bottom right*). (Courtesy of The National Foundation-March of Dimes.)

all the specialists involved, but the pediatrician is the primary manager of the child. The pediatrician can determine the etiology, identify other associated anomalies, and suggest a myriad of laboratory tests that will contribute to the diagnosis. The pediatrician also assesses the overall development of the child and provide for genetic counseling once the etiology is determined. The pediatrician may seek the otologic expertise of the otolaryngologist who may request other information, such as polytomography, computed axial tomography scan or brainstem evoked potential testing.

The audiologist not only contributes baseline audiometry, as well as possible vestibular involvement, but evaluates the

Table 3.4.
Diagnostic Medical Workup of the Child with Hereditary Deafness[a]

History
Detailed family pedigree
Maternal prenatal history

Perinatal and neonatal history
Subsequent medical history

General Physical Examination
Generalized congenital bone disorders
Congenital absence or sparseness of hair and/or nails
Congenital neurologic deficits
Ataxia of gait

Pigmentary disorders
Congenital heart disease

Hand anomalies

Concomitant Head and Neck Physical Findings
Atresia of the external auditory canals
Malformed external ears
Facial anomalies, especially of mandible
Congenital facial nerve paralysis
Branchial anomalies
Heterochromia of the irises
Increased intercanthal distance
White forelock in scalp hair

Retinitis pigmentosa
Rubella retinopathy
Congenital cataracts
Dental anomalies
Short neck; neck anomalies
Goiter
Quality of voice and speech

Routine Laboratory Tests
Family audiometry
Complete blood count

Urinalysis

Special Laboratory Tests where Appropriate
(Age 1 year and under)
Rubella titer
CMV

Other viral titers

Immunoglobulin M
Viral cultures of urine, throat, and nasopharynx for rubella and CMV

(Any age)
Electrocardiogram
Protein-bound iodine
Syphilis serology
Serum pyrophosphate and uric acid
Urine mucopolysaccharide screening

Dermatoglyphics
Karyotype, buccal smear
X-rays as necessary
Petrous pyramid polytomography
Electroretinography
Vestibular testing

[a]Courtesy of LaVonne Bergstrom, M.D.

relationship of the child's functioning to the degree of hearing loss, thus giving information relevant to the diagnosis (Table 3.5). The speech-language pathologist provides a baseline speech and language evaluation that will be used to compare later functioning. During the diagnostic workup, the social worker becomes involved in helping determine where parents are in their process of accepting the problem of the deaf child. Are they in the denial stage, the anger stage, the mourning stage—and how can they be helped to an acceptance of the problem, which will allow them to best nurture the child? It may be necessary, at any given point, to bring in a psychologist for detailed psychologic counseling.

The ophthalmologist is called in for any of the associated eye abnormalities. All hearing-impaired children should have routine vision testing, and those children without a clear syndrome should be checked for retinitis pigmentosa with electroretinography to rule out Usher's syndrome. A renal consultant is obtained in such cases as hereditary chronic nephritis or Alport's syndrome. Cardiologists and neurologists are called in as indicated, and it is found that in such complex cases as Hunter-Hurler syndrome the entire roster of specialists at the hospital may be involved.

Table 3.5.
Hearing Handicap as a Function of Average Hearing Threshold Level of the Better Ear

Average Threshold Level at 500–2000 Hz (ANSI)[a]	Description	Common Causes	What Can Be Heard without Amplification	Degree of Handicap (If Not Treated in First Year of Life)	Probable Needs
0–15 dB	Normal range		All speech sounds	None	None
16–25 dB	Slight hearing loss	Serous otitis, perforation, monomeric membrane, sensorineural loss, tympanosclerosis	Vowel sounds heard clearly, may miss unvoiced consonant sounds	Possible mild or transitory auditory dysfunction Difficulty in perceiving some speech sounds	Consideration of need for hearing aid Lip reading Auditory training Speech therapy Preferential seating Appropriate surgery
26–40 dB	Mild hearing loss	Serous otitis, perforation, tympanosclerosis, monomeric membrane, sensorineural loss	Hears only some of speech sounds—the louder voiced sounds	Auditory learning dysfunction Mild language retardation Mild speech problems Inattention	Hearing aid Lip reading Auditory training Speech therapy Appropriate surgery
41–65 dB	Moderate hearing loss	Chronic otitis, middle ear anomaly, sensorineural loss	Misses most speech sounds at normal conversational level	Speech problems Language retardation Learning dysfunction Inattention	All of the above plus consideration of special classroom situation
66–95 dB	Severe hearing loss	Sensorineural loss or mixed loss due to sensorineural loss plus middle ear disease	Hears no speech sound of normal conversations	Severe speech problems Language retardation Learning dysfunction Inattention	All of the above; probable assignment to special classes
96+ dB	Profound hearing loss	Sensorineural loss or mixed	Hears no speech or other sounds	Severe speech problems Language retardation Learning dysfunction Inattention	All of the above; probable assignment to special classes

[a]ANSI, American National Standards Institute.

Placement Counseling. The decision regarding placement of the child in an educational program must be the parents' prerogative. Unless the parents have made the decision, there will be second thoughts and possibly recriminations at a later date. The parents' decision is based on the following contributions from the congenital deafness team: (*1*) information as to the degree of loss; (*2*) the results of the speech and language evaluations, if relevant; (*3*) an introduction to the types of education available in the community (this would include visits to each of the facilities that are offering programs for hearing-impaired children); and (*4*) encouragement to choose freely and to feel comfortable with making a change at a later date if at any time it appears that another program will better benefit the child.

Monitoring. During the first year or two, the hearing-impaired child should be seen at least every 6 months for periodic reassessment of the etiology of the hearing impairment for the various reasons listed below:

- Repeat audiometry may reveal progression of loss or unsuspected opposite ear involvement.

- Case history review may reveal overlooked historical items such as early history of disease.

- Physical examination may reveal overlooked physical findings or newly developed symptoms, such as thyroid problems, renal problems, and night blindness.

- Repeat family history may show suppressed information or false-positive items.

- An incorrect initial diagnosis may be corrected by reevaluation.

- Progressive concommitant disease may be identified by follow-up evaluations.

- New information, new scientific knowledge, and new technology.

Speech and language evaluations are given to monitor the performance of the child in the particular program in which he or she has been entered. If at any point it is obvious that the child is not making reasonable progress in the system, consideration can be given to looking at a change of program.

Psychosocial reevaluation and monitoring is extremely useful to determine whether or not any help should be given the family in psychologic or social matters. It may be necessary to solicit public funds to help the family's finances in supporting the child in the particular program in which he or she is functioning.

Advocacy. In the children's hearing team's function as an objective advocate of the child, apart from the methodology of the program the child is in, it may be necessary to arbitrate between the family and the system in the following ways:

- If parents believe that the school system has mismanaged the child's placement, it may be necessary for the team to represent the family at hearings called to evaluate the disagreement. Federal law now mandates hearings that the parents can request whenever they believe a change is indicated.

- When college age is reached, the team may be called upon to support the special interests of the student in obtaining a specific type of education.

- The interpretation of new advances, new technologies, or new surgeries can better be done by an objective team in which the parent has confidence.

It is evident that the work of a children's hearing team may be never-ending. It will continue until the client is fully achieving and completely comfortable in the environment that has been chosen.

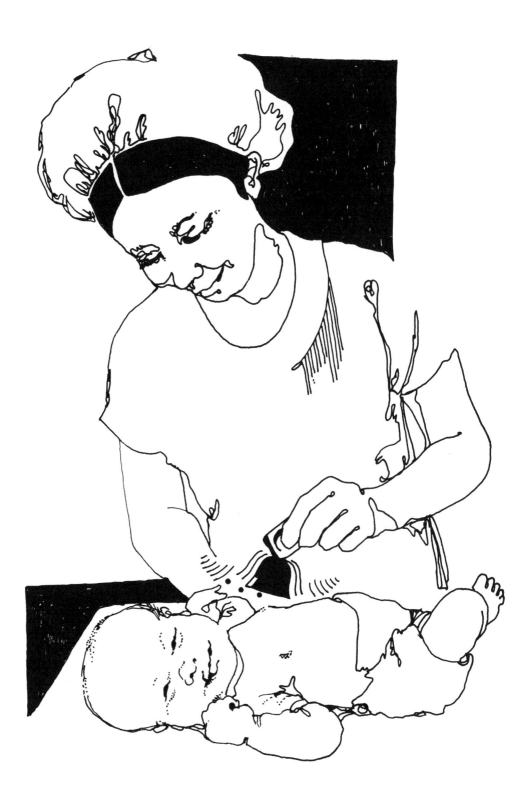

CHAPTER 4

Development of Auditory Behavior

The audiologist has a unique contribution to make to the understanding of how language develops in infants—one that linguists and psychologists cannot offer—and that is the study of the degree to which the acoustic parameters of language learning in the infant are innate, preprogrammed processes and how they influence language learning. There is research evidence demonstrating that there may be special biologic predetermined processes of perception for the various acoustic dimensions of speech. These ideas are reviewed from a number of discipline-specific journals that have made contributions to this field. Once the course of maturation of the auditory response is understood, the hearing testing techniques follow naturally.

PRENATAL AND NEONATAL HEARING

Elliot and Elliot (1964) confirmed physiologically that the human cochlea has normal adult function after the 20th week of gestation. Johansson et al. (1964) were among the first to report testing fetal hearing. Using high-frequency pure tones presented by means of a microphone placed on the mother's abdomen, fetal heart rate increase response to the tones was recorded after the 20th week of gestation. The demonstration of fetal hearing has value in contradicting the theory that the child is born a *tabula rasa* insofar as hearing is concerned. The newborn infant has actually been hearing sounds for at least 4 months—fluid-borne sounds, to be sure—but nonetheless, true auditory signals.

Knowing that the fetus is physiologically prepared to respond to sound is important, but the difficult task is determining how to elicit a response and measure it. Birnholz and Benacerraf (1983) observed the auropalpebral reflex in 236 human fetuses in a study of screening for gross deafness. Stimuli were presented via vibroacoustic stimuli applied to the maternal abdominal wall directly over the fetal ear, and eye clenching was observed with ultrasonic imaging. Their results, confirmed by Kuczwara et al. (1984), indicated that auropalpebral reflexes consistently occur at approximately 24–25 weeks gestational age in normal fetuses

How early does the infant perceive speech and act upon his or her acoustic environment? There is research evidence for the existence of preadaptive processes of perception of the acoustic dimensions of speech. To be sure, the developmental response to sound in the fetus is primarily reflexive in nature, including startle, generalized body movement, possible cessation of activity, and the auropalpebral reflex (involuntary eyeblink).

At birth the infant is able to discriminate his or her mother's voice and to work to produce the mother's voice in preference to the voice of another female. These capacities were demonstrated by DeCasper and Fifer (1980) utilizing the classic sucking paradigm with infants shortly after delivery. Earphones were placed over the ears of the supine infant, and a nonnutritive nipple was placed in his or her mouth. The nipple was connected by way of a pressure transducer to recording equipment that produced only the infant's or the mother's voice. For five randomly selected infants, sucking bursts produced first only the mother's voice on the tape for a predetermined interval and then the voice of another infant's mother.

For another five infants the conditions were reversed. A preference for the maternal voice was indicated if the infant produced it more often than the nonmaternal voice. It was apparent that the infant soon learned to gain access to the mother's voice, since specific temporal properties of sucking were required to produce the maternal voice.

These data of DeCasper and Fifer show that newborns reared in group nurseries that allow minimal maternal contact can discriminate between their own mother's and another mother's speech and, moreover, will work to produce their own mother's voice in preference to that of another.

Is there sufficient acoustic exposure in the uterus to permit such a precocious development? It may be. Bench (1968) has shown that for a 72 dB signal there is the least attenuation of sound going into the uterus at 200 Hz (19 dB); slightly more at 500 Hz (24 dB); more at 1000 Hz (38 dB); and the most at 2000 and 4000 Hz (48 dB). Thus the frequencies of 1000 Hz and below contained the maternal voice that may be heard, if faintly, from the fifth month of gestation when, it has been shown, the fetal ear is capable of analyzing sound.

But a study by Armitage et al. (1980) measured the actual sound level inside the amniotic sac of pregnant ewes by means of hydrophones inside the sac, in the normal fluid environment of the fetus. These investigators found that although sounds from the maternal cardiovascular system were not perceived, the sounds of the mother's eating, drinking, ruminating, breathing, and muscular movements were discernable, as were sounds from outside the mother. They found that the attenuation of sounds measured on a C-weighted scale reached a maximum of 37 dB just below 1000 Hz, but it was reduced below and above this frequency, with its higher frequencies attenuated at about 20 dB up to the highest recorded, 5000 Hz. The amount of attenuation fluctuated, however; conversation at normal levels outside the animal could often,

but not always, be understood when transmitted from inside. Raised voices were almost always distinct. If we make the leap from this animal model to the case of the human fetus, then the mother's and even the father's voices would be heard by the fetus.

Querleu et al. (1981) performed actual intrauterine measures on humans and demonstrated that the fetus could hear the mother's voice and other voices, which were perfectly audible but lacking in tone because the high frequencies were absorbed. When there is no fetal distress the fetus reacts to the sound stimulus by a change in heart rate, often associated with movement. In 1982 Querleu et al. made more careful observations of seven patients during term labor after amniotomy, implanting hydrophones and microphones in the uterine cavity. When external speech was recorded through the uterus, two observers could recognize 64% of the mother's phonemes and 57% of a male's speech.

Apparently a great deal of auditory experience precedes the abilities of the newborn to prefer the mother's voice to other voices. But before such early discriminations can be made, the infant auditory system would have to be preadapted to various acoustic discriminations. Such discriminations have been shown to be present in the newborn, and, assuming a functional ear and central nervous system (CNS), the same capabilities would be present in the 5 month fetus. The innate discriminations that subserve the preference for the mother's voice require the auditory competencies of discriminating rhythm, intonation, frequency variation, stress (suprasegmental aspects of speech), and phonetic components of speech (linguistic aspects).

Neonatal Hearing. *Suprasegmental Speech Activity.* Condon and Sander (1974) reported that neonates move in precise and sustained segments of movements that are synchronous with the articulated structure of speech. Further perception of rhythm in 2 month old infants was demonstrated by Demany et al. (1977) who utilized varied sequences of time bursts in a habituation paradigm relating duration of fixation on a visual figure. Infants were able to perceive intervals of time as subjective links between sounds. Spring and Dale (1977) showed that 1–4 month old babies could discriminate linguistic stress as well as location, fundamental frequency, intensity, and duration. Thus the entire gamut of suprasegmental aspects of speech seem to be available to the infant at birth.

Kimura (1964) has shown that the suprasegmental aspects of speech are handled by the right brain. The segmental, linguistic aspects are located in the left brain, according to Studdert-Kennedy and Shankweiler (1970). But this is not to decry the importance of the suprasegmental aspects of speech in learning its intelligibility. Language learning is not confined to the segmental aspects of speech. Rhythm, intonation, duration, and stress are extremely important to understanding multiple meanings of words, as well as to the meanings of homophones. Many words and phrases contain multiple meanings that are made clear only by intonation, rhythm, duration, and stress. This fact explains a part of the problem of a deaf child in understanding some of the subtle parameters of irony, satire, scorn, implied anger, or humor that convey the sense of multimeaning words or phrases. "You're tired." "You're tired?" are two different sentences depending on the intonation of the rising or falling fundamental frequency. "You drive me up the wall;" "I can't bear it"—make for humorous misconceptions, but it is the kind of thing that is difficult for the concrete-minded deaf child who has not heard the stress and intonations that made the phrases meaningful.

It has been hypothesized that because the fetus is accustomed to listening to the heartbeat of the mother, the fetus wil be quieted effectively by the same sound in the early days in the outer world. Brackbill et al. (1966) found that a tape-recorded heartbeat is no more effective than any other continuous, low-frequency stimulus in lowering the arousal level of the infant. Lowered arousal level means a specific reduction of overt behavior and physiologic patterns: The infant's heart and respiration rates become lower, and the infant cries less and moves about less.

Segmental Aspect. Eimas (1975, 1979) and others have given us evidence that the child is also able to discriminate segmental aspects of speech in a categorical and presumably linguistic manner. He chose to utilize differences in voice onset time (VOT). The categorical perception of VOT has been assumed to be a function of the special processing that the sounds of speech undergo and tends to be a special characteristic of perception in a speech or linguistic mode. Eimas believed that there were special biologically determined processes of perception for this acoustic dimension. In one experiment with 26 infants 1 month old, he employed the classic sucking paradigm in discriminating the differences between the voiced stop /b/ and the voiceless stop /p/ combined with the vowel /a/. His results indicated that infants as young as 1 month of age are not only responsive to speech but are able to make rather fine distinctions in a manner approximating categorical perceptions.

Eisenberg (1970) has demonstrated that most newborns, including those with known CNS abnormalities, can discriminate sound on the basis of frequency, intensity, and stimulus-dimensionality. Thus it is possible that neuronal mechanisms for processing sound pressure levels (SPL) are fully mature at birth.

The processing of frequency differences is described by Eisenberg (1976) as range-dependent. The low frequencies tend to have a soothing or inhibiting effect on the infant. High frequencies have the property of occasioning distress rather than inhibiting it. However, signals in the range below 4000 Hz are 2 or 3 times more response-provoking than those in the very high ranges.

What is particularly significant to the clinician is Eisenberg's finding that speechlike signals seem remarkably effective in producing responses in newborns. This fact is certainly true of the older infant, as will be described later, but to find that the newborn already responds selectively to the dimensionality of human speech gives us directions for clinical testing.

It is intriguing to speculate whether speech dimensional signals are more attention-getting because of some preadaptive auditory reactivity or whether the known frequency-dependent sensitivity of the human ear is operating here. That dependency in itself is intriguing; one wonders which came first, the human ear's greater sensitivity to frequencies in the speech range or the peculiar properties of the human larynx and resonators to produce speech in that particular range of frequencies.

Kagan (1972) suggests that stimulus change is another parameter that should be explored. A 2 day old infant is more attentive to a moving light than to a steady light. The rate of the light change is also important. In the auditory sphere, Kearsley et al. (1962) found that if an unexpected noise of 70 dB reaches maximum intensity within a few milliseconds, a newborn infant closes his or her eyes, starts, and shows an increase in heart rate. If the same sound reaches its maximal intensity in 2 seconds, the infant opens his or her eyes, looks around, and is likely to show a decrease in heart rate. The first reaction is a defensive one; the latter displays interest. Kagan suggests that the attention-getting power of contrast, so evident in the newborn period, diminishes as early as the second month and is succeeded by a different parameter of the stimulus.

Later studies by Morse (1972) confirmed that infants respond in a linguistically relevant manner, showing that categorical perception is present in infants before the onset of speech production. Morse investigated 2 month old infants' abilities to differentiate the voiced stops /b/ and /g/ in a speech context from the same second- and third-formant transitions in a nonspeech context. (The nonspeech context was achieved by eliminating the entire first formant and the steady-state portions of the second and third formants.) With use of the sucking paradigm, he demonstrated that the experimental infants also recovered differentially from the control group who had heard the synthetic patterns. This, he believed, confirmed the linguistic relevance of their distinctions.

The theoretical considerations of the infant's ability to process a segmental unit of speech have occasioned a great deal of speculation. The arguments revolve around the fact that speech is a very complex code; transformation of the acoustic energy signaling speech to the perceptual event may not be a simple conversion mediated by an auditory decoder. Lieberman (1975) states: "The acoustic cues for successive phonemes are intermixed in the sound stream to such an extent that definable segments of sound do not correspond to segments at the phoneme level."

Lieberman believes that the perception of speech signals is mediated in some manner by central neural events, because infants have had no experience in the consistent articulation of phonetic distinctions. Therefore, the ability must be a part of the native endowment of the human organism.

Another theory has been advanced by Stevens and House, who presented an analysis-by-synthesis model presupposing that an internalized or computed auditory pattern is generated and compared with the stored pattern. But for this theory also there is the premise that "perception requires knowledge of phonological rules that can map abstract features into articulatory events" (Eimas, 1975). So all theories lead to the inescapable conclusion that the infant enters this world with considerable knowledge of the phonologic component of language.

Whether the infant's detectors are activated shortly after birth as Eimas has suggested or whether they have become functional during intrauterine life may be a relevant question to his theory. Four months of listening practice might facilitate in a way the categorical perceptions that are evident at birth. We suspect, however, that if the same kinds of experiments could be made on the unborn fetus at 5 or 6 months of gestational age, categorical perception would be present and would demonstrate that detectors need only be activated by hearing speech in order to be fully functional. It remains for some zealous researcher to attempt to replicate these studies during intrauterine life.

That the infant is able to discriminate the acoustic features of speech means that the infant can segment an almost continuous acoustic input into discrete elements. This ability to process language into discrete elements is a basis for full language competence. The infant's ability to do this at the very beginning of language acquisition means that he or she does not have to learn that language is formed by discrete elements. The result is a facilitation of the language acquisition process, and indeed, the ability to break down discrete elementary language may even be requisite to its formation. The audiologist should note that the capacity to process language in discrete units would not be possible were it not for the damping effect of the structures of the cochlea. Were speech sounds—and indeed, any sounds—allowed to reverberate without hindrance in the ear, the hair cells would not be able to discriminate the frequency components of the speech sounds in a manner necessary to language perception.

State. Bench (1971) describes the relationship between the infant's state and response in terms of the law of initial value:

The magnitude of response change is influenced by the state of the individual before stimulation in such a way that the lower the initial or prestimulus state, the greater is the increase in level of activity on stimulation; the higher the initial state, the greater is the decrease in level of activity.

Bench measured the heart rate of 10 normal newborn babies for 10 seconds before and after stimulation by a 95 dB broadband noise. The results indicated that the heart rate change to auditory stimulation was dependent on the prestimulus heart rate. The implication of this work for infant audiometry is that any given baby may show an increase or decrease in activity, or no change at all, depending entirely on his prestimulus state. Bench recommends that babies be tested at low levels of activities, in order to obtain a positive response change.

In another study, Bench and Boscak (1970) applied signal detection theory to infants' responses to three different stimulus levels of 300 Hz (55, 75, and 95 dB). The infants' prestimulus states were rated as 1 (deep sleep), 2 (light sleep), and 3 (limb activity). They found that the signal detection is affected by both the SPL of the stimulus and the state of the baby before stimulation. There was a significant trend for the effect of state in the decreasing order of state 2, state 1, and state 3. A light sleep, then, predisposes to the best response to sound.

Taylor and Mencher (1972) also identified infant state as a significant variable in neonatal testing, reporting that light sleep is the optimal state for evaluating a response to auditory stimuli. They applied single and double presentations of different stimuli at 90 and 100 dB to 225 normal newborn infants. The most common response types observed were eye movement and arousal responses. Stronger responses occurred more often in the light sleep than in the awake and quiet state. The sleep state was defined by touching the examiner's finger to the closed eyelid of the infant. If eye or body movement resulted, a light state was judged to be present; if there was no movement, the deep sleep state was judged.

Active Response. In addition to responding differently in a passive way to stimulus patterns and intensity, newborns can be active in regulating auditory events in their environment. Butterfield (1968) reported that babies made bursts of contingent sucking responses that controlled the onset and offset of tape-recorded music: classical, and popular, and vocal. An instrumental pacifier nipple operated the musical selections. Four 1 day old infants were used in his study, and all responded consistently over several tests. This study leaves no doubt but that newborn infants are not passive in their hearing function. Their feedback loop operates actively at as early an age as study is possible. The availability of such an auditory function strengthens the idea of early application of hearing aids to hearing-impaired infants who have sufficient residual hearing to benefit from them. Eimas et al. (1972) used changes in conditioned sucking rates to measure sound differentiation. By 1 month, infants showed, by changes in sucking rates, that they differentiated the onset time distinction between the phonemes "Pah" and "Bah." By 4 months of age the changes were more marked. Differential perception seems to be well-established in the first few months of life.

Even suprasegmental aspects of speech such as intonational contour can be distinguished by infants as young as 2 months. Morse (1972) showed that some 25 infants 40–54 days old could differentiate changes between phonemes with a falling and those with a rising fundamental contour. This parameter of speech may play an important role in language acquisition.

For the investigator, Eisenberg's (1976) more sophisticated observations on the responses of newborns to sound give substance to the description of responses:

Overt reactions:
  Arousal
  Gross body movements
  Orienting behavior
    Turning of head
    Wide-eyed "what-is-it?" look
    Pupillary dilation
  Motor reflexes
    Facial grimaces
    Displacement of a single digit
  Crying or cessation of crying

To the student of auditory behavior, all of Eisenberg's studies have tremendous significance. It was she who first described differences in habituation to sound as an index of CNS integrity. Newborn infants with known CNS involvement failed to extinguish their responses to repeated acoustic signals. Normal infants habituated to the repeated stimuli in a short time. Sometimes called response decrement, this phenomenon is logical for possible use as a screening tool in identifying CNS problems.

Neonates' sensory habituation to a pure tone was shown by Bridger (1961) using heart rate measures to indicate a startle response to pure tones. All the babies who were tested showed a cessation of marked startle to successive stimuli presentations, provided the interval between the stimuli was less than 5 seconds. Bridger also showed that changing the frequency of the pure tone would renew the startle response after habituation to one tone, showing that babies do discriminate between frequencies.

The hypothesis that CNS-damaged infants will fail to habituate was tested by Schulman (1970) using heart rate changes as the measure of response. An 80 dB buzzer for 3 seconds was used at 20 second intervals. Heart rate was recorded from a cardiotachometer. Five high-risk premature, five low-risk premature, and five normal full-term infants were compared. All risk children were matched for gestational age. Significant habituation occurred in all three groups, although latency of response was significantly longer in the high-risk children. Thus Schulman was not able to confirm the lack of response decrement in the AT RISK child that Eisenberg (1970) and Brackbill and Downs (1969) had reported.

Older Infant. The maturation of auditory processing proceeds after birth in ways that have been demonstrated in research designs. Already at 4 weeks the infant can distinguish phonemic contrasts in sound signals, as measured by heart rate changes. McCaffrey (1970) presented 4–28 week old infants with standard vowel and consonant stimuli, which were then changed to contrasting vowels or consonants. At the point of transition from the standard to the contrasting phoneme, significant heart rate changes were found to occur. Other studies by Jusczyk and Thompson (1978) showed 2 month old infants perceiving phonetic contrast in multisyllabic utterances.

Friedlander (1970) terms these reactions "active critical evaluative processes characterized by creative model-building and formation of hypotheses as to what is likely to happen next." One can conclude that however simple the paradigm, the responses represent some aspect of learning and cognitive processing. This viewpoint is supported by Neisser (1967) who maintains that choices are made of which parts of the incoming information should be attended to. Attending, even in the infant, becomes a constructive, active process rather than an analytic and passive response.

Perception of rhythm in the 2 month old infant was demonstrated by Demany et al. (1977) utilizing varied sequences of time bursts in a habituation paradigm relating duration of fixation on a visual figure. The infants were able to perceive intervals of time as subjective links between sounds, showing that they apprehend a succession of several sounds as a psychologic unit. This ability represents a necessary prelinguistic skill, since language comprehension requires the same kind of process in grasping a semantic unit as a whole despite its sequential character.

Linguistic stress is also discriminated by infants 1–4 months old. Spring and Dale (1977) demonstrated with a high-amplitude sucking paradigm that young infants could discriminate the acoustic correlates of stress, location, fundamental frequency, intensity, and duration. This study completes the number of suprasegmental aspects of speech that have been shown to produce discriminatory responses: intonation, rhythm, and now stress.

Further evidence of the selective listening abilities of infants is given by Friedlander (1970). He devised an ingenious playtest whereby a large pair of response switches are attached to the baby's crib or playpen. The switches regulate a loudspeaker, an electrical control-and-response recording unit, and a stereo tape player with a preprogrammed selection of two-channel audiotapes. Whenever the baby operates either switch, a record is made of the frequency and duration of his or her choice, and the baby turns on one channel or the other of the audiotape. Thus, a record is made of listening preferences. Babies 9–18 months old were studied over long periods. The findings are summarized as follows:

- When sounds and voices are placed under the babies' own control, they display phenomenal productivity in listening responses productivity, ranging from one 9 month old girl's 65,000 seconds of responding in 20 days (3000 seconds per day) to the average response record of 1200–1500 seconds per day of other children. These data indicate that listening to sounds and voices have a hitherto unsuspected potency as a desirable form of activity to babies whose own speech is still very immature.

- Babies show a great range of discriminative listening to a wide variety of natural, disguised, and synthetic language as well as to other auditory stimuli, as the following examples indicate: (*a*) A 12 month old infant preferred to listen to a stranger's voice with bright intonation than to his or her mother's voice speaking in a flat monotone. (*b*) A 14 month old baby could not decide for several days whether to select the stranger's voice or the mother's distorted voice. After several days he made an enormous burst of listening to the mother's voice, and after that he ignored completely the switch that turned on the stranger's voice. This choice is regarded as an "aha" effect with the child ultimately recognizing the mother's voice despite its distortion. (*c*)

Another baby was offered a choice between two tape recordings of animated family conversations: one edited to run for 250 seconds before it was repeated, the other repeated after 20 seconds. The long cycle was considered to have low redundancy and high information; the short cycle had high redundancy and low information. For the first several days, the baby preferred the short tape with high redundancy and low information. After a week he crossed over into a preference for the low-redundancy, high-information selection. This redundancy study was replicated on 11 babies, 9–18 months of age, 7 of whom ultimately chose the low-redundancy, high-information selection.

Exploring the responsiveness of the 0–6 month old infants to various stimuli, Bench et al. (1977) found that both younger infants and 6 month old infants were notably unresponsive to tonal stimuli and even to band widths of 300 Hz. But broad-spectrum noise elicited better responses in the younger infants (1 week and 6 weeks). Six month olds responded most to voice stimuli. Moderate-intensity signals were not effective for awake 6 month olds. The younger infants were mostly in sleep states when studied, so stimuli of 90 dB SPL were necessary for response.

What do these studies mean in terms of differential development in children? A study by Irwin (1952) described the early effects of different kinds of auditory input given to infants. He applied both quantitative and qualitative measures to two groups of infants from the time of birth to the age of 1 year. One group comprised the infants of highly verbal, "white-collar" and professional people; the other group comprised infants of low-verbal, "blue-collar" workers and laborers. The variable was that the first talked a great deal directly to the infant and in its presence; the second group of parents were less communicative both to each other and to the child. The quantity and quality of their vocalizations showed that at about 3 months, something changed the vocalizations of the two groups. The infants of the highly verbal parents began to increase the number of their vocalizations, as well as the quality of the phonemes used, more rapidly than the infants of the low-verbal group. It can be inferred that, by 3 months, the amount and the quality of the auditory input to these infants was already being transformed into commensurate output. The more highly stimulated infants had greater opportunity to select acoustic information and to apply it to their own auditory feedback loop. Active participation and expression resulted, but differentially in the two groups. What more pragmatic proof can there be that infants are active, not passive, in their utilization of incoming acoustic stimuli?

AUDITORY BEHAVIOR AS PRELINGUISTIC ACTIVITY

Concurrent with the maturation of the auditory function are the developing speech and language skills.

It is difficult to determine the absolute age of onset and cessation of various stages of speech development during the first year of life. Although there is agreement about the general order of succession of speech development, the onset of cooing, laughter, and reduplicated babbling is usually more apparent than the onset of vocal play and single-word production. Behaviors typical of one speech development stage may have precursors in a previous stage and may continue into the following stage (Stark, 1980).

The beginnings of language learning occur at birth and—who knows?—possibly before birth. Condon and Sander's (1974) studies showing that the human neonate moves in segments of movements synchronous with the articulated structure of adult speech demonstrate that the infant is a participant in the rhythm of many repetitive speech structures long before use in communication. These rhythms comprise a prelinguistic activity of the human infant even at birth.

The infant's first use of sounds in a repetitive manner indicates the time at which the auditory feedback loop has become effective. By 2 months the baby is beginning to put out certain sounds more than others. The selection of which sounds to repeat seems to depend on the nature of the sound. From 2 to 4 months these sounds are vowel-like. The sequence of use of vowels is presumably from middle (the "schwa" sound /ə/) to front and back vowels (Menyuk, 1972). By 5 months the consonant-vowel (CV) sequences begin. Irwin (1947) states that back consonants (velars and glottals) predominant at 5–6 months of age, with some of the labial (front) consonants entering in. At 9–10 months, the glottal sounds decrease and the alveolar sounds (middle) are frequently used. Menyuk (1972) partially explains this sequence of selection as due to ease of production. It is also possible that the selection is made for them by some differences in the changing vocal mechanism.

Studdert-Kennedy (1976) develops an interesting hypothesis that each infant is born with both an auditory and an articulatory template. For effective function in language acquisition, the auditory template must be "tuned" to specific acoustic properties of speech. The articulatory template is more abstract and includes a range of gestural control, potentially isomorphic with the segmented feature matrix of language. Since persons differ in the precise dimensions of their vocal tract, it would be surprising if they accomplished a particular gesture and a particular acoustic pattern by precisely the same pattern of muscular action. Thus, it seems likely that the articulatory template functions for equivalent vocal tract shapes rather than for specific patterns of muscular action. It is precisely to exploration of his or her own vocal tract and to discovery of his or her own patterns of muscular action that the infant's motor learning must be directed.

Studdert-Kennedy continues his proposal with the statement that neither template can fulfill its communication function in the absence of the other. In short, babble without auditory feedback has no meaning. The infant discovers phonetic meaning by discovering the commands required by his or her own vocal tract to match the output of his or her auditory template, thereby establishing the fact that perceptual skill precedes motor skill.

Although the infant is able to differentiate various speech sounds in the first few months of life, production of the sounds does not develop at the same rate. Berko and Brown (1960) describe the lag between the perception of differences in speech signals and the production of those speech sounds. In the newborn period the infant does not produce phonated sounds, only cries and physiologic sounds. Lieberman et al. (1971) postulated that the reason for this early lack of phonation is that the larynx is positioned relatively high, almost in line with the roof of the palate, limiting the pharyngeal movement that is necessary to speech. In addition, the infant's large tongue fills the oral cavity and prevents the infant from changing the shape of his or her supralaryngeal vocal tract by moving the tongue during phonation.

Lieberman (1975) identifies the range of format frequencies that are necessary to human speech. The well-developed pharynx, with the posterior one third or so of the tongue forming its anterior wall, is the structural arrangement required for a wide range of formant frequencies. In the newborn and in the nonhuman primate, the hyoid bone is high in the throat, so that the tongue lies completely within the oral cavity. There is little or no pharynx. As the larynx and tongue descend, a pharynx is formed and speech sound production becomes possible.

Menyuk (1972) suggests that experimental results comparing primate vocalizations with those of human infants and adults "indicate that speaking is not simply a learned overlaid function on the muscles and structures of breathing and eating, but that man is preprogrammed to develop a vocal mechanism that is specifically adapted to produce speech."

Studies of the development of infant vocalization show a logical, orderly sequence of utterances between the initial sounds made by the baby until the first words are achieved. Regardless of the linguistic community in which they are raised, babies begin by cooing, then produce reduplicated CV syllables and, finally, "variegated" babbling with sentence-like intonational patterns (Oller, 1978, 1980). As the infant's one-word vocabulary grows beginning at about 12 months, the frequency of babbling declines until it is entirely omitted between 18 and 20 months of age.

By 1 month, typical cooing and gurgling sounds are made in addition to the crying; by 3 months, true babbling begins. True babbling consists of the pleasurable repetition of sounds.

Babbling is not easily defined in terms of phonetic or acoustic characteristics. Babbling is defined by Kent et al. (1987) as "an infant's vocal behavior excepting the so-called vegetative sounds associated with respiratory and gastric events and sounds of obvious distress or discomfort (such as cry or fuss sounds)." Stoel-Gammon and Otomo (1986) define babbling as "relative speech-like utterances." The sounds produced by infants include reduplicated syllables, sustained fricatives and trills, prolonged vocalic phonations, prolonged nasal murmurs, gruntlike short vowels, and complex sequences in which variations can be heard in manner, place, voicing, or any combinations of these (Kent et al., 1987).

Up to 5 or 6 months of age, the sounds made by the infant do not seem to be related to the speech sounds he or she hears. The infant's productive capacity for speech lags significantly behind his or her demonstrated ability to perceive differences. From our observations of otherwise-normal deaf infants, their vocalizations are identical with those of normal infants until 5 or 6 months. Furthermore, the deaf infants increase their vocalizations when the parents speak to them, just as normal infants do. It is obvious that the reason for this increase in vocalizations is not the baby's hearing the parent's voice. We postulate that it is a preadaptive, reflexive response stimulated by the presence of the parent's face, much as is the smile response that appears at the same age. The phenomenon of increased vocalization may, indeed, be a milestone that is predictive of eventual communication skills. Certainly the established fact that the auditory feedback loop is present at birth indicates that the elementary babbling sounds have a significant prelinguistic function. The lack of auditory feedback in the deaf child deprives him or her of early prelinguistic experiences.

Maskarinec et al. (1981) compared the vocalizations of a deaf infant with those of normal infants from birth to 32 weeks. They found that during this time the speechlike sounds increased and the nonspeech sounds decreased in the normal infants, while the deaf child's speechlike and nonspeech production both declined with age and showed greater variability.

An important research project was conducted by Stoel-Gammon and Otomo (1986) during which they produced phonetic transcriptions of babbling samples from 11 normal-hearing babies aged 4–18 months and compared their findings with phonetic transcriptions that they obtained from 11 hearing-impaired infants aged 4–28 months. The results of this outstanding study showed that on the average, the normal-hearing babies showed an increase in size of their consonantal repertoires with age in contrast to the hearing-impaired babies who had smaller repertoires that decreased over time. A comparison of multisyllabic utterances showed a general tendency for the hearing-impaired infants to produce fewer multisyllabic utterances containing true consonants and for some of the hearing-impaired babies to produce a high proportion of vocalizations with glides or glottal stops. This study confirms both qualitative and quantitative differences in the babbling development of normal-hearing and hearing-impaired infants.

Because their study included infants with varying degrees of hearing loss, Stoel-Gammon and Otomo noted that although all the hearing-impaired babies' babbling development was different from that of the normal-hearing infants, the magnitude of difference appeared to be smaller for those with moderate hearing loss compared with those with severe-to-profound hearing loss. The parental histories obtained in this study suggested not only that normal prelinguistic and early linguistic development (i.e., onset of babbling and meaningful vocal play) was arrested as a result of sudden onset of deafness but also that the developing speech patterns reverted to behaviors resembling those predominating at earlier stages of development.

This study and others showed the important link between random articulatory movements and the resulting acoustic outcomes to the presence of self-monitoring through the auditory sense. The inability of hearing-impaired babies to hear their own vocalizations prevents them from the acoustic self-stimulation that encourages additional babbling and the consequential expansion of new speech sounds. The results obtained by Stoel-Gammon and Otomo suggest that significant hearing loss affects prelinguistic vocalizations by 8 month of age and possibly earlier. In their analysis of consonantal utterances, the point of divergence between their two groups of subjects was around 6–8 months, implying that at that age hearing loss began to influence the development of the consonantal repertoire.

These self-stimulating sounds strengthen the auditory feedback loop that was earlier demonstrated to be active at birth. The infant begins early to monitor his or her own speech activity, however primitive. The perception and the elementary control of rhythm, intonation, duration, and frequency range of sounds is evident by 4 or 5 months of age.

By 5 months, Chinese children produce the intonation of the Chinese language. Also, by 5 months Polish infants' babbling can be distinguished from the babbling of English infants (Weir, 1966). The later

skills of linguistic organization are undoubtedly dependent upon these early activities.

Reddy and Rao (1977) found that infants between 12 and 21 days of age can imitate both facial and manual gestures. Even sequential finger movement (opening and closing the hand by serially moving the fingers) was imitated. The infant, indeed, enters the world equipped with skills that appear innate to humans.

Even facial expressions can be discriminated, according to Field et al. (1982). They exposed 74 neonates (average 36 hours) to 3 facial expressions—happy, sad, and surprised—and observed diminished visual fixation on each face over trials. The fixations were renewed upon presentation of a different expression. What was surprising was that the babies made imitative facial movements that clued in observers to the expressions of the model, at greater than chance accuracy.

Measurements of the fundamental frequency of the baby's voice (*f*o) have been made by Kent (1976). He showed that during the first 3 weeks of life *f*o is around 400 Hz; then it increases to around 480 Hz by the fourth month where it stabilizes for 5 months. At 1 year it begins to decrease sharply and levels off at 300 Hz at 3 years. Some interest has been shown in the frequency of the cry of abnormal infants. Vuorenkoski et al. (1971) found abnormally high *f*o's in the infants with asphyxia brain damage, and hyperbilirubinemia. A low *f*o was noted in Down's syndrome children.

A most intriguing opportunity and research study presented itself to Kent et al. (1987) when they identified two identical twin boys, one of whom had a severe-to-profound bilateral hearing loss and the other of whom had normal hearing. The etiology of the hearing loss was undetermined, although the infant was first suspected to be hearing-impaired when he failed a routine hospital screening test. His hearing loss was confirmed by auditory brainstem (evoked) response and behavioral testing, and he was fitted with binaural ear-level hearing aids and enrolled in

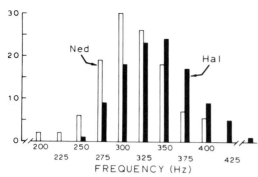

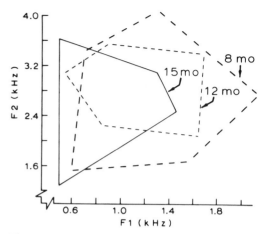

Figure 4.1. Histograms of peak fundamental frequencies of syllable productions of Ned and Hal at 8 months. (Reproduced with permission from R. D. Kent, M. J. Osberger, R. Netsell, C. G. Hustedde: Phonetic development in identical twins differing in auditory function. *Journal of Speech and Hearing Research* 52:66, 1987.)

Figure 4.2. Composite F1-F2 data for Ned's vocalic segments at 8, 12, and 15 months. (Reproduced with permission from R. D. Kent, M. J. Osberger, R. Netsell, C. G. Hustedde: Phonetic development in identical twins differing in auditory function. *Journal of Speech and Hearing Research* 52:67, 1987.)

habilitative services at the age of 3 months. These twin boys offered a rare opportunity to study the effects of hearing loss on vocal development with reasonable control over environmental and genetic factors. The primary objectives of the study conducted by Kent et al. was to obtain longitudinal information on (*a*) fundamental frequency levels and contours, (*b*) formant frequencies of vocalic utterances, and (*c*) spectral characteristics of fricatives and trills. The acoustic data were collected on video and audio while the twins interacted with each other and with an adult (parent or investigator). The twins were evaluated at approximately 3 month intervals, beginning at the age of 8 months, again at 12 months, and again at 15 months.

The results of this unique investigation are presented for syllable shapes, formant patterns, and phonetic inventories obtained from transcriptions of the audiotapes of the twins between 8 and 15 months of age. Histograms of peak fundamental frequencies of syllable productions of the normal-hearing child (called Ned) and the hearing-impaired child (called Hal) at the age of 8 months are shown in Figure 4.1. According to the research team, Hal often showed a phonatory pattern in his utterances that was highly variable, and this hearing-impaired twin had a larger range of peak fundamental fre-

quency values and a higher model value as shown in the histograms. The composite data for vocalic formant frequencies F1 and F2 were determined from spectrograms and plotted as shown in Figures 4.2 and 4.3. The composite F1-F2 results for Ned, the normal-hearing twin (Fig. 4.2), show a configuration of the vowel region over the developmental period. A very different pattern is shown for Hal in Figure 4.3, where the developmental pattern is one of marked constriction such that by the age of 15 months the F1-F2 region is contained within the low-frequency portion of the pattern exhibited at 8 months.

As would be expected from the syllable structure data, Hal and Ned differed markedly in their consonant productions. Of special interest is the fact that unlike the normal-hearing twin—who produced fricatives at several places of articulation, including labiodental, alveolar, palatal, and pharyngeal—Hal was not heard to make even a single fricative sound. Table 4.1 shows the frequency of occurrence data for place of consonant production in the spontaneous vocalizations of Hal and Ned at 24 months. Even though Hal's syllable production was greatly diversified at 24 months compared

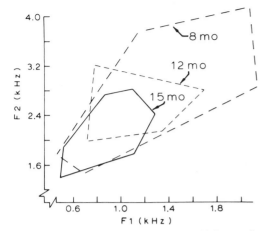

Figure 4.3. Composite F1-F2 data for Hal's vocalic segments at 8, 12, and 15 months. (Reproduced with permission from R. D. Kent, M. J. Osberger, R. Netsell, C. G. Hustedde: Phonetic development in identical twins differing in auditory function. *Journal of Speech and Hearing Research* 52:68, 1987.)

with 8 months, his vocalizations continued to be narrower in range than those of Ned.

In their summary, Kent et al. indicate that the spontaneous vocalizations of the twin boys were clearly different as early as 8 months of age. The hearing-impaired twin's vocal productions were much less variable than the normal-hearing twin, with a fundamental frequency variability that had a wide range extending from a glottal roll to a shriek. The hearing-impaired twin had a restricted range of vowel production and few consonants as late as 15 months of age. This incredible research study has provided the basis of quantitative speech science dif-

Table 4.1.
Frequency of Occurrence Data for Place of Consonant Production in the Spontaneous Vocalizations of Hal and Ned at 24 Months of Age.

Place	Hal	Ned
Bilabial	12 (15)[a]	29 (43)
Dental	1 (1)	9 (13)
Alveolar	60 (77)	15 (22)
Palatal	4 (5)	5 (7)
Velar	0 (0)	5 (7)
Glottal	1 (1)	6 (9)
Total	78	67

[a]Percentages are in parentheses. (Used with permission from R. Kent, M. J. Osberger, R. Netsell, and C. G. Hustedde: Phonetic development in identical twins differing in auditory function. *Journal of Speech and Hearing Research* 52: 69, 1987.)

ferences in a unique study sample—identical twins—where genetic and environmental differences can be assumed to be minimal.

Mother's feedback of the child's sounds lays the groundwork for his or her first production of a word. The sounds the child makes are imitated by the mother, and additional speech improvisations are added by her. Soon the child imitates the mother's imitations, and speech control is under way. Sometimes, the comprehension of the sound sequence precedes the imitation; sometimes, imitation precedes understanding of the meaning of the sound sequence.

The infant begins to practice speech as young as 2 months, according to Trevarthen (1975). Films of babies reveal a kind of "prespeech" activity consisting of a rudimentary form of speaking by movements of lips and tongue, with or without sounds. A specific pattern of breathing is noted with prespeech. Even in the second month the baby may imitate a mouth movement of the mother or a protrusion of her tongue, but this kind of behavior is most often seen after 6 months of age and only after the act is pointedly repeated in a teacher-like way. Trevarthen states that such embryonic speaking confirms the psycholinguistic theory that language is embedded in an innate context of nonverbal communication by which intension and experience are transmitted from person to person. Meltzoff and Moore (1977) have also described both manual and facial imitations in newborn babies.

Bower (1976) described such imitation as occurring at a young age and has photographed tongue-protrusion imitation in an infant 6 days old. He says this ability disappears early, however, reappearing only near the age of 1 year. Bower describes ear-hand coordination, which he says is present in young infants but is soon lost, sometimes permanently. He ascribes the decline to the fact that hearing is a passive situation—one that cannot be controlled as vision can be. Bower tested this hypothesis by fitting a blind infant with an echo-location device that sent out ultrasonic frequencies and converted the echoes to audible pitches. Within a few seconds after the device was put on, the infant reached for objects and showed that he was making sense of the device.

More amazing than imitation is the auditory localization of very young infants observed by Aronson (Bower, 1975). Young babies observed their mother through a soundproof glass screen, with the voice of the mother coming at various positions of a loudspeaker. So long as the sound came from where the mother was, the baby was quite happy. But when the voice came from a speaker in another position, the infants manifested surprise and upset, indicating not only auditory localization but also an expectation that voices will come from mouths. Adults seem to have lost such localization, being unaware for example that voices in movies come from a place other than the screen.

A bimodal representation of speech is present in the infant, i.e., the recognition that the sequence of lip, tongue, and jaw movements corresponds to the sounds we hear. Brown et al. (1982) showed that 18–20 week old infants can detect the correspondence between auditorially and visually perceived speech. They presented the infants with two side-by-side images of a talker articulating, in synchrony, two different vowel sounds, and they recorded by videotape the infants' visual fixations. The infants consistently looked longer at the face that matched the sound. To determine what characteristics of the auditory stimuli were necessary to the detection of the correspondence, the researchers removed the spectral information from the vowels (formant frequencies) while preserving their temporal characteristics (amplitude and duration). Under these conditions, the percentage of fixations to the matched face dropped to chance, indicating that some aspect of the frequency information of the vowel was requisite to produce the effect. The same phenomenon was reported by Kuhl and Hillenbrand

(1979). During the experiments, Brown et al. observed that the 10 infants who heard the vowel stimuli produced babbling utterances, whereas only one of those who heard the pure tone nonspectral information did so. It appears that the intermodal perception of speech is conducive to vocal learning. It follows that (1) communication with an infant should be face-to-face as much as possible and (2) that the intermodal model might well be extended to include tactual information as well as visual for the deaf.

The long period of reception of auditory language symbols is the prerequisite to later language formulation. By the time speech and language emerge, there have been 12–18 months of receiving complex adult spoken language and distilling it into the matrix of the child language structure. This act of refining out of a complex language structure the basic one- and two-word sentences that are the baby's first speech language utterances must rank as creation's noblest day. Chomsky (1966) proposes that the ability to decode and organize these grammatical structures is an innate function, unique to human infants. Lenneberg (1967) prefers to rely on biologic functioning to explain language development. Whichever theory one supports, the important fact is the primacy of reception in the language acquisition of children. Listening to language for a long period of time is essential to the ultimate usage of language. From the studies described above, it is evident that this listening is not a passive process but one in which the infant participates by acting upon the incoming signals.

By the time the child's first meaningful word is uttered, miraculously full-blown at around 1 year, a whole world of listening activity has taken place. Nothing he or she will ever achieve is as intellectually complex as what has preceded that first utterance. Lenneberg states: "By the time language begins to make its appearance about 60% of the adult values of maturation are reached."

OPTIMAL PERIODS

How early is it necessary for the hearing-deprived child to receive language input, to avoid language retardation? The answer to this question is based on whether there exist critical, or optimal, periods for the development of various functions. The theory of critical periods states that there are certain periods in development when the organism is programmed to receive and utilize particular types of stimuli and that subsequently the stimuli will have gradually diminishing potency in affecting the organism's development in the function represented. In the case of audition it means that at a certain developmental stage auditory signals will be optimally received and utilized for important prelinguistic activities, but that once this stage has passed, the effective utilization of these signals gradually declines. An analogous theory for language development holds that language input must be experienced at a certain stage, or it becomes decreasingly effective for utilization in emergent language skills.

The most vociferous opponent of this theory has been Bench (1971) who claims that the concept has no more than heuristic value and that its importance in the field of diagnostic audiology has been greatly overemphasized. Bench requires of the critical period theory that to be thorough, it would demand an irreversibility of the effects: "If a method can be found to change the effects back to normal ('reversing the apparently irreversible'), it is clear that the so-called critical period is not critical after all."

The question of whether intervention after age 3 can produce permanent gains in cognitive ability was addressed by McKay et al. (1978) in a large Columbian population of low socioeconomic status families. At ages 43, 51, 63, and 76 months, treatment was begun for four different groups. A battery of language tests was given at each age, beginning at 63 months and ending at 86 months. The treatment included nutritional, health, and educational interventions. A matched group of privileged children was given the same battery of tests at each period but was given no treatment. The gap between the two groups was dramatically narrowed in the initial period of treatment but tended to fall off with age, despite continued treatment. The significant finding was that the retardation was less amenable to modification with increasing age, bearing out the need to start interventions during early years of plasticity.

Lenneberg (1967) is of the opinion that puberty marks the last milestone for acquisition of language. With regard to the effects of early deprivation, he cites the difference between the congenitally deaf child and the child who acquires deafness through meningitis after a brief exposure to language. He states that those who lose hearing after having been exposed to the experience of speech, even for as short a period as 1 year, can be trained much more easily in all language arts, even if formal training begins some years after they had become deaf. According to Lenneberg: "It seems as if even a short exposure to language, a brief moment during which the curtain has been lifted and oral communication established, is sufficient to give a child some foundation on which much later language may be based."

A classic case in point is that of Miss Helen Keller, whose great achievements in mastering language skills are rightly admired. However, it must be remembered that Miss Keller acquired her deafness and blindness from meningitis at age 2. One cannot expect equal language achievements from a congenitally deaf and blind child, and indeed, one does not see them develop.

Lenneberg (1967) describes in detail the case for the time-locked nature of language learning and concludes:

The inferences we may draw from this material (animal studies on critical periods) is that many animal forms traverse periods of peculiar sensitivities, response-propensities, or learning potentials. Insofar as we have made such a claim for language acquisition, we have postulated nothing that would be extraordinary in the realm of animal behavior. But at the same time we must sound a warning. Merely the fact that there are critical periods for the acquisition of certain types of behavior among a number of species *does not imply* any phylogenetic relationship between them. Age-linked emergence of behavior may be due to such a variety of factors that this phenomenon by itself is of limited heuristic value when it comes to tracing evolutionary origins of behavior. In the case of language, the limiting factors postulated are cerebral immaturity on the one end and termination of a state of organizational plasticity linked with lateralization of function at the other end of the critical period. [With permission from E. H. Lenneberg: *Biological Foundations of Language*. New York, John Wiley & Sons, 1967, pp. 175–176.]

The "Survey of Hearing Impaired Children and Youth" taken in the spring of 1971 by the Gallaudet College Office of Demographic Studies (Series D, No. 9) reports the results of the administration of the Stanford Achievement Test Series to all students in schools for the deaf and hard-of-hearing in the United States. We know from surveys on age of detection of hearing losses that almost all of these children were identified and given beginning training after the age of 2 or 3 years. The highest average reading competence level (paragraph meaning), attained at age 19, was equivalent to grade 4.36. As might be expected, academic reading areas were lowest for those with the most severe degree of hearing loss. Related to the low reading levels of all the students are poor vocabularies and knowledge of word meanings—skills upon which reading ability is built. However, in the nonverbal area of arithmetic computation, the more profoundly deaf students score higher than their better-hearing contemporaries. This fact demonstrates that the lowered degree of language and reading skills of these very profoundly deaf students is not caused by lowered intellectual function in this group.

In an expertly designed study, Templin (1966) compares the language skills of deaf children with the skills of matched groups of normal children. In some of the language areas the deaf showed no systematic improvement in their performance beyond 11 years. At that point such skills as under-

standing of word meanings, sentence construction, and analogies, hit a plateau and remained there without further insights or improvements. The normal-hearing children went on to achieve to the 14 year language level that was the upper limits of the study. It should be emphasized that there was no substantial difference in intellectual abilities between the deaf and the normal hearing group and that the deaf had had intensive language training in their schools. Their rate of learning up to 11 years was comparable with that of the normal-hearing group. But an irreversible language deficit appeared at this age level and precluded further development. The complexity of language forms and of abstract language symbols takes a great leap about this age and leaves the deaf helplessly behind. The blame can be ascribed only to early language deprivation covering many periods optimal for language learning.

The reports of animal research supporting optimal period theory of development are numerous. Reisen (1947) reported that a chimpanzee raised in total darkness for the first 3 months of life never developed adequate vision. But if chimpanzees are raised in light for the first 3 months and subjected to total darkness for the next 6 months, they quickly regain perfect vision when exposed to light. The analogous situation in humans is found in the child born with strabismus of one eye (thrown to a side focus). Ophthalmologists report that unless that eye is forced to be used, through patching the other eye, by the age of 4 no useful perceptions can ever be developed in it despite the fact that organically it is a perfect organ of vision. It is the central perception of vision that, untrained during critical periods, can never regain function. There seems to be no demonstrated reason why auditory perceptions do not fall into the same category as the visual modality.

Reisen (1960) also reported that chimpanzees showed a reduction in the efficiency of auditory learning following early sensory deprivation of hearing. In addition, he found, in cats deprived of visual sensation, three concomitant manifestations: hyperexcitability, increased susceptibility to convulsive disorder, and localized motor dysfunction. This latter experiment has profound implications for the student of deafness. What are the effects on the CNS of early learning deprivation? Many clinicians have described symbolic language disorder, minimal cerebral dysfunction, or other kinds of central involvement in the deaf. Can these disorders be a direct result of the auditory deprivation?

What has not been considered is the effect of the language deprivation on the deaf infant. If biologic theories of language acquisition are correct, then the human infant is just as preprogrammed to develop language skills as to develop motor skills. The effect of early sensory deprivation could then be expected to have far-reaching consequences on CNS functioning in integrative areas of the brain. The concept of language as a biologically predetermined function thus extends the speculation of early sensory deprivation in humans to another plane where animal research cannot apply. It opens up a whole new area of investigation.

Edwards (1968) has summarized concisely the state of the educator's attitude toward optimal periods:

The supremely difficult feat of building language recognition and response which takes place during the first years of life can occur because there is a built-in neurological mechanism for language learning present in every normal human organism. But like the image on the sensitized negative, this potential will not appear as reality unless the proper circumstances develop it. Experience—the right experience—is essential.

Heredity and environment interact. Hereditary possibilities are shaped by the influence that only human culture can provide; they are potentialities that must be developed while the young neurological organism is still rapidly growing, malleable, open to stimulus. If the "critical periods in learning" hypothesis applies to human beings (as we know it does to other creatures—dogs, for instance—and as evidence increasingly indicates it does to us), then the right experience must come at the right time, or

the potential must remain forever unrealized [p. 70].

Edwards' solution to this problem is well worth detailing:

We are going to have to make educational stimulation available from babyhood on for the children whose families cannot provide it for them. Whether tutors should go into the homes, whether children should be brought into carefully planned, well staffed *educational* (as distinct from baby-sitting day-care) programs, we do not now know. Experiments going on in several places in the country should help us decide. But however we do it, intervention by the age of 18 months should be the rule for the children of deprived inner-city or poor rural families. [Reprinted with permission from E. P. Edwards: Kindergarten is too late. *Saturday Review*, p. 77, 1968.]

There have been conflicting arguments about the lasting effects of Head-Start programs. The divergent opinions are summarized by Horn (1981) and Darlington (1981). Horn pointed out that the IQ measures taken on the Head Start children showed large initial gains but that these gains had vanished 5 years after the completion of preschool. He also analyzed Darlington's reports and showed that the beneficial effects of preschool on later school performance past elementary school were no more durable than the preschool effects on IQ. Darlington, on the other hand, states that there is no indication that effects last only through elementary school, when the dependent variable is placement in special education classes rather than a more general measure of failure to meet school requirements. Whichever thesis is true, nonenduring effect on IQ has held up, as well as finding that the most long-lasting effect of any preschool program has been the early mother-child-home projects, birth to 2 years, which showed consistent statistical significance of long-term duration of improved functioning.

Although it is difficult to pinpoint the exact age at which it is optimal that infants be given language stimulation, a report by Dennis (1973) begins to give some guidelines. In an institution for homeless children in Lebanon, he tested the foundlings at all ages, before and after their adoption into homes. Those who were adopted by or before age 2 soon reached normal intellectual functioning, with a mean IQ jump of 50 points postadoptively. But those adopted after age 2 never overcame their preadoptive experiential retardation. Dennis concludes that there is a period near the second birthday that is optimal for complete recovery from the effects of experimental deprivation.

Considered from the physiologic point of view, the infant's auditory system is plastic; i.e., it can be modified not only by anatomical alteration but also by variations of acoustic stimuli. Absent or faulty sound stimuli will result in deviant auditory function. According to Ruben and Rapin (1980), the central and peripheral auditory systems exert reciprocal control over each other. As the inner ear matures, its input is necessary to the development of at least part of the auditory nervous system. By the time the peripheral auditory system is fully developed, its input seems to be necessary for the maturation and innervations of portions of the central auditory system (Webster and Webster, 1977, 1979, 1980; Clopton and Silverman, 1977). Therefore, environmental sounds have the greatest effect in shaping auditory ability from the time the inner ear and eighth cranial nerve first become functional to the time when maturation of the CNS is achieved—roughly from the fifth month of gestation to between 18 and 28 months. The consequences of these findings for intervention programs for the hearing-impaired are strikingly apparent. The time for action is early in the first year of life.

So far as the deaf are concerned, the most definitive study was done by a group of researchers at Lexington School for the Deaf (Greenstein et al., 1976). Thirty severely hearing-impaired children who had been admitted to the school before their second birthdays were studied. Two groups were identified: those who had been admitted prior to 16 months of age and those admitted between 16 and 24 months. Over a period ending when they were 40 months of age, the children were given repeated measures of language skills, including the Receptive-Expressive Emergent Language (REEL) Scale and the Lexington Preschool Oral Language Assessment. In addition, informal measures using observational assessments of mother-infant communication was made. The results indicate that the children admitted prior to 16 months were consistently superior to the later-admitted children in all aspects and at all age levels. Regardless of what caused the differences, its occurrence before 16 months was the variable responsible for the improved speech and language. Here is evidence relating learning ability in the hearing-impaired to time of identification of the hearing loss.

It is often hoped that studies of children who have been socially and sensorally deprived since infancy will shed light on the periods necessary for acquisition of language. The 1797 "wild boy of Aveyron" (Lane, 1977) remained mute and incapable of even subtle communication even after Dr. Itard attempted to teach and socialize him. The report of Genie (Fromkin et al., 1974) who was isolated in a closet for 11 years of her life, states that this is "a case of language acquisition beyond the 'critical period.'" However, Genie's history shows that she was exposed to family life for her first 20 months before being placed in isolation until age 13 years 9 months. The reported language abilities that she acquired after being rescued from a pitiful situation are actually what one could predict for anyone having had 20 months of normal language input. The really critical periods for language during which Genie had exposure laid the matrix from which her language skills could develop.

CENTRAL ORGANIC AUDITORY DISORDERS

Part of the audiologist's task is to determine whether in addition to a peripheral hearing loss there may be another organic disorder of the auditory system. Chapter 5 details the behavioral clues that should alert the clinician to a possible central auditory problem. To understand the central disorders that may produce deviant behavior, it is pertinent to review what is known about the involved pathways and their breakdowns.

The peripheral auditory mechanism extends from the outer ear to the termination of the acoustic nerve in the cochlear nucleus of the brainstem. The neurons leading into the synapse in the nuclei are the auditory input stations for the CNS. A lesion at any point along this system results in reduced auditory sensitivity, represented by decreased thresholds for pure tones and speech.

Beyond the cochlear nuclei in the brainstem lie the neurons of the central auditory system that transmit the auditory information to the brain. Several synapses along the way to the brain begin the coding and analyzing of the information. For example, the neck-turning reflex of the infant to a loud sound is presumed to be mediated at the level of the superior olive. In newborn infants, the reflex can be inhibited by central processing: the normal infant will cease to give a neck turn after several repetitions of the arousing stimulus. The known brain-injured child, on the other hand, once having given this neck-turn response, will be unable to inhibit it on successive presentations of the stimulus (Eisenberg et al., 1976). Even the simple coding system required for inhibiting the reflex will be disrupted by CNS damage.

An excellent historical review of cases of auditory agnosia by Goldstein (1974) shows the sites of lesions that have been reported in autopsies. All lay in the left temporal lobe. In all cases of disordered perception of auditory stimuli the peripheral acuity was within normal range or too slightly reduced to be responsible for the lack of perception.

An example of how long it may take to understand such dysfunction in a child is illustrated by another case history. Brent, a 3 year old boy, the third of eight siblings, presented with a 60 dB sensorineural loss in the right ear and with an 85 dB sensorineural loss in the left ear. He conditioned very well, and retests over many years showed the same hearing levels. Brent sat alone at 6 months but at 7 months developed meningitis. At discharge he was alert, happy, and at first had no evidence of neurologic disorder. After this disease he did not sit again until 9 months of age, and walked at 11 months. He walks with his left toe turned in and drags it slightly.

At 3 years, Brent was fitted with binaural hearing aids and started on an exclusively auditory program. After 6 months he was babbling spontaneously and could localize sounds, but day after day was noted as being "unresponsive to auditory therapy." A Merrill Palmer performance test at this time gave an IQ of 116, and the psychologist noted that although he was visually alert to signs, he had no word comprehension. She felt that there was a specific "auditory comprehension deficit" and noted that "one should not be fooled by his perceptiveness of motor cues and by his perceptiveness of voice inflection into thinking that he understood words."

Six months later, the therapist made exactly the same report as before—no meaningful auditory preceptions had been developed in 1 year's time. A psychometric test at that time showed average intelligence on a Leiter scale and "organic brain damage indications" on a Bender Gestalt test. He could not make simple visual discrimination of forms or perceive and reproduce simple designs.

Brent was then placed in a program emphasizing lipreading and oral training. His teachers reported that he was unable to discriminate any words through lipreading, nor to relate them to reading forms. He mimicked and mouthed words, but only singly. At age 7 he was given an electroencephalogram, which was normal, and another psychometric test. "There were indications that mild neurological dysfunction was interfering with his perceptual motor performance. His nonverbal abilities were good, but his lack of language was the main difficulty." At this time the only method of communication he had was by gesture.

At age 9, Brent was finally sent to the state school to learn signing and fingerspelling, where he has had his only success at learning language—but only through signs and reading. At age 16, he is still not able to fingerspell. He still cannot speak more than single words. Auditory communication is so unrewarding to him that he has not worn an aid for several years. His reading is at the 11 year old level, and it gives him pleasure, which television listening does not.

This case illustrates one of the fundamental principles in differential diagnosis: that peripheral hearing loss and central disorders are two separate entities but that they both may exist in the same individual. If tests for auditory acuity show reduced hearing, it is due to a true peripheral lesion, not to a central one. Brent's final diagnosis was "auditory verbal agnosia and visual agnosia for any rapid denotation movements"—all this in addition to a peripheral hearing loss. Each problem must be treated for its own needs, and the combination of problems should, in this case, have been identified sooner.

Goldstein et al. (1972) state: "It is now well established that unilateral, upper level, central nervous system lesions, regardless of their severity, produce no impairment in auditory sensitivity as long as the peripheral auditory mechanism remains intact." Once this separation between central and peripheral lesions is made clear, one can proceed to test for each problem individually, without confusing the two. In the section on auditory testing (Chapter 5) we describe auditory tests on children with central problems, based on this premise.

By 4 months the localization of sounds begins. This is a primary skill and need not be affected by subtle cerebral dysfunction. When localization does not appear at 4 months of age, it may mean a general retardation of the time schedule. It has been our experience that the infant with central neu-

rologic problems is more apt to give a localization response at this age than at a later age. As such a child grows older, speech becomes meaningless and responses to it unproductive.

It is extremely rare that both localization ability and auditory reflexes will be absent in a very young, centrally disordered child. Even an anencephalic infant will give large startle reflexes to loud sound. In fact, the child will continue to give them ad infinitum without inhibition of the response because of lack of cerebral control. So testing proceeds much the same for the brain-damaged child as for the normal child, and if a lack of response is seen, one must believe that it is due to a peripheral lesion. Too many brain-damaged children have had amplification denied because of the erroneous belief that their audiometric loss was due to a central lesion.

By 6 months the infant localizes to very soft speech; by 8 months the baby imitates some sounds and intonations. To do this, the infant must have a period of auditory differentiation present since birth. Any disruption in the processing of the information disrupts the development of the imitations and of the child's ability to differentiate voice intonations. Usually, the 8 month old child understands the meaning of "no-no" or at least the intonation that accompanies it. When a child is not able to make this differentiation, there begins in the mother the subtle bewilderment that is so often reported by the mothers of centrally involved children. There is a similarity here between the deaf and the centrally involved child: Neither shows the milestones of prespeech and prelinguistic skills. The lack of integrity in responding to human communication puzzles the mothers of both such children. The mother-child relationship depends upon an interplay between the two. When this becomes a one-way street, with the child's responses to mother subtly lacking in meaningfulness, a deterioration of the relationship begins. If a problem of peripheral deafness is discovered early, understanding soon reverses the interpersonal breakdown

(Greenstein et al., 1976). Once the mother recognizes that the child has a sensory loss, but no other deficit, she is able again to "mother" the child appropriately. Such mothering is difficult for the mother of a neurologically disordered child. Often hyperactive to some degree, these are the children whom nobody understands.

AUDITORY LANGUAGE LEARNING DISORDERS

There are many children who appear to have problems in "the processing of auditory material." They are found today in special classes for "learning disorders," "language dysfunction," or "language disabled." A few years ago they were found in therapy classes for "symbolic language disorders"; before that they were labeled as having "minimal brain dysfunction," and before that as the "aphasoid child." Whatever the problem was called, the generic term was "central auditory processing disorder." The only certainty about all this terminology is that it concerns a symptom without a disease. Despite an elaborate system of measuring the symptoms, and a more elaborate treatment protocol, no one has determined the cause or where in the CNS the breakdown might occur.

The type of disorder we are discussing here is not one in which neurologic findings are evident from physical examination or can be inferred from a history of brain trauma or insult. The children so labeled may have no known indications of neurologic involvement; learning disorders are their only symptoms. The learning problems appear to stem mainly from an inability to utilize spoken or linguistic auditory input effectively. Inasmuch as this is deemed to be an auditory problem, the onus is on auditory specialists to determine, if possible, the basis for the symptoms.

Attempts have been made by audiologists to devise auditory tests that will identify children with learning disorders. A sampling of these tests does not, however, give a clear picture of what is being tested.

Stubblefield and Young (1975) used the Staggered Spondaic Word Test (SSW) with learning-disordered children. These children made more errors on the SSW than were considered normal for the test. The SSW test purports to identify the integrity of each ear's function. Willeford (1976) utilized a battery of tests on learning disabled children that included binaural fusion, filtered speech, competing sentences, and alternating speech. Great variability was found on the performance of any given test; however, 8 of 9 learning-disabled children performed poorly on the binaural fusion test. This test involves brainstem function, and Willeford believes that it indicates that normal relationships between the auditory and visual modalities may be disturbed in these children.

Tests have been devised for the prediction of language learning problems. Martin and Clark (1977) used low-pass filtered speech discrimination tests and a combination of dichotic-diotic speech tests to show differences between a normal group of children and a language-learning-disabled group. Although the low-pass filtered speech did not differentiate between the two groups, the test of the difference between a diotic and a dichotic speech presentation identified the language-disordered children. Those who had higher discrimination scores for the diotic presentation than for the dichotic were predominantly in the problem group. This test procedure entails the Word Intelligibility by Picture Identification (WIPI) Test (Ross and Lerman, 1970) and requires only that the child point to the correct picture.

All of these tests diagnose symptoms, not disease. Nowhere can one find a correlation between auditory symptoms and an underlying CNS disorder such as one finds in the literature on adults or children who have had demonstrable trauma or insult to the brain as described in the previous section. In the absence of confirmed lesions in the CNS, there is real doubt as to what is measured in all of the tests for "central auditory processing disorders."

In the area of visual perception and reading there has also been some confusion as to what precisely is measured. Zack and Kaufman (1972) believe that perception is a developmental process, not a unitary event, and state that the evidence that training can alleviate the problem is not overwhelming. Many studies report no real effect on school achievement as a result of special training, and one report shows that special training programs do not seem to influence achievement more than good teaching (Cohen, 1970). Zack and Kaufman (1972) question the method of identification of these children, the definition of their problem, and the techniques of training used. They state: "It would seem that although education begins with an understanding of the strengths and weaknesses of the child, a label derived from a global concept which lacks adequate definition and questionable means for its measurement does not provide a shortcut to good pedagogy."

The tests for auditory learning skills described above, however, do identify the strengths and weaknesses of the child. But the global concept of "auditory processing disorder," without established definition and/or etiology and with the variable measurements, seems to us to be a tenuous concept. A medical model would eschew labeling a disease without clear and tenable diagnosis of etiology or site of lesion. True, it would treat symptoms, but with the recognition always that a workable diagnosis would permit a more knowledgeable application of treatment than mere attention to symptoms. In the realm of auditory learning disorders it may be wiser to attempt to identify etiology if we are to treat symptoms more accurately.

Symptom treatment of auditory learning disorders presupposes that the symptoms have caused the language dysfunction and that isolating the symptoms and treating each one will cure the language learning problem. However, from a developmental viewpoint the specific auditory problems appear to be a result of the language disorder, not the cause of it. Such a developmental approach should certainly be considered. It conforms with the conclusions of Rees (1973) who reviewed studies purporting to show that various "auditory processing disorders," such as auditory memory and auditory sequencing, are responsible for language disorders. She concludes that what the studies show is that instead of having an auditory perception problem the children who were studied had a language disorder.

Rees further points out that the search for the fundamental psychologic unit of auditory processing of sentences has led from the phoneme to the underlying sentence itself. Abbs and Sussman (1971) have shown that individual speech sounds follow one another too rapidly in ordinary speech to allow them to be analyzed separately. Therefore, says Rees, speech perception cannot take place one sound segment at a time. Even the discrimination of paired words such as *bat* and *pat* rests on a linguistic, not merely an auditory, ability. It is the entire sentence that is the basic unit of language, with all its semantic and syntactic implications. Rees agrees with Marquardt and Saxman (1972) that "the importance of any given subskill to speech and language acquisition remains to be demonstrated."

This point of view has been reflected in the 1982 Position Statement on Language Learning Disorders, by the American Speech-Language-Hearing Association, which discounts the view that language-disabled children will succeed in spite of their early manifested problems. Actually, they do not "catch up" but maintain communication problems through adolescence and adulthood. Language disabilities cannot be viewed only as receptive-expressive breakdowns. Such auditory skills as auditory discrimination and auditory sequential memory need to be interpreted within the context of knowledge of language and communication systems; e.g., memory is more than memory for sequences of digits. There must be an interaction between linguistic and perceptual factors; e.g., the ability to discriminate sounds is influenced by the knowledge of vocabulary. In addition, one's ability to remember and comprehend an individual sentence is influenced by the context, one's prior knowledge of the topic, knowledge of linguistic rules, etc.

This approach rejects therapy that is based upon specific disorders in auditory sequencing, auditory blending, and auditory discrimination. It is thus a developmental rather than a unitary approach to auditory processing disorders.

What are the implications of a developmental approach for remediation for auditory learning disorders? Such an approach greatly simplifies the therapy plan, rejecting the training of unitary subskills and concentrating on training language skills rather than isolated functions.

Relevant Research. Many provocative investigations from other disciplines may eventually shed light on the mechanisms involved in organic central auditory dysfunction.

Primacy of Left Hemisphere in Speech and Language, Particularly of the Left Temporal Lobe. Wernicke's area (behind Heschl's gyrus) has been shown anatomically to be larger on the left side in 65% of brains and larger on the right side in only 75% (Geschwind and Levitzky, 1968). The planum temporale is, on the average, one-third longer on the left than the right lobe. This finding correlates with the known specialization of speech and language in the left hemisphere (Penfield and Roberts, 1959; Kimura, 1961; Studdert-Kennedy and Shankweiler, 1970). Right-handedness in most people show the critical nature of the crossover of sensory messages to the opposite side.

Milner et al. (1968) demonstrated in a dramatic experiment that speech processing in both hemispheres is bound to the left hemisphere. Seven patients with midline section of the cerebral commissures including the corpus callosum were given dichotic and monotic competing number tasks. (In dichotic stimulation, each ear received si-

multaneously a different message, usually speech, from a separate channel of a tape recorder, via earphones. In monotic listening, one ear is stimulated at a time by any number of related or unrelated signals.) Milner et al. showed that when each ear of their patients was tested individually on the monotic task with competing numbers, the scores were 100% for both ears. However, when the dichotic mode was presented, there was essentially no perception of speech in the left ear. In other words, the right hemisphere has the ability to perceive speech on a rudimentary acoustic level, but when the right hemisphere is disconnected from the dominant left, the messages that are essential to speech interpretation are not transmitted on to the left hemisphere, resulting in an inability to identify and classify the speech material. Speech information transmission seems to be a one-way street, from the right to the left hemisphere, but not in the opposite direction.

A second task was given to these patients, that of retrieving objects through touch alone when competing messages were given simultaneously in each ear. In this task, the scores for left-handed retrieval were higher for the objects named through the left ear, while through the right ear there was little success in identifying objects. Moreover, when asked to name the left ear items, the subjects commonly gave the names of the items that had been given through the right ear. The specialization of the left temporal lobe for speech in particular, and of the right temporal lobe for tactile identification, seems well-demonstrated here.

Berlin et al. (1972, 1973) have thrown further light on the cerebral dominance of the left temporal lobe in children. Nonsense CV combinations were used in dichotic speech tests on 150 right-handed children 5–13 years old. Precise alignment was made for the simultaneous presentation of a different CV to each ear at the same intensity levels. The results showed that an advantage for the right ear in giving correct responses was already evident in the 5 year olds and did not vary with increasing age. Right-earedness for speech and left temporal-lobedness seem definitely established by age 5, lending strength to Lenneberg's (1967) hypothesis on the age of development of handedness as critical to language learning.

Molfese (1978) and Molfese and Hess (1978) recorded auditory evoked potentials from the left and right hemispheres of 10 adults who were listening to a series of auditory stimuli that varied along linguistic and acoustic dimensions. The brain's electrical responses to these different stimuli were isolated and identified, and it was found that phonetic distinctions based on transitional elements occurred only in the left hemisphere. They also found that the left-hemisphere auditory evoked responses were larger in amplitude than the right-hemisphere auditory evoked responses to speech stimuli for all groups. However, nonspeech stimuli produced larger amplitude responses in the right hemisphere. Molfese and Molfese (1979) looked at neonates in the same way and found that they showed hemisphere differences due to specialized perceptual systems over the cortex that are sensitive to changes in specific acoustic cues. They concluded that early laterality effects are due to the presence of mechanisms within the left hemisphere that detect and analyze specific acoustic cues common to the speech signal.

In 1980, Molfese reported that the right hemisphere diffentiates tone onset time, allowing it as a result to differentiate between voiced and voiceless stop consonants. He suggests that there are basic acoustic systems sensitive to certain acoustic features common to speech sounds that are responsible for the hemispheric differences found in dichotic listening techniques, and he denies the presence of special speech processing mechanisms.

Sperry (1982) points out that the right hemisphere should not be considered word-deaf or word-blind. The right and left hemispheres do not necessarily have different cognitive modes; rather, the right is pri-marily "praxic" or "manipulospatial," and the left mainly processes higher cognition and self-awareness. This view brings an appreciation of the importance of nonverbal components and forms of intellect. Sperry found, in cases of disconnected hemispheres, that there was a normal and well-developed sense of self and personal relationship along with a surprising knowledge-ability in general. It appears that affective components appear to cross at lower brain-stem levels and may affect cognitive processes on the other side.

Nagafuchi (1970) also gave dichotic speech tests to young children and found that by 6 years the adult right-earedness was established. At age 3 a sex difference was found: girls were superior to boys in both dichotic and monotic listening tasks. This finding is in line with known earlier development of speech and language skills in girls.

Tests utilizing speech material show even more clearly the breakdown of the auditory system and have more clinical applicability to children. Kimura (1961) presented different digits dichotically to both ears of temporal lobectomy patients. When the left temporal lobe was the involved site, the total number of digits reported from the contralateral ear, as well as from both ears, was greatly reduced, whereas in the case of right temporal lobectomy the scores were higher. Kimura concludes from this finding that the crossed pathways are the stronger and that the left temporal lobe is more important in the perception of spoken material. This perceptive disruption seems analogous to short-term memory dysfunction but is perhaps dependent upon perception rather than temporal memory.

Temporal Sequence. Temporal sequencing takes place in the temporal lobe and is manifested when breakdowns occur due to lesions in the temporal lobe. Sequencing appears to be critical in auditory processing and has pertinence to children's auditory dysfunction. Efron (1963) tested aphasic patients with high and low tones and with red and green lights. The task was to determine the order in which the tones or the lights were presented. The intervals, were varied between the two tones, as they were for the lights. The aphasic required as much as 500 msec between the two stimuli to make judgments on the order of presentation for both the tones and the lights. Normal subjects required only a few milliseconds to make the same judgment. Normal central processing thus is shown to be crucial in temporal sequencing.

Cat studies confirm the sequencing function specific to the temporal lobe. Neff (1961) and Masterton and Diamond (1964) removed the auditory cortex of cats and found that the cats were then unable to judge sequence and order of clicks; all auditory sequence tasks previously learned could not be retrained. Yet the cats could learn simple frequency difference limen and intensity threshold tasks and could localize a signal to the correct ear.

Dichotic and monotic speech tests using time lags between presentations of two phonemes (time-staggering listening) demonstrate other parameters of the perceptual process. Lowe et al. (1970) systematically separated their CV nonsense syllables by 15, 30, 60, and 90 msec and presented them to normal listeners. In monotic tests, the lead stimulus was more easily perceived by both ears equally at all time intervals, indicating that the precedence of the first signal suppresses the awareness of the second when one ear is stimulated. However, when a dichotic presentation was given, the right-ear scores for both the lead and the lag signals were consistently better than those for the left ear, although the lag syllable was more easily perceived by both ears. Improvement of the lag scores was noted as the time interval increased to 90 msec. By that point the left-ear lag scores approximated the right-ear scores.

The use of time-staggered tests in clinical assessment of recovery after a temporal lobe lesion has been reported by Berlin and Lowe (1972). A patient with a gunshot wound to the superior convolution of the left temporal area was given time-staggered dichotic speech tests. Two months posttrauma there was no lag effect, and the left ear gave the higher scores for both lead and lag positions. One month later the left-ear scores were even higher, and the right-ear scores were lower. Later tests showed further accentuation of the left ear's superiority and the right ear's lowered perception of the speech signals in any position and at any time-staggered intervals up to 500 msec. Berlin and Lowe identify this progression as demonstrating a growth in perceptual capacity for auditory sequence perception in the left ear and suggest the use of such tests in monitoring the growth of the right temporal lobe in perceptual capacity.

These studies have demonstrated that the ability of temporal auditory sequencing is specific to the temporal lobe and that it has primacy in the left temporal lobe. They also cast some doubts on our traditional definition of short-term memory. Instead of being related to disruption of storage of signals, it may be that it is perceptual breakdowns related to temporal lobe functioning that create what we have called defective short-term memory problems.

Specialization of Left Temporal Lobe in Extraction of Linguistic Features of Speech. A group of research reports in which the dichotic listening performance was assessed indicate in detail the further specialization of the auditory temporal lobe. Studdert-Kennedy and Shankweiler (1970) presented consonant-vowel-consonant nonsense syllables dichotically to their subjects, manipulating only one of the sounds of the consonant-vowel-consonant, the initial or final consonant, or the vowel. They found that the right ear of their subjects perceived all consonants better than the left ear but that the right and left ears perceived the vowels equally.

Differences in perception of consonants based on the manner of their production have been reported in several studies. Lowe et al. (1970) and Thompson et al. (1972) found in dichotic speech tests a

marked advantage for the unvoiced consonant over the voiced consonant. In an effort
to determine whether this advantage is
based on some unknown process of selection
in the auditory cortex or on an artifact of
the test condition, Berlin and Lowe (1972)
revised the test condition. They hypothesized that when both bursts of the CVs are
initiated simultaneously, the boundary of
the unvoiced CVs occurs later in time than
that of the voiced onset CVs. They were
able to align the onset of the large-
amplitude vocalic portion of two syllables.
When a voiced syllable competed against an
unvoiced syllable, the alignment gave the
voiced syllable a lag in comparison to the
initial plosion of the unvoiced syllable. The results of this test on normal subjects showed
that the advantage of voiceless over voiced
consonants was markedly reduced.

A dichotic study by Zurif and Sait (1970)
did show right-eared laterality effect with
nonsense sentences that were either structured or unstructured. The structured sentences were modified from a primary
reader, and the connective words were included. These sentences were read with
normal intonation. The unstructured list
was read without intonation, "like a laun-
dry list." The results showed that the structured material produced the larger laterality effect. Whether this effect demonstrates that it is syntax that is better
perceived in the right ear or that rhythm
and intonation are crucial elements in the
learning of speech and language, is a moot
question.

The bold experiments of Penfield and
Rasmussen (1968) of stimulating the exposed cortex with electrical probes give us
an idea of the localization of various auditory functions. Their studies show that only
the temporal lobe close to the fissure of
Sylvius will produce auditory sensory responses. The patients report hearing simple sounds (motor sound, crickets, knock-
ing, buzzing, etc.) The points of stimulation
from which responses were obtained are
shown in Figure 4.4. Penfield and Rasmussen state that the majority of the responses

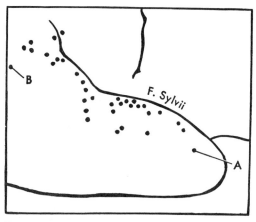

Figure 4.4. Points from which auditory responses
were obtained by stimulation of right and left hemispheres shown above as though all stimulation was
done on the right side. (Reprinted with permission from
W. Penfield and T. Rasmussen: *The Cerebral Cortex of
Man.* New York, Hafner Publishing, 1968.)

were found in Brodmann areas 42 and 22,
the "auditopsychic" area. When stimulation
was given at *point A* in Figure 4.4, the patient reported that he felt as if he were singing. At *point B* another patient heard a
quiet buzzing. These points are considered
out of the primary auditory area. The "audi-
osensory" area (41 of Brodmann) lying
within the fissure of Sylvius on Heschl's
convolution could be stimulated only once,
resulting in a ringing sensation. Whenever
sound was produced at any point, it was
heard in the contralateral ear in most instances. In general, Penfield and Rasmussen believed that stimulation close to the
fissure of Sylvius was more apt to produce
simple tones, ringing, etc., whereas stimulation at a distance on the first temporal
convolution tended to produce some interpretation of sound. Thus they concluded
that interpretive elements are seen in the
secondary auditory area rather than the
primary area.

Penfield and Rasmussen believe that
their studies indicate that there is some degree of intellectual function localized to the
temporal cortex. Only in the temporal regions will electrical stimulation (as well epileptic discharge) activate acquired synaptic
patterns, not in other brain area. There-

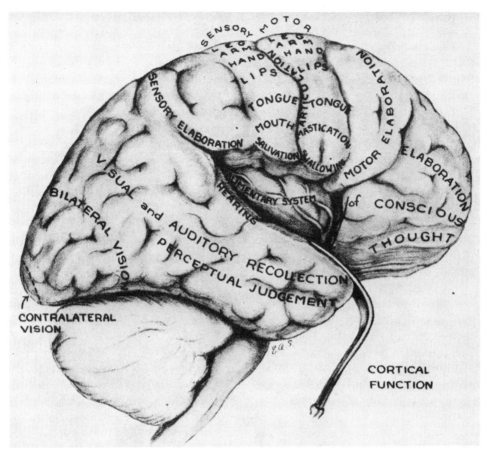

Figure 4.5.   Cortical function. This illustration will serve as a summary restatement of conclusions, some hypothetical (e.g., the elaboration zones), others firmly established. The suggestion that the anterior portion of the occipital cortex is related to both fields of vision rather than to one alone is derived from the results of stimulation. (Reprinted with permission from W. Penfield and T. Rasmussen: *The Cerebral Cortex of Man*. New York, Hafner Publishing, 1968.)

fore, they postulate that the organization of the temporal cortex is evidently different from that of other areas of the brain. For the reader's information, Penfield and Rasmussen's chart of the areas of the brain where various functions are considered to be localized is shown in Figure 4.5.

Fedio and Van Buren (1974) duplicated the Penfield and Roberts experiments and described a functional hierarchy in the left hemisphere with memory as a common process. First, immediate memory is affected when there is minor insult, but with severe interference the basic machinery of naming simple objects is disturbed. The primary memory system is considered to be inti-

mately linked with the anterior temporal lobe, whereas the posterior temporoparietal cortex may support secondary memory.

Midbrain's Function as a Binaural Integration Mechanism and the Mediator of Lateralization Phenomena.   Two-ear fusion was first demonstrated by Matzker (1959) by means of a dichotic integration test. In one ear of normal listeners he presented a speech signal through a 500–800 Hz band-pass filter, and in the other ear the same speech signal through an 1815–2500 Hz filter. Neither band could be discriminated alone, but when both were presented dichotically, frequency fusion occurred and speech sounded normal. When patients with later-demonstrated, postmortem degeneration of ganglion cells through the olivary regions were given these tests, they made many errors. It appears that integration of binaural signals occurs at a low level in the olivary complex.

The psychophysical judgment of sidedness, or localization of auditory stimuli, is mediated at the level of the accessory superior olivary complex, according to Hall (1965). Hall considers that the superior olivary nucleus can be regarded as a transducer that converts differences of interaural time and intensity into differences of the number of cells excited in the left and right accessory nuclei. On anesthetized cats, he measured the spike discharges in the nucleus as related to click stimuli that were presented in various time and intensity configurations. He found that time and intensity configurations did, indeed, affect the number of cells excited in the superior nucleus. The manner of excitation was consistent with results from psychophysical experiments in humans on binaural localization (Deatherage and Hirsh, 1959).

It appears, however, that in humans the interaction of the auditory temporal lobe is requisite to localization-lateralization ability—or that the transaction required in reporting the sidedness sensation depends on an intact temporal lobe. Sanchez-Longo and Forster (1958) showed that patients with diseased temporal lobes had poor abilities in localizing sound in sound field when it arrived first to the ear contralateral to the lesion. Matzker (1959) demonstrated that accurate lateralization of sine wave pulses, presented dichotically under earphones with time leads, occurred in normal listeners when the time delays were as small as 0.018 msec. But in patients with temporal lobe lesions, the lateralization reports were greatly reduced in accuracy.

Cullen and Thompson (1973) confirmed the site of function operative in this test by comparing normal test scores with those of temporal-lobectomized patients. They used word lists at 60 dB SPL and filtered noise at 63 dB SPL in the test ear. This combination reduced the discrimination in normals to 40% and that of the patients to about 33%. (The patients with lesions had poorer discrimination scores in all tests.) But when out-of-phase masking was introduced into the ear contralateral to the test ear, both normals and lobectomized patients showed almost equal gains in discrimination of the words. Cullen and Thompson proposed that this experiment indicates that release phenomena are mediated by two-ear interaction at the subthalamic level, subserved by the same neural mechanisms that play a role in the lateralization-localization phenomena described above. If the auditory cortex were active in suppressing signal pathways for speech, it would be expected that much poorer release scores would be obtained.

Bocca and Calearo (1963) presented classic studies on the use of distorted speech tests in identifying the level of interruption in the auditory pathway. They applied the following tests to normal people and to patients with unilateral temporal lobe tumors.

- *Low-pass filtered speech tests using list of 10 disyllabic meaningful words sent through a low-pass filter that eliminated the frequencies above 800 Hz.* The temporal lobe patients showed markedly reduced discrimination scores in the ear contralateral to the lesion. Normals elicited scores of 70–80%, whereas the patients with tumors gave scores of 50% in the contralateral ear and 65–75% in the ipsilateral ear. The scores for filtered speech tests were consistently lower in the right ear than the left, both preoperatively and postoperatively.

- *Time-compressed speech in which speech is speeded up on a tape recorder, leaving the acoustic spectrum intact.* Although Bocca and Calearo found reduced discrimination scores on this test in ears contralateral to temporal lobe lesions, the results were not as significant as those for frequency-distorted speech.

● *Interrupted speech in which the speech signal is either electronically chopped or blank pieces of tape are interposed between segments of the recorded speech.* Bocca and Calearo found no reduction of discrimination scores on temporal lobe patients who were given this task, indicating that the test assesses brainstem function rather than cortical integration. Berlin and Lowe (1972) indicate that in patients with brainstem lesions, periodic interruption of the speech signal does produce lowered discrimination scores. It is therefore evident that interrupted speech tests provide another tool for assessing brainstem function but that frequency-distorted speech and time-compressed speech stress the cortical level of the auditory pathways.

Dyslexia. That reading is both a simple and a complex task has been brought to our attention by Dr. Sandy Friel-Patti of the Callier Hearing and Speech Center of Dallas. She has been kind enough to share her thoughts and materials with us for this discussion. Learning to read is a major problem for a significant portion of children who, except for their inability to read, appear to have normal cognitive and behavioral abilities. The identification of specific developmental dyslexia from among the population of poor readers is extremely difficult because there is no single clinical factor, nor clear-cut syndrome associated with dyslexia. These children, by definition, represent the extreme lower end of the continuum of reading disabilities (Reid and Hresko, 1981).

A child learning to read must be able to segment words into their phonetic elements and relate them to the graphic symbols. The child must then retrieve the meaning from personal lexicon inventory and assign the syntactic relationship of the word to the other words in the sentence. Finally, the child must use knowledge of the word to make inferences in order to comprehend the text (Snyder, 1980). Thus, the linguistic nature of reading implies that there is some-

thing shared between written and oral language. In fact, the semantic, syntactic, phonologic structures and pragmatic rules are the linguistic core of language used in both print and speech.

Reading ability is understood in terms of the cognitive and linguistic processes involved. Cognitive capabilities set some limits on reading achievement. An important perspective on reading ability is that it reflects essential language processes. The linguistic components of reading are rather intricate: There are both important similarities and differences between spoken and written language that derive from the physical design of the signal and the social design of the message context.

A number of studies have been published to lend strong support to the contention that the best foundation for reading readiness is a good oral language base—which also leads to the conclusion that children with oral language problems are also at risk for problems with written language. For example, Vogel (1974) reported that a group of dyslexic second graders were deficient in oral syntax when compared with normal control subjects. Semel and Wiig (1975) reported quantitative reductions in both the comprehension and expression of syntactic structure for children with learning disabilities. DeHirsch (1974) argued that much of the difficulty youngsters have with reading can be traced to early trouble with the processing of oral language.

The relation between reading dysfunction and auditory skills may be more closely dependent than previously thought. Zigmund (1966, 1973) was able to show that dyslexia may be related specifically to auditory problems. She compared paired associate learning of normal children with that of children with reading disabilities. Her evidence showed that the dyslexic children organized and used psychologic processes in a different way, on the basis of differences in auditory integration abilities.

Evans (1969) found that skill in auditory-visual and visual-auditory sensory integrations was positively correlated with reading achievement; poor readers were significantly impaired in these integrative skills. He suggests that attention should be paid to auditory function in remedial reading classes.

Can one predict reading dysfunction on the basis of any known auditory tests? Some research suggests that it can be done. DeHirsch et al. (1966) found two auditory perception tasks that made a significant contribution to her predictive reading index: the Wepman Auditory Discrimination Test and the Imitation of Tapped-out Patterns Test. Dykstra (1966) found five measures that contribute to a predictive reading index: (1) discrimination between the difference between initial sounds of words (pat-bat), (2) identification of the rhyming elements in the final sounds of words, (3) identification of correct pronunciation of words, (4) use of auditory clues with context clues to identify unfamiliar words, and (5) discrimination between the differences in final consonants and rhymes.

The Illinois Test of Psycholinguistic Abilities (Kirk et al., 1968) subtests on auditory short-term memory and grammatic closure have been shown to identify reading disabilities.

One must appreciate the direct relationship between previous language experience and the learning of reading. When children come to the reading-learning task with inadequate previous language, as many of the hearing-impaired do, reading becomes a laborious process. As Lenneberg (1967) points out, "the deaf come in contact with language at an age when other children have fully mastered this skill and when perhaps the most important formative period for language establishment is already on the decline."

How then should reading be taught to a child who has not had adequate previous language experience? The solution in many schools has been to teach reading through theoretical grammar—the use of sentences learned through the drilling of nouns, verbs, adjectives, and their place in the language structure. Lenneberg calls this "a

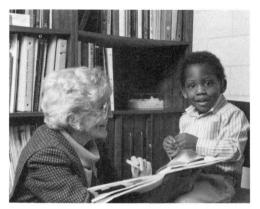

Figure 4.6. Language and speech development is a life-long task for the hearing-impaired child.

situation in which the children are on the one hand quantitatively deprived of a large body of examples, and on the other hand are immediately given a metalanguage, a language about the language which they do not have." Although we know the extent of language retardation in the deaf population at large, the wonder is that their level of achievement is as high as it is (Fig. 4.6).

Geschwind (1962) notes that the brain lesion producing alexia usually destroys color-naming ability but does not affect the ability to name objects and numbers. He suggests that the reason is that objects are learned through multisensory associations including tactile, auditory, kinesthetic, and olfactory sensations. Numbers are learned originally by using our fingers. But both letter-naming and color-naming involve purely arbitrary connections between the auditioned name and the visualized letter configuration. Objects exist as separate entities in the world; letters do not. To make the connection between letters and a name (auditorialized), one must proceed from the purely visual configuration directly to the name—a fairly tenuous pathway from one section of the brain to another. Any slight disruption of this connection could result in dyslexia. But even if the visual-language connections are destroyed, objects can be named because the large numbers of other sensory modes that have been trained allow alternate anatomic routes to be taken.

Confirmation of this theory is found in reports of a few people with brain lesions who had formerly been able to read both English and Chinese ideographic language. These people, posttrauma, lost the ability to read phonetic English but were able to read the ideographic language. The latter uses symbols related to objects and apparently stimulates more learned sensory and motor associations (Gardner, 1973).

Rozin et al. (1971) applied this theory to therapeutic procedures for severely dyslexic children. They gave English meanings to 30 different Chinese ideograms and were successful in teaching eight second-grade children to read them in a few hours. They recommend that these children initially be given characters that represent words rather than sounds and that a transition be made through a system of syllables each representing a phoneme in one configuration.

Etiology of Auditory Language Learning Disorder. Etiology is of utmost significance in any consideration of auditory language learning problems. A review of the possible etiologies may give further direction to planning for therapy.

Organic Lesions. The presence of one or more of the following factors in conjunction with a learning disorder is the only presumptive evidence that organicity may be present.

• History of disease with neurologic insult: meningitis, encephalitis, or diseases with high fever producing neurologic sequelae that are measurable.

• History of neonatal trauma, with neurologic sequelae: anoxia or birth injury producing CNS symptoms that are measurable.

• History of head trauma: actual blow or wound to the head resulting in measurable CNS symptoms.

• Any of the following behavioral symptoms accompanying one of the above histories:

  a. *Disordered behavior.* Overactivity that is characterized by lack of clear direction, focus, or object.

  b. *Short attention span.* Sometimes easily distractible, other times perseverative.

  c. *Emotional lability.* Rapid shifts of mood such as sudden tantrums.

  d. *Social incompetence.* Clumsiness in games with children and aggressive or withdrawal behavior.

  e. *Defective work habits.* Variation in pursuing tasks, either persistently or unevenly.

  f. *Impulsiveness and meddlesomeness.* Inability to keep from touching and handling objects, sometimes destructively.

Environmental Deprivation. Several environmental factors may be present singly or in concert, resulting in a deprivation of language experience during the critical period from birth to 2 years.

• *Lack of adequate stimulation.* As demonstrated by Dennis (1973), and Uzgiris (1970), exposure to low quality of language or reduced frequency of speaking has the same effect on language skills that auditory sensory deprivation has. Yarrow et al. (1971) reported a careful study that identified the great effect that environmental influences in early infancy have on what they call cognitive-motivational functions. We have shown earlier in our discussion of optimal periods that the language deprivation effects of early experiential deprivation appear to be irreversible.

The rat studies of Hebb (1947) confirmed his theory that impaired early experience produces permanent changes in the structure of the cerebral cortex. His studies showed that there is a lasting effect on infant experience in the problem-solving of the adult rat. Forgus (1954) formulated this theory clearly, stating that "the organization of adult behavior is largely determined by the quality of infant experience and learning."

Wachs et al. (1971) stated, as a result of a study of cognitive development of underprivileged children, that "infants raised in slum environments will show significantly slower development at a much earlier age than previously suspected . . . differences that appear as early as 11 months and which increase from 18 months on." They suggest that programs such as Head Start may be reaching these children 3 years too late.

Similar findings were made by Messer and Lewis (1970) who found that not only did lower-class 13 month old children vocalize less than middle-class peers, but they were also less mobile in the playroom. Understimulation produces apathy and reduced language levels. Such children may end up in language learning classes.

- *Sensory overloading.* Lest we become too zealous in stimulating young children auditorally, there is a warning in some studies that too much stimulation is possible. Wachs et al. (1971) found that high-intensity stimulation from which the infant cannot escape and involuntary exposure to an excessive variety of circumstances are responsible for lower levels of cognitive development. In this case, stimulus bombardment rather than stimulus deprivation is shown to be the factor causing developmental problems.

  Another study tested children for auditory discrimination and for reading level and related these scores to the degree of noise levels in their homes (Cohen et al., 1973). Children in the second to the fifth grade who had resided in an apartment complex at least 4 years were compared. The apartments in the upper levels (32 floors) were shown to have 14–16 dB higher noise levels than those in the lower floors, and the children living there had significantly poorer auditory discrimination and reading scores than the children living in the lower levels. The authors stated that "the longer a child must endure noise[,] the more likely he [or she] is to ignore all sounds, whether relevant or not. A consequence . . . is a failure to learn to discriminate speech-relevant clues at a time which may be optimal for such learning."

The reason for reduced discrimination abilities may be found in studies comparing children's auditory thresholds in nonideal testing conditions ("slightly noisy rooms"), with the same tests in sound-treated rooms. Goldman and Sanders (1969) found that high-school graduates from low socioeconomic backgrounds seemed unusually unresponsive to the screening test in the nonideal testing condition. They believed that "the presence of high noise levels frequently found in the disadvantaged home environment might interfere with the acquisition by the child of the ability to extract an auditory signal from a competing background." Nober (1973) identified a relationship between reading skills and discrimination in noise by giving the Wepman Auditory Discrimination Test to three groups of children: normal, speech-deficient, and reading-deficient. The tests were given both in quiet and in 65 dBA of tape-recorded classroom noise. He found that the reading-deficient child performed significantly lower in noise than in quiet.

The theme recurs in other studies, namely, that children raised in noise environments do not respond as well in a distracting situation as their peers from quiet homes (Deutsch, 1964; Clark and Richards, 1966). In effect, such conditions constitute a sensory deprivation just as surely as do hearing loss and the lack of high-quality language stimulation.

- *Malnutrition.* Three appalling sequelae have been reported from malnutrition during early years and even weeks of life.
  a. *Cognitive defects and apathy.* Eichenwald and Fry (1969) showed that chronically undernourished children

scored low on the Gesell developmental quotient as well as on measures of visual, haptic, and kinesthetic integration The same results were shown in a controlled study of two Mexican child populations by Lewin (1975). A group of severely malnourished infants showed significant lag in language and verbal-concept formation by 6 months, as compared with their well-nourished peers, a lag that became larger by 3 years. This finding of increasing differences with age seems to be a constant theme in all deprivation studies, suggesting that if no intervention occurs, the gap between the deprived child and the normal child will continue to widen until adulthood.

b. *Possible CNS effects.* Eichenwald and Fry (1969) state that inadequate feeding of pyridoxal phosphate results in a series of changes in the physiologic function of the brain within 6 weeks. If the deficit continues for a longer period, alterations of cerebral function occur, resulting in severe mental retardation. These data suggest that inadequate protein nutrition or synthesis during brain development could result in changes in function. Crarioto (1966) had made experimental observations confirming these facts.

c. *The possible irreversibility of cognitive and CNS effects.* The Mexican study on malnutrition (Lewin, 1975) observed the children after good nourishment, special training, and care were instituted. The trend line showed that the underfed children remained behind the control group and were not catching up. The one aspect of intellectual development that proved most resistant to special training was short-term memory. This study also analyzed the effects of stimulating home environments versus nonstimulating environment. The results showed the effects of poor stimulation on intelligence, with the greatest deficit coming from both malnourishment and poor environment.

Minimal Auditory Deprivation Syndrome. The impact on language skills of more severe hearing losses is well-known and documented. But the impact of slight hearing loss in early childhood has only recently been recognized. In Chapter 1, we describe this syndrome and its effect on language skills at older ages. What should be considered is the possible permanent effects on the brain of early auditory deprivation. Just as the animal studies on experimental deprivation showed CNS correlates, so do similar studies on sensory deprivation of hearing. Webster and Webster (1977) created conductive hearing losses operatively in mice at 3 days of age. They also deprived litters of mice of sound by surgically closing the mother's larynx and rearing them in a sound-attenuated chamber. These two groups, plus a normal control group, were sacrificed at 45 days, and their brains were examined. Both the operated group and the deprived group were found to have central morphologic defects significantly different from the control group.

Remediation. The question that remains is whether remediation will be effective in restoring or creating CNS connections. What is not indicated is specific teaching of sounds or letters or structures one at a time, for neither phonemes nor words nor phrases are the basic unit of language (Rees, 1973); sentences are the essential unit that should be taught. Nor should linguistic rules be taught formally. Syntactic, morphologic, phonologic, semantic rules are best facilitated, not learned. These rules seem to be innate in the child, just as pecking is innate in chickens. The child has to hear models and act on them in order to construct infinite utterances from the finite rules. Thus the child's language needs not to be taught but to be guided. Contrived language lessons are not useful;

rather, materials and speech from the real world are preferred.

Most logical is the utilization of techniques that will facilitate the child's construction of language:

- *Parallel talk*. Using language within the child's ability to talk about what the child is doing.
- *Expansion*. Taking the child's utterance and expanding it to grammatically acceptable model forms.
- *Modeling*. Responding to the child's utterance with an unrelated linguistic structure that maintains the stream of thought.

The kinds of language structures that are used in such a program should be on a slightly higher level than those in the child's repertoire. A sound knowledge of normal language development is requisite to dealing with children on this basis.

SUMMARY

In summary, we have questioned whether language remediation based on an assumption of specific central brain damage in most of the affected children is a valid base of therapy when CNS symptoms are not present. The various measurable auditory subskills appear to be symptoms of language dysfunction, not the cause. What must be considered is the range of possible etiologies of language dysfunction. When etiologies are considered, a development approach to many of the problems becomes most logical. The presumptive causes of auditory language learning disorders include diagnosed brain trauma or insult, environmental deprivation, and minimal auditory deprivation in early life. Language facilitation emerges as the appropriate therapy when a developmental theory is accepted.

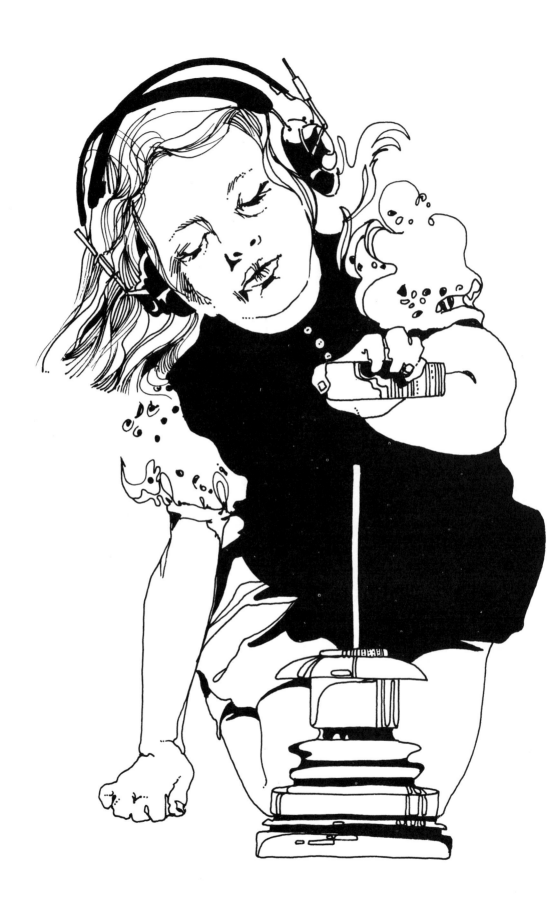

CHAPTER 5

Behavioral Hearing Testing of Children

Modern technology has greatly increased the number of options available to test the hearing of infants and young children. However, regardless of how sophisticated testing techniques become, there will always be need for the behavioral hearing evaluation, since many of the newer procedures require expensive equipment or lengthy time commitment. Audiologists must be cautioned regarding the false sense of confidence provided by hearing test results obtained with physiologic "objective" techniques. Every clinician must be well-versed in the understanding and the application of basic behavioral pediatric audiometry. With experience in pediatric audiology, a battery of special testing procedures becomes available for use in the daily clinical setting, and decisions need to be made for cost- and time-effective protocols to be used with each infant and child. Electrophysiologic tests can be used to estimate auditory sensitivity but are not true tests of hearing and thus should never be a substitute for behavioral audiometry in children.

Auditory evaluation of hearing in children should not be considered "completed" until earphone thresholds are obtained for octave interval frequencies from 250 to 4000 Hz in each ear. All procedures might be needed to obtain this final result, and more than one test session may be necessary to achieve the "completed" hearing examination. Parents may need to be advised that the pediatric hearing examination, especially when hearing impairment is suspected, is an ongoing, age-specific activity, so that as the child grows older, more accurate hearing results can be obtained.

Jerger and Hayes (1976) advocate use of the cross-check principle in pediatric audiometry. They caution that simple behavioral observation of auditory behavior in children can be misleading and result in misdiagnosis of auditory problems and, ultimately, mismanagement of the hearing-impaired child. The cross-check principle uses physiologic test procedures, especially brainstem evoked response (BSER) audiometry and acoustic immittance procedures as a cross-check of behavioral test results. They reason that behavioral test results need to be confirmed by an independent test measure to reduce the potential errors of using behavioral results alone. Jerger and Hayes recommend a pediatric test battery that includes behavioral measurements, BSER audiometry, and acoustic immittance measures. In most cases, thorough immittance audiometry will serve as a cross-check for behavioral audiometry. However, when these two measures are in disagreement, BSER should be used to resolve the controversy. BSER and immittance audiometry are discussed in Chapter 6.

The experience of the clinician is probably the main key to successful evaluation of the difficult-to-test child. A broad test battery approach with children is the best scheme of all, and clinicians who work with pediatric patients must be skilled in a wide variety of testing paradigms utilizing sound field and earphone measurements.

Testing Methods. Considerable progress has been made in recent years to develop better, more accurate means to evaluate hearing in infants and young children. Wilson and Thompson (1984) classified the behavioral audiologic testing of children into two major divisions: (*1*) techniques used without reinforcement, and (*2*) procedures based on reinforcement of the infant or child's responses. Since the early 1970s, considerable research has been devoted to defining the stimulus-response characteristics that may be most effectively used in the assessment of a child's hearing abilities. The techniques utilized that do not incorporate reinforcement principles are known as behavioral observation audiometry (BOA). Procedures that use reinforcement to develop repeatable responses are known as conditioned audiometry, further described by the type of reinforcement used, such as visual reinforcement audiometry (VRA).

BOA is typically limited to infants and young children between 6 and 12 months of age, although the techniques may be used to screen the hearing of children through 24 months of age. Diefendorf (1988) describes BOA as an active response from an infant or toddler passively involved in the task at hand. A typical example of this technique is the presentation of an auditory stimulus to a lightly sleeping infant while observing behavioral changes that are time-locked to the stimulus presentation. Limitations to BOA include rapid habituation of the response, since the reinforcement used and the response magnitude are dependent upon many variables, including state of the infant or child, the parameters of the acoustic stimulus, the definition of what behavior constitutes an acceptable "response," and subjective determination by the audiologist as to whether a "response" occurred or not.

The conditioning approach to assessing hearing levels in infants and children utilizes a stimulus-response-reinforcement paradigm to elicit repeatable responses. In these procedures, the response is clearly defined and cued by the presentation of auditory stimulus. The response is actually strengthened through the use of various reinforcements. In this approach, the infant or child is an active participant in the testing situation. Although studies have shown that infants as young as 6 months can be

evaluated with conditioning techniques, typically these techniques are used with children between 12 and 48 months of age. As an example of a conditioning technique, VRA is used to reinforce the head-turning, localization response of an infant or child with an attractive, illuminated stimulus.

The use of behavioral and conditioning procedures with infants and young children may lack sufficient precision to establish valid auditory sensitivity thresholds. Accordingly, Matkin (1977) suggested the use of *minimum response level* to describe the lowest intensity of auditory stimulus that produces the desired response. Use of the term "minimal response level" rather than "auditory threshold" for pediatric hearing evaluations serves as a reminder that improvement in response behavior might be anticipated as the child matures.

QUESTIONING THE PARENTS

Audiologists can contribute, in addition to the actual hearing test, insight into the auditory and oral behavior of the child. No one understands better than the experienced clinician the effect of a certain degree of loss on the child's behavior and how the history of auditory development relates to the onset and degree of loss. The audiologist's time will most valuably be spent in analyzing these aspects of the child's history. Therefore, the sequence of the audiologic session can be as follows:

1. Question the parents as to the chief concern that precipitated the visit: "Who referred the child?" "Do you believe your child has problems in hearing?"
2. Administer a pediatric audiology test battery to determine if the child has hearing within normal limits or if a hearing loss is present.
3. If a hearing loss appears evident, query the parent as to the child's auditory and oral development:
   - *At 0–4 Months.* When the infant was sleeping quietly, did sudden noises awaken the baby momentarily? Did the infant jump to sudden loud noises?

- *At 4–7 Months.* Did the baby begin at 4 months to turn toward sounds that were out of sight? Did the infant repetitively babble a large variety of sounds at 5 and 6 months? By 7 months did the baby turn directly to sounds or voices that were out of sight? What kinds of babbling sounds were made at 6 and 7 months? Could the infant sit alone at 6 months?
- *At 7–9 Months.* Did the baby turn to find the source of sounds out of direct sight? Did the baby gurgle or coo to voices or sounds that the baby could not see? Did the baby make sounds with rising and falling inflections?
- *At 9–13 Months.* Did the baby turn and find a sound coming from behind? Did the infant begin to imitate some sounds and have a large variety of different sounds? Were some of them consonant sounds (buh, guh, duh)? Did the baby say "ma-ma-ma-ma" or just "mama?" What specific sounds did the baby say?
- *At 13–24 Months.* Did the toddler hear you when you called from another room? Did the toddler make a noise in response or come to you? What other words or sounds than "mama" were made? Did the voice sound normal?

(From this questioning and from listening to the child's present voice quality and speech, the audiologist can derive clues as to the onset of the hearing loss and its degree. If the voice quality at the present time is strident and only vowel sounds are made, an early severe hearing loss would be suspected. If the voice quality is good, in the presence of an evidently severe loss, a later onset would be suspected. Particularly if the child has some words or even sounds in normal intonation, a later onset is suggested. Such clues are helpful in determining the etiology and onset of the hearing loss.)

4. To help in understanding the etiology of the hearing loss, an informal, brief case history may reveal what aspects should be pursued in detail. Table 5.1 contains a list of questions that comprise a basic history that includes the primary items that place a child at risk for hearing loss. Table 5.2 presents a more detailed medical assessment questionnaire for children with sensorineural hearing impairment.

5. Table 5.3 shows the rapid development checklist approved by the American Academy of Pediatrics. Care should be taken in interpreting some of the landmarks as indicative of normal hearing (see Chapter 4 for a discussion of babbling development in normal-hearing and hearing-impaired babies). A deaf infant coos and chuckles quite normally at 2–3 months. He laughs aloud at 4 months, he can babble in two sounds before 6 months, he says something like "ma-ma" at 9 months, and he may have a vocalization that sounds like "da-da" by 12 months. This can be misleading. The parents of one deaf child in our clinic insisted that their boy had normal hearing at 1 year of age because, they reported, he said "mama" and "dada." Yet polytomograms of the child's ears showed congenital gross bony abnormalities of the inner ears that were present at birth and precluded the possibility of any hearing at birth. It is well to view such reports of early speaking with healthy skepticism and in light of documented research studies such as Stoel-Gammon and Otomo (1986) and Kent et al. (1987).

YOU AND THE CHILD

Too often we have heard audiologists say, "I don't like to work with younger children—I can't depend on their responses, and they are too inconsistent to be relied upon." Nothing could be less true. Babies do just what they are supposed to do; the clinician often does not. The clinician has to give the right stimulus in the right structured situation in order to get the right response. There are no poorly responding ba-

Table 5.1.
Audiological Case History Questionnaire for Parents of Children with Hearing Loss

 I. Chief complaint _____
   When was problem first noted? _____
   Extent of problem _____
   Previous examinations and evaluations _____
   _____

 II. Prenatal history
   Exposure to viral diseases during pregnancy? _____
   Which viral disorder? _____
   During which pregnancy month? _____
   Drugs during pregnancy? _____
   Trauma during pregnancy? _____
 III. Birth history
   Gestation age at birth _____
   Birth weight _____ Bilirubin level high? _____
   Asphyxia? _____ Meningitis? _____
 IV. Family history
   Childhood deafness in family? _____
      Relationship to patient _____
   Bith defect or abnormalities _____
      In any other relatives? _____
 V. Developmental history
   Age of first smile response? _____
   Age when sat up alone? _____
   Age when first crawled? _____
   Age of "stranger anxiety?" _____
   Age of walking? _____
 VI. Physical history
   Cleft lip or palate _____ Submucous cleft _____
   Low-set ears _____ Poorly formed ears _____
   High fevers with illness _____ Seizures _____
   Ear infections _____ How many? _____
   Previous treatment for ear conditions? _____
   _____

 VII. What do you (parents) really think caused this hearing problem? _____

   Name of child's pediatrician _____
   Names of other physicians who have seen this child _____
   _____

bies—only inadequately prepared clinicians.

What are the general rules about working with children of all ages? Establish quickly an easy relationship with the parents. Speak pleasantly and relaxedly to them. You will find the child looking back and forth between you two, and finally becoming content that all is well, the child too will relax. In other words, the child absorbs the cathexis between you and the parents and becomes at ease. Many clinicians prefer to work with a child alone without the parents on hand. This is fine if you have enough time to establish a relationship with the child. It may be quicker and easier to use the parents in the testing situation; the child is less apprehensive and stays relaxed during the session. Parents are usually quite cooperative and entirely rational.

Tell the child what you want him or her to do—do not ask. In this respect, the very young and the very old are alike, and one handles them both not by asking whether they would like to do something (they never do) but by telling them firmly and pleasantly that this is what they are going to do. Children do just what you expect of them, and if you firmly expect them to do what you want them to, they usually oblige. Occasionally, of course, a child balks and yells like a banshee anyway—you can't win them all. But give it a try—children are a great deal easier to handle than you think.

Table 5.2.
Sensorineural Hearing-Impaired Child Assessment

Name _____
Age _____
Date of Birth _____
Hospital # _____
Age child identified by M.D. (months) _____
Age suspected of loss by mother (months) _____

FAMILY HISTORY

Were parents relatives before marriage	Yes	No
Family history of kidney disease	Yes	No
Family history of thyroid problems	Yes	No
Family history of progressive blindness	Yes	No
Family history of previous stillbirths or miscarriages	Yes	No
Family history of hearing loss	Yes	No
Another affected child in family	Yes	No
Mother worked outside home	Yes	No
Specify _____		
Father worked during pregnancy	Yes	No
Specify _____		

MATERNAL FACTORS

Drugs (inc. antibiotics)	Yes	No
Specify _____		
Exposure to chemicals	Yes	No
Specify _____		
Exposure to radiation	Yes	No
Specify _____		
Amniocentesis	Yes	No
Rh immunoglobulin given Rh or ABO incompatible	Yes	No
Maternal illness during pregnancy	Yes	No
Specify _____		
Bleeding	Yes	No
Anemia	Yes	No
Diabetes	Yes	No
Toxemia	Yes	No
Paternal illness during pregnancy	Yes	No
Specify _____		

During pregnancy, mother exposed to:

Measles	Yes	No
Mumps	Yes	No
Chickenpox	Yes	No
German measles	Yes	No

During pregnancy, mother diagnosed with:

Syphilis	Yes	No
Herpes virus	Yes	No
Influenza	Yes	No
Cytomegalovirus (CMV)	Yes	No
Toxoplasmosis	Yes	No
Other	Yes	No
Specify _____		
_____		
_____		

DELIVERY/LABOR

Full-term pregnancy	Yes	No
Labor induced	Yes	No
Labor less than 3 hr	Yes	No
Labor longer than 24 hr	Yes	No
Premature membrane rupture	Yes	No
Bleeding	Yes	No
Forceps/assisted delivery	Yes	No
Cesarean section	Yes	No
Other	Yes	No
Specify _____		
_____		

INFANT/NEWBORN FACTORS

Small birthweight (<2 kg/5 lb)	Yes	No
Birthweight (lb/oz) _____		
Apgar low at birth	Yes	No
In an intensive care unit	Yes	No
How long (wk) _____		
Breathing problems	Yes	No
O_2 given	Yes	No
How long (wk) _____		
Bilirubin >15 mg/100 ml	Yes	No
Congenital rubella	Yes	No
Defect of ear, nose, throat	Yes	No
Specify _____		
Congenital heart disease	Yes	No
Drugs (inc. antibiotics)	Yes	No
Specify _____		
Exposure to chemicals	Yes	No
Specify _____		
Exposure to radiation	Yes	No
Specify _____		
Paralysis	Yes	No
Seizures	Yes	No
Septicemia	Yes	No

INFANT/CHILDHOOD HISTORY

Eye problems	Yes	No
Specify _____		
Balance/gait/incoordination		
Dizziness problems	Yes	No
Cerebral palsy	Yes	No
Seizures	Yes	No
Head trauma/skull	Yes	No

Ever hospitalized for:

Meningitis	Yes	No
Encephalitis	Yes	No
Measles	Yes	No
Influenza	Yes	No
Rubella	Yes	No
CMV	Yes	No
Chickenpox	Yes	No
Septicemia	Yes	No
Diabetes	Yes	No
Sickle cell disease	Yes	No
Other (including conductive loss)	Yes	No
Specify _____		
_____		
_____		

Table 5.3.
Rapid Developmental Screening Checklist[a,b]

NAME:	D.O.B.:	1st Visit:

AGE		DATE
1 mo:	Can he raise his head from the surface in the prone position?	Yes No
	Does he regard your face while you are in his direct line of vision?	Yes No
2 mo:	Does he smile and coo?	Yes No
3 mo:	Does he follow a moving object?	Yes No
	Does he hold his head erect?	Yes No
4 mo:	Will he hold a rattle?	Yes No
	Does he laugh aloud?	Yes No
5 mo:	Can he reach for and hold objects?	Yes No
6 mo:	Can he turn over?	Yes No
	Does he turn toward sounds?	Yes No
	Will he sit with a little support (with one hand)?	Yes No
7 mo:	Can he transfer an object from one hand to another?	Yes No
	Can he sit momentarily without support?	Yes No
8 mo:	Can he sit steadily for about 5 minutes?	Yes No
9 mo:	Can he say "ma-ma" or "da-da"?	Yes No
10 mo:	Can he pull himself up at the side of his crib or playpen?	Yes No
11 mo:	Can he cruise around his playpen or crib, or walk holding onto furniture?	Yes No
12 mo:	Can he wave bye-bye?	Yes No
	Can he walk with one hand held?	Yes No
	Does he have a two-word vocabulary?	Yes No
15 mo:	Can he walk by himself?	Yes No
	Can he indicate his wants by pointing and grunting?	Yes No
18 mo:	Can he build a tower of three blocks?	Yes No
	Does he say six words?	Yes No
24 mo:	Can he run?	Yes No
	Can he walk up and down stairs holding rail?	Yes No
	Can he express himself (occasionally) in a two-word sentence?	Yes No
2½ yr:	Can he jump lifting both feet off the ground?	Yes No
	Can he build a tower of six blocks?	Yes No
	Can he point to parts of his body on command?	Yes No
3 yr:	Can he follow two commands involving "on," "under," or "behind" (without gestures?)	Yes No
	Can he build a tower of nine blocks?	Yes No
	Does he know his first name?	Yes No
	Can he copy a circle?	Yes No
4 yr:	Can he stand on one foot?	Yes No
	Can he copy a cross?	Yes No
	Does he use the past tense, properly?	Yes No
5 yr:	Can he follow three commands?	Yes No
	Can he copy a square?	Yes No
	Can he skip?	Yes No

[a]Developed by the Committee on Children with Handicaps, American Academy of Pediatrics, New York Chapter 3, District II.
[b]This checklist is a compilation of developmental landmarks matched against the age of the child. These are in easily scored question form and may be checked "Yes" or "No." "No" responses at the appropriate age may constitute a signal indicating a possible developmental lag. If there is a substantial deviation from these values, then the child should be evaluated more carefully, taking into consideration the wide variability of developmental landmarks. (Adjust for prematurity, prior to 2 years, by subtracting the time of prematurity from the age of the child, i.e., a 2-month-old infant who was 1 month premature should be evaluated as a month-old infant.)

Develop a staunch and fervid belief that when children hear a sound, they will react in a stereotyped way that is consistent with their level of mental functioning. This holds true for the hearing-impaired child as well as for the normal-hearing child. The child with a threshold of 80 dB for a given sound will respond at 85 dB like the normal-hearing child who hears the same sound at 5 dB above the normal-hearing threshold. A 2 year old cognitively impaired child with a mental age of 1 year will respond near his or her threshold in the way a normal-hearing child of 1 year responds near his or her threshold. There is no mystique about observing the hearing-impaired child's responses; the answer, if there is any, is to become confidently familiar with the auditory behavior of normal-hearing children so that the lack of normal responses will be im-

Table 5.4.
Auditory Behavior Index for Infants: Stimulus and Level of Response[a]

Age	Noisemakers (Approx. dB SPL)	Warbled Pure Tones (dB HL)	Speech (dB HL)	Expected Response	Startle to Speech (dB HL)
0–6 wk	50–70	75	40–60	Eye-widening, eye-blink, stirring or arousal from sleep, startle	65
6 wk–4 mo	50–60	70	45	Eye-widening, eye-shift, eye-blink, quieting; beginning rudimentary head-turn by 4 mo	65
4–7 mo	40–50	50	20	Head-turn on lateral plane toward sound; listening attitude	65
7–9 mo	30–40	45	15	Direct localization of sounds to side, indirectly below ear level	65
9–13 mo	25–35	38	10	Direct localization of sounds to side, directly below ear level, indirectly above ear level	65
13–16 mo	25–30	30	5	Direct localization of sound on side, above and below	65
16–21 mo	25	25	5	Direct localization of sound on side, above and below	65
21–24 mo	25	25	5	Direct localization of sound on side, above and below	65

[a]Testing done in a sound room. (Modified with permission from F. McConnell and P. H. Ward: *Deafness in Childhood*, Nashville, Tennessee, Vanderbilt University Press, 1967.)

mediately evident and suggest the need for additional testing.

We would add another principle, at the risk of becoming maudlin—love every child as a human being. The clinician is often hard-put to develop any charitable feelings toward the wall-climber, the temper tantrum expert, the withdrawn child or, in some cases, the syndrome-ridden child with misshapen, contorted face and limbs. The same humanity underlies all these children, the kicker, the screamer, the silent one—all of them humanly acting out their protests at a world that has given them less than it has to others. They too can be loved.

BEHAVIORAL OBSERVATION AUDIOMETRY WITH THE INFANT FROM BIRTH TO 2 YEARS OF AGE

In BOA, the testing of infants and young children is accomplished without reinforcement of responses and rests on the subjective observation of responses under structured conditions. The major advantages to BOA are efficiency in time required and the lack of need for specialized equipment. The disadvantages of BOA include the fact that it is difficult to eliminate tester bias, the responses of infants and young children are quick to reach extinction without reinforcement, and a wide variance of responses are noted in such youngsters. Critics of BOA argue that the technique is useful for initial hearing screening but some form of operant reinforcement audiometry should be used in the establishment of specific hearing threshold data.

The use of noisemakers and sound field signals as acoustic stimuli in evaluating hearing responses in infants and young children is a cornerstone of behavioral observation. Situations and circumstances will exist that require that the audiologist be able to administer and interpret simple behavioral responses to auditory noisemakers. Hearing tests of infants and young children with noisemakers and sound field signals without conditioning and reinforcement is often a first-level indicator of the presence of normal hearing or the suggestion of hearing impairment. Pediatric BOA is certainly the most cost- and time-effective way of evaluating hearing in newborns and children through 2 years of age. The intensity levels and the expected behavioral responses of the normal-hearing newborn to 2 year old child is shown in the Auditory Behavior Index shown in Table 5.4 and in Figures 5.1 and 5.2.

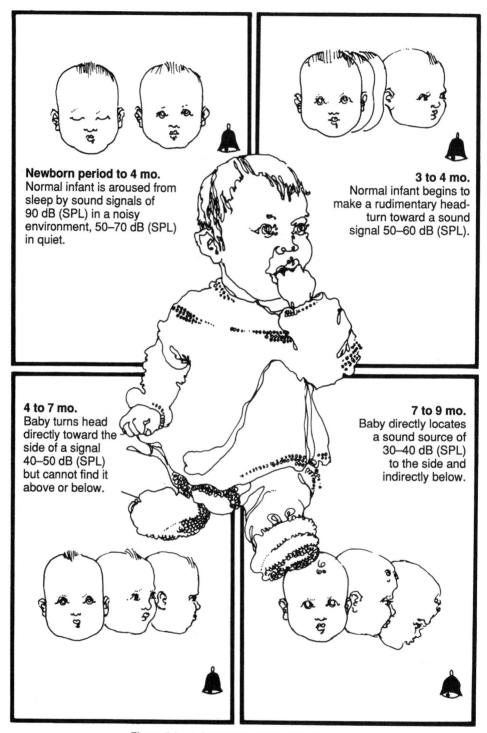

Newborn period to 4 mo.
Normal infant is aroused from sleep by sound signals of 90 dB (SPL) in a noisy environment, 50–70 dB (SPL) in quiet.

3 to 4 mo.
Normal infant begins to make a rudimentary head-turn toward a sound signal 50–60 dB (SPL).

4 to 7 mo.
Baby turns head directly toward the side of a signal 40–50 dB (SPL) but cannot find it above or below.

7 to 9 mo.
Baby directly locates a sound source of 30–40 dB (SPL) to the side and indirectly below.

Figure 5.1. Infant testing: newborn to 9 months.

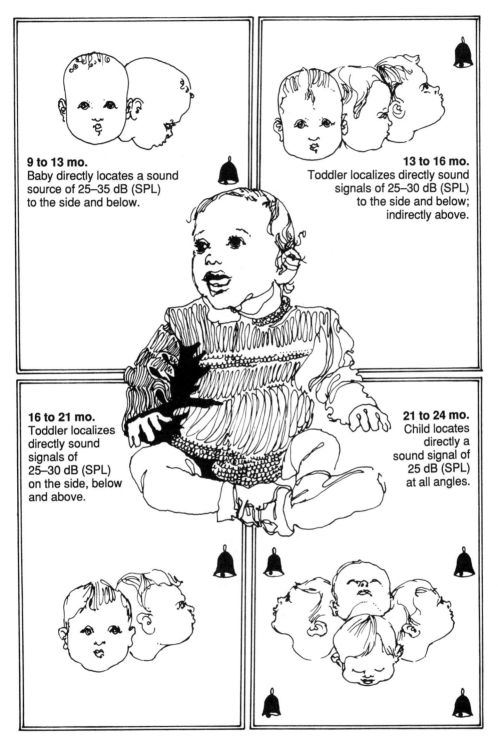

9 to 13 mo.
Baby directly locates a sound source of 25–35 dB (SPL) to the side and below.

13 to 16 mo.
Toddler localizes directly sound signals of 25–30 dB (SPL) to the side and below; indirectly above.

16 to 21 mo.
Toddler localizes directly sound signals of 25–30 dB (SPL) on the side, below and above.

21 to 24 mo.
Child locates directly a sound signal of 25 dB (SPL) at all angles.

Figure 5.2. Infant testing: 9–24 months.

The original concept for an auditory behavior index was developed by Kevin Murphy of Reading, England (1962, 1979). This remarkable observer of infants and children diagrammed the quality of the behavioral responses of children to noisemakers. The value of such an index lies in its description of the normal maturation process that all normal-hearing infants go through during specific periods in their development. Some variability is to be expected around the age periods described for each auditory behavior, but one must be impressed with the consistency and predictability of the age limits at which certain auditory responses are noted.

The auditory responses of infants and young children can also be described in terms of *reflexive* or *attentive* behavior. Reflexive behaviors include the startle (body) response, arm or leg jerks, slow limb movements, the auropalpebral reflex, change in sucking behavior, eye-blinks, and facial twitches. Attentive behaviors are described as quieting responses (decrease in ongoing activity), increase in ongoing activity, breath holding or a change in breathing rate, onset of vocalization, sudden stopping of vocalization, starting or stopping crying, eye widening, searching or localization, head turning as in searching or localizing the sound source, smiling or other change in facial expression, brow furrowing, or shriek of surprise. A commonly seen attentive behavior in response to the presentation of a sound is that the child looks directly at the parent's face as though in expectation of finding the source of the sound.

We urge audiologists not to accept our Auditory Behavior Index as the final word but to work with normal-hearing infants and young children to recognize the expected responses with various noisemakers and sound field auditory stimuli. The value of the Index is enhanced for each clinician by determining individual style of eliciting auditory responses with acoustic stimuli at hand and performing the test on literally hundreds of normal-hearing infants and young children. Only then can the audiolo-

gist feel confident with this simple, but effective, means of separating normal-hearing children from those with possible hearing problems.

For the kinds of responses described above, audiologists generally rely on toy noisemakers or sound field speech and narrowband noise stimuli, with sudden, rapid signal onset. Obviously, the frequency spectrum of such toys is difficult, if not impossible, to control, but the appeal of the sound to youngsters probably has to do with the rich complexity of the frequency spectrum. Some toys, such as a tiny Hindu metal bell, have a higher frequency representation than a baby rattle. Audiologists must be aware that the lack of frequency specificity with toy noisemakers must be recognized as a limitation of this technique. On the other hand, frequency spectrum measurements should be made from each toy noisemaker to define the frequency content of the signal.

Premeasurements of the intensity as a function of distance from the infant's ear is requisite for this procedure. Note that we do not use the term "calibration" of the noisemakers; these toys can obviously not be "calibrated" like an electronic device. However, they must be measured for signal intensity output, at some specific distance typical of the hearing test situation, so that an estimate can be made about the level of the signal necessary to elicit expected behaviors from the infant or child. Typical toys used for auditory localization evaluation include small bells, plastic blocks or rattles with sand inside that can be shaken suddenly, a rubber squeeze toy, and a louder impulse toy, such as a bicycle horn. A commercially available set of preselected noisemakers, with each toy's frequency response and output level measured, is available as shown in Figure 5.3.

A spin-off of the use of the Auditory Behavior Index has been its unexpected value in identifying developmental delay. Zigler (1969) described two theories of childhood maturation in handicapped children that are known as the *developmental theory* and

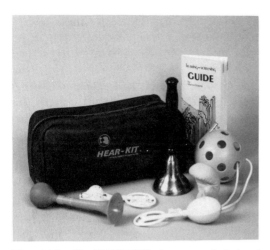

Figure 5.3. The HEAR-KIT features preselected and premeasured toys to use in hearing screening of infants and young children. (Courtesy of BAM World Markets, Englewood, Colorado.)

the *difference theory*. The difference theory predicts that the auditory responsiveness displayed by developmentally delayed children compared with normal children will be unexpected, deviant from the normal, and nonpredictable. The developmental theory assumes that the retarded child passes through the same maturation sequence as the normal child, although much more slowly. Flexer and Gans (1985) have verified the developmental theory for the auditory behavioral testing of multihandicapped children, showing that the expected auditory responses follow the normal sequence of auditory maturation in normal-hearing children but are significantly delayed. Thus, if an 8 month old baby shows only arousal and basic eye-widening to acoustic stimuli but does not show even rudimentary head-turning for localization, his or her auditory behavior is less than expected for the age level. If an 18 month old toddler shows only lateral head-turning localization behavior and does not seek out sound sources presented below or above eye level, the child is performing on a 6–9 month auditory maturation stage.

Further logic suggests that if one can correlate auditory behavior with mental age, with a reasonable level of confidence, then the audiologist who is testing a mentally retarded youngster with a chronologic age of 6 years but a mental age of 2 years or less should be expected to have the auditory responses appropriate to the limited mental age. Thus a 6 year old with an IQ of 60 will not respond with finger-raising behavior but will respond with the auditory localization responses expected from a child of less than 3 years of age. The auditory responses of retarded and developmentally delayed children are much closer to their mental age than to their chronologic age. Wilson and Thompson (1984) state that even though BOA lacks precision as an indicator of hearing thresholds, it is the only available behavioral procedure for some profoundly retarded children. Gans (1987) reports results from BOA minimal response levels used to test 82 profoundly involved handicapped children.

Behavioral Observation Audiometry with the 0–6 Month Old Infant. Typically, infants are presented either in a hospital bassinette or in the arms of a parent. Although reactions to sounds in an awake baby can be observed, as Ling et al. (1970) pointed out, in this condition the chance is too high for observing random responses and judging them to be valid responses to sound. Mencher (1972) reports that the chance of erroneously recording a response from a sleeping baby is about 1%. For these reasons, we prefer to use noisemakers while the infant is in a state of light sleep. It helps, in the observation of responses described below, for the audiologist to be able to see the baby's face clearly, with both ears visible and with all blankets, wraps, coats, etc. peeled off the infant so that responses of the body and limbs will be noted.

In sleeping infants between 0 and 4 months of age, a rather loud sound is usually required to elicit behavioral responses. The only legitimate, acceptable responses to the auditory stimuli need to be easily observable. In clinical practice, the best behavioral response is arousal from the sleep state. By arousal we mean even a brief, transitory movement from the infant that indicates a marked change from the quiet, motionless sleep condition. Acceptable responses include a definite eye-blink immediately following the presentation of the noisemaker stimulus, a slight shudder of the whole body, an opening of the eyes (even briefly), or a marked movement of the body, arms, or legs. The response should be seen within 2 seconds of the noisemaker stimulus presentation in order to be considered valid.

Prior to the presentation of the noisemaker sound, maintaining complete quiet for at least a minute helps to "set the stage" for the sudden onset of the stimulus to evoke a response of large magnitude. Although these noisemaker procedures can be conducted in any situation, the chance for successful observation of clear responses is heightened by performing the evaluation in a quiet background, especially within a sound-treated booth. If the infant is in deep sleep, there is less chance for good behavioral responses than when the baby is in a lighter stage of sleep.

We recommend, following the minute of complete silence, that the toy noisemaker be held motionless within 3 inches of the infant's ear. Naturally, the toy and the motion necessary to create the sound stimulus should carefully be kept out of the baby's visual field. Effort should be made to initiate the sound as quickly as possible, and it may be necessary to maintain the sound stimulus at the same intensity for 2–5 seconds before a response is noted. We follow a specific presentation sequence beginning with the softest (lowest intensity) noisemaker followed sequentially by different and louder noisemakers, ending the test session with the loudest signal to elicit a startle response (Fig. 5.3). The startle response noisemaker is best saved for the final presentation, as this signal may actually frighten the infant into crying (Fig. 5.4). Behavioral responses should be noted with each of the noisemakers, and time should be permitted to elapse between noisemakers to ensure a new, brisk response. If there is

doubt about the presence of a response, the noisemaker can be repeated after a brief period of quiet or can be rotated to be used again later in the sequence. However, these sound stimuli lose their novel effect very quickly, the infants habituate, and their responses soon extinguish. In fact, sometimes a single behavioral response is all that will be made to each noisemaker presentation, so the audiologist must be prepared and alert for accurate observations. If the evaluation with noisemakers takes too long, the baby's sleeping state may change into a deep sleep from which the audiologist must shake the crib, or the infant, to raise the awareness level into the light-sleeping condition again.

It has been our experience that at least 95% of normal-hearing infants—even those at risk for hearing loss—can be quickly identified as having hearing within normal limits during a single test session with careful noisemaker evaluation. Often, babies will "fail" the noisemaker test if conducted in a noise background such as that found in the nursery, but when proper quiet background conditions are established, the same baby will respond briskly and clearly as expected for maturation level.

Thompson and Thompson (1972) had previously noted that for infants of 7–12 months of age, speech and high-pass filtered speech produced the most behavioral responses over other types of auditory stimuli. They recommended the use of the high-pass filtered speech signals as a useful stimulus for assessing high-frequency hearing in infants. They found that with 22–36 month old infants there is no longer an advantage in one auditory stimulus over another.

Samples and Franklin (1978) observed the responses of 7–9 month old infants to speech signals, warble tones, and noise bands. They found that the intensity level required for a response was lower, and the number of responses were significantly higher, to speech signals than to either warble tones or broadband noise stimuli.

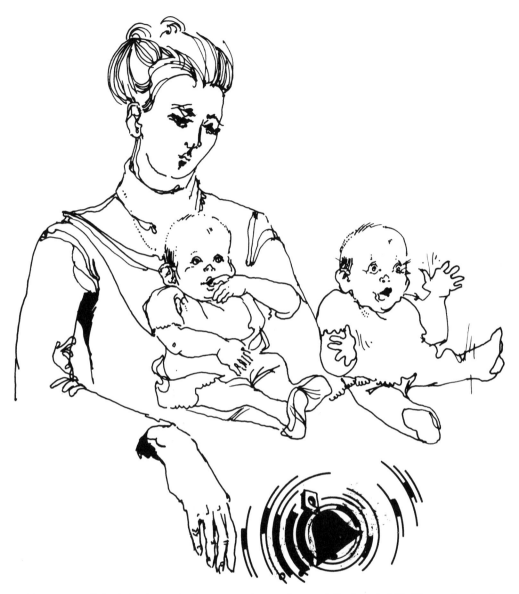

Figure 5.4. Quiet baby shows startle response to sound presentation heard at 65 dB sensation level.

Behavioral Testing of the 4–7 Month Old Infant. Around 4 months of age, the infant takes a giant step toward auditory maturation. Not only does the infant begin to turn toward the sound source, but this response occurs to a lower level of sound than during the first 4 months. From an average minimal response level of 45 dB hearing level (HL) to a sound field speech signal, the baby now becomes aware of speech at about 20 dB HL. During this period of growth, muscle strength and eye-motor coordination also show great improvement. By 6 months of age, the baby now laughs out loud, holds a rattle tightly, reaches for objects and grasps them, can turn over without help, and sits with only minimal support. By 7 months of age, the baby can transfer an object from hand to hand and sit up without support momentarily.

The audiologist should be aware of the visual acuity of the child as testing begins.

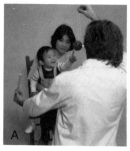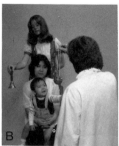

Figure 5.5. Demonstration of BOA with screening noisemakers. **A** shows the testing technique with one tester, while **B** shows the utilization of a two-tester team. (Courtesy of BAM World Markets, Englewood, Colorado.)

Does the baby track a bright object visually from side to side? Does the baby have good eye contact with you for even brief periods? If you smile at the baby and nod your head, is there integrity in the way the infant returns your attentive behavior?

The improved muscular coordination at this age allows the child soon after 4 months of age to begin to turn toward sound with the entire head, but only on a lateral plane. The head turn at 4 months is a wobbly one that is probably not a full 90°. By 6 months of age, the head turn should be stronger and under better control, but the baby will still not find the sound source if it comes from above or below eye level.

The noisemaker localization tests can be accomplished by having the baby sit in the parent's lap, facing you. The audiologist working alone can kneel in front of the baby, with the noisemaker toy array previously set up out of sight (perhaps under the parent's chair), or the audiologist may prefer to stand or kneel unobtrusively behind the parent's chair, totally out of sight of the baby, as shown in Figure 5.5. A small, not-too-attractive, passive toy (such as a book or a soft animal doll) can be given to the baby as an entertaining device. The parent should be instructed not to talk to the baby, not to provide any cues to the baby during the test, and not to make any undue noise. In fact, we sometimes put hearing conservation earmuffs on the parent to ensure

that the parent not participate in any way when the sound stimuli are presented.

Babies at this age will also localize to sound field speech and narrowband noise stimuli presented from loudspeakers. Behavioral observation can be made of the child's responses, or conditioning techniques as described later in this chapter can be included to reinforce the head-turning response. Typically, sound stimuli (speech or narrow bands of pulsed noise) are presented from one loudspeaker at a 45° angle to the child until a head turn response is elicited. Then a similiar or different stimulus is quickly presented from a loudspeaker located 45° on the other side of the child until a head-turn is noted. At this age, an effective speech stimulus is to use the child's name: "Hi, Johnny! Hi, Johnny! Look this way, Johnny." Of course, always find out exactly what name the parents use with the child, as it does little good to say "Hi, Johnny" to John Edwin who is called "Eddie" by his family. As the baby approaches 7 months of age, the infant may now become responsive to a speech stimulus of "bye-bye," and in fact, you may often elicit a voluntary (but somewhat reflexive) wave from the baby. Normal minimal response levels to speech stimuli at this age are approximately 20 dB HL.

Of course, the entire pediatric test battery including acoustic immittance measurements and evoked response testing, if necessary, should be included in the typical hearing evaluation to cross-check the behavioral observations. The startle response at 65 dB HL may also be included at the end of the test period, as shown in Figure 5.4. A sudden onset speech stimulus presented through the sound field loudspeaker system, with the baby seated quietly on the parent's knees as far forward as possible with minimal support, should provide the clinician with a brisk, whole-body startle response as the baby hears the loud speech signal. The lack of a strong startle response following doubtful auditory localization behaviors is suggestive of severe-to-profound hearing loss, and additional hearing evaluation tests including acoustic immittance and auditory brainstem response (ABR) must be accomplished to determine a repeatable minimal response level to auditory stimulation.

Behavioral Observation of the 7–9 Month Old Infant. During the 7–9 month period, the improvement in strength and motor coordination allows the infant to sit steadily and to change position without falling. The child can now manipulate two objects simultaneously and transfers objects hand to hand and hand to mouth. This is the explore-everything-in-the-mouth stage, and the well-advised clinician only gives the infant clean items. This stage is not uncommonly seen in older developmentally delayed children who function at this mental age.

The child of 7–9 months is able to play peekaboo and perhaps pat-a-cake. This age child begins to be initially shy with strangers and may take a few moments to warm up to your presence. The baby probably can respond to "bye-bye" with a wave of the hand and arm but may need some encouragement to perform this act for you. "Dada" and "mama" may be heard in vocalizations but without specific referents. Imitation of gross sounds should be in place by the age of 9 months.

Behavioral observation auditory testing can proceed as described for the 4–7 month old with toy noisemakers or sound field speech and narrowband noise stimuli. Auditorially, the 7–9 month old is now able to find a sound source located below eye level and off to the side but only by looking first to the lateral side and then down to the sound source. This behavior is known as "indirect fixation" of a sound source. The transitional stage of the auditory maturation sequence is clearly evident in this age range. Be warned, however, as this young child is normally visually very alert, and it is difficult to introduce the noisemaker signals without attracting visual attention from the baby before the sound is actually produced. The use of two noisemaker toys,

exactly the same in appearance, with one held in front of the child's face and the other held to the side, permits you to elicit a head turn to the side with the presentation of the auditory signal, without worrying about the child "sighting in" on the stimulus toy.

With soundfield localization stimuli presented from loudspeakers, the minimal response for speech awareness is now approximately 15 dB HL. Usually, a child of this age range will sit quietly in the parent's lap and be mildly amused with a passive toy, book, or a couple of blocks. As in all of the tests with young children, the audiologist needs to develop a calm presence and steady pace and to be fully aware of a "good" moment to present the auditory stimuli. If the child is still exploring the environment, take a few moments to wait until the child is comfortable and relaxed before starting the testing sequence. If the child becomes too engrossed in the toy to be aware of the auditory environment, it may be necessary to change toys (if possible), or you may just have to wait until the enthusiasm for the item diminishes.

The soundfield speech stimuli, alternating from the loudspeakers, may actually turn the child's head from side to side like that of a person watching a tennis match. Not for long, however, without reinforcement of some type, as this is not an interesting enough activity to sustain the child's interest. You may elicit some vocalization response to the speech stimuli, and the child may actually imitate your speech sounds, such as "oh-oh," if presented with singsong inflection. This age child is normally happy and outgoing and very curious about everything going on in the environment. Once again, the cross-check techniques of acoustic immittance and evoked response measurement, when necessary, should be used to confirm your behavioral observations.

Behavioral Observation Audiometry with the 9–13 Month Old Infant. It is normal for the baby of this age to be somewhat afraid of strangers if they come too close or offer to hold the child. "Strangeness" is one of the psychic organizers described by Spitz (1959). In fact, the child who comes easily to the arms of a complete stranger at this age may suffer a lack of psychic development. Permit the parent to handle the child exclusively for the auditory evaluation period. You may need to do your work from outside the sound-treated booth in a darkened room, because as long as the child can see you, suspicion reigns. Without your presence visually, the child will relax and feel secure in the lap of the parent. Normal babies do not object to the quiet of the sound-treated booth, and only occasionally have we seen a youngster object violently to going into the sound-treated booth.

By 11 months of age, the baby is on his or her feet, walking by holding on to furniture or the parents. The child may begin making single-word utterances, perhaps with an appropriate referent. The baby knows its own name easily by now, and a speech awareness response level can be determined by using the name in an ascending intensity approach until the child localizes briskly to the correct loudspeaker. The auditory localization behavior noted during this maturation stage progresses from the indirect to the direct fixation of the sound source on the lower level. By the upper age limit of the stage, at 13 months, the child should also be able to localize with indirect fixation (initial lateral head-turn with subsequent looking up) to auditory stimuli presented above eye level and to the side. Typically, the child in this age range is extremely interested in the environment and will localize rather briskly and quickly to your auditory signals. The average minimal response level at this age is 10 dB HL.

The child of 12 months or older can be conditioned with VRA; accordingly, it is possible to obtain frequency-specific minimal response levels for each ear in the sound field situation. Some audiologists may choose to perform an initial hearing screening with toy noisemakers just to establish some idea of the child's response patterns and behaviors, as well as a means to develop rapport with the child and the parent. Remember, however, the ultimate goal of the hearing test is to obtain as much audiometric frequency-specific information as possible in each ear, verified by speech awareness minimal response levels in each ear, before the child grows tired and becomes irritable about the testing situation. Some time at the end of each test session should be taken to cross-check the behavioral test results with immittance audiometry.

Behavioral Observation Audiometry with the 13–24 Month Old Child. Once the child has reached 13 months, the auditory orientation response is fully mature. Beyond 24 months, the child may actually inhibit response behaviors, especially without reinforcement of some type. It is good to question the parents at this time about the vocalization skills of the child that you can relate to normal speech development milestones. It may also be important to ask the parents about possible previous history of ear infections with medical or surgical treatment and to consider referral for language assessment in children with significant history of recurrent otitis media.

By 18 months of age, the toddler should know a few simple objects well enough to look for them. This skill and ability can be used in the speech stimulus by asking the child, at lower and lower intensity levels, to identify by looking at a few simple toys, such as a "Where is the kitty cat?" or "Where is the doll baby?", or at the appropriate parent, such as "Where is mama (or daddy)?" By 24 months of age, it may be possible to have the child pick up certain simple toy objects and hand them to the parent at your instruction through the loudspeakers. Some children at this age are clever enough to identify simple body parts on your suggestion, such as "Where is your nose?" or "Show me your teeth" or "Show mama (or daddy) your shoes." A final behavioral response may be obtained by asking, "Do you want to go bye-bye?" To establish minimal speech response levels it is necessary to present the carrier phrase in the sound field ("Give momma (or daddy) the ...") at 20 dB speech level and then quickly to shift down to the level you want to test for the keyword ("... doggy"). The minimal response level for speech audiometry in this age child is 5 dB HL for normal hearing.

Do not be surprised when the child suddenly stops responding, as after a certain period of time you will lose the child's interest in this activity. Part of the challenge of pediatric audiology is to learn when the child has had enough and you have exceeded the limits of attention. Then you must be prepared to change the game or activity to reinterest the child so that additional information about the hearing response levels can be obtained. The use of a darkened instrument room is still indicated for children up to 24 months of age. The purity of the child's responsiveness is an unquestioning reaction to the voice signal. At later ages, the child may be confused by the presence of a voice without visualizing a person doing the speaking although between 13 and 24 months the unquestioning obedience of the child serves us well in pediatric speech audiometry.

Be sure to apply the cross-check of immittance audiometry with tympanometry and acoustic reflex measurement to confirm your behavioral observation. Children who appear to have hearing loss should be scheduled for ABR evaluation.

VISUAL REINFORCEMENT AUDIOMETRY WITH THE INFANT AGED 6 MONTHS TO 2 YEARS

Liden and Kankkonen (1961) first coined the term "visual reinforcement audiometry" (VRA), based on a technique described by Suzuki and Ogiba (1961) and termed by them "conditioned orientation reflex" (COR) audiometry. This procedure as currently used employs lighted transparent toys that are flashed on simultaneously with the presentation of the auditory signal during a conditioning period. During the testing phase the light is flashed immedi-

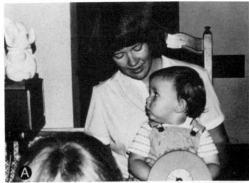
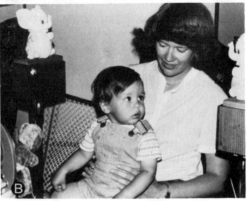
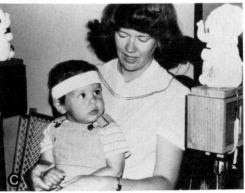

Figure 5.6. VRA. Note head localization to either side when auditory stimulus is heard. Head-turn is reinforced by flashing lighted toy. Bone conduction testing can also be carried out with this technique following the Weber localization concept.

ately following the response of the child looking toward the light (Fig. 5.6).

The technique of VRA is to establish conditioning through the use of a few training trials during which the child's attention should be directed toward the stimulus at the onset of the trial and held there until the reinforcer is presented. Diverting the child's attention toward the stimulus may require prompting or physical assistance, which, it is hoped, can be diminished with each successive training trial. The stimulus and response must always precede delivery of reinforcement; although the "on" time between trials for stimulus presentation should be varied, the reinforcement should immediately follow the desired response, and the stimulus should not be terminated until the response occurs. The training trials will only be successful when the audiologist is absolutely sure that the child hears the stimulus. Therefore, stimulus presentations for a hearing-impaired youngster may, of necessity, be quite loud. Parents or other observers in the test room with the child may wish to wear ear defenders during these loud training trials. Thompson and Folsom (1984) found no difference between 30 dB HL and 60 dB HL conditioning trials prior to exploring minimal response levels in 1 and 2 year old normal-hearing children.

Matkin (1977) found that the technique is useful with earphones and that VRA is successful with 90% of both normal-hearing and hearing-impaired children between the ages of 12 and 30 months. Furthermore, he stated that speech stimuli are more effective than the warble tones. The VRA technique can also be used to test the child's responses with hearing aids.

In sound field, it is apparent that VRA audiometry will test only the better ear in some children, even when loudspeakers on each side of the child produce the signals and the lights for localization. Hodgson (1985) stated that the child with a severe hearing loss will not have learned to localize sound. He suggested that where there is confusion in localization, it is best to use only one loudspeaker in testing. To distract the child from looking constantly at the loudspeaker, an animated toy can be activated in another direction.

Audiologists are aware that children with unilateral hearing loss and one normal hearing ear may have difficulties in localizing the source of a sound, and this is certainly a consideration in children who seem to have difficulty with VRA for no other apparent reason. Children who have unilateral hearing loss can actually localize sound, albeit somewhat slower than normal-hearing children. We believe that localization skills among children vary considerably and seem to be a function of age and the parameters of the stimulus. For example, warble-tone signals are much more difficult to localize than speech or narrowband noise stimuli.

Haug et al. (1967) described a procedure to overcome the problem of testing only the better ear. Their "Puppet in the Window Illuminated Test" (PIWI) was successful in obtaining thresholds in children under 3 years of age. With two loudspeakers, localization responses were reinforced by the appearance of a puppet behind a lighted window. After a conditioning period, earphones were placed on the child, and the puppet again was illuminated every time the child responded to the tone by looking toward the window.

Moore et al. (1976, 1977) affirm the success of VRA in eliciting responses in infants as young as 5 months. A complex noise centered between 1000 and 4000 Hz and maintained at 70 dB was used by them as a stimulus. Each of 60 infants between 4 and 11 months of age were given this stimulus 40 times, reinforced by a toy animal that moved in place. A control trial was also given. The 2–5 month old group and the 7–11 month old group responded significantly more frequently to the signals that were reinforced visually than to the nonreinforced signals.

In testing Down's syndrome infants with VRA, Wilson et al. (1982) found that they did not achieve a high success rate until 10 months BSID (Bayley Scales of Infant Development) equivalent age.

In a previous study, Moore et al. (1977) determined rank order of signals according to their effectiveness in producing VRA localization responses in 12–18 month old infants: (1) an animated toy, (2) a flashing light, (3) social reinforcement, and (4) no reinforcement (Fig. 5.7).

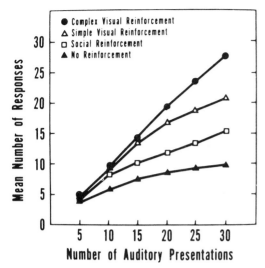

Figure 5.7. Response curves for operant conditioning audiometry. (Reprinted with permission from J. M. Moore et al.: Visual reinforcement of head-turn responses in infants under twelve months of age. *Journal of Speech and Hearing Disorders* 42:328, 1977.)

Wilson et al. (1976) searched for auditory thresholds in 90 infants between 5 and 18 months of age who were divided into groups of 15 according to age. Threshold level was first obtained by using behavioral observations of responses to a complex noise signal. The VRA protocol was begun at that level, with a protocol of attenuating the signal 20 dB after each positive response and increasing it 10 dB after each failure to respond. Threshold was described as the lowest presentation level at which the infant responded at least 3 of 6 times. The results showed the VRA responses to be significantly better than the behavioral observation. Even for the 5 month olds, the 10th and 90th percentile points were 20 and 40 dB sound pressure level (SPL); for the 6–18 month olds, they were 20 and 30 dB SPL.

Eilers et al. (1977) utilized VRA techniques in a speech discrimination paradigm designed to show developmental changes of discrimination ability and termed Visually Reinforced Infant Speech Discrimination (VRISD). They demonstrated that 1–3 month old infants as well as older infants could discriminate certain easier phonemic contrasts such as sa-sa and sa-va but that other contrasts are more difficult for very young children than for older infants as they approach 14 months, e.g., fi-i, sa-za. Thus the use of VRA techniques is extended into the study of the development of auditory prelinguistic skills.

The response modes utilized in the Suzuki-Ogiba COR procedure and the VRA paradigm described by Moore et al. (1975) differ substantially according to Primus (1987). The COR response requires detection of the sound, localization of the auditory image, coordination of auditory and visual space, and subsequent orientation to the appropriate reinforcer with a motor response (i.e., a head-turn). The VRA response requires only a detection of the auditory signal as prerequisite to an appropriate head-turn. The difference between the response modes is that VRA defines one criterion response (i.e., a head-turn toward a single loudspeaker/reinforcer location). The COR response requires that the child localize the test signal to determine which of two reinforcers (left or right) is the appropriate response. Close proximity of loudspeakers and reinforcers is advantageous in both VRA and COR procedures, according to Primus, because most unconditioned children turn spontaneously toward initial presentation of the sound stimulus.

VRA and COR techniques are powerful tools for assessing minimal response levels in young children when used correctly with acknowledged conditioning protocols. These techniques are the evaluation procedures of choice in children between 6 and 24 months of age, although it should be obvious that the older children in this range will condition more easily and quicker than the younger children.

Smith (1987) reports development of a commercially available VRA system with a pair of illuminated and/or animated reinforcement boxes. This system is especially useful for the audiologist working without an assistant as the equipment includes a third (orientation) toy, in front of the child, which can be illuminated between stimulus presentation trials to bring the child's head

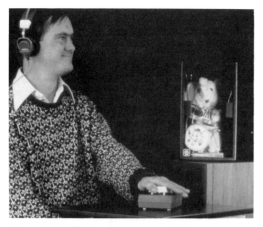

Figure 5.8. VRA system as used with developmentally delayed youngster.

back to the center position in readiness for the next VRA stimulus and head-turn response. Smith states that this VRA system is especially viable for the older, developmentally delayed patient who may be functioning at a level too high for Tangible Reinforcement Operant Conditioning Audiometry (TROCA) but too low for the hand-raising response task (Fig. 5.8).

An automated pediatric audiometer has recently been developed that uses interactive video images as the reinforcement for correct responses in an application of Visual Reinforcement Operant Conditioning Audi-

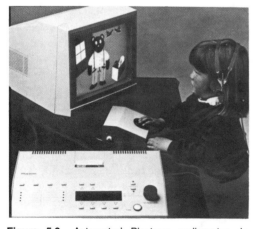

Figure 5.9. Automated Playtone audiometer designed to use interactive video images as the reinforcement for correct responses. (From Life-Tech Instruments, Houston, Texas.)

ometry (VROCA). Keith and Smith (1987) describe the Playtone audiometer designed to facilitate hearing assessment in 3–7 year old children (Fig. 5.9). This computer-controlled audiometer operates in four modes including practice trials, hearing screening, and auditory threshold, both manual and automatic. The child is conditioned during practice trials to depress quickly a bright red button on the response box immediately following presentation of an auditory stimulus. A brief, animated color video presentation occurs following each correct response made within a short time window. False responses produce no visual reinforcement of any kind. This pediatric audiometer adapts the test signal presentation speed to the response speed of the child and in the automatic mode includes several validity checks. Indications from preliminary use of this innovative VROCA audiometer suggests great promise for pediatric hearing assessment.

OPERANT REINFORCEMENT AUDIOMETRY WITH THE CHILD AGED 6 MONTHS TO 2 YEARS

The results obtained by applying operant conditioning principles to populations between 6 and 24 months of age have been particularly encouraging. Stimulus, response, and reinforcement parameters have been studied and evaluated and techniques have been developed to be consistent with each child's developmental level and response capability. The use of reinforcement for responses made to audiometric stimuli strengthens the test paradigm, maintains the child's responses longer, reduces habituation to the stimulus, and thus allows for a more precise estimate of hearing thresholds in young children.

Wilson and Thompson (1984) described two modes of operant conditioning that they termed *operant discrimination* and *conjugate procedures*. In operant discrimination, the stimulus precedes the responses and acts as a discriminative signal that reinforcement is available. In the conjugate procedure, the stimulus follows the response as a consequence. The intensity of a continuously available reinforcing stimulus varies as a function of the rate of the response. Since the stimulus is a consequence of the response, in the conjugate procedure the stimulus itself must have reinforcing value to the child. Since auditory threshold determination is a discrimination task (presence or absence of signal), Wilson and Thompson recommended the operant discrimination paradigm in hearing testing.

An example of a conjugate reinforcement technique is high-amplitude sucking in infants, which was originally developed by Siqueland and DeLucia (1969). This procedure relies on a natural newborn response and capitalizes on the reinforcing properties of the stimulus. The spontaneous behavior (sucking) is brought under stimulus control through the use of response-contingent stimulation. The auditory stimulus is then made contingent upon a criterion-level sucking response, and the auditory stimulus takes on reinforcing properties for the infant. Disadvantages to the high-amplitude sucking response is the heavy physical demand placed on the infant, a baseline criterion level of 20–40 sucks per minute so that criterion level changes may be noted, and the fact that the general length of time required to complete studies is substantial. Eisele et al. (1975) generated threshold hearing data from 100 infants by observing the rate of sucking as a function of stimulus intensity.

Aslin et al. (1983) summarize four versions of the BOA head-turning technique that have been used to evaluate auditory abilities in infants. The first version is a simple auditory threshold procedure in which the infant's task is to respond to any just detectable sound emitted from a single loudspeaker. In a second version, the same task is involved for the infant, except that two sound field speakers are used. The infant is centered between the speaker, and the silence is interrupted by a signal presented from one of the two speakers. The first directional head-turn response is scored and correlated with the location of the sound source.

A third technique is somewhat more complex, as it involves the addition of a background stimulus that is interrupted by the presentation of a different (or target) stimulus. This is then a discrimination procedure to evaluate an infant's ability to differentiate between two suprathreshold auditory stimuli. A "catch trial" is essential in this technique, which consists of informing the observer that a scoring interval is occurring but of not letting him or her know if the target stimulus was included in this tone interval. This is done as an attempt to eliminate experimenter bias. A fourth version of the head-turning technique involves the addition of a trial-to-criterion measure to the basic discrimination response procedure. These discrimination techniques have been used by Kuhl (1979) and Kuhl and Miller (1982) to evaluate speech perception in early infants.

Primus (1987) investigated response and reinforcement features of two operant discrimination paradigms with normal-hearing 17 month old children. He found more success in a paradigm that based the response task on complex central processing skills (i.e., localization and coordination of auditory/visual space) over a simple detection task. His use of animated toy reinforcement resulted in more than a twofold increase in responses. In a 1985 research project, Primus tested the response strength of young children in operant audiometry. One and two year old children reinforced on a variable-ratio schedule of intermittent reinforcement and a 100% schedule demonstrated equivalent response habituation and consistency. Primus reported that the use of novel reinforcement had a strong influence in eliciting conditioned responses from normal-hearing 2 year old children and that an audiologist can delay the habituation of responses by the use of novel (different) reinforcement.

Newer procedures utilizing computer technology can be expected to influence operant conditioning paradigms. Computerized stimulus presentations can include preprogrammed "catch trials" or control presentations when no auditory signal is actually presented. Computerized response criteria can be established to limit the time window of the child's response in other ways and can be used to define the "correctness of response," with the observer(s) blinded as to the presentation of control (no signal) trials.

Tester-Observer Bias.   Response bias by testers and observers is one of the most difficult errors to avoid in the clinical hearing evaluation of children. Several studies have confirmed that there is a tendency for judges to score responses when no auditory signals were presented (Moncur, 1968; Ling et al., 1970; Langford et al., 1975). Weber (1969) suggested using two persons to test the child, with one observer in the room with the child while the tester operates a tape recorder in the control room. The operator selects a randomized stimulus schedule with 20 stimulus presentations—10 of which are heard only by the child. The observer wears earphones and hears all 20 stimulus presentations but cannot tell which sounds are presented to the child under evaluation. The operator and observer each make judgments about the responses of the child, which are compared with the stimulus presentation schedule following the test session.

In our clinic, we have always had one audiologist work with each child during the hearing evaluation process, incorporating the parents' help, when necessary, to shape the child's conditioning behavior. Although we prefer having the audiologist outside the test room, many audiologists prefer sitting in the test room with the child (and parent). Understanding the potential observer bias that can exist with a single tester presenting stimuli and judging the child's responses, our experience has been that this technique is cost- and time-effective and does not significantly alter the results of the hearing test. Gravel (1989) supports this viewpoint of a single audiologist essentially performing all the functions involved in VRA. The audiologist engages the infant's

(or child's) forward attention with a simple toy, selects and presents a test signal, varies its presentation intensity as appropriate, judges the child's behavioral response, and activates directly the reinforcement for correct head-turning. Gravel states, "a careful and thoughtful clinician guarding against these potential hazzards of single-examiner assessment may obtain reliable and accurate audiograms. . . ."

Recently, Gans and Flexer (1982) investigated observer bias in BOA with profoundly involved multiple-handicapped children. Their findings implicated clear observer bias in 85% of the children. At low test intensities, observers aware of the stimulus events tended to score fewer responses than those judges unaware of stimulus intensity. In cases of high sound intensities, judges tend to "see" more behavioral changes to sound than actually occur. Gans and Flexer were disappointed that even when observers were told that they exhibited biased scoring responses, this information did not influence the observer's subsequent scoring tactics.

TANGIBLE AND VISUAL REINFORCEMENT OPERANT CONDITIONING AUDIOMETRY

During operant conditioning paradigms, the stimulus cues the infant or child that a behavior-specific response will immediately produce a positive reinforcement. The positive reinforcement can be a tangible item such as candy, cereal, or a trinket of some sort that is automatically dispensed from specifically designed audiometric equipment. Visual stimulations, in the form of a blinking light array, moving video, or animated puppets and animals may also be used as positive reinforcement. Negative reinforcement (mild punishment), such as "time out" for false positive responses from the child, may also be incorporated into the testing situation. Lloyd et al. (1968) described success with TROCA, using edible positive reinforcement, with a group of developmentally delayed children.

Typically, the child's behavior is conditioned to push a response button whenever a sound is perceived, initially in sound field and subsequently under earphones. The tangible reinforcement item is usually accompanied by an outburst of secondary social approval reinforcement by the audiologist and parents or caretaker. Fulton et al. (1975) reported success using the TROCA technique to assess hearing levels in young children. TROCA is probably most useful with children between 2 and 4 years of age and generally requires more total testing time than traditional conditioning techniques.

CLINICAL TESTING OF THE CHILD AGED 2–5 YEARS

Between 2 and 5 years of age the child grows into the independence of early maturity. The child begins to separate from mother without much fuss and to dress alone, first with supervision and then without. The youngster now becomes a wanderer, so do not turn your back or you may lose the child who is quickly into all your toys and equipment. The child begins to understand some abstract words, such as cold or hungry, and can give a full name when asked. Actually, the child becomes an eager beaver, happy to please you, and as a result, the child may give the clinician a hard time in testing. Once the child knows that cooperation in play conditioning pleases you, they may forget what they are supposed to listen for, in their eagerness to be praised. (Strangely enough, this attitude is often found in older deaf children—even teenagers—who will give false responses in order to please or to give a "good" test.)

The learning of play-conditioning techniques starts at 2 years of age. But do not be deceived by the bright, talkative 2 year old who appears certain to be able to learn the procedure. Play safe, and first get all the information obtainable from the observation of behavior as the child waits in the waiting room, walks into the sound booth, and watches your interaction with the parents. Until the child is 4 or 5 years old, the audiologist's ingenuity is challenged to complete the hearing test. Remember that our

goal is to achieve pure tone thresholds at all test frequencies in each ear. However, do not traumatize the child so much that the youngster will be frightened the next time. There is always another day.

The darkened instrument room should not be forgotten even for these older children. A shy, immature child of 2½ may learn play-conditioning techniques easily, but the odd situation of a stranger's face in the window may create too much distracting stress. The bodyless voice over the speaker can be coped with; it takes the stranger out of the situation. All the necessary instructions to the child can be given through the speech circuit (earphones or loudspeakers) without being seen. So occasionally it will be useful to keep the instrument room darkened.

The description that follows of testing this age group is primarily related to double sound room testing. When the audiometric test is done in the same room with the child, the procedure can be easily adapted. The choice of audiometric testing, whether done in a double sound room or in a single sound room, seems to rest on personal preference. Whatever suits the audiologists style should be elected, but successful rapport with the child is most important in achieving success with the hearing test procedures.

Speech Reception Threshold. We generally begin the hearing evaluation of the 2–5 year old with behavioral speech testing, establishing a Speech Reception Threshold (SRT) for each ear to obtain an initial impression of the hearing levels of the child. We use this beginning because it incorporates the child immediately into the test activity, thereby reducing any apprehension the child has about the test environment. Although the SRT task can be accomplished with the 4 and 5 year old under earphones, we typically start the 2–3 year old by working through the sound field and loudspeaker system to determine a binaural SRT. Once we are sure the 2–3 year old can perform the required task, we attempt to

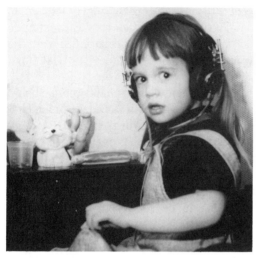

Figure 5.10. Speech audiometry measurement using earphones and toys.

replicate the activity with earphones so that a SRT can be established for each ear.

In the sound-treated room, the armamentarium of the audiologist should include a carefully selected array of toys, the names of which approach spondaic principles as closely as possible. However, to present children with easily recognizable toys, some compromise may be necessary (Fig. 5.10). It is more important for the child to know and recognize the toy than for you to worry if the toy name conforms to the equal-stress-on-each-syllable principle. Typical "spondaic" toys might include an airplane, baseball, toothbrush, hot dog, cowboy, fire truck, etc. Suggestions for nonspondaic toys include a baby (small doll), kitty, doggie, horsie, car, truck, etc. We have found that toys from pet departments are more substantial than variety store items.

No more than four or five of these toys need be used to determine the SRT for the 2 or 3 year old; the 4 or 5 year old can select from among six to eight items. The toys can be presented *via* picture boards, but it is much more interesting to the child if actual toys are involved. We wire the toys to a perforated board and have the parent hold the board while the child responds with a pointing response. Sometimes, very confident and mature 4- and 5 year olds will repeat the SRT words verbally.

With the speech circuit set at 50 dB HL (or as high as necessary to be sure the child can hear you), say, "Hello, there. Can you hear me? Show me the airplane." When the child makes the correct response, use social reinforcement with exaggerated praise. Then descend in 10 dB steps, asking at each level for the child to identify a different toy. When the child no longer responds, ascend 5 dB but set the carrier phrase "Show me . . ." at a 10 or 15 dB higher level and switch quickly to the lower level for the test word. Too long a silent period will lose the child, so when searching for threshold the louder carrier phrase should be given. Accept two valid responses on the ascending presentation and switch quickly to the other ear. Listening at low levels is not easy for a child, and one must work quickly for the sake of holding the child's attention. If discrepancies appear later, a recheck can always be done. It need hardly be said that the tester's mouth should be covered while giving the words.

Thompson et al. (1989) noted a paucity of information about the relative effectiveness of audiometric procedures for testing hearing in 2 year old children. They evaluated 62 2 year old subjects with VRA, VROCA, and play audiometry. Their results indicated that a higher percentage of children could be conditioned to VRA than to either VROCA or play audiometry. However, in terms of response habituation, play conditioning had a longer response activity period. In their conclusions, these researchers noted that under general clinical conditions, the question regarding hearing levels in 2 year olds is whether hearing loss might be a factor in speech/language development. Under this circumstance, VRA is recommended because the vast majority of 2 year olds will readily condition to this task for purposes of hearing screening.

PROCEDURE FOR CONDITIONED PLAY AUDIOMETRY

Place the young child in the parent's lap. The older 3 or 4 year old may prefer to sit alone with a parent nearby in another chair.

The parent's closeness may be important even at the older age.

Sit down and talk to the parents first, developing an easy rapport: "What seems to be Johnny's (or Debbie's) problem?" Let the parents tell you briefly why the child is here, but do not belabor the history. The child is the chief target. Turn interestedly to the child and ask some simple questions. "How old are you?" Comment on the child's clothing, hair, or a toy that the child brought along. Tell the child that you have some special games to play today.

During this period many observations can be made. Listen to the child's voice quality and articulation of words. Does the child substitute for the high-frequency consonants? If they omit or substitute for the unvoiced consonants, either a mild sensorineural or a conductive loss can be suspected. If the child misses the voiced consonants and some of the vowel sounds in addition, a more severe sensorineural loss may be predicted. Is the child able to repeat words readily but not to identify the corresponding toy?

Tell the child what you are going to do, in simple, clear terms that are easily understandable for the language-age of the child. (Do not make the mistake of "asking" the child to play your game.) "Now we're going to play a telephone game. We'll put the telephone (earphones) on you, and you can say hello to me. Hello!" Put the earphones gently but firmly on the child's head, saying "Hello, how are you? Now wait, and I'm going to telephone to you from the other room." Try to get out before the child balks at the phones, but if the child does, do not fight it. Take off one phone and have the parent hold it to the ear "like a real telephone." With the very young and the shy child it may be preferable not to start with earphones at all. Do a trial run in sound field first, allowing the child to become familiar with the situation, then the placement of earphones may be attempted.

Another way to start the test session is to put the earphones on yourself. Have available a number of sets of motivational toys geared to different ages: plain blocks for building a tower; a graduated ring tower; beads to throw into a container; and a peg board with colored peg (put a horse or a car in the center and build a fence or a garage). A popular game is to drop pennies into a bank.

Other motivational games can be devised by the ingenious audiologist. Usually, one is sufficient to accomplish the task, but you must be ready to switch to another one at the first sign of boredom. It is largely the enthusiasm of the clinician that keeps the child attending, but occasionally novelty must be employed.

Show the child what the game is about. In fact, the audiologist can communicate all instructions without talking much. Facial expression, body language, and clear demonstrations can transmit even to the nonverbal child what is to be expected. Or you can talk to the child and say, "We're going to hold this peg (or block, etc.) up to our ear and listen for a little bell. Oh! I hear it, so I can put the peg in the board. Now I'm going to listen for a little one. Oh! I hear it, so I put the peg in. Now you can do it, and build a fence for the horse." In the case of the 2 and 3 year old, instruct the parent to hold the child's hand with the peg at the test earphone (or ear if using sound field) and to guide the hand to the peg board when the sound is heard. Then practice it through sound field even to the extent of establishing a quick threshold for a 2000 Hz tone or narrowband noise stimulus so you can be sure the task is understood. Three or four trials should be sufficient for the child to learn.

Now tell the child to do it all alone, preferably with earphones. Present the tone at 40–50 dB above the expected threshold. Praise the child for a correct action by switching quickly to the speech circuit. Instruct the parent to have another peg ready to give to the child the moment the child has responded accurately. Descend in intensity as rapidly as possible from 40 to 50 dB HL in 10 or 15 dB steps, indicating that the child is to listen for a "tiny little bell (or beep)." Again, work quickly to obtain threshold, accepting two responses on the ascending presentation.

Select 2000 Hz as the first frequency to be presented. It is the most important one so far as a sensorineural loss is concerned. If the SRT was not normal, be sure the initial practice tone is loud enough for the child to hear. Sometimes a child will seem to be cooperative at first but will soon forget what to do. In this case, recondition the child, with the parent's help, at levels you are certain the child can hear. Several reconditioning periods may have to be run during a test. Do not give up until it is quite apparent that the child is not about to stay with the task.

The next frequency to test is 500 Hz, significant in a conductive loss. Then switch to the opposite ear and obtain thresholds at 2000 and 500 Hz. If by this time you have lost the child, at least you have some minimal valuable information. If the child stays with the task nicely, fill in the 1000 and 250 Hz thresholds and then 4000 Hz threshold for each ear. Know when to stop, because the bone conduction test is still to be done, and there must be some reserve of attention to carry the child through it.

It should be noted that when the child persistently refuses to wear even one earphone, resort to sound field audiometry. Warbled pure tones or narrow bands of noise precalibrated to the location where the child is sitting should be presented by utilizing the play-conditioning techniques. The thresholds will represent the hearing in the better ear only but will give essential information about how the child is hearing, at least in the better ear.

Repeat with the Bone Conduction Receiver.

Next, fit the child with a bone conduction receiver, saying: "We're going to use another kind of telephone—one that goes behind the ear. But you can hear the sounds just like the other telephone. That's like airplane pilots (or astronauts) use!"

Repeat the test as above, doing the more important frequencies first and filling in with the others where possible. If there is any doubt about the bone conduction thresholds, do the SRT through the bone conduction receiver just as for the air conduction. It is assumed that the bone conduction SRT has been precalibrated on normal-hearing people. The average normal threshold is generally around 35–40 dB on the dial of most instruments. Merely switching of the "microphone" input and the "bone conduction" output puts the speech circuit into the bone conduction receiver on most audiometers. If SRTs are all that can be obtained on a child, the difference between air- and bone-conducted speech thresholds gives significant information. In addition, the bone-conducted speech can be masked effectively in the opposite ear without affecting the validity of the child's responses. The bone-conducted speech test is one of the most useful of the audiologist's tools. At the end, praise the child or reward him or her with some token. This is insurance for future cooperation. You may have to see this child many times, so lay the groundwork for a happy return visit.

Verify Audiometric Impressions with Immittance Audiometry and the Cross-Check Principle.

The immittance test battery consists of tympanometry, acoustic reflex measurement, and physical volume measurement (see Chapter 6). When test results are still confirmatory or question exists about the child's actual hearing levels, a referral for ABR evaluation may be in order. We should make it very clear, however, that we do *not* incorporate ABR evaluation into every pediatric patient's workup. Because of the time and expense associated with ABR evaluation, this technique is reserved for those children whose hearing levels cannot be precisely determined through any other method.

Table 5.5.
Selected Pediatric Speech Audiometric Procedures[a]

Test[b]	Materials	Message Set; Response Mode	Task Domain	Minimum Age (yr)
SERT	30 environmental sounds (train, telephone)	Closed; picture identification	Unrestricted: 4 alternatives	3
ANT	Numbers 1 through 5	Closed; picture identification	Restricted: 5 alternatives	3
NU-CHIPS	50 monosyllabic words (food, school)	Closed; picture identification	Unrestricted: 4 alternatives	3
PSI	20 monosyllabic words (dog, spoon)	Closed; picture identification	Restricted: 5 alternatives	3
PSI	10 sentences, 2 syntactic constructions (Show me a bear brushing his teeth.) (A bear is brushing his teeth.)	Closed; picture identification	Restricted: 5 alternatives	3

[a]From S. Jerger: Speech audiometry. In: J. Jerger (ed.): *Pediatric Audiology*. San Diego, College Hill Press, 1984.
[b]SERT, Sound Effects Recognition Test (Finitizo-Hieber et al., 1980); ANT, Audio Numbers Test (Erber, 1980); NU-CHIPS, Northwestern University Children's Perception of Speech (Elliott and Katz, 1980); and PSI, Pediatric Speech Intelligibility (S. Jerger et al., 1980, 1981).

SPEECH DISCRIMINATION TESTING IN YOUNG CHILDREN

Speech discrimination testing (Table 5.5) in children is an area that has yet to be fully developed, although research is currently underway to rectify this situation. As Olsen and Matkin (1979) point out, the selection of receptive vocabulary competency, the designation of an appropriate response task, and the utilization of reinforcement are primary factors that may affect the reliability and validity of pediatric measurements. The results obtained during speech discrimination measures may actually be more a reflection of the child's interest and motivation for the task at hand than a real indication of higher auditory speech discrimination abilities.

There is no standard technique or test of auditory discrimination in children. Although numerous tests have been developed for this purpose, apparently none of them "fits the bill" well enough for all clinicians to agree generally on which is most suitable for clinical work. One major problem with most current speech discrimination procedures is that the data base underlying the development of the test has not been standardized well enough on a broad spectrum of children of varying ages and backgrounds, and few implications can be generalized between normal-hearing and hearing-impaired children.

Many children are too shy to speak in the test room environment, and, of course, articulation problems are common in children, so it may be difficult for the audiologist to score speech discrimination tests as we do with adults. The most practical method of testing auditory discrimination in children has been to use some form of picture identification task. The child hears the test word and attempts to identify an appropriate picture.

Susan Jerger (1983) published an excellent discussion and review of current speech audiometry materials for children. She points out in her paper that two basic principles have been important in the history of speech testing in children—vocabulary restriction in the selection of test material and limited response set definition. To these basic tenets she adds two more important considerations necessary in pediatric speech test development and administration: (*1*) the need to control the influence of receptive language ability on test performance, and (*2*) the need to consider the effect of extra–auditory (cognitive) factors on children's performance.

Probably the most widely used speech discrimination test for children currently comprises three lists of phonetically balanced words selected from the spoken vocabulary of kindergarteners. These lists were developed by Haskins in 1949. This is an open-ended set of stimulus words usually administered live-voice or via tape recording and known as the PBK-50 word lists. It must be kept in mind that these words are from a kindergarten level vocabulary, and without task-oriented or play techniques, children younger than 4½ years may not do well. Smith and Hodgson (1970) did show that tangible reinforcement (i.e., candies, toys, pennies, etc.) was an effective method of maintaining the interest of young children in the PBK-50 test. In fact, token reinforcement created significant improvement in speech discrimination scores from these children aged 4–8 years. Olsen and Matkin (1979) recommend that clinicians use caution with this test unless there is relatively good assurance that the receptive vocabulary age of the youngster under evaluation approaches at least that of a normal-hearing kindergartener.

One of the earliest attempts was the Discrimination by Identification of Pictures (DIP) test developed by Siegenthaler and Haspiel in 1966. Their test consists of 48 cards with two pictures on each card. One can quickly surmise that chance selection would produce fairly high scores, since only two choices were involved in each presentation. Of interest is the fact that these investigators selected test words on the basis of contrasting acoustic dimensions rather than the traditional phonemic balance approach. The test was standardized on 295 normal-hearing children between the ages of 3 and 8 years and was administered at sensation levels of 0, 5, and 10 dB.

Ross and Lerman (1970) developed a picture identification test for hearing-impaired children known as the Word Intelligibility by Picture Identification (WIPI) test. They evaluated the test on 61 hearing-impaired children of ages 5 and 6 and caution about the use of the test with children younger than 5 years of age. The test consists of 25 picture plates with six pictures per plate used as test stimuli. The test is thus a closed-response set. The lists are reported to have high reliability coefficients, and the tests are simple and rapid to administer.

In 1976, Sanderson-Leepa and Rintelmann compared the speech discrimination performance of 60 normal-hearing children on the WIPI test, the PBK-50 test, and the Northwestern University Auditory Test No. 6 (NU-6). The children were in groups by age, 3½, 5½, 7½, 9½, and 11½ years. They found that the WIPI test yielded the highest discrimination sources; the PBK-50 test, intermediate scores; and the NU-6, the lowest scores. Their inclusion of the NU-6, although an adult speech discrimination test, was to determine the lowest chronologic age for its appropriate use. They recommended that the WIPI was the test of choice for the 3½-year-olds, the WIPI and the PBK-50 were appropriate for the 5½-year-olds. For children 7½, 9½, and 11½, the NU-6 was more difficult than the PBK-50 test. Clinicians must be cautioned that this study was conducted on normal-hearing children, and the same age recommendations might not be appropriate for hearing-impaired children.

Erber (1980) noted that the traditional speech discrimination tests developed for children are often inadequate for real diagnostic purposes or too difficult for children with severe hearing impairment. He developed a simple auditory test to determine whether a young hearing-impaired child can perceive spectral aspects of speech or only gross temporal acoustic patterns. Known as the Auditory Numbers Test (ANT), this live voice test required the child to identify counted sequences and individual numbers. The ANT requires only that the child be able to count to five and be able to apply these number labels to sets of from one to five items. Picture cards are used that are color-coded and depict groups of one to five ants with the corresponding numerals. Erber recommends this test for rapid evaluation of speech perception in young severely and profoundly hearing-impaired children to aid in the planning of auditory training and habilitation activities.

The Northwestern University Children's Perception of Speech (NU-CHIPS) test developed by Elliott and Katz (1980) uses 50 monosyllabic words that were documented to be in the recognition vocabulary of normal children older than 2½ years of age. The test includes 65 word pictures and interchanges 50 words as test items and foil items. Simple words, such as "food" and "school," are represented in a four-alternative picture set, and the child responds by "picture painting." Chermak et al. (1984) question the reliability of the NU-CHIPS when it is administered in a noise background.

Finitzo-Hieber et al. (1980) described the development and evaluation of a Sound Effects Recognition Test (SERT) to use in the pediatric audiologic evaluation. They point out that such a test may be the only available standardized measure of auditory discrimination in children with limited verbal abilities. The test is comprised of three equivalent sets, with each containing 10 familiar environmental sounds (such as a dog barking, a toilet flushing, a mother singing, hammering, a cat meowing, and a baby crying). The authors indicated that the SERT is not intended to be a substitute for traditional speech discrimination tests but is expected to supplement them, especially when the child has very limited verbal abilities.

In a review article regarding the effects of noise on perception of speech by children, Elliott (1982) points out that quite young children have poorer levels of performance than do adults when listening at low levels in quiet, to words that are well within their receptive vocabularies. When the NU-CHIPS test is used, in order for normal hearing 3 year olds to perform with nearly 100% accuracy, the words had to be presented at levels more than 10 dB greater than the level at which 5 year olds score 100%, approximately 15 dB greater than the level at which 10 year olds score 100%, and nearly 25 dB greater than the level at which adults score 100%. These differences occurred even though the words and pictures had been developed to be well within the receptive vocabularies of 3 year old children when presented at comfortable listening levels. Her data warn that environments for children, such as classrooms, etc., need to be designed for very low ambient background noise.

S. Jerger et al. (1980, 1981) described their use of realistic speech materials to control the receptive language factor in children by incorporating the actual responses of normal youngsters between the ages of 3 and 6 years in the new Pediatric Speech Intelligibility (PSI) test. The children composed both monosyllabic word and sentence test items elicited by picture stimulus cards selected from lists of words and actions comprising children's early vocabularies. The PSI test is composed of 20 monosyllabic words and a 10-sentence procedure. The word lists include simple nouns such as "dog" and "spoon" and two types of sentence construction identified as Format I and Format II. An example of a Format II sentence is, "A bear is brushing his teeth." The different sentence formats represent the different speech patterns of normal children between 3 and 6 years of age. The test materials are applicable for children as young as 2½ or 3 years old.

The Jerger group has worked long and hard to establish a strong data base and to evaluate a number of influencing variables that control a child's performance on speech discrimination/intelligibility tasks. Their carefully designed approach to PSI test development has documented information regarding the utilization of the test items in the presence of a competing message and the definition of performance-intensity functions for children of varying chronologic and receptive language age groups. Their results have confirmed the ability of children to perform these tasks that were previously applied only to adults. They have focused attention on the importance of variables such as predetermination of receptive language ability and cognition skills, rather than considering only chrono-

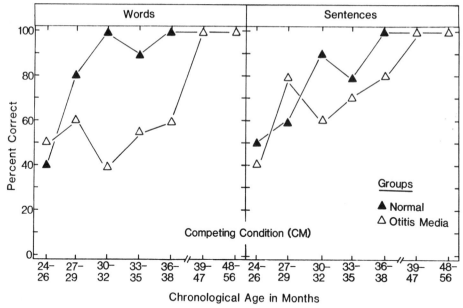

Figure 5.11. Data from the Pediatric Speech Intelligibility (PSI) test with a competing message condition for a group of normal-hearing children and a group of children with otitis media. Note the disparity between the two groups, shown with the word materials. Although the sentence materials also bring out perceptual differences between the two groups, the poorer performance by the otitis media group is especially evident with the word test. (Courtesy of Susan Jerger, Baylor School of Medicine, Houston, Texas.)

logic age. The PSI test is commercially available (Figs. 5.11 and 5.12).

Mackie and Dermody (1986) developed a monosyllabic adaptive speech test for use with children of 3 years or older. In this procedure, test stimuli are familiar monosyllabic words presented as a closed set with a picture-pointing response and using

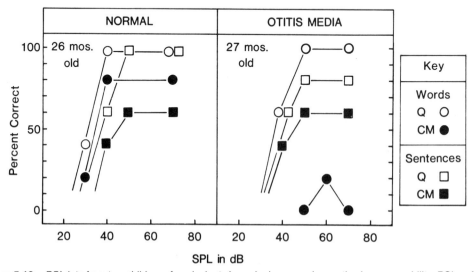

Figure 5.12. PSI data from two children of equivalent chronologic age and receptive language ability. PSI performance-intensity functions in quiet (*Q*) look quite similar between the two patients, but note the performance-intensity function for the otitis medial child when words are presented with a competing message (*CM*) background. (Courtesy of Susan Jerger, Baylor School of Medicine, Houston, Texas.)

a simple up-down adaptive procedure to establish speech threshold. Their initial research results indicate that the monosyllabic adaptive speech test procedure provides an accurate estimate of the 50% point on the rising portion of the performance-intensity function for speech recognition of monosyllables.

Several studies have reported that people with language-learning disabilities have poorer auditory discrimination than their normal-hearing peers. Recently, Elliott and Hammer (1988) showed that children between 6 and 9 years of age with language-learning problems, despite having normal intelligence and normal hearing, showed poorer auditory discrimination than normal-hearing children. Their experimental protocol required "fine-grained" auditory discrimination that demanded careful listening for small acoustic differences.

TESTING THE CHILD AGED 5–16 YEARS

By 5 years of age the child of normal intelligence can cooperate in the standard adult pure tone techniques and can repeat simple words. The youngster will attend for fairly long periods of time to the hand-raising technique, given sufficient praise and encouragement. Do not give too much encouragement, however, as the child may begin to give false responses in order to please. The normal-hearing child can cooperate with the speech recognition tests willingly.

The pure tone audiometric technique that is chosen is a matter of preference, so long as it fulfills the requirements of the descending-ascending bracketing technique. Carhart and Jerger (1959) described the most commonly accepted techniques for obtaining thresholds.

A method proposed by Berlin and Catlin (1965) has some advantages over the traditional procedures. The initial tone presentation is given at 0 dB HL and ascends in 10 dB steps until the level is reached where the subject responds. Another signal is given at 5 dB above that level to confirm its

validity, and then another presentation is given at 10 dB below the previous one. An ascent is then made. If a response is given, the next tone is presented at 10 dB below that level, and the next tone ascends 5 dB. Three "no" responses must be found at 5 dB below the level of "threshold," and three responses must be found at 5 dB above the level of "threshold." Two or three responses must be seen at "threshold." Advantages to this method are: (*1*) it structures the bracketing of threshold; (*2*) it confirms the first response at a higher level; (*3*) it eliminates the taking of false responses as the threshold, by confirming the lowest response level through a 5 dB higher level; (*4*) it accustoms the child immediately to listen for softer tones rather than louder tones; and (*5*) in the case of a functional hearing loss, it minimizes the "measuring stick" of the child by the presentation of lower hearing levels at the start.

Whether this precise method is used, the experienced clinician will routinely employ the confirmatory procedure of presenting a 5 dB higher level than the presumed threshold. False responses can be rapidly spotted through this maneuver.

Aged 5–10 Years. The younger child in the 5–10 year age group requires motivation to keep his or her attention on the test. Usually this can be done by social approval: smiling, nodding the head, clapping the hands, etc. The time spent in gaining rapport with the child is worth the effort. Talk to the child briefly about clothes, interests, toys, activities, etc. Display a real interest in each youngster. During this time, make useful observations about the voice quality, articulation, the extent of vocabulary, and the degree of cooperation you can expect.

Explain to the child exactly what is going to happen, telling the child what you are going to do—not "will you do this for me?" Be sure particularly to explain that the child is to raise his or her hand (or finger) even when the tone sounds very faint and far away. Stress that the child must listen hard for these "little tiny sounds," because they are "a long way off."

Always make certain of the mental age of the child. If a 5 year old has a known IQ of 70, do not expect normal 5 year old behavior. Many children over 5 are labeled "untestable" merely because the clinician failed to apply the test procedure appropriate for the mental age level represented.

Aged 10–16 Years. Very few modifications of standard audiometric procedures are ever required for the 10–16 age group. The development of rapport, the complete explanation of the test procedure, and the use of mild motivational techniques are usually sufficient for a valid test. However, there are a few precautions to take at this age, which are given below.

If the clinician has been presented with an audiogram from elsewhere showing a 30–60 dB loss, yet the youngster responds perfectly well to soft speech levels, be prepared to conduct the hearing tests very carefully. In this case, start with a slow, ascending presentation of both pure tones and speech. Time will be saved in arriving at an accurate understanding of the hearing problem.

The hard-of-hearing child of this age must be handled carefully. Often the hearing-impaired child overresponds when no sound is actually heard, in an attempt to appear to have more favorable hearing than really exists. It is best not to let such children see you during the test presentation. Face them completely away from you, because they can catch even a raised eyebrow out of the corners of their eyes. During the test, give them long periods of silence occasionally, and if they respond falsely, reprove them for the false response. Perhaps the clinicians who have tested such a child have been overeager to motivate the child, and the child responds by merely trying to please. Gentle reprimands are sometimes necessary to counteract this behavior.

At this and younger ages, the child has a right to understand what it means to have a hearing loss, providing the child has any receptive language at all. Too often we tend to "talk over" the child to the parents, in words that the child does not understand. In the meantime, the child is sitting there, wondering what is wrong. The clinician should take time to explain in words that the child can understand about the hearing loss, how severe it is, and what is going to be done about it. Often the clinician's explanation of the problem will ease the way toward accepting the amplification and habilitation that will follow. Parents may be unable to explain these things to the child or may try to gloss over the facts, leaving the child bewildered and sometimes antagonistic. The child may be worried over what the other children will think and say in school. Explain that the hearing loss does create special problems but that you are going to be sure that the child can do everything the "other kids" can do and that the child will now be able to hear your friends and the teacher better.

USING A TESTER ASSISTANT

Although many audiology clinical settings require that the audiologist work alone, the hearing testing of children is often enhanced by the use of an extra observer or an assistant to the tester. This tester assistant remains in the test room with the child to help control the test paradigm, to monitor and direct the behavior of the child under evaluation, and to communicate with the tester as necessary. Guidelines are in order so that the tester assistant can be of maximum use in the audiologic evaluation.

To be a successful team, the tester and the assistant must have clearly defined roles and areas of responsibility understood before the testing begins. One person is identified as the "tester" and typically is the person responsible for the task at hand. The other person is the "assistant" and follows the directives of the tester. Both are in continuous contact by earphones and the talkback circuit of the audiometer, or through the sound field system, or even by closed circuit video. The designated responsible person has the task of all major communication with the parents. It is very disruptive to have both the tester and the assistant talking to the parents at different times during the test session appointment.

The assistant is in charge of the test room as much as possible and maintains the behavior of the child and the parents. It may be appropriate for the assistant to talk briefly to the parents during the session to warn them of what is about to happen in the test sequence, or to guide their communication with the child, or to caution them about influencing the responses of the child unless specifically asked to do so. The team must often make an educated estimate about whether or not to include the parents in the sound room during the test session, based on a number of observations including the behavior of the parents, the relationship between the parents and the child, the number of accompanying relatives, friends, neighbors, and siblings.

Prior to the start of the test session, the sound room environment needs to be well-organized. Toys must be kept out of sight until they are ready to be introduced to the child, one at a time, under control of the assistant. The test room should be as visually bland as possible to keep distraction at a minimum. Careful consideration must be given to the arrangement of chairs, tables, sound field speakers, visual reinforcers, position of the parent(s), assistant, and child, all with thought so that the tester will also have an unobstructed view of the child under evaluation.

The parent's chair should be oriented so that the infant or child is at a 90° angle to the visual reinforcer. The infant must be held, or the child seated, in such a way that if they turn to "find" the parent for reassurance, the head-turn will be away from the reinforcer. The situation should be organized so that when the child seeks the reinforcer light and/or toy, a clear head-turn response will be required.

The test session should be started when the infant or child is showing a moderate amount of interest in a quiet toy used as a distractor. The timing of the test signal presentations, and the time interval between signal presentations is very important to the success of the test session. Generally, the initial test presentations are slow, and as the child's performance improves, trials can be generated with much shorter intertrial intervals. "Time out" may be utilized following false responses from the child, allowing the youngster to "settle down" again. One of the most common errors made by inexperienced testers is to run through the test session too quickly too soon. Well-trained infants and children can perform quite well with rapid trial presentations, but the tester must be sure that the desired response relative to the stimulus presentations has been adequately shaped.

The assistant's task is to keep the child in a moderate state of alertness—not so absorbed in the toys that he or she will not be responsive to the auditory stimulus, yet not so uninterested that he or she will continuously visually search the room or fixate on the reinforcer. It is to be expected that there is tremendous variability among children's behavior in the test room environment. There is also wide variation in the child's attention level during the test session. The real challenge is for the assistant to judge precisely and anticipate the state of the child and to have an ability to manipulate and maintain the child's state at the desired level.

Obviously, the choice of toys is important. Toys vary in how much attention they demand from children. Sometimes a child will have no preconceived idea of what a specific toy is supposed to do, so the imagination of the assistant has much to do with how successful a toy can be during the test session. Beware of toys that generate noise and of action toys that become too intriguing. Introduce only one toy at a time, and keep all other toys out of sight. Put finished toys also out of sight and out of reach. Toys in use should be kept directly in front of the child to eliminate false head-turns. The manipulation of the toys by the assistant is very important to the timing and the eventual success of the hearing evaluation.

CENTRAL AUDITORY TESTING

Children with either organic lesions of the central auditory pathways or auditory perceptual and language disorders often benefit from tests of central auditory function. In the 1990s, the ability to test for these problems is a necessary skill for all audiologists. A complete discussion of this topic is beyond the scope of this section, and the reader is referred to a number of textbooks that include additional information and references. They include *Handbook of Central Auditory Processing Disorders in Children* (Willeford, 1985), *Central Auditory and Language Disorders in Children* (Keith, 1981), and *Assessment of Central Auditory Dysfunction* (Pinheiro and Musiek, 1985).

A number of problems exist that continue to make the topic of central auditory testing somewhat "fuzzy." One of the major problems is the lack of data on the cause-and-effect relationship of auditory-preceptual deficits and language, reading, and learning disorders. The lack of standardized terminology and diagnostic techniques raises doubt about the validity of remediation for such problems. The development of adequate remediation programs for children with auditory processing disorders continues to be a problem for those who work with this population. One indication of the multidisciplinary nature of this problem is that no professional specialty has stepped forward to claim this area as their own, and remediation programs are best developed through group interaction. Communication specialists and educators agree that central auditory processing disorders of varying difficulty exist in their students. Classroom teachers look to speech-language pathologists and audiologists for guidance in managing children with these problems.

Keith (1986) has defined an auditory processing disorder as "impaired ability to attend to, discriminate, recognize, remember, or comprehend information presented auditorily[,] even though the person has normal intelligence and hearing sensitivity. These difficulties are more pronounced when listening to low redundancy (distorted) speech, when there are competing sounds, or when there is a poor acoustic environment." Keith states further that in the normal child, auditory processing abilities develop in a parallel or reciprocal relationship with language abilities and that children with auditory processing disorders are a subset of children with receptive and/or language disorders. Keith (1988) hypothesizes that some basic auditory-perceptual skills, e.g., appreciation of frequency, intensity, and duration of sounds, exist in every child and serve as building blocks of audition, leading to language development through imitation. As language skills are acquired, children also acquire other linguistically dependent auditory-perceptual skills, such as memory, discrimination, closure, and blending. In addition, as the child's neuroanatomic pathways mature, the ability to cope with higher level auditory tasks such as dichotic listening, binaural release from masking, and other nonlinguistically based listening skills begins to improve. A number of available tests are designed to measure these auditory abilities. It is necessary to select carefully the appropriate test for the ability to be measured and to evaluate the results against appropriate normative standards. Recent developments in electrophysiologic techniques indicate promising approaches to assessing central processing abilities in children in the future. These techniques, including middle latency responses and various other cortical evoked potentials, will require substantial investigation before they can be applied for clinical purposes.

Keith (1988, page 1218) defines the most common central auditory abilities that test developers attempt to measure and presents examples of these tests in Table 5.6.

Table 5.6.
Examples of Tests That Attempt to Measure Certain Auditory Abilities in Children[a]

Auditory Abilities	Test
Localization	Sound Field Localization
Binaural synthesis	Rapid Alternating Speech Perception
	Binaural Fusion Test
Figure ground	Goldman-Fristoe-Woodcock Test of Auditory Discrimination (GFW)
	Flowers-Costello Test of Central Auditory Abilities
	Kindergarten Auditory Screening Test (KAST)
	GFW Selective Attention Test
	Composite Auditory Perceptual Test (CAPT) Figure-Ground Test
	Kindergarten Figure Ground Tests
Binaural separation	Willeford Competing Sentence Tests
	Dichotic CV Identification Test
	Staggered Spondaic Word Test
Memory	Illinois Test of Psycholinguistic Abilities (ITPA): Auditory Sequential Memory
	Wepman Auditory Memory Span Test and Auditory Sequential Memory Test
	GFW Auditory Memory Test
	Lyness Auditory Perception Test
Blending	ITPA Sound Blending Test
	KAST
	GFW Test of Sound Blending
	Rosewell-Phall Auditory Blending Test
Discrimination	KAST
	Wepman Auditory Discrimination Test
	GFW Auditory Discrimination Test
	Lyness Auditory Perception Test
Closure	Flowers-Costello Test of Central Auditory Abilities
	Filtered Speech Subtest: Willeford Battery
	Time Compressed Speech
	ITPA Test of Auditory Closure
Association	Competing Environmental Sound Test
Cognition	Wechsler Intelligence Scale for Children (WISC)
	Carrow Test of Auditory Comprehension of Language

[a]From R. W. Keith: Central auditory tests. In N. J. Lass et al. (eds.): *Handbook of Speech-Language Pathology & Audiology.* Philadelphia, B. C. Decker, 1988, p. 1229.

Localization. The ability to locate auditorily the source of a sound. This ability requires binaural stimulation.

Binaural Synthesis. The ability to integrate centrally incomplete stimulus patterns presented simultaneously or alternately to opposite ears.

Figure Ground. The ability to identify a primary signal or message in the presence of competing sounds. Auditory figure-ground can be a monaural or a binaural task.

Binaural Separation. The ability to listen with one ear while ignoring stimulation of the opposite ear. Dichotic listening, as a binaural separation task, requires the listener to attend to and report back different signals presented simultaneously to two ears.

Memory. The ability to store and to recall auditory stimuli, including length or number of auditory stimuli, and sequential memory or the ability to recall the exact order of auditory stimuli presented.

Blending. The ability to form words out of separately articulated phonemes.

Discrimination. The ability to determine whether two acoustic stimuli are the same or different. In speech, auditory discrimination is the ability to recognize fine differences that exist among phonemes.

Closure. The ability to preceive the whole (word or message) when parts are omitted.

Attention. The ability to persist in listening over a reasonable period of time.

Association. The ability to establish a correspondence between a nonlinguistic sound and its source.

Cognition. The ability to establish a correspondence between a linguistic sound and its meaning. Cognition is the highest level of auditory perception and results from a summation of all auditory (and all sensory) tasks.

CHILDREN WITH UNILATERAL DEAFNESS

Unilateral deafness is not an uncommon problem among children with a prevalence of 3–13 in 1000, depending upon the degree of hearing loss in the abnormal ear (Berg, 1972). Often due to mumps, the unilateral hearing loss may develop in every early childhood or as the sequela to subclinical mumps with no obvious symptoms. In many instances, the child is unaware of the problem, and the parents do not discover the loss until some sequence of events suggests the unilateral hearing loss. Parents will note that the child can only hear on the telephone with one particular ear, or the child cannot be awakened when the normal-hearing ear is pressed into a pillow.

Once the unilateral hearing loss is confirmed, the audiologist should take time to explain the ramifications of the problem. Studies of adults with severe-to-profound unilateral hearing loss have confirmed that these patients have difficulties in localizing the source of a sound, with pronounced difficulties in listening in backgrounds of noise, and they lose the binaural summation effect provided by two ears, creating general communication difficulties.

Until recently, children with unilateral deafness have been considered education-ally handicapped. Studies by Bess and his associates (1984, 1986) at Vanderbilt University, however, have brought renewed attention to the child with only one normal-hearing ear. They identified 60 children with unilateral hearing loss who were enrolled in the Nashville Metropolitan School System and closely examined their educational records. They found that approximately one third of this group had *failed* at least one grade during their school years and nearly 50% of the group needed special resource assistance in the schools! In a series of research studies conducted by Bess, with 25 of the unilaterally hearing-impaired children matched with 25 normal-hearing children, the children with unilateral hearing loss performed much poorer on localization tasks and syllable recognition tasks. Based on his studies, Bess concluded that children with unilateral hearing loss experience considerably more difficulty in communication and in education than was previously supposed.

Oyler et al. (1987, 1988) challenged the Vanderbilt data on unilateral hearing loss by conducting a similar study in a large school district of Tucson, Arizona. They found a remarkably similar academic failure rate, proving again that children with unilateral hearing loss are at a risk factor approximately 10 times greater than that for the general school population of academic difficulties resulting in grade failure. Of special interest in both the Nashville and Tucson studies, the recurring profile among the unilateral hearing loss students who experienced academic difficulties included (*a*) early age of onset, (*b*) severe-to-profound hearing impairment, and (*c*) right-ear impairment.

Recommendations for Management. Oyler et al. (1987) suggested several management recommendations for supporting the child with unilateral hearing loss. Actually, these recommendations are equally applicable for communicating with all children who have hearing loss:

- Gain the child's attention before beginning to speak.

- Use familiar vocabulary and less complex sentence structure.

- Rephrase statements that are misunderstood, rather than just repeat them verbatim.

- Provide visual supplement to the communication to improve understanding.

- Give students preferential classroom seating to take advantage of the better hearing ear.

- Minimize noise interference generated from within or outside the classroom.

- Routinely monitor the child's speech and language development and academic progress.

- Consider use of the CROS (cross routing of signal) hearing aid fitting.

- Consider use of a personal FM or the classroom amplification system to enhance the signal-to-noise ratio.

- Give hearing conversation rules to protect the good ear:
  (*a*) Stay away from loud noises.
  (*b*) Get prompt medical care for any ear infection.
  (*c*) Avoid putting anything into the ear.
  (*d*) Avoid ototoxic drugs unless absolutely necessary.
  (*e*) Take special care of general health, especially during flu seasons.
  (*f*) Have an otologic and audiologic check once a year.
  (*g*) Do not get advice on treatment from anyone except qualified otolaryngologists and audiologists.

NONORGANIC HEARING LOSS IN CHILDREN

The child who presents with a nonorganic, or functional, hearing loss is a quite different problem from the adult with a nonorganic loss. The child is a much less sophisticated feigner of poor hearing than the adult, and the underlying motives, what-

ever the impelling factor, are sometimes more obscure. The needs that drive the child to give an inaccurate hearing test are probably more honest, and certainly engender more sympathy, that those that drive the adult.

Any child who presents with a functional hearing loss has a problem, whether it be a minor transient difficulty or a deep-seated permanent disorder. It is a symptom of something, just as a runny nose or a fever is a symptom of something. It should never be disregarded or passed off as a temporary foible. It may represent a cry for attention, an apology for poor performance, or a rebuff to a hostile world.

Children who have some basic need that is unfulfilled may choose from a variety of symptoms that are available to them, ranging from the conscious to the psychosomatic. They may complain of stomachaches, headaches, poor vision, poor hearing, or specific pains. They may act out their needs in aggressive behavior or in withdrawal. Their symptoms may enter the psychosomatic realm, with disorders such as eczema or chronic stomach problems. Even psychosis may be present. When their behavior becomes outwardly aggressive and approaches delinquency, their disturbance becomes a threat to their families and to society.

The large majority of children who present with such problems are referred because of failure on the screening test in school. Johnny sees that Joe, who has failed the hearing test, is given special treatment—he is excused from school to have further examinations, and he is given special seating and attention in school. It is like having headaches or stomachaches—it gives an excuse for poor performance and a chance to bid for sympathy.

It should be recognized that this discussion of nonorganic hearing loss does not include those children who did not understand the instructions given them during a previous test. It should be obvious when the child has responded only to the loudness level of the first tone he heard. However, this is also strategy used by the child with true nonorganic hearing loss, so care should be taken to ensure that the child has completely understood the directions.

Leshin (1960) reported a screening program that identified a number of cases of nonorganicity in children. He investigated the social dynamics of each case and instituted a remedial program that would fulfill the needs of the child that impelled him or her to a symptom such as hearing loss. Such a program can be highly recommended.

The audiologist should recognize the nonorganic hearing loss child by a number of presenting symptoms. One should be on alert for all types of exaggerated behavior, such as verbosity, brashness, over-withdrawal, lack of personal affect, exaggerated straining to hear the test tones, inconsistent intratest results such as poor PTA (pure tone average of thresholds at 500, 1000, and 2000 Hz) and SRT agreement, and audiometric threshold variation of 15–25 dB at the same frequency. Often, better behavioral thresholds may be obtained with careful and slow ascending technique.

Of course, in the final analysis, immittance and audiometric techniques and ABR measurement will reveal the true state of hearing in the child with nonorganic hearing loss. Normal tympanograms and the presence of bilateral acoustic reflexes rule out any possible conductive hearing problem, and the ABR threshold exploration procedure can be used to estimate normal or near-normal hearing sensitivity. It is rare that any of the classic auditory tests for functional hearing loss used with adults need to be used on children. The naiveté of young children in responding at normal levels with speech audiometry and exaggerated threshold levels with pure tones makes identification of the nonorganic hearing problem obvious. Occasionally, in the case of a monaural feigned hearing loss, the Stenger test can be used to estimate the level of hearing in the supposed "bad" ear.

Once the inconsistencies have been identified, hostility and threats toward the child from the audiologist will only make matters worse. When the child realizes that you are suspicious of the responses, priorism for "saving face" is an important step toward resolution of the problem. Use statements such as "perhaps you didn't understand my instructions clearly," or "the results of this hearing test are not coming out correctly, and I would like you to listen again as carefully as you can." Take your time in the presentation of pure tones, and be prepared to "wait the child out." If normal hearing levels can be established through traditional behavioral techniques, time and effort are streamlined. If the child's responses are just not forthcoming as correctly as you believe they should, the next option is to schedule an ABR hearing evaluation.

In terms of general management of the nonorganic hearing loss child, it is best to refer actual psychologic problems to the professionals best trained to deal with abnormal behavior. The continuum of severity of emotional causes of nonorganic medical problems runs a gamut from mild, transient behaviors to severe malingering. Transient, isolated instances describe most children's attempts to feign hearing loss and, when resolved, usually cause no additional concerns. As the nonorganicity of hearing loss appears to be somewhat more entrenched in the child's daily behavior, certainly the audiologist needs to talk frankly with the parents about the child's problem and to suggest professional counseling. Given truly bizarre behavior including total noncooperation from the child in the hearing test situation, the main task of the audiologist is to establish the organic hearing levels of the youngster; and psychiatric counsel should urgently be advised with the agreement of the managing physician. The cry for help that is inherent in the presentation of nonorganic hearing loss in a child should not be taken lightly by the audiologist.

TESTING THE DIFFICULT-TO-TEST CHILD

The judgments the clinician makes on children's hearing abilities often necessarily involve a differential evaluation. In the presence of other disorders the child's behavior or level of functioning may be so erratic that standard techniques of audiometry cannot be used. To apply appropriate tests for hearing, the clinician must be able to recognize the dysfunction present and to adjust the tests to it. The classical disorders to be differentiated are mental retardation, cerebral dysfunction, and autism (Myklebust, 1954). More than one of these may be present in one child. The clinician trained in evaluating any of these disorders may also test the child's functioning in that specific area, as well as in the hearing area. But at the very least the audiologist has the responsibility of recognizing the disorder that exists and of being able to apply the proper tests for hearing and to make referral for diagnosis and treatment of the other disorder.

In discussing the entities that must be recognized, it is necessary to reiterate an important fact; i.e., neither cerebral dysfunction, nor central auditory disorders, nor mental retardation, nor autism itself results in a decrease of auditory acuity as represented by the audiogram. The responses that can be elicited certainly require more ingenuity to obtain. But when credible responses reveal reduced hearing for pure tones and speech, a peripheral hearing loss is present, in addition to any central disorder that may exist (Goldstein et al., 1972; Kleffner, 1973). The clinical audiologist's task is to choose the appropriate test procedures that will reveal the presence or absence of peripheral hearing loss and/or central auditory disorder. It is not always a simple task to make this distinction.

Multihandicapped Children.

Multihandicapped children present the difficult testing problems for audiologists. By definition, profoundly multihandicapped children cannot function independently at the most basic skill levels including self-presentation, self-care, mobility, and communication (Baker, 1979). When viewed within the context of developmental theory, the profoundly multihandicapped child responds to the same stimulation parameters as the normal child of the same developmental age (Kamhi, 1982). The developmental theory implies that the retarded child passes through the same auditory developmental states as the normal child, except that the retarded child develops more slowly and with less potential.

The evaluation of hearing in profoundly multihandicapped children requires the utmost in audiologic skills and the cross-check principle of physiologic tests such as ABR and immittance evaluations, along with behavioral audiometry if possible. Although the ABR procedure is usually required for definitive hearing assessment, these patients cannot always be successfully tested with ABR because their problems are often confounded by central nervous system drainage and severe neurologic abnormalities. Accordingly, behavioral measurement of hearing must be included as a basic component of the auditory evaluation. On occasion, the uncontrollable behavior of the multihandicapped child makes it extremely difficult to structure the testing situation properly (Table 5.7).

In the most severe cases of multiple involvements, including blindness and retardation, we have found it useful to rely on the simplest of behavioral commands, presented through the sound field speaker system, of "sit down," "stand up," various orienting stimuli, and observation of quieting responses to specific stimuli presentations. At the most rudimentary level, these response behaviors may suggest the presence of near-normal hearing, although the absence of consistent responses can, in no way, be interpreted as the presence of hearing loss.

Flexer and Gans (1985, 1986) have studied the auditory responsiveness of profoundly multihandicapped children and report that their results support the practice

Table 5.7.
Suggestions for Audiologic Testing of the Multihandicapped Child[a]

Concern	Adaptation
These children vary in their capabilities for selective attention.	May need to reduce extraneous visual or auditory distraction to avoid "overload"; e.g., reduce demands for motoric or visual activity when eliciting auditory response.
State of arousal may vary during interaction.	If child becomes lethargic, change in positioning may heighten arousal; e.g., rock from supine to sitting position. Parent or teacher may suggest strategy.
Child often requires more than the usual amount of response time.	Careful pacing of stimulation to allow for latent responses.
Interfering self-stimulatory behaviors.	Provide alternative action. Ask parent and teacher for input regarding methods for reducing these behaviors.
Tactile defensiveness may affect interaction with examiner.	Inquire and observe for incidence of this behavior. Approach the child carefully if touch is nonreinforcing.
VRA response requires many prerequisites that may not be in the child's repertoire.	Note if the child has self-regulated looking, sufficient head-neck control, cognitive prerequisites. Explore adaptive positioning (can the child lie on the floor and roll to sound source? While in standing board, can the child shift eye gaze to light stimulus?) Are the visual and auditory stimuli reinforcing enough?
Child may exhibit subdued or noncharacteristic behavior in new environment.	Observe the child in a natural setting (school or home) if possible. Allow "visits" to the suite before testing. Provide warm-up/exploration time and sufficient practice trials.

[a]Adapted from M. P. Moeller: *Sensory Organizational Issues: Multi-Handicapped Child*. Omaha, Nebraska, Boys Town National Institute, Coordinator for Aural Rehabilitation, 1988.

of determining auditory evaluation of these children in relation to their development age. These researchers noted that narrow bandwidth auditory signals are simply not as effective in eliciting responses from infants and profoundly multihandicapped children as are broader bandwidth stimuli (including speech), because in all likelihood the broader bandwidth signals sound "louder." Flexer and Gans also found that profoundly multihandicapped children display relatively more reflexive than attentive behaviors and exhibit fewer behaviors per response than do normal children.

An interesting examination of classical conditioning utilizing an air puff as the unconditioned stimulus in order to perform hearing assessment with multihandicapped children and adolescents was described by Lancioni et al. (1989). Their findings indicate that the classical conditioning paradigm was successful in 21 of 23 children, whereas operant conditioning with VRA succeeded in only 15. The auditory thresholds obtained with the classical conditioning

air puff technique were equal or within 10 dB of the VRA established thresholds.

Accurate assessment of hearing level in developmentally delayed persons is crucial to optimal efforts at rehabilitation, intervention, and follow-up. A comparative study of audiometric testing techniques with 61 moderately and 103 profoundly mentally retarded from a large institution was conducted by Benham-Dunster and Dunster (1985), who compared BOA with visual reinforcement, Sensitivity Prediction with the Acoustic Reflex (SPAR) test technique, and ABR (sedation administered as required—66% of moderately delayed and 91% of profoundly delayed).

The study corroborates the general wisdom that accurate assessment of hearing loss for the profoundly delayed is far more difficult than for normal populations or even moderately delayed populations. BOA appears to be more reflective of developmental capabilities than of hearing loss, especially among the profoundly delayed. The SPAR method tends to overpredict hearing loss and is problematic with profoundly delayed persons because of uncooperative behavior.

ABR seems to hold promise for the accurate measurement of hearing loss among the profoundly delayed. For a thorough investigation of the auditory mechanism and hearing in the developmentally handicapped, a full battery of tests offers the most complete assessment. A wide range of data helps overcome gaps in information that result from difficulties inherent in testing developmentally delayed individuals (Gans and Flexer, 1982).

Mental Retardation. One principle should be kept in mind when dealing with the mentally retarded child: If generalized developmental retardation is the only disorder, the child will behave in all areas at the level of his or her age. This principle will hold up in all cases except those in which autistic behavior or cerebral dysfunction is superimposed upon the general retardation. Then the testing problem is further compounded, although not insoluble. Of course, this group of difficult-to-test children are prime candidates for the auditory brainstem evoked potential (ABR) and acoustic immittance measurements described in Chapter 6.

Younger Child. During the younger years the mentally delayed child has not yet developed the social behaviorisms, the self-stimulating activities, or the inattention patterns typical of the older mentally delayed child. In the first few months of life the child will sleep a great deal, giving an opportunity for good observations of responses to sound stimuli in a sound room.

After 4 months the retardate can be identified through his or her auditory behavior as well as through the developmental landmarks present. If by 5 months the child is not making even a partial head-turn towards the sound, determine developmental milestones such as reaching and holding objects and laughing aloud. The mentally delayed child may not hold the head erect or be able to follow a moving object—behavior

that would place the child below the 3 month level of functioning. In this case one can expect only the auditory responses listed for a child under 4 months old.

The same observations of auditory behavior and developmental behavior should be made of the older child, referring to the developmental landmarks. If all behaviors are consistent for a certain age level, and the auditory indices are within the normal limits listed for that age level, the hearing level is judged to be normal. For example, if a 15 month old child's behavioral landmarks are at the 8 month level, a speech awareness level of 15–20 dB and pure tone awareness of 45–55 dB are considered to be normal hearing. Of course, ABR testing and acoustic immittance measurements would be used to confirm this impression.

If previous developmental scales or IQ test results are available, the clinician will have no difficulty in correcting the auditory test results for mental age. It is when the intellectual status is unknown that the clinician must apply his or her own observations of developmental landmarks. If these are not consistent at a certain age level, another disorder should be suspected. The 5 year old who has normal motor coordination and good personal-social adjustment for age, yet is unable to identify all of a group of familiar toys, should be evaluated further, providing that his or her hearing test is normal.

Among the audiologic and otologic studies on the prevalence of hearing loss and ear disease in institutions for mental retardation, the percentages of loss range from about 10% to 45% or greater. Lloyd (1970) presented a review of the literature on the audiologic aspects of mental retardation in which a summary of the various reported incidences is given. Each percentage is affected by the chronologic and mental age of the population tested, by the testing procedures used, and by the criteria for failure that are applied.

Dahle and McCollister (1983) have reviewed all of the procedures for evaluating mentally retarded children, including an appropriate review of the physiologic tests of hearing. They point out that normal ABR tracings in this group of children give valuable information about their auditory peripheral sensitivity. However, when the ABR is abnormal, and a central nervous system abnormality is obvious, the ABR results are ambiguous (Worthington and Peters, 1980).

Older Child. A large number of older developmentally delayed children will have a level of functioning that permits behavioral conditioning or speech audiometry tests to be used. If their mental age is over 2 years, the tests described for children of that age can be applied. Play-conditioning techniques often are successful with the older retarded child when standard techniques fail.

A period of pretest observation will reveal what can be expected of the youngster. Present the child with toys and see how familiar he or she is with them. Can the child hand them to you on a command? If the child recognizes most of the toys and can give them to you on command, you can probably expect to obtain both a speech reception threshold and play-conditioned thresholds. If not, the routine observations of behavioral responses can be made. Depending on the degree of accuracy required during the hearing test, the audiologist must be prepared to cross-check the subjective auditory thresholds with additional independent tests. When precise thresholds are desired in such a borderline functioning child, the techniques of VRA, immittance audiometry, and ABR should be used.

The Centrally Disordered Child. The suggested techniques for testing the brain-damaged child rest on two basic assumptions:

- Any reduction in auditory acuity for pure tones, speech, or other signals is caused by lesions in the peripheral auditory system, not in the midbrain or higher pathways (see our discussion in Chapter 4 on "Disorders in Auditory Learning"). No real evidence has ever been presented that unilateral lesions central to the cochlear nuclei result in reduction in auditory sensitivity.

- Only in the extremely severe centrally damaged child with gross motoric involvement will we see the complete absence of all of the four basic auditory reflexes: head-turn, eye-blink, startle response, and arousal from sleep.

The first rule in testing such a child is to determine the level of behavior through some means of pretesting. Sit and talk quietly and play with the youngster in the sound room. Can the child attend for any length of time to anything you say or do? Can the child give his or her name, age, or other appropriate information? Can the child hand you toys or repeats words on request? In the case of a very young child, as well as an older one, is the eye contact steady, and does it have integrity? Can the child sit still for any length of time? Is the child hyperactive, and does the child throw things around?

The child who has auditory perceptual dysfunction may be able to sit quietly and attend to visual stimuli but not be able to repeat words or to pick up objects on command. Such a child may, however, be perfectly able to do play-conditioned audiometry with pure tones and speech signals. Do not give up on formal testing unless it is proved to be ineffective.

If it is evident that formal testing techniques will not be successful, it is best to start at the lowest level of testing procedure, as has been described for the infant from 4 months on. The entire battery of observations should be made, from localization procedures to startle reactions. Remember that this child may be inconsistent in responses to various stimuli and at various times. The startle or the eye-blink response to a loud stimulus may confirm the observation of inconsistent reactions to soft levels.

It is rare for all of the behavioral auditory reflexive responses to be absent in a child. These auditory behavioral reflexive responses are mediated at the level of the brainstem and are usually intact in the presence of higher cortical dysfunction. Auditory reflexes only tell us about the integrity of the peripheral auditory system and the central auditory system through the brainstem. They tell us nothing about the higher orders of perception and integration.

Only in the presence of degeneration of the brainstem at the olivary complex can the absence of the head-turn and eye-blink be expected. Even then, the startle reflex, mediated at a low brainstem level, should be active, unless there is widespread motoric damage that prevents the muscular system from coordinating. Although the startle or eye-blink reflexes to a 65 dB (speech level) signal do not eliminate the presence of a sensorineural loss, it is likely that the hearing loss is not of a degree that would produce severe degree of symptoms found in a child with profound or total deafness.

An extensive study of tympanometry on nearly 900 institutionalized developmentally disabled persons found that the general prevalence of conductive disorders is higher than that of a normal population, thus emphasizing the importance of detecting conductive pathology in this population (Zoller et al., 1985). This study noted a trend for prevalence of conductive disorders to increase with (*a*) mental retardation, as indicated by tympanometry, possibly as a reflection of increasingly poor aural hygiene, and (*b*) a decrease in the patient's ability to convey information about hearing disability as the degree of retardation increases.

Stein et al. (1987) evaluated 122 profoundly retarded children from a single residential institution over a 4½ year period. Most of the children were nonambulatory and had multiple handicapping conditions. The children ranged in age from infants to 18 years with a mean age of 7.8 years. By definition, this group represented the most profoundly retarded subpopulation of the retarded described as untestable or difficult-to-test by behavioral audiometry. This study noted that 32% of the population showed hearing loss, by ABR testing, of 20 dB or greater in one or both ears, with 12% conductive loss and 20% sensorineural hearing loss. Some 8% of the study sample showed bilateral severe-to-profound hearing loss. Although the authors caution that the data reported are limited in generalization to the *institutionalized profoundly retarded*, nonetheless this study confirms the presence of a high incidence of hearing loss in such populations. Six of nine children in this group fitted with hearing aids accepted and appeared to benefit from the use of personal amplification.

Autistic-Like Child. It is seldom that one sees the purely autistic-like child, but when one does, the bizarre behavior displayed can be recognized almost immediately: refusal to meet any person's eye gaze, disregard of all human speech stimuli, long-term fixation on some object, and refusal of physical contact with humans. This child will consistently fail to attend to any speech stimulus, yet will attend to some other acoustic signals. One such child will look for pure tone signals at low intensities, another will search for a novel sound field speech signal at soft levels, and another will localize to a white or a complex noise signal. All will startle or eye-blink to a 65 dB HL voice in a structured sound room situation if hearing is normal. All the stimuli described for testing from birth on should be tried. Some stimulus will likely produce a response if the hearing is normal, even if it is only a startle response.

The real testing problem arises when autistic behavior is superimposed on central dysfunction. Indeed, one wonders whether all brain damage is not accompanied by some degree of autistic behavior. The symptoms are often so similar that they defy separation. In addition to the behavior described above, there may be the heightened activity and lashing out at humans. If such a child is difficult for the neurologist and psychiatrist to understand, so too is the child for the audiologist.

The testing procedures described for mental retardation and for central nervous system disorders are applicable here. Keep in mind that autistic symptoms are sometimes found in the deaf child, so do not let anything mislead you in the search for peripheral hearing loss. The cross-check principle is especially important in the evaluation of hearing in these children. The physiologic tests, such as ABR and immittance measurements, with special attention to acoustic reflex thresholds, are extremely valuable.

Deaf-Blind Child. In our opinion, evaluation of hearing in deaf-blind children is the most difficult task faced by the audiologist. These cases are most often confounded by central nervous system damage that makes it difficult to structure the testing situation properly.

In severe cases of multiple involvements, we have found it most expedient to rely again on the auditory reflexes, on orientation responses, and on quieting responses. In the absence of speech and language, one must apply the tests as for the infant, proceeding to the upper limits of the auditory abilities present. The audiologist must be prepared to perform or to refer such patients for, auditory evoked potential evaluation. The immittance test battery is an important part of the auditory evaluation of every deaf-blind child.

An excellent report on the neurologic handicaps, degree of hearing and visual disability, and the level of language and developmental characteristics of a young deaf-blind population was published by Stein et al. (1981). These authors reviewed data from 141 deaf-blind children evaluated at their clinic between 1972 and 1979. Of the 141 "deaf-blind" children seen for diagnostic evaluation, 38 were found to have normal or near-normal hearing and, therefore, were technically not "deaf." The diagnosis of normal hearing in most of these difficult-to-test children was accomplished only

through the use of the ABR technique (Stein et al., 1981). The previous diagnosis of deafness given these children was based largely on behavioral testing—and these children simply failed to respond behaviorally to sound. This finding is not uncommon in groups of "deaf-blind" children.

Stein et al. summarize the findings in their study as follows:

- A high incidence of neurologic handicapping conditions are associated with congenitally deaf-blind children, including neuromuscular disorders.

- Severe hearing disability was more common than severe vision disability in their sample of deaf-blind children. Sixty-eight percent of the children had so little usable hearing that the potential benefit of wearable amplification is minimal at best.

- Many of the "deaf-blind" children referred for evaluation proved to have normal peripheral hearing without normal behavioral responses to sound. The use of the ABR as part of the audiologic evaluation is thus an absolute necessity with these children.

- The combination of hearing and visual problems together with neurologic handicapping conditions has a profound effect on the language level, cognitive skills, and general development of these children.

- The severe hearing loss and neurologic problems will require that most, if not all, of these children will require supervised care for the rest of their lives.

It is the audiologist's responsibility to make the decision about the multihandicapped child's hearing abilities. It must, perforce, be a bold decision, for any equivocation is not useful to the child. The conservative hearing aid trial with careful observations by all concerned during a diagnostic therapy period may be helpful. Hesitance may deprive the child of critical time for learning auditory skills and thus do him or her a disservice. Little textbook information or standardized developmental scales are available regarding techniques for evaluating the hearing response in these children. It is often useful to the audiologist to discuss the hearing potential of deaf-blind children with the parents and teachers who are with the child for long periods of time.

PARENT MANAGEMENT

Often it is the audiologist who must inform the parents that they have a deaf or hard-of-hearing child. It is always best to have the parents observe the child's responses in a free-field situation so that they can see for themselves that the child does not hear normally, as well as note what their child can and cannot hear. Although in many instances the parents have a strong suspicion that their child has a hearing problem, confirmation of the handicap may still be an extremely traumatic situation for them. Whether the parents show grief openly or contain it within themselves, you may be sure that they will be deeply distubed over the knowledge. The audiologist must find ways to help them over this initial shock.

Stein and Jabaley (1981) have published an excellent chapter on parent counseling in their textbook, *Deafness and Mental Health*, in which they describe their conclusions based on 15 years of talking with parents of hearing-impaired children. They state that the two most common factors in the environment of deaf children that can account for their emotional or behavioral differences are (*1*) the lag in language development and its effect on family communication and socialization, and (*2*) the psychologic response of parents to the diagnosis of hearing handicap in their child. Stein and Jabaley describe three stages of parental responses: (*1*) an initial expression of anger toward the professionals who diagnose the deafness in their child; (*2*) subsequent expressions of anger toward the child as they find it increasingly difficult to deny the existence of the hearing loss; and finally (*3*) the acceptance of the hearing-impaired child by the parents, which marks the transition from sadness and anger to the development of adaptation and coping behaviors. They urge the development of a working relationship with the involved parents to reduce the high prevalence of emotional and behavioral problems, while helping to establish the important parent-infant bond.

It is the usual tendency of parents to want to find out immediately everything that concerns the future of the child and his or her functioning. One must resist the temptation to go into great detail about the prognosis for the child's development. Whatever is said will be only half-absorbed and largely distorted on the first visit. One should limit the amount of information to the relative degree of loss that seems to be present—mild, moderate, severe, or profound—and concentrate on the implications of the loss and what is going to be done for the child. If the parents press the question as to whether the child will speak, what kind of school he or she will go to, or whether the child will ever communicate, assure them that you will be able to answer these questions but only after a period of diagnostic therapy. No one can ever guarantee what a child will be able to do with training; only the results will demonstrate that.

There is perhaps no way to cushion the shock of finding out that a child is hearing-impaired. Any attempt to minimize the problem would be a disservice and would avoid the reality of the situation. But a sympathetic attitude and an understanding of the parent's feelings will help as much as possible: "You probably feel pretty upset about this news," or "It's perfectly natural for you to feel badly about this." Let them air their questions and fears. Allot sufficient time for them to express their feelings. Offer to be available for any questions that they might have, and let them feel that you will work with them closely on finding out what their child can do with this loss. Emphasize that he or she is a child first, has a hearing loss only secondarily, and is just as lovable as any other child.

Wherever possible, parents' groups under qualified psychologic counselors should be organized in order to provide ongoing guidance. If further help seems indicated, psychiatric or psychologic counsel should be sought for the individual parents. The audiologist should be aware of his or her limitations in providing psychotherapy for parents who cannot handle their problems.

In his or her relationship with the parents, the audiologist's responsibility includes the following:

- A complete explanation of what the audiogram means, and what the child can and cannot hear.

- A description of the type of loss, whether conductive or sensorineural, and what it means in terms of whether medical treatment may or may not be possible.

- A thorough explanation of the educational programs that are available for the child: auditory, oral, or total. The parents should be directed to visit each program so that they may participate in the decision as to which program will be chosen. With proper guidance, they should be able to make this decision themselves.

- Psychologic support. This may take the form of a one-to-one relationship, or the parents may require group programs or even individual psychiatric counseling. The audiologist should remember that in this difficult role he or she can and should seek counseling both for oneself and for the parents if he or she believes the parents are unable to cope adequately with the situation.

All students of audiology, as well as practicing clinicians, should read the excellent book written by David Luterman, Ph.D., *Counseling Parents of Hearing-Impaired Children* (1979).

AUDIOLOGIST'S SELF-UNDERSTANDING

In his or her zeal to help the hearing-handicapped child and the child's parents, the audiologist often overlooks his or her own motivations and how they will affect relations with the parents. These relations may be critical to the parents' acceptance of the problem. Quite without meaning to, he or she may leave the parents with fears and with pent-up emotions that can adversely affect the habilitation process. At some point the audiologist must look inward to see what his or her own feelings are in relation to the way information is given to the parents and how he or she handles them. If the audiologist has entered the audiologic profession with an emotional zeal for "do-gooding," he or she may see himself or herself as the authoritarian figure who directs the lives of people and thus will not permit the parents to express themselves, because he or she is in charge of operations. If the audiologist has entered the field through an objective interest in the scientific manifestations of hearing, he or she may shrink from becoming emotionally involved and committed to the parents' problems.

So the audiologist, too, may have problems in feeling comfortable in his or her role as protagonist in the drama of the parent-clinician interplay. This subject deserves extensive coverage because it is vital to the ultimate emotional health of the child. A most meaningful exposition of the subject has been written by two experts in parent management, Dr. Brian Hersch, a psychiatrist, and Carol Amon, an instructor of deaf children. We are indebted to them for permission to use their analysis of the dynamics of the parent-clinician relationship (Hersch and Amon, 1973), presented below.

To parents who are anxious to hear that their idealized child is perfect, the statement that "Your child has a hearing impairment" may be painful words. Those words can cause many emotions . . . shock, bewilderment, depression, anger, guilt, or anxiety. If these emotions are outwardly expressed by the parents, the audiologist, too, will experience feelings which may also be painful.

In order to avoid this uncomfortable experience, many audiologists today choose a painless method of reporting the diagnosis—a way that, although it is painless for themselves, may have devastating effects on the parents and their child. After listening to many parents relate their experiences and frustrations, we began to realize that the act of reporting the diagnosis was not only of paramount importance, but also that it was the beginning of a process that would include the habilitation and education of the child as well as the crucial involvement of the parents. This process could be enhanced or interfered with, by the interpersonal relations of the initial contact.

An approach toward lessening the trauma of the initial contact is proposed. It is an outgrowth of an idea that an interdisciplinary approach to understanding hearing-impaired infants and their families (the disciplines being audiology, deaf education, and psychiatry) is far superior to an isolated fragmented approach of one profession (Schlesinger and Meadow, 1972).

Schlesinger and Meadow describe three ineffective professional stances which are often seen today in the reporting of the diagnosis:

1. *The "hit-and-run" approach.* The diagnosis is reported very quickly and matter-of-factly in passing. "Your child didn't respond too much today . . . his hearing loss is probably severe to profound. I'll see you in 6 months for another evaluation." The parents are left with their feelings of bewilderment as to what to do next. The reporting of the diagnosis appears to be a dead end with no source of help.

2. *Minimizing the problem.* The clinician infers that there is really nothing to worry about. "In this day and age, deaf children can be given hearing aids and go to regular school just like any other child." These words give false hope to the parents, but the audiologist says them in order to make the parents feel better.

3. *The objectivity approach.* Many audiologists are hidden behind objectivity, using the "big word" technique. In 1 hour's time, they report the diagnosis, explain the audiogram and the hearing mechanism, and how their child differs from normal, describe methods of habilitation, demonstrate the use and maintenance of a hearing aid, and schedule the child for the first habilitation session. The audiologist does most of the talking, often using professional jargon which leaves parents confused and feeling lost. The audiologist avoids listening.

4. *The action-oriented approach.* This fourth approach is also a popular one. The audiologist states the problem, and almost before he completes the reporting of the diagnosis he tells the parents what they are going to do to take care of the problem. The action part is essential, but only if there is adequate provision for exploring the feelings of the parents.

Such approaches by the audiologist greatly interfere with the process of acceptance of the handicap. A lack of acceptance prohibits the parents from helping their child grow both emotionally and educationally. The parents may deny the information and shop around for a professional who will tell them that their child is normal. Beck (1959) and Meadow (1968) have pointed out that parents are more likely to listen and to integrate painful and unpleasant information from interested and "feeling" individuals.

The ineffective approaches used by the audiologist stem from a number of complex variables. First, he may lack knowledge and understanding of the habilitative process, and of the effect of his initial report. Second, he may be uncomfortable with the range of emotions that these parents may feel. Often audiologists state that they simply do not have the time to devote to reporting. This reasoning, however, may actually be a way of avoiding a more significant factor . . . that is, the audiologist has not yet worked out in his own mind what it means to him to tell someone some painful news. It is natural for people to avoid pain. The audiologist and the parents in a way become secretly and jointly involved in an agreement to avoid dealing with feelings.

There is no painless way to inform parents that they have a child with a hearing loss. However, pain does not have to be regarded negatively. It is part of a process that facilitates and encourages a family's involvement. Even though there is no way of softening the blow, there is a way to help parents accept the realities of the situation and to make use of the resources available to them. The goals of this important first discussion of the diagnosis are multifold.

1. *Statement of the facts.* Initially, it is important to state the facts as clearly and as emphatically as possible. These parents want up-to-date and accurate scientific information about their child's problem presented to them authoritatively, but in language they can understand. If an alliance is going to be created with these parents, it is most important that the audiologist admit any lack of information or knowledge about the problem that he has, doing so confidently and without strain. Throughout the giving of this information, the audiologist must convey a true interest in this family. The tone of voice and non-verbal behavior of an audiologist can convey callousness, or it can convey concern. It is essen-

tial to convey concern rather than the idea that you are just doing your job.

2. *Support through listening.* Perhaps the most important goal is to provide support through listening. By listening patiently and nonjudgmentally, you may be able to bring some of the parents' feelings out into the open—feelings of which they may not have been aware. Many parents have indicated during the initial conference that they had been anxious about their child for a long period of time, but had never shared that anxiety with anyone, not even the spouse. This may be the first opportunity they have had to express what they have been feeling for months.

In order that these feelings be expressed by both parents together, they should both be present to discuss the diagnosis unless it is physically impossible. During this discussion, we can begin to assess the parents' interactions and begin to decide whether they have the kind of relationship that will provide support to one another or whether they will require some help from outside. It is important that the audiologist note and report his initial impression of the parents, as these notes may be valuable to others involved with the family.

3. *Giving the parents a role.* Another important goal of this first contact is to convey to the parents that they have a great deal to offer, even though they may have little formal knowledge about hearing loss and child development. Focusing on the parents' interaction with their child during that initial contact can give them some confidence. "You seem to sense Joey's needs very well." "That's beautiful, you called Joey's attention to that sound." "That's one of the most important ideas you will learn and you already appear comfortable with it." You can provide initial reinforcement of attributes that the parents are already equipped with, that will help their child's development.

During the initial discussion, the parents need to be made aware of the resources available to them—not only resources for habilitation and educational programming, but also resources available to help with emotional needs. Ideally, the audiologist will remain in contact with the family periodically, in order not only to give repeated evaluations, but also to act as a coordinator of professionals working with this family. It is vital that there be an interface between the person delivering emotional supportive services and those people primarily responsible for the habilitation program. This interaction will provide an opportunity to share and be aware of mutual concerns and will prevent the traditional approach of professionals working in isolation of each other.

In order for these goals to be realized, four criteria need to be present: First, the clinical audiologist must have some knowledge of the rehabilitative process; second, he must be comfortable dealing with feelings; third, adequate time must be provided for the reporting; and fourth, an atmosphere of mutual respect must be created.

For many years, the clinical audiologist has accumulated experience in diagnosing and fitting hearing aids, but has known little about the habilitation process. There is a trend today to provide audiologists with more information about habilitation, a trend which we see as positive. Perhaps as audiologists become more familiar with rehabilitative methods, they can objectively direct parents toward programs suited to their child's needs and alleviate the emotional controversy of the deaf.

Many audiologists are sensitive and concerned about their role in helping these families, but this does not necessarily mean that they feel comfortable in dealing with feelings. Sensitivity in raw form can potentially be a valuable tool and an asset for the audiologist, but just because the potential is there does not mean that it will automatically be used in a facilitative way. To learn how to use one's sensitivity effectively is a delicate process and cannot be taught. This exemplifies the necessity for an interdisciplinary approach where the audiologist who is uncomfortable in this area may take advantage of the mental health professions that deal with feelings routinely.

A seemingly minute detail in the criteria for effective reporting of the diagnosis is the allotment of time; however, this is probably an essential factor in reporting. One of the most consistent complaints of parents in their dealings with audiologists initially is that the situation was regarded lightly and not enough time was devoted to this important problem. It is our feeling that the audiologist must allocate a minimum of 45 min to this initial reporting. Should this not be possible, or should both parents not be available during this initial session, it is critical that an appointment be scheduled within the next 24 hours to discuss the problem thoroughly. As was indicated earlier, parents may experience a number of feelings at the outset, the most frequent being shock. Then may come anger, guilt, or depression. It is very important not to tell parents what they may feel because people experience different emotions. It is important to provide an open-ended approach, however, such as, "Today I have told you about your son's hearing loss. Over the weeks and months to follow, you may or may not experience some uncomfortable feelings as many parents naturally do. We will be available to you to discuss whatever feelings you may be having. Let's plan to talk again in a month or anytime before that, should you desire."

The approach to effective reporting of the diagnosis is not only dependent upon the audiologist's knowledge, his comfortable feelings and the allotment of adequate time but also upon the atmosphere created. It is the universal observation of those who have constructed programs for special groups of young disabled children that unless the parents' emotional needs are adequately dealt with, the programs themselves have limited benefit for the children (Mindel and Vernon, 1971). Thus, it is critically important that an atmosphere of mutual respect and honesty be created— an atmosphere which allows the expression of feelings in nonjudgmental and accepting ways.

Often the atmosphere of mutual respect is interrupted when the parents' depression explodes into external anger which sometimes is directed at the audiologist. If the audiologist does not understand that this expression of anger is only an indication of the parent's internal struggles, he may become defensive. The parents will be aware of his defensiveness even if it is only conveyed nonverbally, and thus the climate of mutual respect is destroyed.

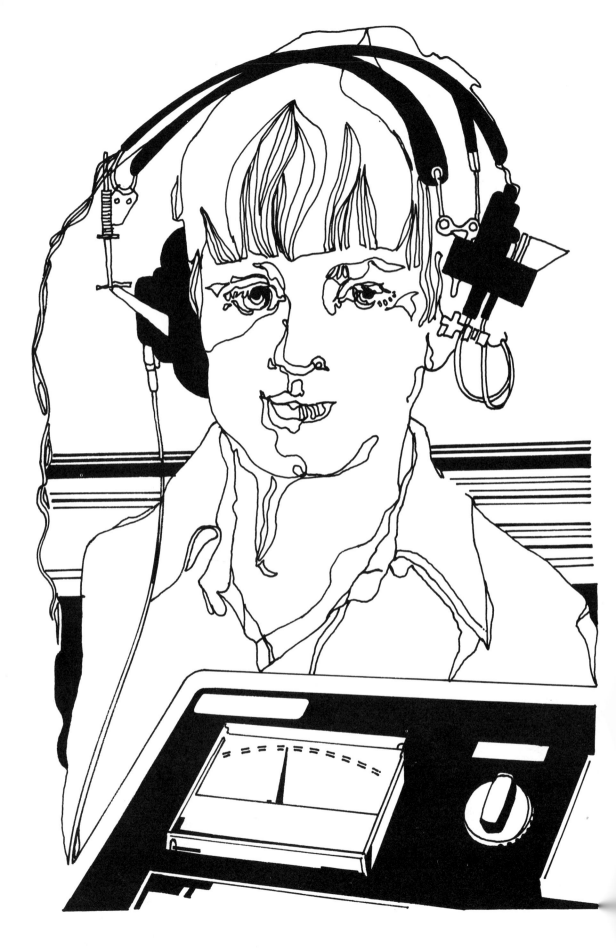

CHAPTER 6

Physiologic Hearing Tests

Nothing can be more frustrating to an audiologist than to work with a 2 year old child who needs to have his or her hearing evaluated but who refuses to cooperate with any of the testing procedures. It seems impossible that a youngster who sat quietly and politely in the patient waiting area can suddenly turn into a crying, yelling, totally uncooperative subject in the sound-treated booth. And what causes a child, who has been happily playing while waiting for his or her hearing test, to suddenly become an overly self-conscious, introverted, and unworkably shy patient? How does a clinician establish rapport with a youngster who is hidden in mother's skirt or wrapped around father's leg? Every clinician ultimately faces the child who cannot be tested. There are, indeed, means of handling such children, but the skills necessary to evaluate the hearing in uncooperative children are gained through experience and insight.

One may expect the behavior of "normal" children occasionally to be obstinate. What about testing the hearing of a hyperactive, mentally retarded child? How does one elicit cooperation and establish play-conditioning techniques with an autistic or mentally disturbed youngster? Can you fit earphones on a child with hydrocephaly? Play-conditioning techniques are obviously not possible with a child who will not even sit down! Just when the audiologist thinks that every conceivable situation has occurred, a child will show up who baffles every attempt to evaluate his or her hearing. Audiologists continue to seek a simple and accurate objective hearing test that can be used with any uncooperative child much like the early Spanish explorers continued to hunt for the Fountain of Youth! Almost no other aspect of audiology stimulates interest in the same manner as a new report describing a promising objective hearing test to solve problems associated with testing the hearing in difficult-to-deal-with children.

To deal with these difficult-to-test patients, the field of audiology has worked long and hard in the development of "objective" tests of hearing. An objective hearing test is one that defines a patient's hearing ability without the patient's active participation or cooperation. In the case of children, many factors may influence the child's ability to cooperate. The child may not have the mental or physical capabilities to cooperate fully or to attend to the hearing test task required by the clinician. The child's interest span may be too short. A clinician's skill in evaluating the hearing of these children often depends on the ability to establish rapport with the youngster and, at the same time, make an accurate evaluation of the child's capabilities in performing some task. A false start with these children may alienate them toward the testing situation, making additional test sessions necessary and possibly more difficult.

Many "objective" hearing tests, usually related to an autonomic physiologic response, have been suggested and reported. The Ewings of England in the early 1940s (Ewing and Ewing, 1944) observed eyeblinks, squinting, involuntary jumping, and sound localization with body or head movements while testing young children. Froeschels and Beebe (1946) evaluated the cochleopalpebral reflex (also known as the auropalpebral reflex)—defined as the involuntary closing of eyelids due to acoustic stimulation—in children and infants.

New objective hearing tests are formulated with older children or cooperating adults, and these results are then generalized to young children. Somehow, the generalization that such procedures, which work well with adults, therefore should apply also to children comes to a sudden lack of credibility when the clinician comes face to face with a severely multiply-handicapped 3 year old child.

We should pause to reflect that the presence of some physiologic response, seemingly related to the presence of an auditory signal, does not ensure that the child does indeed "hear." Hearing, in this sense, implies meaningful interpretation of the sound so as to produce thought and language with verbal or nonverbal encoding and decoding. The toughest test for a new clinical procedure is to withstand clinician criticism by proving itself to be reliable, quick, easy to administer, inexpensive, and worthwhile over a long period of time.

IMMITTANCE AUDIOMETRY

The clinical application of acoustic impedance measurements has come to be known as immittance audiometry. The terms "impedance" and "immittance" are used interchangeably. The testing techniques are especially well-suited for children, since they are objective, accurate, quick, easy to administer, and create little discomfort to the patient. Children who will not cooperate with conventional audiometric techniques may not object to the immittance test battery. Immittance audiometry results are of special benefit to the physician who is unable to perform adequate otoscopic examination on a youngster, as well as to the audiologist who has difficulty in establishing valid hearing thresholds on an uncooperative child.

Vast numbers of children have been tested with the immittance technique and a wide variety of normative immittance test values are available. Studies by Brooks

(1968, 1971) and Jerger (1970) have validated the tremendous benefits of immittance audiometry in children.

Northern (1978c, 1980c) published comprehensive reviews of the use of impedance audiometry in special populations of children, including the profoundly deaf, the retarded, the deaf-blind, those with cleft lip and palate, those with Down's syndrome, and those with craniofacial disorders.

The clinical impedance technique in the evaluation of the auditory mechanism was originally proposed by Metz in 1946 and has been used routinely in Scandinavia since that time. North Americans, however, were slow to accept the clinical utility of this testing procedure until Alberti and Kristensen (1970) and Jerger (1970) independently published articles exalting impedance audiometry as a valuable routine procedure for assessing the nature of hearing loss in patients. Jerger succinctly stated the significance of impedance audiometry by commenting. "We frankly wonder how we ever got along without it." Immittance audiometry is now included as routine testing technique in many otologic and audiologic clinics, and we have found it to be particularly useful in the evaluation of hearing in children.

By definition, immittance audiometry is an objective means of assessing the integrity and function of the peripheral auditory mechanism. The electroacoustic immittance meter may help determine existing middle ear pressure, tympanic membrane mobility, eustachian tube function, continuity and mobility of the middle ear ossicles, acoustic reflex thresholds, and nonorganic hearing loss. The electroacoustic immittance meter is equally practical for private office work and institutional clinics.

The electroacoustic impedance technique is based on the principle that sound pressure level (SPL) is a function of closed cavity volume. A diagram of the impedance meter is shown in Figure 6.1. An air-tight seal is obtained with a small probe inserted into the external auditory canal of the patient. The probe has three small holes.

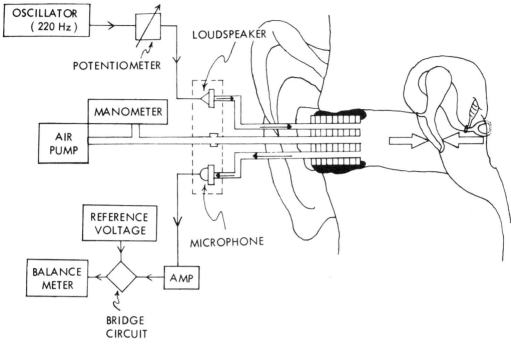

Figure 6.1. Electroacoustic immittance meter. Note probe sealed into external auditory meatus with three holes for (a) probe tone from oscillator, (b) air pressure system, and (c) pickup microphone to compare SPL in the cavity between the eardrum and probe tip with the reference voltage of immittance bridge. (Reprinted with permission from J. Jerger: Clinical experience with impedance audiometry. *Archives of Otolaryngology* 92:311–324, 1970.)

From the hole the probe tone is emitted; a second hole is an outlet for an air pressure system capable of creating positive, negative, or atmospheric air pressure in the cavity between the probe tip and the tympanic membrane; the third hole leads to a pickup microphone that measures the SPL of the probe tone in the canal cavity.

The SPL of the probe tone in the external auditory canal cavity is determined by the compliance of the tympanic membrane and integrity of the middle ear system. The pickup microphone quantifies the SPL of acoustic energy that is reflected back into the external auditory canal. A high amount of reflected energy is measured when the middle ear system is stiff or heavy as in such pathologic conditions as ossicular fixation, otitis media, or cholesteatoma. In contrast, discontinuity of the middle ear system creates a flaccid tympanic membrane that absorbs most of the probe tone sound

energy and reflects very little sound back into the external auditory meatus.

The continuing development of new immittance equipment reflects the widening market and increased demand for easy-to-use instruments. There are currently more than 20 commercially available immittance meters ranging from micro processor-based clinical units with data storage capabilities to miniaturized hand-held screening devices. Although this increase in the number of instruments has led to automated and easy-to-use test equipment capable of recording an automatic tympanogram as well as measuring an ipsilateral acoustic reflex in a matter of seconds, the lack of agreement in manufacturing standards is readily apparent. Few if any validating studies exist for the majority of immittance meters currently available for clinical use (Schwartz, 1986).

The immittance test battery includes tympanometry, static immittance, the ear

Table 6.1.
Summary of Immittance Audiometry Applications in Children

Tympanometry
  Objective measurement of tympanic membrane
    mobility
  Measures middle ear pressure
  Confirms patency of ventilation tubes in tympanic
    membrane
  Estimates static compliance
Static compliance
  Differentiates middle ear fixation from disarticulation
Acoustic reflex threshold
  Objective measure of cochlear pathology
  Validates nonorganic hearing loss
  Validates conductive hearing loss
  Differential diagnosis of conductive hearing loss
  Objective inference of hearing sensitivity
Ear canal physical volume test
  Identifies nonintact tympanic membrane,
    perforation, and patency of ventilating tubes

canal physical volume test (PVT), and acoustic reflex threshold measurement. Although each of the test procedures can provide significant information, their diagnostic capabilities are strengthened when results from all four procedures are considered together (Table 6.1). The entire battery of four tests can easily be administered by an experienced person in 60–90 seconds per ear.

Clinicians using immittance measurements must learn to follow three general rules: (1) recognize overall patterns in the tests of the impedance audiometry battery, (2) pay little attention to the absolute value of any of the immittance test battery results, and (3) beware of the implicit diagnostic conclusions based only on the immittance test battery (Northern, 1980b). Jerger and Hayes (1980) state that in the "diagnostic application of immittance audiometry there are no absolutes; . . . the results of any single immittance measurement are usually ambiguous and have little individual value."

Tympanometry. Tympanometry is an objective technique for measuring the compliance or mobility of the tympanic membrane as a function of mechanically varied air pressures in the external auditory canal. The general term, tympanometry, refers to methods and techniques for measuring, recording, and evaluating changes in acoustic impedance (or resistance of the auditory mechanism) with systematic changes in air pressure. The compliance of the tympanic membrane at specific air pressures is plotted on a graph known as a tympanogram.

Tympanic membrane mobility is of particular interest, since almost any pathology located on or medial to the eardrum will influence its movement.

Children with middle ear effusions are typically identified by physicians through an otoscopic examination. Physicians vary in their ability to examine visually the tympanic membrane (Stool and Anticaglia, 1973). Otologists teach that pneumatic otoscopy is an absolute necessity to identify the presence of middle ear effusion, yet only 25% of physicians use the pneumatic otoscope (Howie and Ploussard, 1974). In a study of the accuracy of otoscopic diagnosis, 15–20% of ears in children under 3 years of age with effusions were missed clinically (Paradise, 1976a).

Tympanometry, however, is more objective than the otolaryngologist's eye, and the air pressures involved with the technique are very small compared with the air pressures created with a pneumatic otoscope. Often, eardrums noted to have normal mobility by pneumatic otoscopy examination can be shown to have abnormal mobility with tympanometry.

The compliance of the tympanic membrane is at its maximum when air pressures on both sides of the eardrum are equal. That is, the eardrum achieves its best mobility when the air pressure in the external auditory canal is exactly the same as the existing air pressure in the middle ear (Fig. 6.2). The electroacoustic impedance meter permits the compliance of the eardrum to be evaluated under systematic variance of air pressure, which is controlled by the clinician. Thus, when the clinician finds the air pressure value where the eardrum reaches its maximal compliance, he or she can then infer that the middle ear pressure is the same as the ear canal air pressure. The air

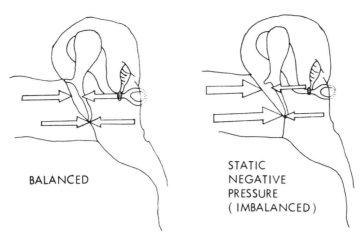

BALANCED

STATIC
NEGATIVE
PRESSURE
(IMBALANCED)

Figure 6.2. Compliance of the tympanic membrane is at its maximum when air pressure is equal on both sides of the tympanic membrane as shown on the *left*. When air pressure on either side of the eardrum is unequal, as shown on the *right*, the tympanic membrane does not move well, and a conductive-type hearing loss can often be noted.

infer that the middle ear pressure is the same as the ear canal air pressure. The air pressure at the point of maximal compliance is also the middle ear air pressure.

The knowledge of middle ear pressure is important clinical information. When the process of aeration in the middle ear is halted, as in closure of the eustachian tube, the now static air in the middle ear space is absorbed by the blood vessels in the mucosal lining. This situation produces negative air pressure in the middle ear space, causing transudation of fluid and retraction of the tympanic membrane. If the aeration process of the middle ear cavity is blocked for an extended period of time, fluid may totally fill the middle ear space. Thus, the early identification of negative middle ear pressure may permit the physician to practice preventive medicine and avoid the condition of otitis media.

The presence of unequal pressures on either side of the tympanic membrane usually occurs when negative pressure exists in the middle ear space. This may be sufficient to cause a retraction of the eardrum accompanied by mild conductive hearing loss in spite of the fact that no fluid may be observed in the patient's middle ear. The most explicit

example of this occurs when air pressures are changed in the passenger cabins of commercial aircraft. A normal-hearing passenger will first experience discomfort due to unequal air pressure in the middle ear cavity and external ear canal. When the passenger forces open his or her eustachian tube in order to alleviate this discomfort, the passenger will notice that when the air pressures are equalized and the eardrum is again in a most compliant condition, the environmental sounds in the aircraft become suddenly louder. This may be a practical explanation of the numbers of children seen by audiologists to have mild conductive hearing loss, and they are found by the examining physicians to have no evidence of otologic problem.

Jerger (1970), Liden et al. (1970), and Paradise et al. (1976) have described basic tympanogram patterns and related them to conditions of the middle ear. Jerger's classification system of tympanometry curves, which he also calls "pressure-compliance functions," is summarized in Figure 6.3. For simplicity, Jerger ascribed alphabetical letters to each type of curve. This classification is convenient, but it may be more explicit to describe each tympanogram in

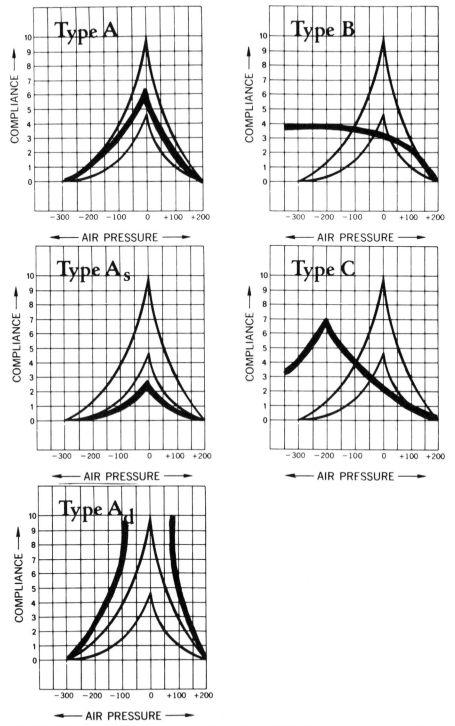

Figure 6.3. Classification of tympanograms according to Jerger (1970). See text for clinical significance of each type of tympanogram.

terms of its dynamic compliance and the air pressure at which maximal compliance is noted.

Types of Tympanograms. *Type A.* Type A curves are found in patients with normal middle ear function. The curve shows adequate relative compliance and normal middle ear pressure at the point of maximal compliance. Some controversy exists concerning the limits of normal middle ear pressure values. Alberti and Kristensen (1970) recommended the use of ± 50 mm H_2O as normative values, but we have noted many instances of negative middle ear pressure as great as -150 mm H_2O in patients who demonstrated normal audiograms and normal otoscopic examination. Brooks (1969) evaluated 1053 children in England and determined "normal" middle ear pressure from a statistical distribution to be from -170 mm H_2O to 0 mm H_2O. Decisions regarding "limits of normal" in terms of middle ear pressure will undoubtedly vary depending on the clinical situation and circumstances.

Type A_S. This pressure compliance function is characterized by normal middle ear pressure and limited compliance relative to the mobility of the normal tympanic membrane. This type of curve may be seen in cases of otosclerosis, thickened or heavily scarred tympanic membranes, and some cases of tympanosclerosis. The subscript "S" nomenclature is indicative of "stiffness" or "shallowness" of the tympanogram.

Type A_D. This curve is represented by large changes in relative compliance with small changes of air pressure. The A_D curve is noted in middle ears where discontinuity of the ossicular chain has occurred or the eardrum demonstrates a large monomeric membrane. The significance of this curve is its representation of an extremely flaccid eardrum, with the subscript "D" indicating "disarticulation" or a "deep" tympanogram curve.

Type B. The type B tympanogram is characterized by a function representing little or no change in compliance of the middle ear as air pressure in the external ear canal is varied. Often no point of maximal compliance is observable with air pressure as low as -400 mm H_2O. This curve is seen in patients with serous and adhesive otitis media and some cases of congenital middle ear malformations (Northern and Bergstrom, 1973). This pattern is also noted in patients who have perforations of the tympanic membrane, ear canals totally occluded with cerumen, or with a patent ventilating tube in the eardrum.

Type C. This tympanogram is represented by near-normal compliance and middle ear pressure of -200 mm H_2O or worse. This curve may or may not be related to the presence of fluid in the middle ear, but one can conclude that the eardrum still has some mobility. Bluestone et al. (1973) reported a very low incidence of middle ear effusion in children with type C tympanograms upon whom they performed myringotomies. Paradise et al. (1976) published an impressive set of data dealing with the use of tympanometry and detection of middle ear effusion in infants and young children. They report that a poorly compliant negative pressure tympanogram is approximately 3 times more likely to be associated with middle ear effusion than a negative pressure tympanogram that is highly compliant.

Persistence of the type C tympanogram infers poor eustachian tube function in the presence of an intact tympanic membrane. Sometimes, patients can be instructed to "pop their ears" or perform the Valsalva procedure (patient holds nose and forces positive air pressure into the middle ear cavities). If the patient can open his or her eustachian tube, a repeat tympanogram may show that the type C curve has changed to the type A curve. Youngsters with upper respiratory infections, however, seldom can alleviate the type C tympanogram with the Valsalva maneuver.

A major drawback to the use of such categories to classify tympanograms is that the clinician inevitably comes across a tympanogram that does not clearly fit into one of the expectant categories. Such tympanograms may be few, but they do exist. In addition, various categorical systems do not always agree on the same nomenclature for the tympanogram patterns. The clinician should describe the mobility of the eardrum in terms of compliance and middle ear pressure or can draw a simple picture of the tympanogram, if possible. Margolis (1979) suggested that we express acoustic immittance clinical results in quantitative physical measurements rather than in arbitrary units.

Tympanogram Procedure. The technique for obtaining a tympanogram is quite simple. The eardrum is put into a position of known poor mobility with an air pressure of +200 mm H_2O pumped into the cavity created by the meter's probe tip and the patient's tympanic membrane. Then the positive air pressure is removed, and relative changes in the compliance of the eardrum are noted. The compliance change is actually measured by the electroacoustic meter as a decrease in the SPL of the enclosed cavity. When the compliance of the eardrum is permitted to increase, with the release of air pressure, more of the sound energy is transmitted through to the middle ear, creating a decrease in the SPL of the enclosed cavity.

As the air pressure variation approaches the point of maximal compliance, the mobility of the tympanic membrane increases. Maximal compliance is, of course, achieved when the air pressure in the external auditory canal equals the existing air pressure in the middle ear space. The clinician continues to reduce the air pressure in the enclosed cavity, which unbalances the equalized air pressure on either side of the tympanic membrane, and therefore creates a decrease in eardrum compliance again as shown previously in Fig. 6.2.

Tympanometry can be used to follow the entire progression and resolution of serous otitis media in children. Typical tympanograms obtained under such circumstances are shown in Figure 6.4. Imagine a 2 year old youngster who demonstrates a type A tympanogram under healthy conditions. As the otologic disease process begins with a closed eustachian tube, negative pressure is created in the middle ear space that produces a type C tympanogram. As fluid develops medial to the tympanic membrane, the compliance of the eardrum is decreased, and a type B tympanogram will be demonstrated by the child. If prescribed medications are effective and the fluid condition of the ear begins to resolve, we would expect to see the type C tympanogram once again and, finally, the type A tympanogram when the middle ear is back in its normal healthy condition (Northern, 1978b).

Paradise (1982) published an editorial retrospective review of tympanometry in which he states that tympanometry has instructional, practical, and intellectual value for the physician. Tympanometry serves the primary care provider in three ways: (*1*) separating infants and children not easily examined otoscopically into two subgroups, those with suspected or nearly certain disease who require careful examination and those virtually certain to be free of disease; (*2*) refining and clarifying doubtful otoscopic diagnoses; and (*3*) objectifying the follow-up evaluations of patients with diagnosed middle ear disease. However, Paradise indicates that it is for the clinical researcher that the value of tympanometry has become most firmly established, since in investigations that in any way involve otitis media, diagnostic accuracy is critical to the validity of the findings.

Studies have been conducted to show the influence of negative middle ear pressure (identified with tympanometry) to elevate hearing thresholds. Cooper et al. (1977) examined 1133 children with middle ear pressures between −150 and −400 mm H_2O and found their hearing thresholds to be elevated as much as 25 dB. An orderly relationship exists between the degree of negative middle ear pressure and hearing threshold shift, with an approximately 8 dB shift in the speech frequency range and middle ear pressure of −100 mm H_2O, in-

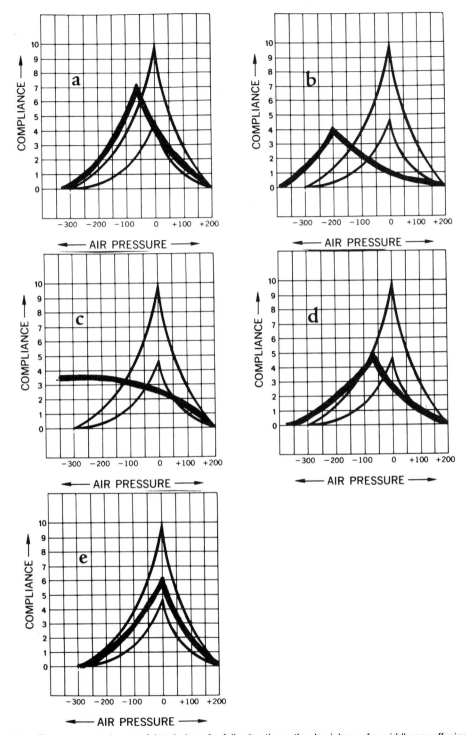

Figure 6.4. Tympanometry is a useful technique for following the pathophysiology of a middle ear effusion. **a.** A near-normal tympanogram. **b.** Negative middle ear pressure and reduced compliance often accompany an upper respiratory problem. **c.** Middle ear effusion. **d.** and **e.** Return of the middle ear to its proper normal control condition.

creasing to at least a 20 dB shift when middle ear pressure is -400 mm H_2O.

Static Immittance. The concept of acoustical impedance, or static immittance, is a direct outgrowth of applications made by electrical engineers and physicists to describe the willingness of an electrical system to permit electron flow and the ease with which a mechanical system moves.

The impedance of any mechanical system involves a complex relationship between three factors—the mass, friction, and stiffness of the system. In the middle ear mechanical system, mass is represented primarily by the weight of the three ossicles. The weight of the three ossicles, however, as is immediately obvious to one who has ever held the ossicles in his or her hand, constitutes very little mass. Friction in the middle ear is due primarily to the suspensory seven ligaments and two muscles that support the ossicular chain. This intricate suspension of the ossicles, however, lends to ease of mobility; thus friction as a factor in mechanical impedance constitutes meager influence in the impedance of the middle ear. The third element of impedance, stiffness, has a much more prominent role in the middle ear. The stiffness element has been identified as occurring at the footplate of the stapes, where a large resistant component must be overcome to move the fluids of the cochlear ducts. Thus, the impedance of the middle ear mechanical system is stiffness-dominated (Zwislocki, 1963).

Compliance is technically the inverse of impedance. A system with a great deal of mobility, or high compliance, has very little resistance to motion, or low impedance. Likewise, a poorly mobile system has low compliance and high resistance. This small equivalent volume in cubic centimeters of compliance is equal to a large impedance in acoustic ohms, and vice versa. In the middle ear pathologies, serous otitis media, for example, creates a middle ear system of very low compliance or very high impedance. On the other hand, a disarticulated ossicular chain in the middle ear creates a condition of high compliance or low impedance.

Static immittance is actually tested by making two equivalent volume measures with the tympanic membrane under specific conditions. The first volume measurement (C_1) is made with the eardrum clamped with $+200$ mm H_2O pressure. The second volume measurement (C_2), which is really an equivalent volume measure, is done with the eardrum in its most compliant air pressure condition. The two volume measures have little actual significance individually because they include the volume of the external ear canal. However, simple subtraction of the two volumes, C_2–C_1, cancels out the contamination of the ear canal from both measures and gives an answer equal to the static immittance of the middle ear.

The major weaknesses of static immittance is its wide variance in values related to specific pathologies of the auditory mechanism. In clinical patient populations, the variation in static immittance values create considerable overlap among normal middle ears, otosclerotics, and ears with discontinuity. Stach and Jerger (1990) find the usefulness of static immittance to be limited to differentiate only between normal and extreme pathologic conditions.

As a guideline, the middle ear can be considered abnormally stiff when the static compliance is less than 0.28 cc of equivalent volume and abnormally flaccid when the static compliance is greater than 2.5 cc of equivalent volume. Serous otitis media often creates poor compliance of 0.1 cc of equivalent volume or less. S. Jerger et al. (1974) found static compliance to be the least informative test of the impedance battery in children under 6 years of age.

Physical Volume Test. Since the immittance meter is able to measure volume in cubic centimeters, information about the absolute cavity size medial to the probe tip can be quite significant. The immittance meters rely on the physical principle that the intensity of a sound trapped in a closed cavity is a direct function of the cavity size.

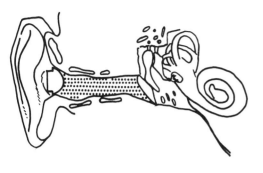

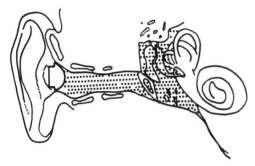

Figure 6.5. Utilization of the immittance meter to estimate volume. *Top scheme* shows volume between probe tip and intact eardrum; *bottom view* shows greater volume measurement when eardrum is perforated or has a patent ventilating tube in place. (Reprinted with permission from J. L. Northern: Clinical measurement procedures in impedance audiometry. In J. Jerger and J. L. Northern (eds.): *Clinical Impedance Audiometry*, ed. 2. Acton, Massachusetts, American Electromedics Corp., 1980b, Chap. 2.)

Thus, a signal of fixed intensity introduced into a large cavity and into a small cavity will produce two different SPLs in the two cavities. The larger cavity will have a lower SPL, the smaller cavity will have a higher SPL.

In the presence of an intact eardrum, the typical enclosed ear canal cavity between the probe tip and the tympanic membrane should be 0.65–1.75 cc in an adult or 0.5–1.0 cc in a child. In infants the PVT value may be as small as 0.5 cc. This value may vary depending on how far the probe tip cuff is inserted into the ear canal or how large or small the diameter of the external canal might be (Fig. 6.5). Ear volume estimation is a routine component of most current commercially available immittance instruments (Hall, 1987).

Table 6.2.
Tympanometry and the Physical Volume Test in Children

Tympa-nogram	Physical Volume	Etiology
Type A	0.8–1.0	Normal middle ear
Type B	<0.3	Cerumen or canal wall
	0.8–1.0	Serous otitis; middle ear congenital anomaly
	>2.5	Tympanic membrane perforation or patent ventilation tube
Type C	0.8–1.0	Negative middle ear pressure; inadequate eustachian tube function

When the physical volume size is considerably greater than these norms in light of an hermetically sealed probe tip and cuff, the clinician can reasonably assume that the cavity includes the external ear canal, middle ear space, and possibly even the mastoid air cells and entrance to the eustachian tube orifice. In circumstances of a nonintact tympanic membrane, PVT value may be 3 or 4 times greater than normal volume values, often exceeding 5.0 cc. We use the PVT as a means to rule out a nonobservable perforation behind an exaggerated anterior canal wall overhang or beneath an adherent crust on the eardrum. The PVT can be used to identify obstruction of ventilation tubes as well as blind attic retraction pocket perforations.

Knowledge of the physical volume in cubic centimeters will help clarify the etiology responsible for type B tympanograms. Nonmobile tympanic membranes with volumes larger than 2.0 cc in children are usually indicative of a perforation or patent ventilation tube; type B tympanograms with normal volume measurement are indicative of a nonmobile intact tympanic membrane; and abnormally small physical volumes may be related to cerumen occluding the external canal or probe tip, or perhaps the probe tip is pressed against the canal wall (Table 6.2).

Acoustic Reflex Thresholds. The acoustic reflex test in the immittance battery is the determination of the signal threshold level at which the stapedial mus-

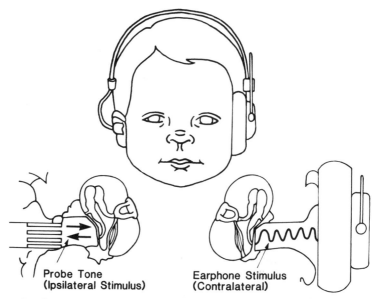

Probe Tone
(Ipsilateral Stimulus)

Earphone Stimulus
(Contralateral)

Figure 6.6. Acoustic reflex measurements may be made with a contralateral stimulus from an earphone or with an ipsilateral stimulus presented through the probe tip.

cle contracts. Metz (1952) and Jepsen (1963) reported that in normal-hearing persons, a bilateral acoustic muscle reflex can be elicited by stimulating the person's test ear with pure tone signals between 70 and 100 dB hearing threshold level (HTL) and approximately 65 dB HTL for white noise. The lowest signal intensity capable of eliciting the acoustic reflex is the acoustic reflex *threshold* for the *stimulated* ear.

Since the stapedial muscles contract bilaterally in response to an appropriate acoustic stimulus represented in either ear, both an *ipsilateral* (uncrossed) and a *contralateral* (crossed) acoustic reflex may be measured (Fig. 6.6). Most current immittance meters will measure the acoustic reflex in ipsilateral or contralateral mode. In ipsilateral reflex measurement, the eliciting acoustic stimulus is presented through the probe tip itself and the acoustic reflex is monitored in the same ear. Under conditions of contralateral acoustic reflex measurement, the acoustic stimulus is presented through an earphone to one ear while the resultant change in immittance is verified by the probe tip in the opposite ear. Regardless of whether measuring ipsilat-

eral or contralateral (crossed or uncrossed) acoustic reflexes, it is standard practice to *record* the acoustic reflex for the stimulated ear—noting in writing, of course, as to which lateral mode (contralateral or ipsilateral) was used for the measurement.

The major advantage of ipsilateral reflex measurement is that confusion is eliminated regarding which ear is being tested. Utilization of ipsilateral reflex techniques virtually eliminates the need for the cumbersome headband-earphone arrangement used in contralateral reflex measurement. Thus, a whole new family of hand-held probe tips, without headband, are appearing on portable immittance meters. The use of ipsilateral reflex measurement and the hand-held probe tips should be especially useful in immittance measurements in hearing screening programs. Research reports that compare acoustic reflex threshold sensitivity between contralateral and ipsilateral stimuli have been published, indicating that ipsilateral thresholds are 3–6 dB more sensitive than contralateral thresholds (Moller, 1962; Fria et al., 1975).

The function of the stapedial muscle is still open to question, but the classical in-

Table 6.3.
Interpreting Crossed and Uncrossed Acoustic Reflexes with the Audiogram to Identify Site of Lesion of Hearing Impairment[a]

Reflex Pattern	Audiogram	Predicted Site
Neither crossed nor uncrossed can be elicited from either ear	Bilateral air-bone gap	Middle ear
Neither crossed nor uncrossed can be elicited from either ear	Bilateral severe sensory loss	Cochlea
Neither crossed nor uncrossed can be elicited from either ear	Normal	Brainstem

[a]Reproduced with permission from B. Stach and J. Jerger: Immittance measures in auditory disorders. In J. Jacobson and J. Northern (eds.): *Diagnostic Audiology*. Boston, College-Hill Press, 1990, p. 118.

terpretation offered by Wever and Lawrence (1954) is that the stapedial muscle reflex is responsible for protection of the inner ear from loud sounds. Anatomically, the stapedial muscle is attached from the neck of the stapes to the posterior wall of the middle ear cavity. When the stapedial muscle contracts, it pulls posteriorly on the ossicular chain, thereby decreasing the compliance of the middle ear system and attenuating the intensity of the sound that actually reaches the cochlea.

Acoustic reflex threshold testing should be carried out at frequencies of 500, 1000, 2000, and 4000 Hz. However, acoustic reflex responses at 4000 Hz are often absent for no apparent reason even in normal-hearing patients, so pathologic conclusions may not be valid if only the 4000 Hz reflex is not present. Acoustic reflex thresholds are difficult to interpret in isolation, since absence or elevated acoustic reflex thresholds may occur for a wide variety of conditions. Comparison of contralateral (crossed) and ipsilateral (uncrossed) acoustic reflexes increases confidence in interpreting the audiogram and immittance audiometry results (Table 6.3).

Much emphasis has been placed on the clinical value of the acoustic reflex measurement. Since the acoustic reflex is mediated by loudness, it is a sensitive indicator of cochlear pathology. The acoustic reflex

threshold level in patients with cochlear pathology usually occurs at sensation levels less than 60 dB above the auditory pure tone threshold. The patient with cochlear pathology hears the test signal as though it were much louder, as a result of abnormal appreciation of loudness. Thus, the acoustic reflex threshold provides an objective, simple technique to identify the site of pathology to the cochlea.

The ability to establish the presence of the loudness recruitment phenomenon permits the clinician to localize the site of auditory lesion to the cochlea. Anyone who has ever attempted the traditional psychophysical loudness balance procedures on a youngster under 6 years of age to identify a cochlear site of lesion will immediately appreciate the simplicity and objectivity of this technique.

The informed audiologist can achieve considerable diagnostic information through the subtleties of acoustic reflex interpretation. For example, the acoustic reflex sensation level shows an inverse relation to the degree of sensorineural hearing loss. The acoustic reflex sensation level decreases from approximately 70 dB for patients with a 20 dB sensorineural hearing loss to approximately 25 dB for patients with an 85 dB sensorineural hearing loss. Jerger et al. (1972) concluded that as long as the cochlear hearing loss is less than 60 dB, there is a 90% likelihood for the presence of the acoustic reflex being observed. As the sensorineural loss increases above 60 dB, chances of observing the acoustic reflex grow less. With an 85 dB hearing loss, the chances are only 50% of observing the acoustic reflex; if the loss is 100 dB hearing level (HL), only a 5–10% chance exists of the reflex being present. Thus, the presence of acoustic reflex thresholds, in light of hearing loss, provides a powerful indication for sensorineural diagnosis. In patients with unilateral cochlear hearing loss less than 85 dB, the acoustic reflex should be easily observable bilaterally.

In children with conductive hearing problems, the contralateral acoustic reflex can be observed only in mild *unilateral* conductive hearing loss. When the unilateral conductive hearing loss exceeds 30 dB HL, the acoustic reflex is typically obscured bilaterally. Thus, when the stimulating sound is presented to the conductive hearing loss ear, the 30 dB + hearing loss is sufficient to prevent the signal from being perceived loudly enough to elicit the acoustic reflex. Then when the earphone is on the normal ear and the probe is in the unilateral conductive loss ear, the mechanism causing the conductive loss prevents the eardrum from showing a change in compliance. Naturally, in a bilateral conductive loss, the acoustic reflexes will be absent bilaterally because the pathology in *each* ear prohibits the probe from noting a compliance change when the opposite ear is stimulated with sound. The ipsilateral acoustic reflex will also be absent bilaterally.

Since conductive-type pathology precludes tympanic membrane compliance change, the acoustic reflex can be expected to be absent when the probe tip is in a conductive loss ear, regardless of how small an air-bone gap exists. The presence of a small air-bone gap of only 10 dB is sufficient to obscure the reflex to the probe ear *80%* of the time (Jerger et al., 1974b). Conversely, if acoustic reflexes can be noted in the probe ear, it is virtually impossible for a conductive hearing loss to exist in that ear. Thus, even a *very mild* conductive hearing loss will obscure the acoustic reflex. Interpretation of acoustic reflexes in hearing loss can be diagnostically important, and of particular value when the patient is a youngster in whom audiometric masking is impractical or impossible.

Clinical Application of the Immittance Battery with Children. While tympanometry, static compliance, the ear canal physical volume measurement, and the acoustic reflex threshold each provide some information about the function of the auditory system, their results become more meaningful when relationships between the three tests are considered. Diagnostic judg-

ments and patient referral are made with greater authority and assurance when the overall pattern is considered. Tympanometry alone is useful to only a limited degree, static compliance norms are too variable for accurate diagnosis, and the absence of the acoustic reflex may occur from several factors. When considered together, however, the limitations of each test are reduced while their combined implications are enhanced (Table 6.4).

Examples of the immittance test battery and its relation to clinical diagnosis are shown in Figures 6.7 and 6.8. Immittance test results from a case of negative middle ear pressure in a youngster's right ear are demonstrated in Figure 6.7. The audiogram shows a mild hearing loss with a 20 dB air-bone gap on the patient's right ear and normal hearing in the left ear. The audiogram gives no clue as to the etiology of the unilateral conductive hearing loss. The tympanogram for the left ear is superimposed on the normal tympanogram pattern, while the tympanogram for the right ear shows slightly reduced compliance and middle ear pressure of -200 mm H_2O. Static compliance is reduced in the right ear, suggesting stiffness, thereby corroborating the reduced compliance noted in the tympanogram. Static compliance in the left ear is within the normal range. The contralateral acoustic reflexes are present but show elevated thresholds when the stimulating earphone is on the involved ear. The 20 dB air conduction hearing loss in the right ear is not severe enough to prohibit loudness from eliciting the acoustic reflex when the earphone is on this ear. When the earphone is placed over the normal-hearing left ear, the acoustic reflexes are absent. The probe tip is now in the involved conductive loss ear, and the conductive loss element prohibits compliance change in the right tympanic membrane. Knowledge of only the immittance test battery results, accompanied by experience in test interpretation, would permit a close estimation of this patient's audiogram if audiometry could not be successfully accomplished.

Table 6.4.
Use of Immittance to Help Confirm Audiometric Impression in Evaluation of Young Children[a]

Tympanometry	Static Compliance	Acoustic Reflex	Confirm Behavioral Audiometric Impression
Type A bilaterally	Within normal range bilaterally	Normal bilaterally	Bilateral normal hearing or bilateral mild-moderate sensorineural hearing loss or unilateral mild-moderate sensorineural hearing loss
Type A in one ear; type B or C in other ear	Normal in A ear; low in B or C ear	Absent bilaterally	Unilateral conductive loss
Type B or C bilaterally	Low bilaterally	Absent bilaterally	Bilateral conductive loss

[a]From J. Jerger: Clinical experience with impedance audiometry. *Archives of Otolaryngology* 92: 311–324, 1970.

Figure 6.8 demonstrates findings in a patient with unilateral otitis media. The audiometric results show a stiffness-type air conduction curve with an approximate 30 dB air-bone gap in the right ear. Hearing in the left ear is normal. The tympanogram on the involved right ear shows a type B pattern, substantiated by a rather low static compliance measure. These results ensure the presence of a stiffness component to the etiology of the right conductive hearing loss. That the contralateral stapedius reflex is absent bilaterally, in view of a unilateral hearing loss, confirms that the loss must be

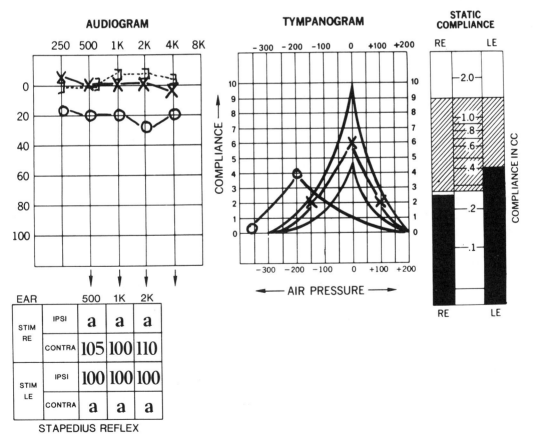

Figure 6.7. Audiometrics and immittance results accompanying a right-sided conductive hearing loss caused by significant negative middle ear pressure. Note contralateral and ipsilateral acoustic reflex findings. See text for full explanation.

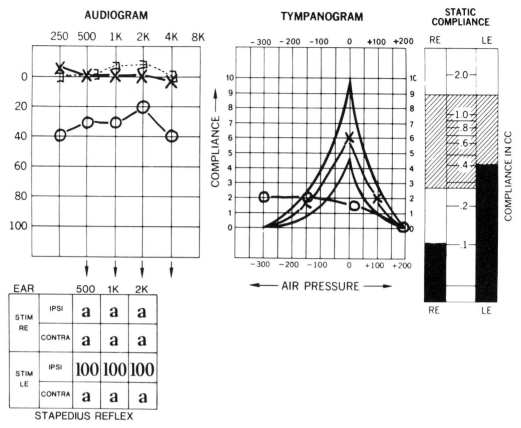

AUDIOGRAM

TYMPANOGRAM

STATIC COMPLIANCE

EAR		500	1K	2K
STIM RE	IPSI	a	a	a
	CONTRA	a	a	a
STIM LE	IPSI	100	100	100
	CONTRA	a	a	a

STAPEDIUS REFLEX

Figure 6.8. Audiometrics and immittance results in a unilateral conductive hearing loss of otitis media etiology. Note contralateral and ipsilateral acoustic reflex findings. See text for full explanation.

conductive in nature. This overall pattern could also represent cerumen packed in the right ear canal, a perforation of the right tympanic membrane, or otitis media. Diagnosis is in the realm of the physician, but these immittance test findings, even without the audiogram, would suggest referral of this child to a physician.

Bluestone et al. (1973) compared air conduction audiometry and tympanometry in 84 youngsters with concurrent or recent middle ear disease to determine which procedure could better predict the presence of middle ear effusion. They concluded that tympanometry is far more sensitive than air conduction audiometry for detecting common conduction defects in children. They caution, however, that tympanometry cannot detect sensorineural hearing loss and thus cannot be substituted for pure tone audiometry as a screening technique. They suggest that tympanometry in combination with air conduction audiometry appears to constitute the best method available for detecting middle ear disease and hearing impairment in large groups of children.

Immittance and Infants. There is contradictory evidence in the literature regarding the merits of performing acoustic immittance measurements in infants as shown by Northern's reviews of studies of immittance in infants (1981 and 1988). Margolis (1978) described the situation with a statement that impedance measurements in infants have provided results that are "both promising and perplexing." In an effort to determine whether immittance could be effectively used with newborns, Keith (1973,

1975) tested healthy infants from the newborn nursery. Keith reported normal tympanograms in 33 of the infants and a "W-shaped" tympanogram in 7 infants. Keith also examined stapedial reflex measurements in these 40 infants, using a 220 Hz probe tone with stimulus presentations of 100 dB HTL at 500 and 2000 Hz. He reported that stapedial reflex responses were often contaminated by behavioral movement of the infants. In fact, from 160 stimulus presentations, only 33% resulted in clear stapedial reflex responses. No acoustic reflex responses were noted in 26% of the stimulus presentations, and 4 of the 40 infants showed no acoustic reflex in either ear initially, although all 4 babies were later confirmed to have normal hearing responses.

The authors warned that immittance findings cannot stand alone and that immittance should only be interpreted in combination with some independent assessment of hearing sensitivity level. Unfortunately, this warning has been largely unheeded.

Immittance utilization with infants seemed to be a reasonably well accepted clinical tool until the publication of an article by Paradise et al. (1976). Their evaluation of 280 children ranging in age from 10 days to 5 years showed a high positive correlation (86%) between tympanometry and otoscopy for subjects over 7 months of age. Poor correlation, however, was found between the two measures in infants less than 7 months of age. In fact, from 43 infants less than 7 months of age, 40 of 81 ears had confirmed middle ear effusion (determined by myringotomy), yet 24 of the 40 abnormal ears displayed *normal tympanograms*. The authors concluded that although the use of tympanometry had much to offer in the diagnosis of middle ear effusion, its use (tympanometry) was not recommended in infants less than 7 months of age.

In contrast to the studies that question the efficacy of tympanometry with infants, successful tympanometric results with 91 infants between 4 weeks and 17 months were reported by Groothuis et al. (1978,

1979). These clinicians used otoscopy and tympanometry in 549 evaluations to study the pathogenesis of acute and chronic otitis media. Normal tympanograms and normal otoscopy findings correlated highly in 92% of the evaluations; flat tympanograms and abnormal otoscopy findings were correlated 93% of the time. However, the intermediate negative pressure tympanograms and otoscopy correlated only 59% of the time. Groothuis et al. reported that the tympanometric examination took about 45 seconds. The authors reported that *no* flat tympanograms were found in otitis-free infants.

The Groothuis studies provide some especially interesting findings. First, because of the report of Paradise et al. (1976) regarding the shortcomings of tympanometry in infants less than 7 months of age, Groothuis et al. examined their data separately for infants older and younger than 7 months. They found that the high correlation of tympanometry and otoscopy findings were similar in infants *above* and *below* 7 months of age. Second, when a nonmobile tympanogram appeared in an asymptomatic infant in the study who had not previously had otitis media, acute otitis media developed within one additional month. Third, the resolution of otitis media was often prolonged as long as 6 months in 60% of the infants. The authors concluded that tympanometry is a most useful tool and may be utilized for the earlier identification and more accurate follow-up of acute otitis media in infants.

Reichert et al. (1978) examined 878 3 month old infants with otoscopy and tympanometry. All infants were examined tympanometrically while being held in their mothers' arms and being comforted with a pacifier or bottle. The authors concluded that tympanometry produced a low diagnostic specificity (accuracy in identifying nondiseased individuals) with a high number of false positive results—16 "flat" tympanograms were found in ears that were otoscopically normal. In their discussion, Reichert et al. recognized that inclusion of the measurement of the acoustic reflex may have provided different results than were obtained only with the use of tympanometry.

Keith (1978) summarized the situation by stating it is imperative that tympanometry and stapedial reflex testing always be done together. To do less, according to Keith results in erroneous statements that "tympanometry is neither accurate nor reliable for use in screening infants." Keith expressed concern that such statements will be interpreted by some as indicating that the immittance *battery* is not valid or reliable for infants under 7 months of age.

Studies published by Orchik et al. (1978a, 1978b) clearly show that prediction of middle ear effusion on the basis of tympanometric data alone is difficult at best, unless the tympanogram is a flat, nonmobile pattern where a 90% occurrence of effusion is present. Wright et al. (1985) followed 210 infants during the initial 2 years of life with routine pneumatic otoscopy and immittance at each physician encounter. Tympanometry proved to have high predictive value (86%) for confirming normal ears but relatively poor predictive value (58%) for detecting abnormal ears. In general, the tympanometrically abnormal ear often appears normal during otoscopic examination. The problem is the determination of which procedure is really the criterion against which the other procedures should be compared. Otoscopy is most often accepted as the criterion test against which to compare other screening techniques, although it is well-known that the accuracy of otoscopy is only as valid as the person behind the otoscope (Paradise et al., 1976). Since otoscopy is so subjective, it can be argued that immittance should be the criterion procedure because of its objectivity and test-retest reliability. Generally speaking, otoscopy used as the criterion (as reported by Wright et al., 1985) produces higher sensitivity agreement, since fewer subjects "fail" otoscopy, while many subjects may "fail" tympanometric screening.

Schwartz and Schwartz (1978a, 1980) published data that supported the combined use of tympanometry and acoustic reflex measurement to identify middle ear effusion in infants. They conclude that while a normal tympanogram cannot be considered evidence of a mobile tympanic membrane or effusion-free middle ear, the presence of an acoustic reflex with a normal tympanogram supports normal middle ear function. Freyss et al. (1980) also found that the presence of the acoustic reflex provided a higher sensitivity than tympanometry for separating normal dry middle ears from middle ears with fluid.

Acoustic Reflexes in Infants. An intriguing finding concerning infant acoustic reflexes was reported by McCandless and Allred (1978), who showed that with a 220 Hz probe tone only 4% of 53 infants less than 48 hours of age demonstrated an acoustic reflex. But when the probe tone was increased to a frequency of 660 Hz, an astounding 89% of the same infants had an acoustic reflex. McCandless and Allred opened the door for subsequent research on immittance measurements in infants by suggesting that although a 220 Hz probe tone was superior for infant tympanometry tracings, the 660 Hz probe tone was clearly better for acoustic reflex evaluation.

In a series of studies of acoustic reflexes in infants, Bennett and Weatherby (1979, 1982; Weatherby and Bennett, 1980) used a two-component variable probe tone immittance meter to record contralateral acoustic reflexes in newborns. Their studies show that as the probe tone frequency is raised, the prevalence of the reflex increases while the threshold of the acoustic reflex decreases. With a maximum intensity of 96 dB SPL, no reflexes were detected with a 220 Hz probe, whereas with probe tones above 8000 Hz all newborns exhibited acoustic reflexes. Bennett (1984) pointed out that calibration of the contralateral earphone stimulus in infants is important because of the smaller volume of newborn ear canals and that differences in SPLs between adults and infants under earphones can easily exceed 6 dB. Bennett found the optimal probe tone frequency for detecting acoustic reflexes in neonates to be 1400 Hz.

In a thorough study of tympanometry and acoustic reflexes in neonates, Sprague et al. (1985) reported 80% observable reflexes with the 660 Hz probe tone and 50% observable reflexes with a 220 Hz probe tone with ipsilateral and contralateral activating stimuli. Instead of a standard earphone cushion for the contralateral stimulus, these researchers used insert receivers and found lower acoustic reflex thresholds than previously reported in other studies. McMillan et al. (1985) investigated ipsilateral and contralateral acoustic reflexes in neonates with probe tones of 220 and 660 Hz. Their results indicated that ipsilateral and contralateral reflexes to pure tone activators occurred 3 times more frequently with a 660 Hz probe tone (76%) than with the 220 Hz probe tone (24%). In their review of research papers dealing with acoustic reflex measurements in infants, Hodges and Ruth (1987) conclude that "the acoustic reflex mechanism is functional for infants as young as 9 hours after birth, and both crossed and uncrossed acoustic reflex thresholds can be measured."

Wright et al. (1985) followed 210 infants during the initial 2 years of life with routine pneumatic otoscopy and immittance at each physician encounter. Tympanometry proved to have high predictive value (86%) for confirming normal ears but relatively poor predictive value (58%) for detecting abnormal ears. In general, the tympanometrically abnormal ear often appears normal during otoscopic examination. The problem is the determination of which procedure is really the criterion against which the other procedures should be compared. Otoscopy is most often accepted as the criterion test against which to compare other screening techniques, although it is well-known that the accuracy of otoscopy is only as valid as the individual behind the otoscope (Paradise et al., 1976). Since otoscopy is so subjective, it can be argued that im-

mittance should be the criterion procedure because of its objectivity and test-retest reliability. Generally, otoscopy used as the criterion (as reported by Wright et al., 1985) produces higher sensitivity agreement, since fewer persons "fail" otoscopy, while many persons may "fail" tympanometric screening.

Practical Pediatric Impedance Considerations. Nearly anyone can be trained to turn the dials and read the meters of an immittance meter. And most clinicians have little difficulty testing cooperative adults. But the real challenge occurs when the clinician is face-to-face with an uncooperative youngster! A prime requisite for impedance clinicians faced with a difficult youngster is *confidence*. Persistence has its reward when working with children and impedance, so do not give up easily if difficulty is encountered—a second, third, or fourth effort may yield important results. The clinician who manages each child with a matter-of-fact attitude of self-assurance will often triumph!

On occasion, the clinician must be willing to compromise the entire test battery for less than optimal information. While it is desirable to complete the immittance test battery whenever possible, with some difficult-to-manage children the clinician may have to settle for a quick tympanogram and a single acoustic reflex measurement in each ear. Clinicians must be prepared to work rapidly and efficiently; a smooth, effective initial effort is often surprisingly successful.

The main limitation of immittance measurements in young children is that the test battery cannot be completed while the youngster is vocalizing—speaking, crying, yelling, or any combination of these noises. Acoustic reflex contraction and eustachian tube changes during vocalization cause the compliance of the tympanic membrane to alter wildly, thereby making immittance measurements impossible. The clinician's most challenging task is to make the youngster stop vocalizing for just the few neces-

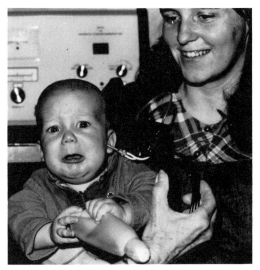

Figure 6.9. Acoustic immittance testing is an essential part of every pediatric hearing evaluation.

sary moments to obtain impedance data. Each clinician must devise his own techniques to momentarily distract the screaming child (Fig. 6.9).

For children less than 3 years of age it is helpful and essential that a second or even third person be utilized for obtaining impedance measures. Practice and coordination of these personnel are helpful, and they must be in constant communication during all aspects of the test to ensure rapid and reliable results. It is difficult for one person to manipulate the ear insert while operating the pressure pump and other dials on the immittance devices. It is preferable to have one person operate the impedance instrument while a second stabilizes the child's head and inserts the probe tip. This latter person must be appraised at all times as to whether or not a seal has been obtained or the pressure manometer must be in a position to be observed directly by him. Sometimes it works well to hold the probe tip in place by hand after insertion, and the head is stabilized by the assistant during the entirety of the test to prevent a loss of pressure seal due to head movement.

The age range between 2 and 12 months presents one of the most difficult periods in which to obtain immittance tests. The chil-dren are not old enough to understand the test or to respond to verbal enticements, yet they are old enough to react (sometimes decisively!) both to the test situation and to the insertion of the probe tip in particular. We have found that it is most effective to employ a distractive technique to redirect the youngster's attention from the test. The form of distraction is relatively unimportant so long as it is sufficiently novel to compel the infant to disregard the insertion of the probe tip. The external stimuli can be visual, tactile, auditory, or a combination of these. Prior to assuming a distractive procedure to be essential in immittance testing, one should try first to place the probe tip quickly, but gently, in the ear. Frequently this takes the child by surprise, and further games are not necessary. Often, the entire immittance battery can be completed before the child really has time to react or respond; however, at the first hint of reaction from the child the clinician should be prepared to present a visual distraction. If habituation to one mode of distraction occurs, instantly alter or introduce other diversionary tactics. If the diversions fail, it may be possible to apply passive restraint of the child's body, head, or hands to complete the test.

The following are examples of the many possible distractive techniques that can be used with children under the age of 3 years. The number and type of devices are limited only by the ingenuity of the examiner.

- *Animated Toys.* Introduce animated toys only as required at critical times necessary to complete the test. Avoid movement artifacts by keeping the toy well out of the reach of the child.

- *Cotton Swab.* Gently brush the back of the child's hand, arm, or leg in a slow even motion. Make the distraction visual as well as tactile by making oscillatory or exaggerated movements of the swab.

- *Pendulum.* Using a bright and unusually shaped object, make a pendulum with about an 18 inch string. This technique is highly effective if the examiner will swing the pendulum about in various motions within various areas of the infant's vision.

- *Mirror.* To an infant less than 1 year who is capable of reacting and attending to faces, a large mirror is sometimes irresistible.

- *Toys Which Produce Sounds.* Toys or other devices that elicit intense sounds should be avoided if at all possible, since they may evoke an acoustic or other reflexive response from the child. Toys that produce softer sounds in no way interfere with the test and can therefore be used effectively.

- *Watch.* In front of the child, simply remove one's wrist watch, manipulate or wind it well out of reach of the child, or point to it.

- *Shoe.* A simple, yet effective, technique is to begin lacing and unlacing a child's shoe either on or off his foot. Move slowly and methodically and do not appear to have any objective in mind except to lace and unlace or tie and untie the shoe.

- *Action Toys.* A variety of toys are available that perform repetitive actions.

- *Wad of Cotton or Kleenex.* A cotton ball or pledget can facilitate effective passive attention by balancing the cotton on the hand, arm, or knee of the subject or on the hand of the assistant. It can be squeezed or otherwise manipulated; it can be blown or allowed to fall repeatedly from the hand. A Kleenex can also be used as a parachute, torn slowly into strips, rolled into small balls and be placed in the child's hand, waved, punctured, etc.

- *Tape.* A roll of adhesive or paper surgical tape has been found to be one of the most effective distractive devices available in the clinic. Bits of tape can be torn off or stuck on various parts of the child's or examiner's anatomy. The child can be allowed to pull the tape off, objects can be picked up with the adhesive side of the tape, fingers can be bound together, links can be made with small strips, rings can be formed, fingernails covered, and innumerable other totally nonmeaningful manipulations can be performed.

- *Miscellaneous Devices.* Tongue blades, cotton swabs, colored yarn, or similar devices are all effective as distractive devices. They are best utilized when manipulated or "played with" by the examiner. If the child insists, he or she can be allowed to manipulate tape or string, etc. But care must be taken to permit only passive action so as to reduce movement artifact while the test is proceeding.

The audiologist should beware of a too-elaborate array of toys or gadgets because the child may want to play with the toys and not be bothered with the test procedure. For impedance testing, extensive entertainment is usually not warranted.

There is no way to predict the behavior or reaction of children between 1 and 3 years of age. Their reaction to the test situation is influenced by past exposure to other tests, to "doctors," by their age, by their personalities, and by their general evaluation of what they see is about to happen to them. In many instances they are most concerned whether or not the procedure will be painful. For these reasons some general rules apply when testing children in this age group. First, never ask a child for permission to perform impedance tests; calmly assume you are going to administer the test and proceed to do so. Second, avoid undue explanation regarding the test procedure. Instructions to the child contribute nothing to the test results unless it helps reduce physical movement. Besides, the child would not understand explanations even if given. It is sufficient to say something like, "here, listen to this," or "hold still," or "listen to this radio," then proceed with the test. Most often it is better to say nothing unless the child reacts to placement of the headset or insert. Explanations usually take longer than the test itself!

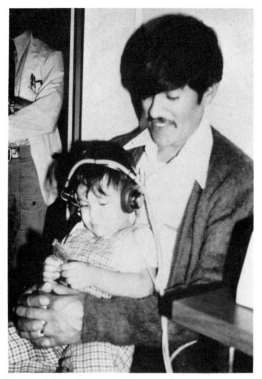

Figure 6.10. Successful acoustic immittance testing in children requires a perceptive and experienced clinician.

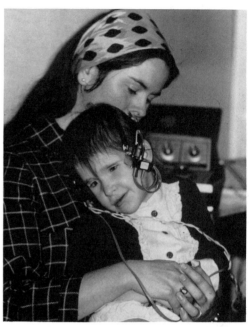

Figure 6.11. Immittance testing can be accomplished with difficult-to-test patients such as this mentally retarded rubella youngster.

For most children older than 3 years of age, no special distraction is required when applying immittance measures unless the child is particularly apprehensive in an unfamiliar clinical situation. Only a few children in this age category will demonstrate adverse reactions to immittance testing. Where necessary one can reduce anxiety by saying simply, "we are going to test your hearing, please hold still," or other uncomplicated statements of reassurance. Most 3 year olds can be tested with a single examiner. Allowing the child to observe other children or adults being tested helps to allay any fears that a pain will occur. With these children as with the younger group, refrain from asking permission to perform the test. Distractive techniques are viewed with suspicion, so treat this age category essentially as you would adults except for mild and occasional words of instruction or encouragement (Fig. 6.10).

Impedance Audiometry with the Mentally Retarded. The evaluation of hearing in the mentally retarded patient presents a most difficult task. Many retarded children do not condition well to pure tone play audiometry. They may not have sufficient maturation to perform auditory localization tasks or may lack consistent startle response. They may be too hyperactive to cooperate or too lethargic to be aware of changes in the environment (Fig. 6.11). Incidence studies have established that there is a higher incidence of hearing impairment among the retarded than among the nonretarded (Lloyd, 1970; Rittmanic, 1971). Yet the retarded are excluded from traditionally recommended screening techniques because of their limited capacity for responding.

Brain damage in these children often makes physiologic auditory responses unreliable. Yet, accurate assessment of hearing function or middle ear status of these children may be critical for educational placement or medical/surgical treatment. Sometimes, even a tympanogram or acoustic reflex measure can be a valuable result, since the clinician can then make reasonably accurate assumptions regarding the presence or absence of middle ear problems and the need for medical referral. Immittance measurements are also valuable in the evaluation of the severely mentally retarded "mattress care" children, who are virtually impossible to test with any other testing procedure. These institutionalized youngsters are certainly at high risk for developing chronic middle ear disease.

The earliest acoustic impedance studies with retarded children were published by Lamb and Norris (1969, 1970) and Borus (1972). Although it was reported that considerable variability in reflex thresholds was noted among the mentally retarded persons, the authors noted that the retarded persons were easily tested, and they recommended that the immittance battery should be included as a part of the audiometric test battery.

Jordan (1972) pointed out that even a mild degree of hearing loss may have a disproportional impact on the mental retardate because he or she is less capable of compensating cerebrally with the aid of other senses. Mentally retarded children now considered to be educable were "mattress cases" 25 years ago. Standards set forth by the Accreditation Council for Facilities for the Mentally Retarded in 1971 require that all residents of institutions must be given audiometric screening at regular intervals. Audiologists in such facilities find themselves faced with great numbers of retarded patients of all ages and functioning levels, for auditory screening. We see no alternative for auditory evaluation of such patients without immittance audiometry.

Immittance with the Congenitally Deaf Child. The workup of patients with substantial sensorineural deafness will usually not identify superimposed middle ear anomalies. Immittance audiometry provides a useful means of evaluating the conductive hearing mechanism in patients with sensorineural hearing loss (Northern, 1980c).

Children attending schools for the deaf are not routinely evaluated by otolaryngologists. These deaf children seldom complain about their ears or of changes in their hearing sensitivity due to otologic pathology. Bone conduction measurements are of limited usefulness in this special population with severe-to-profound sensorineural hearing impairment. Only a few published articles are available describing immittance measurement results from children attending schools for the deaf (Rubin, 1978; Ruben and Math, 1978; Rood and Stool, 1981).

Rossi and Sims (1977) reported the use of acoustic reflex measurements in the severely and profoundly deaf in an effort to evaluate the validity of audiometrically determined air-bone gaps. They conducted immittance studies of 85 deaf students, showing that some 80% of the "air-bone gaps" produced by audiometry were, in fact, invalid. They recommend the use of the acoustic reflex to resolve the ambiguity of responses due to probable tactile-vibratory stimulation with the audiometric bone oscillator from true conductive components.

These studies show that immittance provides a useful means of evaluating the conductive mechanism in patients with profound deafness. The Brooks (1975) study brought out an important additional fact about the increase in hearing loss that accompanies middle ear problems. In deaf children this additional hearing loss may have significant deleterious effect on hearing aid performance. If the child is mature enough to recognize the need to turn up the hearing aid gain, problems may be created with distortion and feedback; if the child is too young to note the change in hearing, poor performance with the hearing aid may also result. Immittance audiometry should, by all means, be a routine procedure for children attending schools for the deaf.

Hearing Loss Prediction by the Acoustic Reflex. A revolutionary application of impedance audiometry was developed by Niemeyer and Sesterhenn (1972) to determine air conduction hearing thresholds from stapedial reflex measurements. They noted that the acoustic reflex threshold for white noise was lower than the acoustic reflex threshold for pure tones and that the difference in decibels between the two thresholds is related to the degree of sensorineural hearing impairment. They verified their results on a large group of normal-hearing and hearing-loss persons and concluded that their technique provided an objective means to predict hearing levels within 10 dB in just a few minutes without extensive equipment expenditures.

Two years later, Jerger et al. (1974b) simplified the procedure into a test he called Sensitivity Prediction with the Acoustic Reflex (SPAR). SPAR is an attempt to ascertain sensorineural hearing loss within four categories of impairment (normal hearing, mild loss, severe loss, or profound loss). The Jerger technique calls for establishment of pure tone acoustic reflexes at 500, 1000, and 2000 Hz and broadband noise threshold difference to predict the degree of hearing loss. In a series of over 1000 patients, Jerger et al. (1974b) reported that the predictive error of SPAR was clinically insignificant in 63% of the group, was moderate in 33%, and was serious in only 4%.

The success of the SPAR procedure has inspired a number of innovative approaches to predict hearing loss with acoustic reflex measurements. Hall and Bleakney (1981) divide these approaches into three general categories—SPAR, regression equations, and the bivariate plot system. All depend, in one fashion or another, on the noise-tone difference in acoustic reflex thresholds and have been reviewed in detail by Hall (1980) and Popelka (1981).

In general, the regression equations predict HTL by assigning acoustic reflex threshold data for pure tones and noise in differentially weighted equations. These formulas are based on statistical regression techniques. The bivariate plot coordinate system simply differentiates those patients with normal hearing from those with sensorineural hearing loss. According to Hall and Bleakney (1981), the SPAR methods, regression equations, and bivariate plot system all appear to estimate, or identify, hearing loss with accuracy rates in excess of 60%. Silman et al. (1987) state that the bivariate plot method has the greatest utility with children of the acoustic reflex-based methods for hearing loss evaluation.

Hearing loss prediction from the acoustic reflex is apparently influenced by a number of variables including chronologic age, minor middle ear abnormalities, and audiometric configuration. Fortunately, for those of us involved in pediatric audiology, predictive accuracy with the SPAR test is more successful in children (ages 0–10 years) and grows less accurate in older children and adults. Jerger et al. (1978) conclude that the best approach to predicting the presence of hearing loss of any degree is to rely on the broadband noise and pure tone acoustic reflex difference, whereas the absolute acoustic reflex threshold level for broadband noise stimuli is used to predict the degree of hearing loss. In the Jerger et al. (1978) study, 100% of the children predicted to have normal hearing did, indeed, show normal audiograms. Severe hearing loss was accurately predicted in children 85% of the time. Prediction of moderate hearing loss in children was somewhat less accurate (54%).

The prediction of hearing loss with the acoustic reflex is a valuable asset to those clinicians involved with hearing evaluations in children. Objective prediction of hearing loss in children has numerous applications in daily clinical testing, and all clinicians should be familiar with and able to implement the technique when appropriate. Successful use of these procedures with children have been reported by Jerger and Hayes (1976), Keith (1977b), Niswander and Ruth (1977), Silman (1984), and Northern (1988). According to Hall (1980), there is reason for optimism about the potential of acoustic reflex hearing level predictions. In

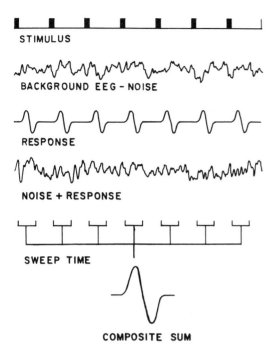

STIMULUS

BACKGROUND EEG – NOISE

RESPONSE

NOISE + RESPONSE

SWEEP TIME

COMPOSITE SUM

Figure 6.12. Signal-averager computers utilize a summation technique to cancel out random ongoing background physiologic "noise," which creates an improved signal-to-noise condition to enhance specific, time-locked potentials of small magnitude. (Courtesy of Laszlo Stein, Ph.D., Northwestern University.)

very young children, acoustic reflex prediction methods clearly offer the most rapid objective measure of hearing sensitivity—even with the "difficult-to-test" child.

EVOKED AUDITORY RESPONSE AUDIOMETRY

Nearly 45 years ago Davis (1939) noted that the electrical activity of the brain as indicated by electroencephalographic recordings showed a change when the subject heard a loud sound. This led numerous clinicians to attempt to use the standard electroencephalographic technique as a test for hearing acuity. Results, however, were disappointing. The electrical response in the cortex to auditory stimuli is so small that it is difficult to see in the normal ongoing electrical activity of the brain, particularly when the stimuli are low-intensity pure tones.

In the early 1960s a number of special purpose computers appeared on the commercial market. These computers, known generally as signal-averager computers, utilized a summation technique to cancel out random ongoing background physiologic "noise." This created an improved signal-to-noise condition to enhance specific, time-locked potentials of small magnitude. These computers store and average potentials related in time to the onset of a stimulus. The "random" noise consists theoretically of an equal number of positive and negative electrical potentials and is averaged out. Thus, only the wanted potential activity summates in the computer (Fig. 6.12).

The averaged evoked response is not a unitary response but rather is a composite response reflecting various activities from the auditory pathway. An idealized auditory evoked potential is presented in Figure 6.13, which shows the component potentials as they are commonly described in terms of latency. Davis (1976) identified these potentials in terms of their latency "epoch" as *first components* (0–2 msec, including the cochlear microphonic and summating potential); *fast components* (2–10 msec, the acoustic nerve and auditory brainstem responses); middle latency components (8–50 msec, thalmus and auditory cortex activity); *slow components* (50–300 msec, primary and secondary areas of the cerebral cortex); and the *late components* (300 msec and longer from the primary and association areas of the cerebral cortex).

The amplitude of these auditory evoked responses is generally related to the intensity of the stimulus; the more intense the stimulus, the larger the average evoked response to a certain point. The growth in amplitude of the wave is accompanied by a decrease in latency of the peak components. As the stimulus signal is decreased toward threshold levels, the presence or absence of the averaged evoked response becomes difficult to separate from the biologic baseline activity. The clinical applications of evoked potential measurements are quite varied and include auditory, visual, and somatosensory evaluations. Evoked potentials may also be used for surgical monitoring by otolaryngologists, ophthalmologists, and orthopedic surgeons.

The evoked potential literature has absolutely grown by leaps and bounds during the 1970s and 1980s. These studies were the beginning of a tremendous change in the field of physiologic evoked potential measurements. Improvements in equipment and computer technology have helped clarify the various evoked potentials in humans and, in turn, have influenced greatly the field of audiology.

The application of auditory evoked response evaluations in special populations has been an important asset to pediatric audiologists. Stein and Kraus (1988) describe the use of auditory evoked potentials (AEPs) as tests of both hearing and neurologic dysfunction common to many pediatric disorders including mental retardation, deafness-blindness, hydrocephalus, meningitis, and infantile autism. The authors comment that although the audiologist is primarily interested in AEPs as tests of hearing, abnormal neuropathologic conditions may hinder the diagnosis of hearing loss. Thoughtful interpretation of AEP results must take into account the effect of potential peripheral hearing loss and neurologic condition.

Most audiology and otolaryngology textbooks now include complete materials devoted to descriptions of AEPs. Our task will be to present a current overview of the early evoked potentials and their application in the clinical evaluation of hearing in children. Our discussion has drawn heavily from the materials of Fria (1980), Jerger et al. (1981), and Jacobson (1985).

Auditory Brainstem Evoked Responses. In 1967, an important discovery was reported by two Israeli physicians, Sohmer and Feinmesser, who used click stimuli to evoke a polyphasic response recorded with electrodes on the vertex of a human subject. This evoked potential was

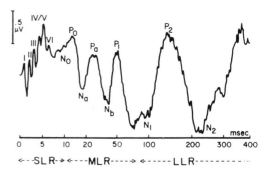

Figure 6.13. An idealized full AEP representing the short-latency response (*SLR*), the middle-latency response (*MLR*), and the long-latency response (*LLR*). (From American Speech-Language-Hearing Association: *The Short Latency Auditory Evoked Potentials.* Rockville, Maryland, American Speech-Language-Hearing Association, 1987, p. 29.)

of very short latency, within the initial 12.5 msec poststimulus and consisted of a specific pattern with five positive-direction waves. In 1970, Jewett noted seven positive peak waveforms, occurring within the initial 10 msec poststimulus, that had remarkable stability and consistent waveform latencies (Fig. 6.14).

Auditory brainstem evoked response (ABR) measurements provide information regarding the identification of site of lesion in the auditory brainstem pathways, including acoustic nerve tumors, assessment of auditory function in patients with stroke or trauma, infant hearing assessment, predicting hearing sensitivity in difficult-to-test children, evaluation of aided versus unaided auditory performance, neurologic disease and/or dysfunction, and central auditory processing information. ABR measurements are utilized by audiologists as well as other medical specialists such as otolaryngologists, neurologists, ophthalmologists, neurosurgeons, anesthesiologists, and orthopedic surgeons (Chiappa and Ropper, 1982).

Jewett and Williston (1971) systematically recorded the early ABR human responses to varying stimulus and recording parameters. They labeled their seven positive peaks from I to VII as shown in Figure 6.14. Waves VI and VII have subsequently been found to be not always readily appar-

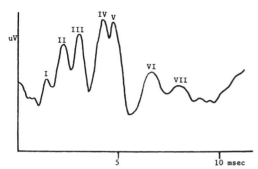

Figure 6.14. An idealized example of the peaks in the early component evoked response according to Jewett and Williston (1971).

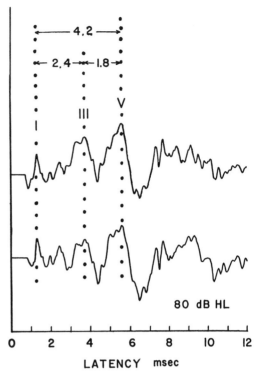

Figure 6.15. Typical latency measurements and interwave latency measurements for a high-intensity ABR. (Courtesy of Laszlo Stein, Ph.D., Northwestern University.)

ent, and general clinical interpretation has focused on waves I through V. Wave V has proven to be the most prominent component of the response pattern and is often seen combined with wave IV to form the "IV–V complex." The normal latency of each wave is about 1 msec longer than its designated number, so wave I has a latency of about 2 msec, while wave V has a latency of about 6 msec, as shown in Figure 6.15. Although the amplitude of the waves is easily influenced by numerous variables, the latency of the peaks is very stable.

The neural generators for the ABR were postulated to be the peripheral acoustic nerve and the various nuclei of the ascending auditory brainstem pathway. Experimental studies in animals and studies of ABR in human patients with confirmed lesions have led to the general conclusion that wave I represents the auditory nerve site and that waves II and III are associated with the medulla and pons, specifically the cochlear nucleus and superior olivary complex. Changes in the wave forms of IV and V are associated with lesions affecting midbrain auditory structures, the lateral lemniscus and the inferior colliculus (Fig. 6.16). Although controversy exists over the exact specification of origin sites for each wave of the ABR, Picton et al. (1974) suggested that waves I through IV represent activity from the auditory nerve and brainstem auditory nuclei, but that the total wave pattern is also influenced by the composite contribution of multiple generators. J. Jerger

et al. (1981) point out that with such a "far-field" recording technique with electrodes on the scalp, it is too simple to assume site specification of each wave to a unique generator. It is more reasonable to assume the ABR represents a "complex interplay and interaction of evoked potential activity from multiple overlapping dipoles involving all the structures of the auditory system."

The clinical attributes of the ABR were summarized by Davis (1976) to include waveform consistency, easy recordability with proper equipment and technique, and optimal latency—slow enough to avoid confusion with the cochlear microphonic, yet fast enough to avoid being masked by muscle reflexes. The ABR is widely known for its freedom from the effects of central nervous system state and the replicability of the waveform pattern. In fact, the validity of an ABR tracing is usually verified by repeating the test and comparing both runs.

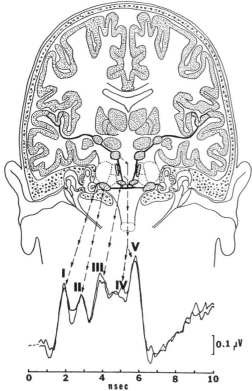

Figure 6.16. Diagrammatic representation of the auditory brainstem response waves and their generator sites. Wave I is associated with the auditory nerve, wave II comes from the cochlear nucleus, wave III comes from the superior olivary complex, wave IV is thought to come from the area of the lateral lemniscus, and wave V is from the inferior colliculus. (Courtesy of Laszlo Stein, Ph.D., Northwestern University.)

Shimizu (1981) points out that the technique with children is attractive because the ABR is relatively unaffected by the physiologic state of the patient, the measurement is accomplished as a nonsurgical test, with excellent results in both awake and sleep stages.

Auditory Brainstem Evoked Response Parameters. The ABR is optimally recorded differentially from the vertex scalp to the ipsilateral mastoid or earlobe with an electrode on the contralateral mastoid serving as ground. The ABR is usually evoked with click stimuli, repetitively presented ($N = 2000$) at 30 clicks per second and summated by computer analysis. Click stimuli

provide a sufficiently short rise time to ensure a synchronous neural burst from the auditory system (Hecox et al., 1976). Therein, however, is the main shortcoming of the ABR technique—the lack of frequency-specific information about the hearing of the patient. The spectral energy of the transient click stimulus is shaped by the earphone resonant characteristics and the duration of the click. Because clicks fail to allow frequency specificity in the auditory system, the ABR reflects predominantly the basal turn of the cochlea or hearing information between 1000 and 4000 Hz.

Several techniques have been developed with stimuli other than clicks to enable ABR results to be more frequency-specific. Tone pips, filtered clicks, or the subtractive masking procedure can be used as frequency-specific stimuli, although there is some question about the spread of energy around each of these transient sudden onset signals. The use of these frequency-specific stimulus techniques are typically more demanding and time-consuming than the use of unmasked tone bursts or filtered clicks. An excellent discussion of stimuli spectrum has been published by the American Speech-Language-Hearing Association (1987).

Stockard and Stockard (1979) have shown that stimulus factors can have an interactive influence on the ABR waveform, but varying individual parameters of the stimulus will also exert modification of the wave pattern. Increasing stimulus intensity influences the ABR waveform by increasing the amplitudes and decreasing wave latencies. The relationship between stimulus intensity and wave peak latencies is used to plot "latency-intensity functions" for each of the waves. Figure 6.17 demonstrates typical latency-intensity functions as used in differential diagnosis of hearing losses, compared to the normal range of latency-intensity responses.

The latency-intensity function is usually plotted for waves I, III and V, and it is important to know that the pattern of all three functions is approximately parallel. This

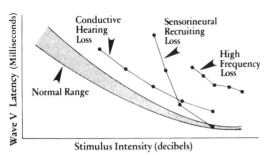

Figure 6.17. Characteristic latency-intensity functions obtained with normal listeners and various types of hearing loss patients. (Courtesy of Nicolet Biomedical, Madison, Wisconsin.)

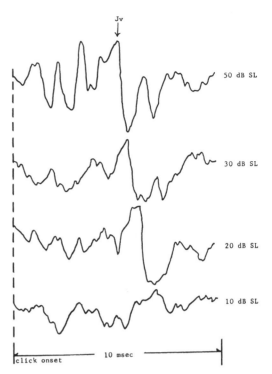

Figure 6.18. Summed brainstem evoked responses at decreasing intensities. Each response represents 2048 click presentations. (Courtesy of Steven Staller, Ph.D., Cochlear Corporation.)

also indicates that the interpeak intervals (sometimes called interwave latency intervals) are relatively constant over the entire intensity range. Thus, the interpeak intervals (i.e., I–III, III–V, or I–V as shown in Fig. 6.15) can be measured at any intensity level without concern that the measurement will be affected. In general the I–III interpeak interval is about 2 msec, the III–IV interpeak interval is approximately 2 msec, and thus the I–V interval is about 4 msec.

At high stimulus intensity (80 dB HL or greater), all five waves are usually seen with clarity in normal persons. As stimulus intensity is decreased, below 60 dB HL for example, waves I, II, and IV tend to become difficult to identify with certainty. When stimulus intensity nears auditory threshold, wave V is often the only remaining landmark in the response tracing. In this fashion, as shown in Figure 6.18, ABR is used to estimate auditory threshold. The tester must keep in mind the lack of information provided from traditional audiometric test frequencies below 1000 Hz. Likewise, the ABR is very sensitive to peripheral high-frequency hearing loss and central auditory pathway disorders. These conditions, either singularly or together, can make the ABR waveform difficult to interpret.

Gorga et al. (1985) compared ABR responses with pure tone audiograms obtained from patients with cochlear hearing loss. The click-evoked ABR thresholds were most closely related to behavioral audiometric thresholds at 2000 and 4000 Hz, with poor agreement at 1000 and 8000 Hz. The ABR latency-intensity function slope was related to the configuration of the hearing loss so that high-frequency sensorineural hearing losses had steeper slopes than patients with flat hearing losses or normal hearing.

An increase in the stimulus click rate increases the latency and reduces the amplitude of the ABR waves. The amplitude of wave V is constant up to 30 clicks per second, although the peak latency of wave V may change about 1.0 msec as stimulus click rate is increased from 10 to 100 clicks per second. These technical considerations make it mandatory that all clinical facilities that wish to perform ABR establish their own norms for their particular test parameters and procedures prior to testing patients.

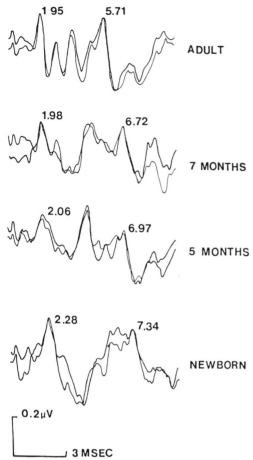

1 95   5.71

ADULT

1.98   6.72

7 MONTHS

2.06   6.97

5 MONTHS

2.28   7.34

NEWBORN

0.2 μV

3 MSEC

Figure 6.19. Maturation of the auditory brainstem response from postnatal newborn period to adulthood. (Reprinted with permission from K. Hecox and J. Jacobson: Auditory evoked potentials. In J. L. Northern (ed.) *Hearing Disorders*. Boston, Little, Brown & Co., 1984.)

Another important variable in the interpretation of ABR tracings, especially in premature infants, is the effect of maturation on the waveforms. The effect of maturation in infant populations is significant, and without proper normative standards, misinterpretation of peak wave latencies can easily occur. However, between the ages of 18 months and 25 years of age, the ABR shows little change in latency or amplitude. Figure 6.19 shows the general maturation of the ABR from newborn to adulthood (Jacobson et al., 1982).

Gorga and associates (1987) have contributed substantially to the establish-

ment of ABR normative standards in infants and young children. A comprehensive study of 585 graduates of an intensive care nursery showed small, systematic decreases in response component latencies occurring with increasing age. The normal distribution of results, therefore, makes it possible to identify an individual infant's wave V latency or interpeak latency difference that might fall below the 5th or 10th percentile of the respective cumulative distribution. Their results also confirmed the importance of taking chronologic age of the infant into account when evaluating ABR latencies.

As an extension of the above-described study of ABR with intensive care nursery infants, Gorga et al. (1989) reported normative data on 535 normal-hearing children from 3 months to 3 years of age. Wave V latency decreased as age increased, at least to 18 months of age, while little or no change was noted in wave I latencies over the same age range. Interpeak wave latency differences followed the same developmental time course as wave V. More information on the maturation effect in premature infants may be found in Chapter 7 (ABR in infant screening).

Binaural stimulation is often useful when testing children (Fig. 6.20). Binaural stimulation with clicks produces waveforms that are about 1½ times greater in amplitude than noted with monaural stimulation of either ear. The latencies of the waves are essentially the same for monaural and binaural stimulation. The binaural stimulation technique is good for approximating auditory threshold, since the response to binaurally presented clicks is the same as the response to monaurally presented clicks in the better hearing ear.

A major disadvantage in ABR with children is that most children between the ages of about 6 months and 4 years must be sedated for the duration of the testing session. This requires the use of a professional medical staff to be on hand during the session. We allow a minimum of 1 hour for each test session, although we are always pre-

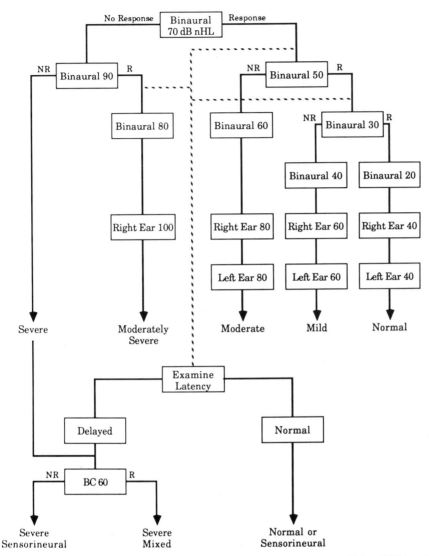

Figure 6.20. Flow diagram of Jerger's "binaural strategy" technique to obtain time-efficient ABR hearing threshold estimates in children. (From J. Jerger, T. Oliver, and B. Stach: Auditory brainstem response testing strategies. In J. Jacobson (ed.): *The Auditory Brainstem Response*. San Diego: College-Hill Press, 1985, pp. 371–388.)

pared to carry on longer if necessary to obtain adequate information about the hearing of the patient. Most children older than 4½ can be entertained during the session or will sit fairly quietly until the test is completed.

Jerger and Hayes (1976) have brought out the value of the cross-check principle in young children who may yield a behavioral audiogram, the validity of which is under question because of conflicting speech audi-

ometry results or impedance audiometry findings. No ABR study should be undertaken without first attempting behavioral audiometrics and impedance audiometry. Shimizu (1981) warns that ABR is only a part of the whole diagnostic process for clinicians whose responsibility must cover history taking, traditional audiometrics, evaluation of the patient's overall communicative abilities, parent counseling, and overall case disposition. Fria (1980) states emphat-

Table 6.5.
Candidate Pediatric Populations for ABR Tests[a]

Age Group	Definite Candidates	Possible Candidates
Newborns (0–2 mo)	Conditions leading to intensive care nursery admission	
	Conditions leading to high-risk register enrollment	
	Failure of behavioral hearing screening in normal nursery	
	Meningitis	
Infants (3–23 mo)	Meningitis	Recurrent apnea
	Congenital atresia	Failure to thrive
	Persistent otitis media with effusion	Infantile autism
	Sepsis and ototoxic drug therapy	Developmental delay
	Delayed speech	
	Parental suspicion of hearing loss	
Children (24 mo +)	Mental retardation	Autism
	Emotional disturbance	Developmental delay
	Learning disability	Sudden and progressive sensorineural hearing loss
	Suspicion of retrocochlear lesion	
	Meningitis	

[a]From T. Fria: The auditory brainstem response: background and clinical applications. *Monographs in Contemporary Audiology* 2(2): 37, 1980.

ically that the ABR cannot test "hearing" in the perceptual sense, nor can it identify a specific neurologic lesion at a given location (Table 6.5). Consequently, the ABR results cannot stand alone and must be interpreted in the context of other clinical information. J. Jerger et al. (1980) cite overinterpretation of ABR as the most common error made by clinicians and/or failure to consider other test findings in the whole clinical picture.[a]

Auditory Middle-Latency Evoked Responses. The auditory middle-latency evoked responses (MLRs), so called because their latency lies between that of the early or brainstem evoked responses and the late cortical evoked responses. The latencies of the MLR peaks are found between 12 and 60 msec poststimulus. The discovery and the major investigation of auditory middle-latency evoked potential are associated with Goldstein and Rodman (1967), Mendel and Goldstein (1969), and Mendel (1980).

The site of generation has not been identified precisely, although Beagley and Fisch (1981) believe it to be situated in the auditory radiations in the thalamic region and in the primary auditory cortex in the temporal lobe.

Hood (1975) describes the nature of the MLR to be two major positive peaks, P_o with a latency of 12 msec and P_a with a latency of 32 msec, and three negative troughs, N_o, N_a, and N_b, occurring at 8, 18, and 52 msec, respectively. Hood suggests, based on the works of Goldstein and associates, that with the finding of close agreement between MLR thresholds and behavioral thresholds for the same stimuli, the MLR may serve to be an indicator of auditory sensitivity (Fig. 6.21).

Mendel and Goldstein (1971) showed that the amplitude of the MLR is influenced dramatically through various sleep stages and wakefulness. Subsequent studies have verified the sleep effect on the MLR (Liden et al., 1985). Recent work by Kraus et al. (1989) shows that wave P_a detectability is especially poor during certain stages of sleep. Jerger et al. (1986) point out that since young children must typically be sedated to carry out evoked response testing, the effects of natural and/or induced sleep are a crucial factor in limiting the MLR in pediatric applications.

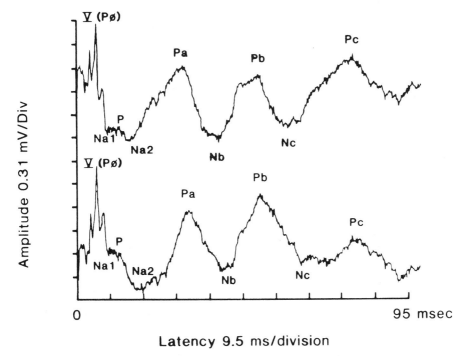

Figure 6.21. Normal MLR curves. *Upper waveform* was recorded with standard-phase shift settings, while *lower waveform* was recorded with zero-phase shift (filter setting = 15 Hz, 24 dB/octave). (From K. T. Kavanagh and W. D. Domico: High pass digital and analog filtering of the middle latency response. *Ear and Hearing* 8(2):102, 1987.)

Kraus et al. (1989) states that the occurrence of MLR in children ages 4–9 years is not haphazard and that the MLR in children can be reliably obtained during certain states of arousal. These authors routinely measure simultaneously the ABR and the MLR in children to obtain a measure of low-frequency hearing. When MLRs are present, they provide a useful test of auditory threshold estimation at 500 and 1000 Hz. But because of the inconsistency of the detectability of the MLR in children, absence of the MLR cannot be interpreted as an indication of hearing loss in the low frequencies.

Kavanagh et al. (1989) compared low-intensity ABR and MLR in a group of 48 mentally handicapped persons. Although the ABR measurement generally showed less test-retest variability than the MLR, several of the retarded persons with hearing loss were noted to have recordable MLRs when no ABR could be detected. These authors suggest that this is evidence that the

ABR and MLR have different neurologic centers and that perhaps a loss of neuronal synchronization may result in the absence of the ABR but still allow recording of the low-frequency MLR.

Although early investigations reported MLRs in babies, attempts to use the MLR for infant hearing screening have been unsuccessful. Jerger et al. (1988) point out that the MLR is observed in babies only under very slow stimulus rates and is a "very fragile" response at best. The Jerger group concludes that the MLR parameters (large number of average responses, slow rate of data acquisition, and the dependence of stimulus rate) limit the clinical value of this evoked potential.

Ozdamar and Kraus (1983) published a study of auditory MLRs and ABRs in the same persons. They found that mild sedatives did not appear to affect either MLR or ABR and that MLR differed from ABR in their stimulus-related properties, implying that the neuronal mechanisms underlying

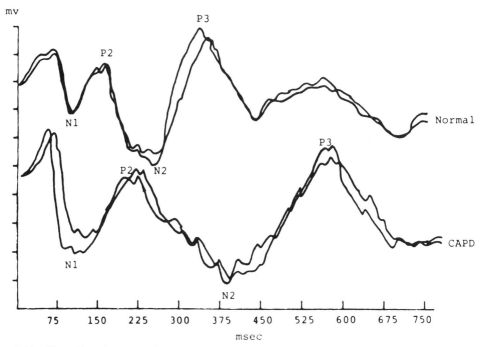

Figure 6.22. Normal long-latency auditory potentials from a normal control group (*top*) and a group of children with central auditory processing disorders (*CAPD*) (*bottom*). Note shift in P_3 component latency. (From J. Jirsa and K. Clontz: Long latency auditory event-related potentials from children with auditory processing disorders. *Ear and Hearing* 11(3):225, 1990.)

their generation are not the same. In contrast to previous studies (Mendel et al., 1975), they found that MLR wave components were not as readily identifiable at low stimulus levels as the ABR wave V, and they concluded that the ABR appears to be the test of choice when hearing sensitivity is in question. Finally, they suggest that MLR are likely to be most clinically useful in patients with neurologic or central auditory processing disorders.

Late Auditory Evoked Potentials. The late auditory evoked potentials have had a long and colorful history beginning in the 1960s. In fact, during the mid-1960s, the late evoked potentials were being hailed as "the answer" to audiometric testing problems and the difficult-to-test patient. The success of the technique was related to the fact that under the best of conditions, auditory thresholds obtained with this "objective" procedure agreed within 20 dB of adult auditory behavioral thresholds!

Unfortunately, the late potentials are extremely sensitive to even minor alterations in subject state of awareness, level of consciousness, and changes in stimulus parameters. Technical problems, equipment expense, and lack of clinical precision made routine use of auditory late potentials impractical for most clinical facilities. Thus, efforts to use late cortical potentials in clinical measurements were largely abandoned in the early 1970s.

The cortical evoked response results from generalized electrical activity on the cortex because of the presentation of various sensory stimuli including light, vibrotactile stimuli, and sound. In fact, the presentation of any sensory stimulus of sufficient intensity or the abrupt change of any stimulus produces a widespread evoked potential from the human brain during the 300 msec following the stimulus presentation (Fig. 6.22).

The late cortical potentials are currently under renewed interest because of their

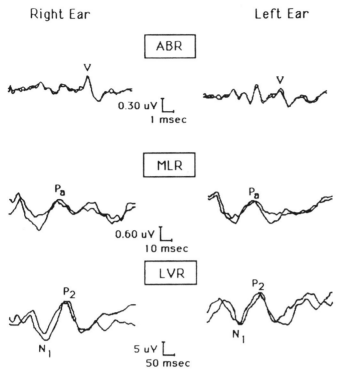

Right Ear   Left Ear

Figure 6.23. Auditory evoked potential series from a child with delayed speech and language development. Auditory evoked potential testing included the auditory brainstem response (*ABR*) to a click presented at 70 dB nHL, the middle-latency response (*MLR*) to a click presented at 70 dB nHL, and the late vertex response (*LVR*) to a 500 Hz tone burst presented at 50 dB nHL. All auditory evoked potential components were of normal latency, amplitude, and morphology. (Courtesy of B. Stach, Ph.D., Baylor School of Medicine, Houston, Texas.)

presumed relationship to the perceptual attributes of sound and interhemispheric differences and because of their various neurologic and psychiatric applications (American Speech-Language-Hearing Association, 1987). One particular wave, the P300 component, has been studied in various cognitive tasks and is thought by some to hold promise for investigating how the brain "processes" information (Mendel, 1985). At present, however, the late cortical potentials are not used in routine clinical audiometric evaluations (see Figures 6.23 and 6.24).

ELECTROCOCHLEOGRAPHY

Investigators have long been intrigued by the electrical potentials generated within the auditory system. Clinicians have made many efforts through the years to utilize these auditory potentials in some form of clinical procedure. These measurements were termed "electrocochleography" (ECochG) by Lempert et al. (1947). The electrocochleogram (ECochGm) consists of more than one auditory electrical potential including the whole nerve action potential (AP), the cochlear microphonic (CM) and the summating potential (SP). The AP is the most obvious and easily recorded component of the ECochGm (Fig. 6.25).

The electrical potential from the auditory nerve is the AP, noted initially by Derbyshire and Davis (1935). The AP consists of nerve impulses in the eighth nerve triggered by the CM. The AP response consists of a well-synchronized volley of impulses called N_1, which may be followed by smaller waves known as N_2 and N_3. Although initial clinical attempts to use auditory electrical potentials centered around the CM, the compound AP response is currently proving most valuable in clinical use.

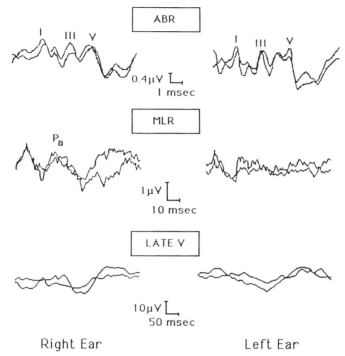

Figure 6.24. Auditory evoked potential series from a child with a diagnosis of central auditory processing disorder. Auditory brainstem response (*ABR*) to a click presented at 70 dB nHL, the middle-latency response (*MLR*) to a click presented at 70 dB nHL, and the late vertex response (*Late V*) to a 500 Hz tone burst presented at 60 dB nHL. *Wave V* is identifiable at normal latencies on the ABRs, and *peak P_a* is identifiable on the right-ear MLR. The P_a on the left ear was degraded. No waveform peaks were identifiable on the LVRs. (From B. A. Stach, L. H. Loiselle, J. F. Jerger, S. L. Mintz, and C. D. Taylor: Clinical experience with personal FM assistive listening devices. *The Hearing Journal* 40(5):24–30, 1987.)

The compound AP has a latency of about 2 msec when the cochlea is stimulated by an abrupt sound stimulus. Although the individual AP in each auditory nerve fiber is a diphasic spike potential, the response of the whole auditory nerve is a compound potential that gives information from the basal turn of the cochlea and, to a lesser extent, from the middle turn (Beagley and Fisch, 1981).

The CM originates from the hair cells in the organ of Corti as originally described by Wever and Bray (1930). The CM reproduces faithfully the waveform of the stimulating auditory signal and is usually measured by an electrode from the round window niche. The CM has no "threshold" other than the lower limits of the recording apparatus; i.e., the CM is produced to any auditory signal, no matter how slight.

Simmons and Glattke (1975) state that the ECochG is the most powerful electrophysiologic index of cochlear integrity—

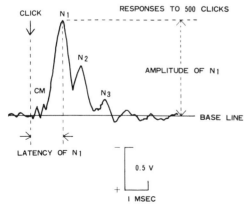

Figure 6.25. Electrocochleographic (ECochG) averaged response as recorded by Yoshie and Ohashi (1969) from an electrode in the wall of the external auditory canal. This figure illustrates the definition of N, latency, and amplitude.

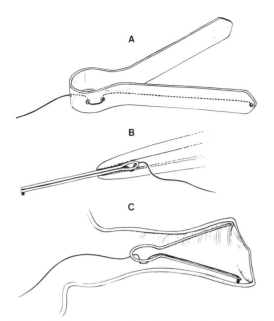

Figure 6.26. Example of special electrode developed for recording from the external ear canal silver ball electrode (**A**), electrode assembly held by forceps for placement into ear canal (**B**), and placement in the ear canal (**C**). (From A. C. Coats: On electrocochleographic electrode design. *J. Acoustic Society of America* 56:79, 1974.)

when a response is present, there is at least some residual hearing at the end organ, and when there is no response, one can be reasonably certain that no residual hearing exists. With transtympanic recording (through the tympanic membrane with the needle electrode positioned on the otic capsule) the large promontory responses require relatively few samples to obtain useful data, an entire input-output function for click stimuli can be generated very quickly. In fact, most early work with ECochG involved inserting a needle electrode through the tympanic membrane, touching the promontory of the otic capsule. This "surgical" invasive procedure obviously limited greatly the clinical utilization of the technique in the United States.

More recently, it has been shown that electrodes placed in the ear canal, touching or very near to the tympanic membrane, may yield acceptable ECochGm results. A variety of extratympanic electrodes have been described by Coats (1986) and are

shown in Figure 6.26. The extra tympanic electrodes can be used in children with appropriate sedation, and current auditory evoked potential recording systems allow for either independent or simultaneous recording of ECochG and ABR potentials.

Ear canal ECochG has not proven particularly useful for auditory threshold estimation and, in fact, has largely been replaced in the United States with widespread use of the ABR. The ABR requires less technical expertise, is less expensive and less traumatic to the patient, and offers more extensive information about the auditory system and hearing threshold estimation.

Excellent descriptions of the ECochG technique and clinical application have been published by Ferraro (1986), the American Speech-Hearing-Language Association (1987), and Staller and Lunde (1988).

Otoacoustic Emissions. Otoacoustic emissions (OAEs) are low-level, inaudible sounds produced by vibratory motion in the cochlea (Zizz and Glattke, 1988). Spontaneous OAEs apparently occur naturally in many normal-hearing persons and may be detected with special measuring equipment. Evoked otoacoustic emissions (EOAEs) may be elicited from normal-hearing persons as a release of sound energy from the cochlea in response to external acoustic stimulation.

Kemp (1978) was the first to show that EOAEs could be detected in the human external ear canal following stimulation with clicks. Using a miniature microphone and a sound source sealed in the external ear canal, Kemp recorded an acoustic response beginning 5 msec following the click stimulus onset. Subsequently, a number of carefully controlled experiments proved the origin of the EOAEs to be cochlear in origin, probably related to activity of the outer hair cells (Kemp, 1980; Kim, 1980).

The presence of EOAEs is evidence of a normal functioning cochlea and are reduced or abolished by the presence of a conductive hearing loss or cochlear hearing loss (Anderson and Kemp, 1979). Cope and Lutman

Table 6.6.
Electrophysiologic Response Classifications[a]

Response Latency Classification	Site of Origin	Response Waveform	Response Latency (msec)	Amplitude (μV)
Electrocochleography	Auditory nerve	Fast	1–5	0.1–10
Early	Brainstem	Fast	4–8	0.001–1
Middle	Brainstem/primary cortical projection	Fast	8–50	1.0–3
Late	Primary cortical projection and secondary association areas	Slow	50–300	8.0–20
Very Late	Prefrontal cortex and secondary association areas	Very slow	300 and beyond	20–30

[a]From P. Skinner and T. J. Glattke: Electrophysiologic response audiometry: state-of-the-art. *Journal of Speech and Hearing Disorders* 42:180, 1977.

(1988) have shown that 80–90% of normally hearing ears can produce EOAEs, but that these emissions can seldom be recorded from persons with hearing loss in excess of 20–30 dB HL (Kemp et al., 1986). Consequently, according to Lutman et al. (1989), the presence of a click EOAE can be taken as a powerful indicator of relatively normal hearing. Collet et al. (1989) confirmed, with a study of 76 subjects with sensorineural hearing loss, that OAEs are never found when hearing loss at 1000 Hz exceeds 40 dB HL and the mean audiometric hearing loss at 500, 1000, 2000, and 4000 Hz exceeds 45 dB HL.

In a fascinating clinical application of EOAEs, Bonfils et al. (1988) described a study of infant hearing screening wherein auditory thresholds obtained with traditional ABR technique was determined in 30 ears from normally hearing infants and 16 ears from infants with sensorineural hearing impairment. From the same infants, EOAEs were elicited to a click stimulus of 20 dB HL. EOAEs were always present when ABR wave V threshold was equal to or below 30 dB HL. Infants with sensorineural hearing loss and ABR wave V thresholds greater than 40 dB HL never produced EOAEs. The authors reported that the recording of EOAEs required approximately 5 minutes per ear, while ABR threshold measurements took 40 minutes average duration. The suggestion of using EOAEs as an objective, noninvasive, and

quick screening procedure as an infant hearing screening technique holds tremendous promise for the future and may be the most important development in recent years to solve the problems of early identification of hearing loss in newborns.

Electrophysiologic Auditory Testing.
Skinner and Glattke (1977) present an excellent overview article on electrophysiologic response audiometry (Table 6.6). They categorize evoked responses that occur within a latency range of 1–5 msec as originating from the cochlea and auditory nerve. Responses in the 4–8 msec latency range have the brainstem as their origin. Responses with latencies from about 8–50 msec presumably arise from the upper brainstem and primary projection areas. Slow wave responses from 50 to 300 msec originate as a secondary discharge from the primary cortical projection areas and surrounding secondary and association areas. The longest latency potentials, about 300 msec, are slow shifts that appear to arise from the prefrontal and secondary or association areas of the cortex. Skinner and Glattke summarize that the early, or brainstem, potentials will find the widest application, since they can be easily and reliably detected in young individuals and are not affected by sedation. The MLRs may be of secondary importance, and late potentials are not reliable for use with young children and are markedly affected by sedation.

They indicate that ECochG remains the most reliable of all electrophysiologic techniques but should only be considered after behavioral and other electrophysiologic tests have proven inconclusive.

The widespread use of such diagnostic tests could make the hearing loss description of "sensorineural" archaic—we can describe hearing loss as either "sensory" deafness or "neural" deafness, depending on the procedures. Knowledge of the exact anatomic location of a child's deafness is very important to the overall management of the individual. Research into the prevention and treatment of nonconductive deafness must depend on our ability to identify accurately the anatomical location of the disorder.

Sedation for Auditory Evaluation. On occasion, it may be necessary to consider the use of sedation to quiet down an uncooperative youngster for auditory physiologic evaluation including immittance, ABR evaluation, or ECochG. Chloral hydrate or secobarbital are often used because of their ease of administration and general effectiveness. The action of chloral hydrate and secobarbital is such that drowsiness, quieting, and sometimes deep sleep is achieved within an hour. Following the auditory evaluation, the youngster can be aroused and taken home. The major disadvantage to chloral hydrate and secobarbital is that both drugs are long-acting sedatives. Acoustic reflexes can be observed in patients sedated with chloral hydrate or secobarbital, but researchers have shown the acoustic reflex thresholds to be elevated (Robinette et al., 1974; Mitchell and Richards, 1976).

Clinicians must be aware that a child's reaction to such medication is not always as expected. Children vary considerably in their response sensitivity to sedatives, and the recommended dosages may not be sufficient to induce the desired effect. The same dosage in other children may actually increase activity and excitement levels so that the desired impedance study is still not possible.

Mentally retarded children are often maintained on medication for management of behavioral or convulsive disorders. Thus, the absence of acoustic reflexes in this population may be drug-related. Richards et al. (1975) evaluated immittance findings in 10 functionally retarded normal-hearing children on phenobarbital. These authors reported that low-level amounts of phenobarbital have no effect on the acoustic reflex threshold.

Immittance evaluation under conditions of general anesthesia is usually unsuccessful. Results are influenced by the anesthesia technique and drug agent. Middle ear pressure is increased under inhalation of some gases such as nitrous oxide, thereby decreasing the compliance of the tympanic membrane and obscuring the acoustic reflex (Thomsen et al., 1965).

EVALUATION OF CHILDHOOD DIZZINESS

There is a scant array of literature regarding vestibular evaluation of children with complaints of dizziness and/or vertigo. Considerable time and effort are exerted on the problem and prevention of hearing loss in children, yet we often ignore concurrent or subsequent vestibular disorders. This neglect could be due to several factors, perhaps the most common being the fact that vertiginous crises in childhood are often attributed to behavior problems. When vertigo is described by a youngster (in addition to suspicion of a functional disorder) the possibility of epileptic seizures, brain tumor, or brainstem lesion are considered. Hence, the child with vertiginous complaints may be subjected to a series of lengthy and expensive medical tests.

More attention should be directed to the likelihood of peripheral disturbances in children suffering from vertigo and/or disequilibrium. Basser (1964) described a syndrome called "benign paroxysmal vertigo of childhood." He reported that it was quite common in children but differed significantly from the benign paroxysmal vertigo found in adults. The distinction rests on the childhood prevalence and on the pure paroxysmal nature of the attacks, their brev-

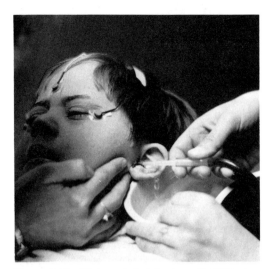

Figure 6.27. Water caloric irrigation with ENG electrodes in place on cooperative youngster.

ity, recurrence, absence of any prolonged disequilibrium, and the absence of the febrile illness or upper respiratory infection at the onset. Utilizing electronystagmography (ENG) (Fig. 6.27), Basser successfully documented vertiginous complaints from children. Koenigsberger et al. (1970) also reported successful application of ENG testing in children with benign paroxysmal vertigo. An excellent overview and discussion of pediatric vestibular evaluation was published by Cyr (1983).

Within the population of vertiginous children we evaluate are postmeningitis patients and those with combined renal dysfunction and decreased visual acuity, as in Alport's syndrome. Children displaying visual and vestibular disturbances are of particular concern because of the risk of permanent damage to two of the three systems necessary for maintenance of balance. We also test children who have received long-

term and/or high doses of ototoxic drugs that are particularly toxic to the vestibular portion of the inner ear, i.e., gentamicin and streptomycin.

The development of a clinically feasible battery for evaluating vestibular function in infants and preschool children has been described by Cyr et al. (1985). Their procedures involve modifications of standard ENG testing and the use of the low-frequency rotary chair. They report that the vestibular test battery with children is easy to administer, takes a minimal amount of time, and is not adversive to most patients. The test battery includes pediatric ocular motor testing, positional testing, caloric testing with simultaneous binaural bithermal stimulation through a closed-loop irrigation system, and computerized rotational chair testing (harmonic acceleration). Infrared video technology can also be employed to provide ongoing monitoring of the child's head and eye position in a darkened test enclosure during the examination.

An ENG should be performed on any child for whom there is strong suspicion of vestibular dysfunction. The child who develops bilateral vestibular weakness in infancy or childhood will often be asymptomatic and may adapt to the loss in a few days. But when this child is left in the dark, begins to swim underwater, or grows up to be a deep-sea diver or a construction worker on high buildings, the loss of vestibular function will very quickly and suddenly become apparent. It is our responsibility to recognize and understand the implications of vestibular dysfunction in childhood and to be prepared to undertake appropriate evaluation and/or referral.

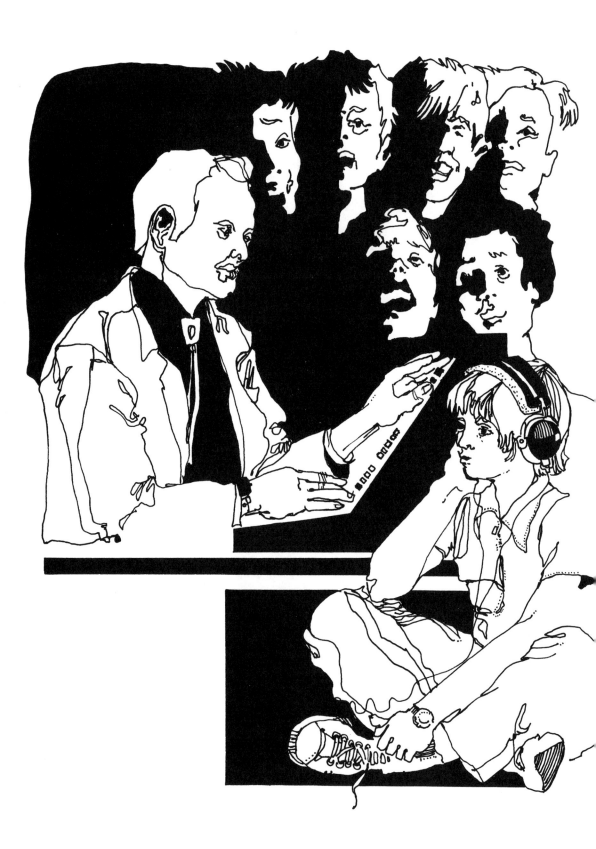

CHAPTER 7

Screening for Hearing Disorders

HEARING SCREENING IN CHILDREN

Screening is the process of applying certain rapid and simple tests, examinations, or other procedures, to generally large numbers of persons, that will identify those persons with a high probability of a disorder from those persons who probably do not have the disorder. A criterion measurement cutoff point is always involved, below or above which the persons are suspect. Screening is not intended as a diagnostic procedure; screening merely surveys large populations of undiagnosed and typically asymptomatic persons in order to identify those who are suspected of having the disorder and who require more elaborate diagnostic procedures. Persons who are identified with positive or suspicious findings must be referred to their physician for diagnosis and, if necessary, appropriate treatment (Last, 1983).

Since hearing impairment is relatively invisible, hearing screening tests have been in use for at least 60 years to identify children for further auditory evaluation. Screening for hearing loss in the public schools of the United States has been in practice since the 1930s, and nearly every state has some sort of mandated hearing screening program to identify the child with an educationally handicapping hearing impairment. The literature of audiology abounds with descriptions of various group and individual hearing tests designed for use in schools dating from the introduction in 1927 of the Western Electric 4-C group speech test (McFarlan, 1927).

In the past 25 years, hearing screening programs for newborn babies have been established in an effort to identify early the presence of severe-to-profound hearing loss so that habilitative measures can be instituted as soon as possible. Again, we see the historical development of hearing tests for infants from the early behavioral observation techniques to today's sophisticated auditory evoked response screening procedures. Screening for disease as early as possible in the child's life is now an accepted public health mandate. Out of 3,700,000 live births in the United States during 1987, it was estimated that some 7–12% of babies born were "at-risk" for severe-to-profound sensorineural, congenital hearing loss (Wegman, 1987).

A more difficult problem has been the development of simple, efficient, and valid hearing screening techniques for young children between 2 and 4 years of age. The effect of mild-to-moderate hearing impairment in this age group has been shown to be detrimental in speech/language development in some of these children, but no hearing screening technique has gained universal acceptance for use in Head Start Programs, primary care physician offices, or public or private preschool grades.

Inasmuch as we present a wide variety of material relative to all aspects of screening hearing in children, it is useful to look at the philosophy of screening from the vantage point of all the health sciences, as well as to examine the construct and evaluation procedures for individual screening procedures. A great deal of effort has been expended by public health agencies and epidemiologists to analyze the performance characteristics of all types of screening procedures. Such discussion will help us generally to evaluate the present status of our approaches to children's hearing screening

Table 7.1.
Yield in Screening Tests[a]

Disease Screened	Yield
Phenylketonuria	1 in 15,000 births
Combined immunodeficiency disease	25 in 3 million births
Maple syrup urine disease	1 in 300,000 births
Neonatal hyperthyroidism	1 in 6,000 births
Neonatal hearing screening, high-risk register	1 in 50 to 100 births

[a]From M. P. Downs and K. P. Gerkin: Early identification of hearing loss. In N. Lass et al. (eds.): *Handbook of Speech-Language Pathology and Audiology*. Toronto, B.C. Decker Inc.; 1988, Chap. 43, p.1191.

programs and specifically to provide the tools to critique individual hearing screening tests.

THEORIES OF HEARING SCREENING

Let us look at some theories of screening and how they relate to hearing conservation programs. Two aspects of screening philosophy are relevant: (*1*) the selection of the disorder or disease that should be screened, and (*2*) the evaluation of the screening procedures.

Which Diseases Should Be Screened?

The first question that must be asked is whether a certain disease should be screened. Certain criteria should be applied to the selection of disorders to screen (Frankenburg, 1975; North, 1976).

Occurrence Frequent Enough or Consequence Serious Enough to Warrant Mass Screening. How prevalent is the disease in the population to be screened? Some balancing of cost with the numbers of children who have the disease must be made. Cunningham (1970) has stated: "From the point of view of a public health program, in order to justify a mass screening program, the condition must be reasonably frequent or if rare it must have serious consequences if not detected." In the case of hearing, screening neonates for congenital deafness can be justified on the basis of its severity and resultant disastrous consequences; the screening of the young child can be justified

on the basis of numbers alone, as well as on consequences. The comparison of the yields of various newborn screening programs is shown in Table 7.1 and illustrates the relative status of hearing screening. Hearing screening not only yields the highest returns among these diseases but also is more productive of results once the problem is identified.

Amenability to Treatment or Prevention That Will Forestall or Change the Expected Outcome. What would be the prognosis for the person if treatment is instituted or if it is not instituted? It perhaps matters little if such a disorder as color blindness is detected early, as no treatment will change it. But the tragic consequences of untreated hearing losses are all too commonly seen: the complete lack of speech or language development at ages when these functions should be well-implanted; the deterioration of the parent-child relationship into subtle rejection or bewildered overprotection; and personality deviations of a wide variety, ranging from autistic-like withdrawal to hyperactivity and acting out. So long as a disease state can be accurately identified, its severity should at the very least be lessened by treatment if we are to regard mandatory screening as a profitable endeavor. There is no question that the sequelae of a true hearing loss can be ameliorated if the disorder is given proper treatment.

Availability of Facilities for Diagnosis and Treatment. If a child is identified as being a suspect for a disorder, can the child be properly assessed and treated, without too much expenditure in money and effort? This question largely concerns the state of the art and the number of trained professionals that can be depended upon to produce accurate evaluations and remediation for the child. If 1 year old Johnny is found in a rural area to have profound deafness, there may not be a facility for his diagnosis and training for hundreds of miles. And even in a big city the facilities available may be viewed with a jaundiced eye by critical fellow professionals. When these situations occur—and they doubtless do—can we justify screening for the disorder in that location? The concerned professional must answer "yes" to that question.

Cost of Screening Reasonably Commensurate with Benefits to the Individual. Is the screening equipment costly to purchase and to keep up? Do the personnel administering the screening tests require expensive training or high-level salaries? We are hard-put to designate any costs as excessive where the health and welfare of many individuals are at stake, but there are sometimes limitations to the funds available in any area. Fortunately, most of the audiometric equipment necessary to screen at any age ranges from $350 to $1500. Such equipment can continue to be used for long periods of time and for many thousands of tests before any repair or calibration is required. And, as the trend toward the use of nonprofessional aides continues, the cost of screening continues to decrease.

Cooper et al. (1975) published data regarding efficiency and cost of school screening programs. They reported that the ongoing rate for audiometric screening was about 5 minutes per student, or 12 students per hour. They also reported data for immittance screening to be about 1.1 minute per child, or 21 children per hour. Cooper and associates determined the cost of their screening program by establishing an index of cost per accurate referral of failures. To compute the cost per accurate referral, the following formula was developed:

$$\text{Cost/child} = \frac{S}{R} + \frac{C + (M \times L)}{(N \times L)}$$

$S =$ salary of person screening, in dollars per hour
$R =$ screening rate in children per hour
$C =$ cost of equipment in dollars
$M =$ annual maintenance cost of equipment in dollars
$L =$ lifetime of the equipment in years

$N =$ number of children screened per year.

Queen et al. (1981) used the Cooper formula to evaluate their immittance screening program in Kansas City, Missouri.

The cost analysis of screening the infant and preschool population also varies, but in no case would it be considered unfeasible when compared with the benefits accrued.

Screening Test Performance Characteristics. The success of a screening program depends on the effectiveness of the measures used to identify those who are likely to have the target disorder and to pass over those who do not have the target disorder. It is no longer sufficient to evaluate a test procedure critically by simply reporting the percentage of positive results in patients with the "disease" and the percentage of negative results in patients without the disease (S. Jerger, 1983). More rigid and critical performance characteristics must be applied to each screening test to evaluate fully its effectiveness in the overall attempt to identify infants and children with hearing problems. John and Claire Jacobson (1987) provide an excellent discussion of screening test performance characteristics, and we are grateful for their permission to utilize their material as the basis for the following discussion.

Keep in mind that the principle objective of any hearing screening program is to correctly identify hearing loss in those persons who truly have a problem, while ruling out hearing loss in normal-hearing persons. Screening tests should identify high-risk persons who are predisposed to develop disease or who are asymptomatic (undiagnosed), so that they can be effectively treated. Thus, the validity of a screening test is based on the proportion of test results that are confirmed diagnostically. If a hearing screening test too often passes infants or children who, indeed, have hearing impairment or it too often mistakenly identifies normal-hearing infants or children as

Table 7.2.
Matrix Analysis for Test Performance Characteristics[a]

Test Results	Impaired[b]	Normal	Total
Positive	TP	FP	TP + FP
Negative	FN	TN	FN + TN
Totals	TP + FN	FP + TN	TP + FP + FN + TN

[a]From J. Jacobson and C. Jacobson. Application of test performance characteristics in newborn auditory screening. *Seminars in Hearing* 8(2):133–141, 1987.
[b]TP, true positive; TN, true negative; FN, false negative; FP, false positive.

Table 7.3.
Matrix Analysis for Hypothetical Test Results[a]

Test Results[b]	Impaired	Normal	Total
Positive	70	180	250
Negative	30	720	750
Totals	100	900	1000

[a]From J. Jacobson and C. Jacobson. Application of test performance characteristics in newborn auditory screening. *Seminars in Hearing* 8(2):133–141, 1987.
[b]Sensitivity: 70/100 (70.0%); specificity: 720/900 (80.0%); predictive value of positive test: 70/250 (28.0%); predictive value of negative test: 720/750 (96.0%); overall: 790/1000 (79.0%); incidence: 100/1000 (10.0%).

hearing-impaired, the screening test will not stand up to critical performance evaluation and should be considered invalid and economically unfeasible.

Decision Matrix Analysis. A decision matrix is typically a 2 × 2 table that describes the results of a test procedure to the actual presence or absence of the disease, i.e., hearing impairment (Table 7.2). The four components of the matrix table are: *true positive* (TP), the number of hearing-impaired persons correctly identified by the test; *true negative* (TN), the number of persons with normal hearing who are correctly identified; *false positive* (FP), the number of persons with normal hearing incorrectly labeled as hearing-impaired; and *false negative* (FN), the number of persons truly impaired but incorrectly identified as normal. A screening test of choice would result in a high proportion of true positive rates and in a low proportion of false positive rates, because those with the disease would be identified, whereas healthy participants would pass the screen. It is the formulation of actual screening pass-fail results to this decision matrix that allows the calculation of test performance validity.

The validity of a screening test that is dependent on diagnostic confirmation for every person under consideration is determined by the relationship of three components: (*1*) sensitivity, the ability of a test to correctly identify patients with the disease (hearing loss); (*2*) specificity, the ability of a test to correctly identify those without the

disease (normal hearing); and (*3*) disease prevalence, the total number of diseased patients in a given population. Thus, it is the actual test results that define these terms.

Sensitivity. When a test operates at a 70% sensitivity rate, only 7 of every 10 patients who are hearing-impaired are correctly identified. The remaining three impaired patients are improperly classified. This concept is illustrated in Table 7.3, which uses a hypothetical group of 1000 screened newborn infants. In this example, a total of 100 babies are truly hearing-impaired; however, only 70 (70%) were correctly identified as diseased. Thus, for this example 70% (70/100) represents the true positive rate, whereas 30%, the misclassified (passed the screen), represents the false negative rate.

In auditory screening it is most desirable to use a test that gives the highest possible rate of sensitivity. For example, if an infant passes a hearing screen but presents with significant impairment, the abnormality may hold serious behavioral, developmental, and educational consequences if it goes undetected even for a short period early in a child's life.

Specificity. If all children with normal hearing passed a screening, the test would perform at a 100% specificity rate. However, as the test begins to fail normal-hearing children, the rate of specificity decreases. For example, if 8 of 10 infants were correctly identified as normal hearing, the test would operate at 80% specificity. The remaining two incorrectly classified normal-hearing infants would be subjected to subsequent diagnostic follow-up. In Table 7.3, 720 of 900 normal-hearing babies passed the screen, resulting in 80% (720/900) test specificity. Those 180 normal-hearing newborns who were incorrectly classified rendered a 20% false positive rate. This situation may result in parental stress and anxiety; however, misdiagnosis is usually ameliorated by further diagnostic assessment.

Table 7.3 demonstrates that the terms sensitivity and specificity represent the true positive and true negative rates, respectively. It is evident that a reciprocal relationship exists between sensitivity and the false negative rate and, similarly, between specificity and the false positive rate.

Prevalence versus Incidence. Both of these characteristics describe disease frequency rate. Prevalence rate is a census measure that expresses the presence of diseased patients per 100,000 population at the time of investigation. The rate of prevalence is calculated by dividing the number of diseased patients in the population at a specified time by the number of individuals in the population at that specified time. In contrast, incidence rate is the frequency of new outbreak of a disease condition in a population for a given time period. To calculate incidence rate, two variables must be defined: (*1*) the beginning and end of the time period under study, and (*2*) the population at risk for developing the disorder under study. Incidence rate is calculated by dividing the number of new diseased patients in a population during a specified time period by the number of persons exposed to the risk of developing the disease during that same period.

The relationship between prevalence and incidence is clarified by the following example. The incidence of an acute disease such as middle ear effusion in high-risk infants may be high, because a large number of neonates contract the disease during convalescence. The prevalence is usually low,

however, because the disease has a relatively short duration. Conversely, the incidence of a chronic disease such as sensory hearing loss may be low in newborns, but the prevalence in the population may be high. Although only a small percentage of babies are identified as sensory-impaired each year, sensory hearing loss is irreversible and therefore cumulative. Thus, the incidence of sensory hearing loss in children increases cumulatively as the average age of the sample cohort grows older.

Predictive Value. Performance characteristics define the ability of a test to estimate disease or nondisease in a given population accurately and, therefore, are of primary importance in the selection of a screening test. In contrast, predictive values, which are related to disease prevalence, examine the percent of patients correctly labeled diseased or healthy by the test and provide information about test result interpretation. The predictive value of a positive test (PVP) is defined as the percent of all positive results that are true positive when the test is applied to a population containing both healthy and diseased subjects (TP/TP + FP × 100). The predictive value of a negative test (PVN) represents the percent of all negative results that are true negatives (TN/TN + FN × 100).

It is important to recognize that predictive values are dependent on test performance characteristics and disease prevalence in the population under study. Once measures of sensitivity and specificity are tabulated, it is then possible to establish probability statements regarding the presence or absence of disease, because predictive values relate directly to test outcome. Predictive value measures can be derived from Table 7.3. Of the total 250 patients who failed the screen, 70 were true positive. The remaining 180 patients were false positive, leaving a PVP of 28% (70 of 250). The PVP results mean that approximately three fourths (180 of 250) of all patients who failed the test were false positive. The PVN result was 96% (720 of 750), meaning that

Table 7.4.
Effects of Disease Prevalence on Predictive Values when Sensitivity (90%) and Specificity (90%) Remain Constant[a]

Test Results	Impaired	Normal	Total
Disease prevalence 5%			
Positive	225	475	700
Negative	25	4275	4300
Totals	250	4750	5000
PVP = 32.1%			
PVN = 99.4%			
Disease prevalence 1%			
Positive	45	495	540
Negative	5	4455	4460
Totals	50	4950	5000
PVP = 8.3%			
PVN = 99.9%			
Disease prevalence 0.1%			
Positive	4.5	499.5	504
Negative	.5	4495.5	4496
Totals	5	4995	5000
PVP = 1.0%			
PVN = 100%			

[a]From J. Jacobson and C. Jacobson. Application of test performance characteristics in newborn auditory screening. *Seminars in Hearing* 8(2):133–141, 1987.

this test correctly identified 720 of the normal-hearing population. Thus, for persons who were determined to have passed the screen, only 4 of every 100 negative results were false negative. Finally, the overall efficiency, i.e., a measure of the percent of all true positive and true negative results, was 79%.

Disease prevalence within a target population will influence predictive values. Table 7.4 presents a hypothetical example of such an effect. By decreasing the prevalence of the disease from 5% (50/1000) to 1% (10/1000) to 0.1% (1/1000) while maintaining relatively high performance characteristics (sensitivity 90%, specificity 90%), predictive values change correspondingly. The PVP result decreased from 32.1% to 8.3% to less than 1.0%, whereas the PVN result in this case remained stable. When disease prevalence is 0.1% (1/1000), it is similar to that reported in mass auditory screening. The false positive rate is 99.1%. This example clearly points to the importance of applying screening tests to high-prevalence populations (such as high risk for hearing loss and intensive care nursery (ICN) in-

fants). If not, the false positive rate will be so great that it may be indefensible.

Pass-Fail Criteria. Given the inherent differences in biomedical investigation, it is unlikely that any test, screening or diagnostic, will be designed that can separate all patients with disease from those without disease. The result is that there will always be those screened who are inaccurately labeled. This integration of normal and pathologic patients has been addressed by Thorner and Remein (1967) in the theory of overlapping distributions. The selection of a cutoff point within the overlapping distribution will directly influence the anticipated yield (incidence) of identified patients with disease as well as affect test performance characteristics. The determination of pass-fail criteria is a critical factor in the establishment of eventual test outcome.

Figure 7.1 illustrates the concept of overlapping distribution. In this hypothetical hearing screening population, a cutoff score was initially established. Using this stated pass-fail criteria (i.e., a predetermined intensity level), a certain proportion of patients passed the screen,

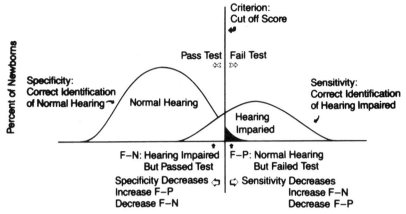

Figure 7.1. Graphic representation of a hypothetical newborn screened population. Illustration displays an overlapping subject distribution and its effect on specific operating characteristics. (From J. Jacobson and C. Jacobson: Newborn auditory screening. *Seminars in Hearing* 8(2):139, 1987.)

whereas others did not. Depending on individual test outcome, measures of sensitivity and specificity, false positive rates, and false negative rates were established. However, if the cutoff score was adjusted either up (higher intensity level) or down (lower intensity level), performance values would change correspondingly. If the cutoff score was increased so that more hearing-impaired persons pass the test, sensitivity would decrease because the false negative rate (hearing-impaired persons who pass the test) would increase. Conversely, as sensitivity decreased, specificity rate would increase as a result of the reduced number of false positive (normal-hearing persons who fail the test) results. If, on the other hand, the cutoff point was lowered, fewer hearing-impaired persons would pass the test, and the false negative rate would decrease. By doing so, specificity would decrease as the false-positive rate would increase. The result is a reciprocal relationship between sensitivity and specificity; as sensitivity increases, specificity decreases, and as specificity increases, sensitivity decreases.

A cutoff score is an arbitrary point that can be set to favor specific test outcome. The PVP and PVN results also change as the pass-fail cutoff point is manipulated. Since the predictive value is influenced by both test performance characteristics and disease prevalence, an increase in the cutoff point will reduce the "overall incidence" of hearing impairment. And finally, the overall test efficiency will be influenced, since the cutoff point may also determine the correct identification of hearing-impaired and normal-hearing persons.

The ideal hearing screening test would correctly differentiate, 100% of the time, between normal-hearing and hearing-impaired persons. Unfortunately, the development of such a hearing screening test that would meet the requirements of objectivity, ease of administration, rapid and simple technique, as well as economic feasibility, is unlikely. Therefore, as each specific population targeted for hearing screening is determined, the selection and implementation of a hearing screening tool must depend heavily on the various measures of test validity and desired performance characteristics. The use of sensitivity, specificity, and their reciprocal counterparts can provide information about the number of persons correctly identified as hearing-impaired or normal-hearing as measures against predetermined pass-fail criteria. Predictive values that are dependent on the prevalence or incidence of hearing disorders describe the test's ability to separate correctly true positive and true negative results in those with and without hearing

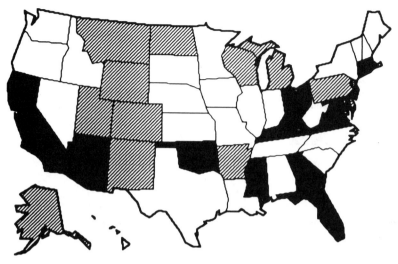

Figure 7.2. Statewide neonatal hearing screening programs. *Black*, states with mandates for neonatal hearing screening; *lined*, states with no legal mandate but with neonatal screening programs widely in place; *white*, no statewide screening program in place. (From P. E. Blake and J. W. Hall III. The status of state-wide policies for neonatal hearing screening. *Journal of the American Academy of Audiology* 1:68, 1990.)

loss. And, of course, the final validation of any screening test measure must account for the diagnostic confirmation of *all individuals screened*, regardless of initial test outcome.

NEONATAL HEARING SCREENING

Needs and Recommendations. It is the urgency of securing language input for the infant that makes it mandatory for any congenital hearing loss, whether severe or mild, to be detected at birth. Even the slight loss due to otitis media has been shown to cause auditory language learning problems if it occurs in the first 2 years of life. So otitis media will be one of the pathologies sought, in addition to the embryologic-related pathologies, the genetic pathologies, and the congenital acquired pathologies. We cannot settle for any lesser goal than detection of hearing loss in the first months of life, nor can we settle for any lesser targets than mild as well as severe congenital hearing losses. In their description of a community-based high-risk register for hearing loss, Fitch et al. (1982) state that the greater value of such programs may lie in the identification of increased

numbers of children with mild-to-moderate conductive losses that are amenable to treatment (see Figure 7.2).

In 1969 a National Committee was formed of representatives from the Academy of Pediatrics, the Academy of Ophthalmology and Otolaryngology, and the American Speech and Hearing Association, charged with making recommendations for newborn infant hearing screening. The Committee at that time addressed itself to the use of behavioral observation hearing screening tests that had been developed and described by Downs and Sterritt (1964) and Downs and Hemenway (1969). The Committee also addressed attention to the development of a high-risk register for deafness that identified five criteria that would put newborn infants at risk for having severe hearing impairment. These factors would be identified by examining the medical records of each infant to see whether there was any history or physical finding that would give a high probability of hearing loss. The Downs and Sterritt project mass-screened 17,000 newborns in the city of Denver to identify 17 infants with profound hearing loss, and the high-risk register approach

Table 7.5.
Confirmed Hearing Loss on High-Risk Register (January 1982 to December 1986)[a]

High-Risk Factor	Number	Degree of Loss	Type of Loss
Family history	4	Severe/profound (2)	Sensorineural
		Moderate/severe	Sensorineural
Defects of head & neck (syndromal abnormalities)	6	Severe/profound (1)	Sensorineural
		Severe/profound (2)	Mixed
		Moderate (2)	Conductive
		Moderate/severe (1)	Mixed
Cytomegalovirus	1	Moderate/severe	Sensorineural
Low birthweight	1	Moderate	Sensorineural
Low Apgar, hyperbilirubinemia	1	Severe/profound	Sensorineural
Low Apgar, hyperbilirubinemia; family history of unilateral loss	1	Profound (unilateral)	Sensorineural

Total Births: 12,739
High risk: 1,399 (11%)
Hearing loss requiring habilitation: 14 (1 in 100 high-risk babies)

[a]From M. Downs and K. Gerkin: Early identification of hearing loss. In N. Lass et al. (eds.): *Handbook of Speech-Language Pathology and Audiology*. Toronto, B. C. Decker Inc., 1988, Chap. 43, p. 1192.

was an attempt to focus attention on those infants most likely to have significant hearing loss.

Richards and Robert (1967) stated that a high-risk register, to be efficient, should identify a disease that is 14 times more prevalent in the register than in the general population. Significant hearing loss in high-risk infants has a prevalence of approximately 1 in 50, which is easily more than 14 times greater than seen in the general population. A typical yield from a high-risk program is shown in Table 7.5, which shows that 11% of the high-risk infant population born in one hospital had confirmed significant sensorineural hearing loss during a 4-year period. The high-risk concept assumes that one can identify a small group of children whose history or physical condition identifies them as possessing a high chance of having the target handicap.

The recommendations for a high-risk register were further buttressed by a national Maternal and Child Health Conference that delineated Guidelines for Early Screening (Conference on Hearing Screening Services for Preschool Children, 1977). The conference reaffirmed the Joint Committee's program and made some supplementary suggestions:

1. That audiologic follow-up of the high-risk infants be made "as soon as possible, but certainly by 7 months"

2. That the mother-child relationship in the first 4 months be safeguarded by education and careful information

3. That informed consent be obtained

4. That information on what to look for in later infancy be given

5. That the development and implementation of adequate identification and diagnostic procedures related to hearing impairments be undertaken by public health agencies

The Joint Committee on Infant Hearing met again in 1982 and in 1990 to propose new position statements relevant to practices of identifying the hearing-impaired neonate and infant. The Joint Committee on Infant Hearing (1990) represented the American Speech-Language-Hearing Association (ASHA), the American Academy of Pediatrics, the American Academy of Otolaryngology–Head and Neck Surgery, the Council on Education of the Deaf, and the directors of Speech and Hearing Programs in state health and welfare agencies. The 1990 Joint Committee statement is presented below:

I. Background
The early detection of hearing impairment in children is essential in order to initiate the medical and educational intervention critical for developing optimal communication and social skills. In 1982, the Joint Committee on Infant Hearing recom-

mended identifying infants at risk for hearing impairment by means of seven criteria and suggested follow-up audiological evaluation of these infants until accurate assessments of hearing could be made [Asha, 1982]. In recent years, advances in science and technology have increased the chances for survival of markedly premature and low birth weight neonates and other severely compromised newborns. Because moderate to severe sensorineural hearing loss can be confirmed in 2.5% to 5.0% of neonates manifesting any of the previously published risk criteria, auditory screening of at-risk newborns is warranted. Those infants who have one or more of the risk factors are considered to be at increased risk for sensorineural hearing loss.

Recent research and new legislation (P.L. 99-457) suggest the need for expansion and clarification of the 1982 criteria. This 1990 statement expands the risk criteria and makes recommendations for the identification and management of hearing-impaired neonates and infants. The Joint Committee recognizes that the performance characteristics of these new risk factors are not presently known; further study and critical evaluation of the risk criteria are therefore encouraged. The protocols recommended by the Committee are considered optimal and are based on both clinical experience and current research findings. The Committee recognizes, however, that the recommended protocols may not be appropriate for all institutions and that modifications in screening approaches will be necessary to accommodate the specific needs of a given facility. Such factors as cost and availability of equipment, personnel and follow-up services are important considerations in the development of a screening program [Turner, 1990].

II. Identification
  A. Risk Criteria: Neonates (birth-28 days)
     The risk factors that identify those neonates who are at-risk for sensorineural hearing impairment include the following:
     1. Family history of congenital or delayed onset childhood sensorineural impairment.
     2. Congenital infection known or suspected to be associated with sensorineural hearing impairment such as toxoplasmosis, syphilis, rubella, cytomegalovirus and herpes.
     3. Craniofacial anomalies including morphologic abnormalities of the pinna and ear canal, absent philtrum, low hairline, et cetera.
     4. Birth weight less than 1500 grams (3.3 lbs.).
     5. Hyperbilirubinemia at a level exceeding indication for exchange transfusion.
     6. Ototoxic medications including but not limited to the aminoglycosides used for more than 5 days (e.g., gentamicin, tobramycin, kanamycin, streptomycin) and loop diuretics used in combination with aminoglycosides.
     7. Bacterial meningitis.
     8. Severe depression at birth, which may include infants with Apgar scores of 0-3 at 5 minutes or those who fail to initiate spontaneous respiration by 10 minutes or those with hypotonia persisting to 2 hours of age.
     9. Prolonged mechanical ventilation for a duration equal to or greater than 10 days (e.g., persistent pulmonary hypertension).
     10. Stigmata or other findings associated with a syndrome known to include sensorineural hearing loss (e.g., Waardenburg or Usher's Syndrome).
  B. Risk Criteria: Infants (29 days-2 years)
     The factors that identify those infants who are at-risk for sensorineural hearing impairment include the following:
     1. Parent/caregiver concern regarding hearing, speech, language, and/or developmental delay.
     2. Bacterial meningitis.
     3. Neonatal risk factors that may be associated with progressive sensorineural hearing loss (e.g., cytomegalovirus, prolonged mechanical ventilation and inherited disorders).
     4. Head trauma especially with either longitudinal or transverse fracture of the temporal bone.
     5. Stigmata or other findings associated with syndromes known to include sensorineural hearing loss (e.g., Waardenburg or Usher's Syndrome).
     6. Ototoxic medications including but not limited to the aminoglycosides used for more than 5 days (e.g., gentamicin, tobramycin, kanamycin, streptomycin) and loop diuretics used in combination with aminoglycosides).

7. Children with neurodegenerative disorders such as neurofibromatosis, myoclonic epilepsy, Friedreich's ataxia, Huntington's chorea, Werdnig-Hoffmann disease, Tay-Sach's disease, infantile Gaucher's disease, Niemann-Pick disease, Charcot-Marie-Tooth disease, any metachromatic leukodystrophy, or any infantile demyelinating neuropathy.
8. Childhood infectious diseases known to be associated with sensorineural hearing loss (e.g., mumps, measles).

III. Audiologic Screening Recommendations for Neonates and Infants
  A. Neonates
  Neonates who manifest one or more items on the risk criteria should be screened, preferably under the supervision of an audiologist. Optimally, screening should be completed prior to discharge from the newborn nursery but no later than 3 months of age. The initial screening should include measurement of the auditory brainstem response. Behavioral testing of newborn infants' hearing has high false-positive and false-negative rates and is not universally recommended. Because some false-positive results can occur with ABR screening, ongoing assessment and observation of the infant's auditory behavior is recommended during the early stages of intervention. If the infant is discharged prior to screening, or if ABR screening under audiologic supervision is not available, the child ideally should be referred for ABR testing by 3 months of age but never later than 6 months of age.

  The acoustic stimulus for ABR screening should contain energy in the frequency region important for speech recognition. Clicks are the most commonly used signal for eliciting the ABR and contain energy in the speech frequency region. Pass criterion for ABR screening is a response from each ear at intensity levels 40 dB nHl or less. Transducers designed to reduce the probability of ear-canal collapse are recommended.

  If consistent electrophysiological responses are detected at appropriate sound levels, then the screening process will be considered complete except in those cases where there is a probability of progressive hearing loss (e.g., family history of delayed onset, degenerative disease, meningitis, intrauterine infections or infants who had chronic lung disease, pulmonary hypertension or who received medications in doses likely to be ototoxic). If the results of an initial screening of an infant manifesting any risk criteria are equivocal, then the infant should be referred for general medical, otological, and audiological follow-up.

  B. Infants
  Infants who exhibit one or more items on the risk criteria should be screened as soon as possible but no later than 3 months after the child has been identified as at-risk. For infants less than 6 months of age, ABR screening is recommended. For infants older than 6 months, behavioral testing using a conditioned response or ABR testing are appropriate approaches. Infants who fail the screen should be referred for a comprehensive audiologic evaluation. This evaluation may include ABR, behavioral testing (<6 months) and acoustic immittance measures.

IV. Early Intervention for Hearing-Impaired Infants and Their Families
  When hearing loss is identified, early intervention services should be provided, in accordance with Public Law 99-457. Early intervention services under P.L. 99-457 may commence before the completion of the evaluation and assessment if the following conditions are met: (a) parental consent is obtained, (b) an interim individualized family service plan (IFSP) is developed, and (c) the full initial evaluation process is completed within 45 days of referral.

  The interim IFSP should include the following:
  A. The name of the case manager who will be responsible for both implementation of the interim IFSP and coordination with other agencies and persons;
  B. The early intervention services that have been determined to be needed immediately by the child and the child's family.

  The immediate early intervention services should include the following:
  1. Evaluation by a physician with expertise in the management of early childhood otologic disorders.
  2. Evaluation by an audiologist with expertise in the assessment of young children, to determine the type, degree, and configuration of

Table 7.6.
Mother's Interview

MOTHER'S NAME: _____

ROOM NO.: _____

1. Do you know any of the baby's relatives who now have a hearing loss which started before the age of <u>five</u>?

   Think hard about all of your family and the baby's father's family ....

   Yes _____ No _____

   A. If <u>no,</u> proceed to question No. 2.

   B. If <u>yes,</u> ask the following:

      (1) Who were they? (relationship to baby)

         (A). _____ (B). _____ (C). _____

      (2) Do you know what caused the loss? ....

         Yes _____ No _____

         (A). _____ (B). _____ (C). _____

      (3) What makes you think the onset of the hearing loss was before age 5?

         (A). _____ (B). _____ (C). _____

      (4) Did he/she wear a hearing aid before age 5? .... (A) _____ (B) _____ (C) _____

         Does he/she still wear an aid? .... (A) _____ (B) _____ (C) _____

      (5) Did he/she attend a special school for the deaf? .... (A) _____ (B) _____ (C) _____

         Did the person attend public school? .... (A) _____ (B) _____ (C) _____

      (6) Did he/she have a speech problem? .... (A) _____ (B) _____ (C) _____

2. During your pregnancy did you have 3-day measles, German measles, rubella, or a rash with a fever? ......

   .... Yes _____ No _____

   WHEN: First 3 mo. _____ Middle 3 mo. _____ Last 3 mo. _____

3. During your pregnancy, were you around anyone who had 3-day measles, German measles, rubella, or a

   rash with fever? .... Yes _____ No _____

   WHEN: First 3 mo. _____ Middle 3 mo. _____ Last 3 mo. _____

4. Do you have any reason to be concerned about your baby's hearing? .... Yes _____ No _____

   If yes, why? _____

5. What pediatrician or clinic will be caring for your baby when he/she leaves the hospital? _____

   _____

   Approximate location _____

6. Nearest relative or friend: Name: _____

   Address: _____

   Phone: _____

---

the hearing loss, and to recommend assistive communication devices appropriate to the child's needs (e.g., hearing aids, personal FM systems, vibrotactile aids).

3. Evaluation by a speech-language pathologist, teacher of the hearing-impaired, audiologist, or other professional with expertise in the assessment of communication skills in hearing-impaired children, to develop a program of early intervention consistent with the needs of the child and preferences of the family.

4. Family education, counseling and guidance, including home visits and parent support groups to provide families with information, child management skills and emotional support consistent with the needs of the child and family.

5. Special instruction that includes:

   a. the design and implementation of learning environments and ac-

tivities that promote the child's development and communication skills;

   b. curriculum planning that integrates and coordinates multidisciplinary personnel and resources so that intended outcomes of the IFSP are achieved; and

   c. ongoing monitoring of the child's hearing status and amplification needs and development of auditory skills.

● *Application of High Risk Register.* The detailed procedures that are used in identifying the infants in the high risk categories are as follows:

● *Identification Through Query of the Mother.* The questions used in the mother's interview are shown in Table 7.6. Although the questions may be easily asked verbally, the form may also be used as a written questionnaire. The mother's answers are recorded on the form by the interviewer, and serve as an important initial sort for the high risk register.

This questionnaire should be given to all new mothers in the hospital at some time after the baby is born. It should be prefaced with an explanation that "We are conducting a survey of all babies born in this hospital, to see how many families have certain hearing problems. We would appreciate your help in this survey. There is nothing to worry about if you answer yes to any of the questions, so do the best you can with them."

- *Identification Through Visual Observations of the Infant. Cleft Lip or Palate, Including Submucous Cleft.* The cleft lip is an immediately observable malformation, but cleft palate—and particularly submucous cleft—will be searched for by a physician. A bifid uvula always accompanied submucous cleft, but the cleft may be present without this symptom. Submucous cleft has been found to be associated with congenital middle ear anomalies, so it is important that the palate be carefully examined.

   Malformations of the Ears. Abnormal pinnae may be obvious, but they also can be very subtle. Atresia, with partial formation of the pinna, or a small tab of skin where the pinna should be are easily observed. Often however, the ears are merely low-set, or they may not have complete formation of helix, antihelix, tragus, or antitragus. A small tab of skin known as a pre-auricular tag may occur in front of the pinna, on the cheek, with an otherwise normal-looking ear. Sometimes these symptoms are accompanied by cranial malformations of the nose, eye orbits, maxillae, or cranial bones, so any odd looking feature may be a clue.

- *Identification Through Search of the Medical Records and Physical Examination.* Whoever is assigned to examine the mothers' and infants' medical records must be well trained in interpreting doctors' abbreviations and terminology. The items to be searched for are shown in Table 7.7.

- *Implementation of the High Risk Registry Program.* The implementation of a high risk registry program for infants will vary from location to location according to situational needs. Several methods and systems are in use around the United States. In general, the high risk for deafness program should be supervised by a qualified audiologist. It is not necessary for the audiologist to perform all of the functions inherent in the program, but the audiologist is really the one professional who can be responsible for ascertaining the quality of each part of the program. Remember that the hearing screening portion of the program is only one half of the task; the identification of hearing-impaired infants is useless unless there is a formalized strategy for insuring that adequate follow-up of each child is performed to completion. All the best of intentions of infant hearing screening efforts are lost without a strong system in place to insure additional hearing evaluation for those babies who fail the hearing screening, as well as a habilitation program or referral source to take charge of the special needs of a hearing-impaired infant and the associated family or care-providers.

   Trained Volunteers. Individual volunteers, or volunteers from various community service groups, can be trained by the audiologist to perform many of the functions required in an infant hearing screening program. Not all volunteers actually want to test the hearing of the babies, or even be in the intensive care nurseries of the hospitals, but the personnel support from such groups can be effectively directed to interviewing mothers, reviewing hospital medical records, conducting record-keeping and other administrative tasks, telephoning to insure that follow-up care is provided

Table 7.7.
Chart Review

MOTHER'S ROOM NO. _____
BABY'S NAME: _____
BABY'S HOSP. NO.: _____
BIRTHDATE: _____ SEX: _____
DISCHARGE DATE: _____
NURSERY LOCATION: MR.   HR.   NB
CARD PUNCHED: Yes   No

INFANT CHECK LIST

Mother's Name _____ Hosp. No. _____ Father's Name _____
Home Address _____ City _____ State _____ Zip _____ Phone No. _____
Pediatrician/Follow-up Clinic _____ Location _____
Birth Weight _____ Birth Length _____ Head Circumference _____ Gestation Age _____
Volunteer _____ Chart Review Dates _____ / _____ / _____

HIGH RISK CRITERIA

	YES	NO
1. Birth weight (B/W) less than 1500 g or/over 5000 g.		
2. Apgar 7 or less at 5 minutes. (Severe asphyxia—arterial pH level lower than 7.25, coma, seizures or the need for assisted ventilation.)		
3. Jaundice-hyperbilirubinemia: history of exchange transfusions. B/W — Bilirubin Level 1000-1250 — 10.0 1251-1500 — 13.0 1501-2000 — 15.0 2001-2500 — 17.0 >2500 — 18.0		
4. Any of the following conditions: Skeletal and cranial defects _____, skull abnormalities _____, short neck _____, absent clavicles _____, dwarfism _____, malformations of extremities and digits _____, cleft lip _____, cleft palate (overt or submucous) _____, underdeveloped maxillae or mandible _____, external ear abnormalities _____.		
5. Family history of deafness.		
6. Rubella, rubella exposure.		
7. Cytomegalic inclusion disease (CMV), herpes, toxoplasmosis, syphilis, meningitis.		

REMARKS:
_____
_____
_____

and secured by the involved families for the suspect infant, and in running the day to day detail of various aspects of the program. When volunteers are used in hospital situations, it is suggested that appropriate steps be taken to insure legal protection and legal clearance for these nonprofessional people to examine medical charts, move babies from the nurseries to the audiologic test area, interview new mothers, etc. The advantage to the use of volunteers is the low cost for supportive manpower; the major disadvantage of using volunteers is often a progressive lack of interest in this particular project, or a change-over in the club's officers or a change in direction of the service organization's activities. The audiologist dependent upon a volunteer staff to perform the infant hearing screening program must be a master of working with people to obtain high quality support, as well as ingenious at maintaining the volunteer enthusiasm for the project at hand.

Public Health Agencies. Some states and regions use public health agencies or facilities to conduct high risk screening programs. For example, the Colorado State Department of Health has enlisted private hospitals in rural areas throughout the state to compile lists of infants

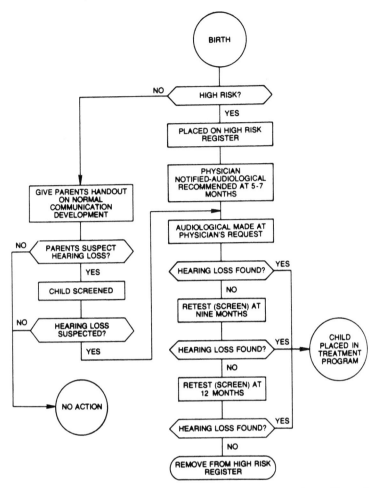

Figure 7.3. Flow chart diagram of a community high-risk registry program for deafness. (Reproduced with permission from J. L. Fitch et al.: A community based high risk register for hearing loss. *Journal of Speech and Hearing Disorders* 47:373–375, 1982.)

born with high risk factors for deafness. Nurses in the newborn nurseries fill out the appropriate questionnaire and search the medical charts to identify infants born under high risk factors. Regional audiologists perform the appropriate hearing screening and follow-up audiologic evaluations, and work with the parents of infants found to have hearing impairment (Weber, 1987). The state of Utah is unique in its use of each newborn's birth certificate to record high risk deafness factors (Mahoney, 1984).

Private or Community Agencies and Audiologists. Some infant hearing screening programs are conducted through contracts developed by hospitals with community agencies (i.e., hearing, speech/language centers, group health agencies, etc.) or with private audiologists. These contracted services are provided on a fee-for-service basis and may rely on portable hearing testing equipment to test high risk infants in the medical facility. An excellent flow chart of a community based high risk register for hearing loss is shown in Figure 7.3.

High-Risk Factors for Deafness. The high-risk register for deafness should be the basis of any infant hearing screening program. Knowledge of these factors is extremely helpful in eliciting history about children who are discovered to have hearing impairment. A wealth of information is available from studies of various aspects of the high-risk register. The clinician should be familiar with this background, since an infant with any of these factors in his or her neonatal history has an increased chance of having hearing impairment. Although the factors themselves are easily memorized, audiologists often overlook their significance or do not fully understand the medical implications of each category.

Accordingly, the following discussion presents material on each of the high-risk categories. Note that the sequence of the factors is presented in a mnemonic order known as the "ABCs of high-risk deafness."

A. Asphyxia. Asphyxia (hypoxia or anoxia) is a condition in which there is a lack of oxygen and an increase in carbon dioxide in the blood and tissues. With the introduction of intensive care treatment for very sick babies has come increased skill and technology in resuscitation and mechanical breathing. Short spells without breathing (known as apneic attacks), however, are not uncommon during the neonatal period. Asphyxia may be the single most important factor causing developmental sequelae.

The clinical definition of asphyxia varies somewhat among authors. Scheiner (1980) suggests the use of multiple measures in determining clinically significant asphyxia, including the length, degree, frequency, and severity of the episodes. The occurrence of asphyxia is commonly related to a number of other medical conditions, so it is difficult to absolutely establish asphyxia as the single cause of a specific case of deafness. MacDonald (1980) points out that a preterm infant is more likely to experience anoxic episodes than a full-term infant. Infants with anoxia may also have low Apgar scores at 1 minute and 5 minutes following birth, low arterial pH level, coma, seizures, or the need for resuscitation with oxygen by mask or intubation.

The Apgar method of evaluation has proven most practical as a guide to prognosis and the need for particularly close observation or care in the delivery room and nursery (Apgar, 1953; Apgar and James, 1962). Sixty seconds after the complete birth of the infant, five objective signs including heart rate, respiratory effort, muscle tone, response to catheter in nostril, and color are noted, and each is given a score of 0, 1, or 2 as shown in Table 7.8. A total score of 10 indicates an infant in the best possible condition. Low Apgar scores taken at 1 minute and 5 minutes is an index of asphyxia and an excellent indicator of the need for assisted ventilation (American Academy of Pediatrics, 1986). The 5 or 10 minute scores are a more accurate index of likelihood of neurologic involvement such as cerebral palsy (Vaughan et al., 1979).

D'Souza et al. (1981) conducted hearing, speech, and language studies in 26 children who survived severe perinatal asphyxia. Although only 1 child had sensorineural hearing loss, nearly one third of the children in their sample had deficits of speech and/or language. Simmons (1980a) implicates anoxia as the single high-risk factor that dominates all others in the medical histories of hearing-impaired babies.

B. Bacterial Meningitis. Bacterial meningitis develops in approximately 1 of 2500 live births and is a leading cause of acquired hearing loss in infants and children. Neonatal meningitis may develop in utero or following infection at the time of, or subsequent to, delivery. In neonates the infecting bacteria are usually acquired from the mother during delivery. However, bacteria may spread from infant to infant via nursery personnel or contaminated equipment. With the advent of antibiotics, treatment of meningitis is usually successful, although bacterial meningitis is still responsible for 1–4% of neonatal deaths.

The clinical manifestations of neonatal meningitis are often subtle and deceptive, so that suspicion by the attending physician, coupled with verification by appropri-

Table 7.8.
Apgar Evaluation of the Newborn Infant[a]

Sign	0	1	2
Heart rate	Absent	Below 100	Over 100
Respiratory effort	Absent	Slow, irregular	Good, crying
Muscle tone	Limp	Some flexion of extremities	Active motion
Response to catheter in nostril	No response	Grimace	Cough or sneeze
Color	Blue, pale	Body pink, extremities blue	Completely pink

[a]From V. Vaughan et al.: *Nelson Textbook of Pediatrics*, ed. 11. Philadelphia, W. B. Saunders, 1979, p. 393.

ate laboratory studies, provides the only means of diagnosis in newborns (Feigin and Dodge, 1976). The degree of hearing loss associated with meningitis usually ranges from severe to profound, but mild-to-moderate hearing loss is also seen. Finitzo-Hieber et al. (1981b) reports an incidence of 35% sensorineural hearing impairment in 94 infants and children following meningitis. In their study, the highest percent of hearing impairment was associated with H. influenzae type meningitis at 55%.

C. Congenital Perinatal Infections. This group of infections is known by the acronym "TORCH" to draw attention to the problem that they are difficult to diagnose because they present with minimal nonspecific symptoms and yet create devastating developmental complications. The TORCH infections may be acquired by the embryo or fetus during gestation or by the newborn at time of delivery. In the acronym, *T* stands for toxoplasmosis; *R*, for rubella virus; *C*, for cytomegalovirus (CMV); *H*, for herpes simplex virus (HSV); and *O*, for other bacterial infections, especially syphilis, that result in hearing impairment. The classic paper on the TORCH complex was published by Nahmias in 1974.

TORCH infections are often clinically inapparent, and when the infections are identified, their associated signs and symptoms are nearly indistinguishable. A subclinical infection can result in the same serious defects as one that is clinically apparent. Prognosis for the involved infant is usually grim. Nahmias estimates that 1–5% of all deliveries are infected by one of the TORCH agents, and each year in the United States a minimum of 400 infant deaths result, and at least 2000 additional children are left with significant sequelae.

Nahmias stated that the lack of symptomatology in the pregnant woman makes the diagnosis in TORCH infections very difficult. Even when symptoms are manifest, the diagnosis cannot be confirmed without special laboratory tests. *Toxoplasma* infections and cytomegalovirus rarely cause a clinically definable syndrome in the pregnant woman; the rash associated with rubella is not specific enough to differentiate it from other entities. In the case of herpes simplex infections, it is not the readily diagnosable cold sores or fever blisters that are of particular concern, but it is the less discernable genital infections that are often missed at the cervix, the primary site of involvement.

There is no clear-cut pattern in the sensorineural hearing loss attributed to TORCH complex infections. The hearing loss can be progressive and range from mild-to-profound, and cases of both bilateral and unilateral losses are well-documented. Virus excretions may remain active for several years following birth, constituting a contributing factor in the degenerative process. In terms of infant follow-up, it is important to realize that any pattern and degree of hearing loss may occur with the TORCH complex. The screening technique of choice with these infants is auditory evoked potentials, since the chance of detecting a mild-to-moderate loss is possible. The potential for progressive hearing loss requires follow-up testing within shorter time intervals than when following a child with a nonprogressive risk factor. An audiologic evaluation each 6 months would be appropriate for the first year.

Toxoplasmosis. This is a parasitic infection transmitted by pregnant women to their unborn children. Most adults who are infected with the parasite have no symptoms. However, the infected child with congenital toxoplasmosis is typically manifested by chorioretinitis (inflammation of the choroid and retina of the eye), cerebral calcification, psychomotor retardation, hydrocephalus or microcephaly, and convulsions. Although reports of hearing disorders related to toxoplasmosis are in fact sparse, the congenital infection is so serious that there is no doubt that it may cause hearing loss. Active congenital infection may be fatal in days or weeks or become inactive with residuals of medical problems in varying degrees and combinations. The full impact of the infection may not become evident until some weeks or months after its apparent cessation. Apparently, the later in pregnancy the infection occurs, the less severe the clinical symptoms. *Toxoplasma* may be responsible for premature birth, cerebral palsy, blindness, and mental retardation (Vaughan et al., 1979). Some afflicted newborns appear normal but develop blindness, epilepsy, or mental retardation in later years.

Pregnant women acquire toxoplasmosis as an active disease at a rate of 2–7 per 1000, and 30–40% of these women have infected infants, making toxoplasmosis one of the most common causes of birth defects in the United States (Babson, 1980). Humans are typically contaminated in one of three ways: (*1*) by eating raw or insufficiently cooked food; (*2*) by direct contact with cat feces, since the house cat is a carrier; and (*3*) by eating fruits and vegetables soiled by animal carriers (Robillard and Gersdorff, 1986).

Campbell and Clifton (1950) described childhood progressive hearing loss of three or four family members with acquired (not congenital) toxoplasmosis. An infant with toxoplasmosis as a risk factor should be followed for hearing every few months until the age of 1 year or until normal speech development is assured.

Syphilis. Technically speaking, syphilis is a bacterial infection that produces similar manifestations as the viral infections of the TORCH complex, but it can be diagnosed with routine laboratory tests—so it is not usually considered part of the TORCH family. However, we include it so that this infection is not overlooked in the high-risk register for deafness.

Early manifestations include nasal discharge (snuffles), rash, anemia, jaundice, and osteochondritis. Later manifestations include saddle nose, saber skin, Hutchinson teeth, mulberry molars, and other dental anomalies. Congenital syphilis may demonstrate a multitude of central nervous system abnormalities including vestibular dysfunction, sensorineural hearing loss and, occasionally, aortic valvulitis. Possible accompanying mental retardation depends on severity of neurologic damage.

Auditory impairment may not be present at birth. Onset of hearing loss is generally in early childhood, usually sudden bilaterally symmetrical hearing loss causing severe-to-profound impairment. The hearing loss is usually not accompanied by marked vestibular manifestations. Poor hearing function and limited use of hearing aid can be expected as a result of neural atrophy. The general treatment of congenital syphilis consists of prompt treatment of infant with penicillin.

Rubella. The devastating effects of the rubella epidemic of the 1960s that left 10,000–20,000 children with handicaps is well-known. Although deafness is one of the most common manifestations of rubella with an incidence of 50%, associated problems include heart disease (50%), cataract or glaucoma (40%), and psychomotor/mental retardation (40%) (Cooper, 1969). The present crop of congenital rubella syndrome (CRS) youngsters are now adults, and there appear to be a number of late-onset medical disorders including diabetes, glaucoma, endocrine pathology, and central nervous system infections (Vernon and Hicks, 1980).

With public awareness of the 1960s rubella epidemic, immunization programs developed and the number of congenital rubella cases decreased quickly. As cases of any endemic disease decrease, however, so does public concern, resulting in a reduced number of immunizations. A recent concern is that in some women the vaccine seems to provide immunity to rubella for only 8–12 years. Thus, women who were vaccinated during their prepuberty stage may again become susceptible to rubella during their childbearing years. Rubella virus is generally acquired by airborne distribution and enters the maternal respiratory tract (Vernon and Klein, 1982).

The gestational age of the embryo or fetus is the critical factor in determining the outcome. Prior to the eighth week of gestation, between 50% and 80% of fetuses exposed to maternal rubella virus become infected; and finally during the third trimester, infection of the fetus is fairly uncommon, with a rate of 6–10% (Pumper and Yamashiroya, 1975). Live rubella virus, however, may persist for extended periods of time in the newborn infant and serve as a source for spreading the infection to susceptible pregnant women (Vaughan et al., 1979).

Congenital rubella may range from mild, subclinical infection to severe disease. Infants of a mother with known or suspected rubella should be followed carefully throughout childhood, since asymptomatic infants may subsequently develop defects later in life. The most commonly delayed manifestation of CRS is progressive sensorineural hearing loss. An excellent monograph has been assembled by Stuckless (1980) on the status of deafness and rubella.

It is often difficult to verify rubella exposure during pregnancy in the postpartum mother, who may actually have had such a mild, subclinical infection that it remained unrecognized. Children with a suspected history of rubella or rubella exposure should be followed with hearing tests until 18–24 months of age, keeping in mind the potential late-onset and progressive nature of rubella hearing loss.

Cytomegalovirus. CMV is a major cause of prenatal subclinical infections and is the most common of the TORCH complex of infections. Nahmias (1974) estimated that although 20% of pregnant women may have CMV, only 2% of infants are infected at birth, and some 10% of infants are infected by the age of 3 months. Gershon (1981) estimates that 1.2% of infants born in the United States are congenitally infected, but he verifies that less than 10% of these infected infants develop severe symptoms.

Cytomegalic inclusion disease is a systemic illness characterized by enlargement of the liver and spleen, jaundice, petechial rash, chorioretinitis, cerebral calcifications, and microcephaly. In contrast to toxoplasmosis and rubella, the visual system is less commonly involved.

Infection of the fetus may be intrauterine, i.e., caused by exposure to the virus as the baby passes through the infected birth canal. There is also strong evidence that CMV may be transmitted transplacentally prenatally or postnatally through infected urine, saliva, breast milk and perhaps feces or tears or through blood transfusions from infected donors.

The effects of CMV vary between severe central nervous system destruction to asymptomatic carrying of the virus. In its most severe form, CMV causes global central nervous system infection involving the cerebral cortex, brainstem, cochlear nuclei, and cranial nerves as well as the inner ear.

Some authors believe that fetal risk is related to both the time of infection in utero and to the immune status of the mother (Panjvani and Henshaw, 1981). However, while it is documented that infants with clinically apparent CMV at birth will manifest more significant sequelae, undetected virus has been shown to lead to late-appearing sequelae, namely hearing defects.

Pass and Stasno (1980) reported the incidence of hearing loss to be 30% in symptomatic cases of CMV. Reynolds et al. (1974)

reported hearing loss in 9 of 16 patients who had inapparent or subclinical CMV, while Stagno (1977) found hearing defects in 17% of children with subclinical CMV. Hanshaw et al. (1976) verified bilateral hearing loss in 5 of 40 children who had evidence of antibody against CMV, including 3 with profound deafness.

Herpes Simplex Virus. HSV is rapidly becoming one of the most common sexually transmitted diseases. The most common mode of transmission of HSV to the fetus is during the birth process if the mother is actively infected. HSV is rarely placentally transmitted (Gershon, 1981). However, if HSV is transmitted in this manner it may produce intrauterine malformations of the fetus.

HSV may cause a severe generalized disease in the neonate, with high mortality and devastating sequelae. HSV infects the genital tracts of an estimated 20–25% of the population according to *Medical World News* (1980). HSV infections in the newborn are rarely subclinical or asymptomatic. The majority of cases are thought to be acquired during passage through the birth canal. A cesarean section delivery is indicated for mothers with a known genital infection at the time of delivery. When HSV infection does occur in the neonate, more than 50% are fatal. According to Nahmias and Norrild (1979), only 4% of neonatally infected HSV infants survive without sequelae. Unfortunately, this sexually transmitted infection is apparently on the increase with no cure or effective treatment current available.

D. Defects of the Head and Neck. Anomalies associated with craniofacial and skeletal abnormalities range from the very obvious to slight, subtle defects. Infants at risk for deafness in this category manifest anatomical malformations involving the head, neck, mouth, ears, etc.

Typical indications of a neonate with head and neck defects include babies with craniofacial syndromal abnormalities, malformed, low-set, or aberrant pinna configu-

rations, such as microtia and/or atresia, preauricular or postauricular tags and pits, cleft lip and/or palate (including submucous cleft palate), first- and/or second-arch anomalies including mandibular and maxillary variants, and branchial cysts.

It must be remembered that not all infants with such defects will have hearing impairment. The presence of such abnormalities, however, increases the risk of hearing problems in that particular child.

E. Elevated Bilirubin. Hyperbilirubinemia ("jaundice") occurs when there is an excess amount of bilirubin in the blood. Rh or ABO incompatibility between mother and child may be associated with hyperbilirubinemia, although other physiologic problems may also be responsible.

There are two types of bilirubin, conjugated and unconjugated, which are sometimes referred to as direct and indirect bilirubin, respectively. As red blood cells break down, unconjugated bilirubin is routinely released into the plasma serum. This is observed during the healing of a bruise when the surface area under the skin becomes yellow (or jaundiced) due to the presence of unconjugated bilirubin.

The unconjugated bilirubin is bound to plasma albumin and transported to the liver where an enzyme "conjugates" it. That is, the potentially toxic unconjugated bilirubin is joined together with a substance in the body to form a detoxified product. The now "conjugated" bilirubin is normally excreted from the body through the small intestine. When bilirubin cannot be conjugated, it builds up in the serum until it crosses the plasma membrane and is deposited in the brain. Kernicterus is a neurologic syndrome resulting from the deposition of unconjugated bilirubin in brain cells, causing motor and sensory deficits, mental retardation, or death.

The Joint Committee on Infant Hearing (1982) suggests that those infants with a bilirubin level that exceeds indications requiring a blood exchange transfusion are "at risk" for hearing impairment. The Com-

Table 7.9.
Serum Bilirubin Level for Exchange Transfusion (mg/100 ml)

Birth Weight (g)	Normal Infants	Abnormal Infants
100	10.0	10.0
1001–1250	13.0	10.0
1251–1500	15.0	13.0
1501–2000	17.0	15.0
2001–2500	18.0	17.0
2500	20.0	18.0

mittee on Fetus and Newborn (1982) of the Academy of Pediatrics suggests the serum bilirubin level needed for exchange transfusion is a function of the infant's birthweight (see Table 7.9). The values in this table may be used as a guide in deciding whether or not to place an infant on the high-risk register for deafness. Newborns often have some degree of jaundice following birth because their immature liver function does not adequately handle the normal breakdown of red blood cells.

The level of bilirubin is not the only deciding factor in determining the need for an exchange transfusion. Consideration is given to several other factors including perinatal asphyxia respiratory distress, metabolic acidosis with pH levels less than or equal to 7.25, hypothermia, low serum protein levels, birthweight less than 1500 g, and/or signs of clinical central nervous system degeneration (Levine, 1979). In his sample of hearing-impaired newborns, Simmons (1980a) cited hyperbilirubinemia as the most common sequela of anoxia causing deafness. Vernon and Klein (1982) suggest that although Rh incompatibility was once a major cause of deafness in today's adult deaf population, increased skill in transfusion technology should reduce this factor as a cause of childhood deafness from the current 3–4% to about 1% in the future.

Nwaesei et al. (1984) conducted auditory brainstem evoked response (ABR) evaluation, before and after exchange transfusion, in an effort to determine whether hyperbilirubinemia is associated with acute effects on brainstem function of neonates. Acute brainstem toxicity appears to be reversible with exchange transfusion, as they cite

three infants whose evoked wave absence before exchange transfusion was followed by the appearance of the waves after the exchange transfusion.

F. Family History. Congenital deafness may be "passed on" or "inherited" from other family members who were deaf or hearing-impaired in childhood. The various patterns of inheritance are described in Chapter 3. Obviously, an infant with a family history of hearing-impaired blood relatives is "at risk" for inheriting that same trait.

Not so simple, however, is the task of eliciting family history from the baby's parents. Unfortunately, family history information is sparse beyond the infant's grandparents. Often, only one parent is available for interview, so that little information is available from the "other side" of the family. Information about handicapped relatives is often glossed over by relatives, so that considerable uncertainty exists about the true nature, degree, onset, or diagnosis of the condition. And finally, the interview technique may bring forth unexpected responses. A parent told us that no deafness existed in his family, although a cousin did attend the state deaf school. The parent was quick to add that the cousin was not "deaf"; he "wore a hearing aid and could hear normally." Another parent implicated his uncle, who "was not hearing-impaired since childhood . . . but he was totally deaf since birth."

Questions must be phrased carefully to avoid misunderstandings or erroneous responses. We ask, "Do you know any of the baby's relatives who now have a hearing loss which started before the age of 5 years? Please think hard about all of your family and the baby's father's family." If the answer is "yes," we proceed to ask who they were (relationship to baby). "Do you know what caused the hearing loss? What makes you think the onset of the loss was before the age of 5? Did he or she wear a hearing aid before age 5? Does he or she still wear a hearing aid? Did he or she attend a special school for the deaf? Did he or she attend public school? Did (or does) he or she have a speech problem?"

When the family history information is positive, the infant is identified as "at risk" for hearing impairment. It is important to remember the potential progressive nature or possible late onset of hereditary hearing loss. Careful follow-up and thorough parental counseling is advised for those babies who are "at risk" but who pass the initial hearing screening test.

G. Gram Birthweight Less than 1500.
In the past few years, with the aid of sophisticated medical equipment, premature babies so small that they fit into an adult's hand now have good chance for survival. Low-birthweight infants are more likely to have congenital defects, neurologic disorders such as cerebral palsy and seizures, gastrointestinal disorders, and respiratory problems. In the past, low-birthweight infants often were stillborn or died during delivery or soon after. Low birthweight is still the major factor associated with infant death. Compared with normal-weight infants, low-birthweight infants are almost 40 times more likely to die during their first 28 days of life, and very low birthweight infants are more than 200 times as likely to die during this period. Black women are more than twice as likely as whites to have a low-birthweight infant. This higher rate is the major factor contributing to higher mortality among black infants.

Some babies survive at a cost of significant disabilities. The current lowest limit of viability is 24 weeks (out of full-term or 40 weeks) gestation with a minimum weight of 500 grams (just over one pound). Infants this small have a 5–20% chance of survival. Breathing must be accomplished with a ventilator, since the babies lungs are not capable of breathing without mechanical aid.

"Preemies" (technically any baby born more than 3 weeks early) have about a 70% chance of survival if they weigh under 2 pounds; 90% of preemies weighing between 2 and 3 pounds survive. Improvement in

technology in the neonatal intensive care unit (NICU) has resulted in an increased survival rate of premature, high-risk infants. A study conducted by Kenworthy et al. (1987) with a sample of 266 high-risk infants with extreme immaturity revealed that approximately one third of the population exhibited hearing impairment and/or speech/language problems. Kenworthy et al. recommend that such infants should be routinely assessed for communication development and hearing sensitivity at various age levels during childhood.

Infants delivered prior to 37 weeks are considered to have a shortened gestation period and are *premature* or *preterm*. Historically, prematurity was defined by low birthweight. In essence, however, prematurity and low birthweight are usually concomitant, particularly among infants weighing 1500 g or less at birth (about 3 pounds), and both factors are associated with increased neonatal morbidity and mortality. It is difficult to separate completely the factors associated with prematurity from those associated with low birthweight (Vaughan et al., 1979).

It has been well-documented that hearing loss occurs in relatively higher incidence in preterm infants than in full-term babies. The problem of ascertaining the etiology of hearing loss is difficult because preterm infants often have associated medical complications. Simmons (1980a) states that while it is true that the incidence of prematurity is higher in hearing loss babies, it is unlikely that prematurity per se causes the deafness; rather, neonatal anoxia is the underlying factor. In addition to anoxia, problems associated with the premature infant include hyperbilirubinemia and an increase in bacterial/viral infections. Treatment for infant septemic infection often includes antibiotics, which are themselves potentially ototoxic.

The hearing loss associated with low-birthweight infants tends to be sensorineural with a steep high-frequency component. Clark and Conry (1978) studied 204 low-birthweight babies and found 5% to have sensorineural hearing loss—each of whom also had elevated bilirubin levels at birth. Abramovich et al. (1979) evaluated the hearing of 111 perinatal care survivors with birthweights of 1500 g or less. They found 10 patient (9%) with sensorineural hearing loss, 1 (1%) with congenital conductive hearing loss, and 21 (19%) with middle ear effusions.

Other High-Risk Factors. Other neonatal hearing risk factors have been suggested and are currently under consideration by the 1990 Joint Committee on Infant Hearing Screening. These potential high risk factors for deafness include fetal alcohol syndrome (Church and Gerkin, 1987), persistent pulmonary hypertension (Naulty et al., 1986), length of stay in the ICN and gestational age (Helpern et al., 1987), severe neonatal sepsis (Feinmesser and Tell, 1976), and parental consanguinity (Coplan, 1987). Some published reports advocate hearing screening for all infants in NICUs (Galambos et al., 1984; Jacobson and Morehouse, 1984).

TECHNIQUES OF INFANT HEARING SCREENING

Behavioral Observation Screening. Inasmuch as many audiologists believe there is virtue in behavioral observation hearing screening for at-risk infants, an overview of this technique is described. The recommended procedure for behavioral screening includes the following salient points (Mencher, 1976).

1. The stimulus should be 90 dB (sound pressure level) in intensity and with a low frequency attenuation of 30 dB per octave below 750 Hz.
2. The infant should be asleep, with eyes closed and no body movement, for at least 15 seconds before the stimulus is presented.
3. The only acceptable response is a generalized body movement involving more than one limb and accompanied by some form of eye movement.

4. Scoring should be done by two observers, independent of each other. Two (of eight maximum) stimulus responses should be positive to score as a pass, and failures should be retested at least once.

Expected Responses. The kinds of responses one looks for are age-specific, depending on the maturation of the infant, as shown in Figure 7.4.

Birth to 4 Months. At this age auditory responses are largely reflexive. In a very quiet environment one may see an eye-blink or eye-widening response to the softer noisemakers, but these responses are not standardized. The only reliable response is a startle or eye-blink to the loud noisemaker. At 3 or 4 months the infant may begin to turn his or her head toward a sound, but this response also is not yet reliable.

4–7 Months. By 4 months the infant will begin to turn his or her head toward the sound source in a wobbly way, and by 7 months there will be a direct turn toward the side. It will not be a direct localization of the sound at the lower level, however; it will only be a turn toward the side.

7–9 Months. Between 7 and 9 months the infant will begin to find the sound source on the lower level, locating it directly by 8–9 months. The infant will not yet look directly at a sound on a higher plane, i.e., above eye level.

9–13 Months. By the end of 13 months the infant will be able to localize sounds directly in any plane. Full maturation of the child's auditory development has been attained.

13–36 Months. The same responses will be seen in the 13–36 month period, i.e., localization in all planes. Other factors begin to enter into the testing in this period and must be considered. For example, a 2–3 year old may hear the sound but will inhibit the orienting response, since the child may suspect that the examiner is making the sound. Skill and experience must prevail with this age child to be sure any responses

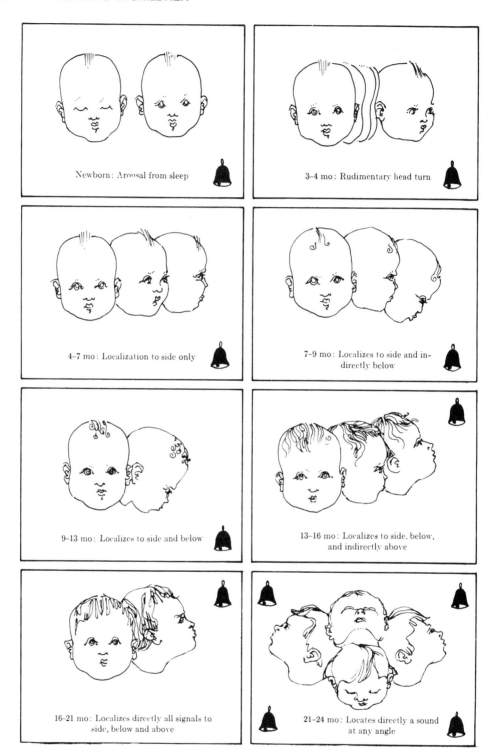

Figure 7.4. Normal maturation of the auditory localization response.

noted are specific to the presentation of the auditory stimulus *only*.

Questionnaires for Parents. It is useful to get some idea from the parents as to how the child is functioning. A communication questionnaire (Table 7.10) may bring out facts that are not evident in the hearing test findings. The questions presented in Table 7.10 cover both auditory behavior and developmental milestones. If either is deficient, the child should be referred for appropriate evaluation. The parent can be questioned either by written questionnaire or by oral query, depending upon which suits the needs of the population served. The questionnaire includes information on developmental status and communication abilities in addition to the questions concerning hearing status. It is recommended that this kind of questionnaire be used as a screening device to identify other problems that might benefit from treatment at an early age. The hearing questions are separated from the developmental questions because most of the commonly used developmental milestones are found to be present in otherwise-normal deaf babies and, therefore, would not identify a hearing loss.

Some knowledge of the attributes of the deaf is necessary in order for the questioner to understand why the questions are worded as they are. For example, a deaf child will look around or will wake up when a door slams, when someone stamps a foot on the floor, when a large truck rolls by on the street, or when a loud airplane flies low overhead. Therefore, if the parent states that the child awakens to a loud sound, the parent must be asked to specify the type of sound.

Another characteristic of the deaf infant is that he or she is unusually visually alert and attends to movement in peripheral vision. Therefore, if the parent reports that the child turns around to an interesting sound or name, the parent must be asked if the sound is out of the child's peripheral visual field.

Until the age of 6 months the deaf infant sounds to the uninitiated person much like the normal infant; the deaf baby babbles just as much, increases vocalizations when the parent appears, and coos just as the normal child, and only an expert phonetician could identify the subtle qualitative differences in the babbling sounds that the deaf child makes. Therefore, great care has been taken in the questionnaire not to assume that the baby's vocalizations are any index of ability to hear.

A very misleading indication is a parent's report that the baby says "mamma" at around the age of 1 year and that, therefore, the baby must be hearing at that point. Oddly enough, the parents of most deaf children make just such a report, and it is universally true that a profoundly deaf infant will apear to be saying "mamma" at around 1 year of age. Actually, what the baby is saying is "amah," which is the most primitive sound that can be made, involving as it does the almost animal-like "ah" vocalization plus the coming together of the lips. It has been postulated that one of the reasons for its development is that in infancy the baby is carried close to the mother, feels the vibrations or hears low frequencies of the mother's voice, and thus is stimulated to perpetuate the sounds. At any rate, the sounds soon drop off, and nothing remains except the "ah" vocalization in a strident voice.

Auditory Brainstem Evoked Response as a Screening Technique in Infants. The application of brainstem evoked response to auditory screening represents a relatively new dimension in the early identification of hearing loss. The rapid development of ABR procedures has resulted in the pursuit of evidence for effective application as a screening technique. Several leading laboratories have evaluated both neonatal normal and high-risk populations with ABR techniques in an attempt to determine the reliability, sensitivity, and accuracy of the procedures (Fig. 7.5).

Gorga et al. (1988) reported ABRs from 89 infant graduates of an ICN who were fitted with insert earphones and who were

Table 7.10.
Questions to Ask the Parent at the Well-Baby Examination[a]

2 MONTHS		
Hearing		
1. Have you had any worry about your child's hearing?	Yes	No
2. When he's sleeping in a quiet room, does he move and begin to wake up when there's a loud sound?	Yes	No
Developmental and Communication		
3. Does he lift up his head when he's lying on his stomach?	Yes	No
4. Does he smile at you when you smile at him?	Yes	No
5. Does he move both hands together in the same way?	Yes	No
6. Does he look at your face without your making gestures to him?	Yes	No

4 MONTHS		
Hearing		
1. Have you had any worry about your child's hearing?	Yes	No
2. When he's sleeping in a quiet room, does he move and begin to wake up when there's a loud sound?	Yes	No
3. Does he try to turn his head toward an interesting sound or when his name is called?	Yes	No
Developmental and Communication		
4. Does he lift his head up to 90° and look straight ahead?	Yes	No
5. Does he touch his hands together and play with them?	Yes	No
6. Does he laugh and giggle without being tickled or touched?	Yes	No
7. Does he coo to himself and make noises when he's alone?	Yes	No

6 MONTHS		
Hearing		
1. Have you had any worry about your child's hearing?	Yes	No
2. When he's sleeping in a quiet room, does he move and begin to wake up when there's a loud sound?	Yes	No
3. Does he turn his head toward an interesting sound or when his name is called?	Yes	No
Developmental and Communication		
4. Does he lift up his head and chest with his arms?	Yes	No
5. Does he keep his head steady when sitting?	Yes	No
6. Does he roll over in his crib?	Yes	No
7. Does he reach for objects within his reach and hold them?	Yes	No
8. Does he see small objects like peas or raisins?	Yes	No

8 MONTHS		
Hearing		
1. Have you had any worry about your child's hearing?	Yes	No
2. When he's sleeping in a quiet room, does he move and begin to wake up when there's a loud sound?	Yes	No
3. Does he turn his head directly toward an interesting sound or when his name is called?	Yes	No
4. Does he enjoy ringing a bell or shaking a rattle?	Yes	No
Developmental and Communication		
5. Does he support most of his weight on his legs?	Yes	No
6. Can he sit alone unaided for 5 minutes?	Yes	No
7. Can he sit and look for objects that have fallen out of sight?	Yes	No
8. Can he pick up two objects, one in each hand?	Yes	No
9. Can he transfer an object from one hand to the other?	Yes	No
10. Can he feed himself a cracker?	Yes	No
11. Does he make a number of different sounds and change their pitch?	Yes	No
12. Does he clap his hands in imitation and make noises at the same time?	Yes	No

10 MONTHS		
Hearing		
1. Have you had any worry about your child's hearing?	Yes	No
2. When he's sleeping in a quiet room, does he move and begin to wake up when there's a loud sound?	Yes	No
3. Does he turn his head directly toward an interesting sound or when his name is called?	Yes	No
4. Does he try to imitate you if you make his own sounds?	Yes	No
Developmental and Communication		
5. Does he play peekaboo with you?	Yes	No
6. Can he stand for at least 5 seconds, holding onto a crib or chair?	Yes	No
7. Does he try to hold a toy when it's pulled away?	Yes	No
8. Is he shy or afraid of strangers?	Yes	No
9. Can he pull himself to standing position alone?	Yes	No

Table 7.10.
(Continued)

12 MONTHS		
Hearing		
1. Have you had any worry about your child's hearing?	Yes	No
2. When he's sleeping in a quiet room, does he move and begin to wake up when there's a loud sound?	Yes	No
3. Does he turn his head directly toward an interesting sound or when his name is called?	Yes	No
4. Is he beginning to repeat some of the sounds that you make?	Yes	No
Developmental and Communication		
5. Can he pick up a raisin or a pea?	Yes	No
6. Can he get to a sitting position without help?	Yes	No
7. Does he wave bye-bye or pat-a-cake when you tell him to?	Yes	No
8. Can he say "mamma" or "dadda?"	Yes	No

[a]The pronouns "he," "him," and "his" as employed in this table are not meant to convey the masculine gender alone. Use of these terms in their generic sense, to denote persons of both sexes, is intended solely to avoid redundancy and awkwardness in expression.

compared with infants fitted with circumaural earphones. Equivalent threshold levels and ABR wave latencies were similar once the delay introduced by the sound delivery tube for the insert earphones was considered. Insert earphones are recommended for use with infants to prevent erroneous conductive hearing waveforms due to collapse of the external ear canals, a common occurrence when circumaural earphones are used.

Hecox and Galambos (1974) evaluated 35 infants, aged 3 weeks to about 3 years, with the ABR technique. They found the latency of wave V to be a function of both click intensity and the age of the subject. The latency at a given signal strength shortens postnatally to reach the adult value (about 6

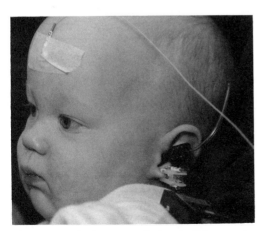

Figure 7.5. Brainstem evoked potential screening being performed on neonate with the use of insert receiver earphones.

msec) by 12–18 months of age. At this time, Hecox and Galambos suggested, the reliability and lack of variability of ABR could provide an objective method for assessing hearing in infants.

Schulman-Galambos and Galambos (1979) used ABR as an auditory screening procedure in three groups of newborns. One group consisted of 220 normal-term infants who were within 72 hours of birth and in whom no hearing abnormalities were detected; the second group consisted of 75 ICU newborns, 4 of whom were found to have severe sensorineural hearing loss at the time of hospital discharge. The third group consisted of 325 infants, 1 year or older, who had previously been discharged from the intensive care unit (ICU). Of these infants, an additional 4 showed sensorineural hearing loss. The authors estimated the incidence of hearing loss in the ICU population to be 1 in 50 and concluded that ABR is a cost-effective screening test.

A number of investigators have compared ABR between normal and high-risk infants in early postnatal life. Salamy et al. (1980) indicate that infants born "at risk" but free of severe auditory defects and major neurologic difficulties can be distinguished from healthy (age-matched) controls in terms of the brainstem averaged potential throughout the first postnatal year. Barden and Peltzman (1980) evaluated 61 newborns to study the potential influence of perinatal risk factors for hearing impairment and/or asphyxial brain damage. Their results, although not conclusive, suggest that birth asphyxia and/or low birthweight may be associated with shortened latencies in evoked potential waveforms.

Routine screening of infants from the newborn ICU for auditory impairment with auditory brainstem potentials has been recommended by Marshall et al. (1980) as a clinically feasible and useful procedure. In their study, infants with a gestational age of 24–43 weeks and a birthweight of 530–2338 g were classified as pass or fail, depending on the presence or absence of wave V at a latency of 7–11 msec in response to clicks of 60 dB above the normal adult threshold. The failure babies were not correlated with excessive noise exposure or ototoxic medications, but nearly all the babies who failed had intracranial hemorrhage.

Marshall et al. (1980) suggested that the smaller, younger babies failed the ABR screening because of the physiologic immaturity of the small infants and the pathologic severity of the patient's diseases. Starr et al. (1977) reported ABR studies on infants as young as 28 weeks of gestational age and believed that the brainstem response wave complexes could be identified if the stimuli were sufficiently loud.

Schwartz et al. (1989) studied the relationship between peripheral and central auditory maturation with ABR in preterm infants. Their study found wave I latency and amplitude to be equivalent to those of adult subjects, while waves III and V did show prolongation. They also recommended the use of rarefaction stimuli for greater amplitude of waves I and III over condensation stimuli. Schwartz et al. conclude that any prolongation in wave I latency is typically correlated with a diagnosis of otitis media with effusion.

Galambos et al. (1982) conclude that because of the high incidence of hearing loss in infants discharged from the tertiary ICN, ABR techniques are the most reliable, sensitive, and accurate of the newborn hearing tests available at the present time. In their

evaluation of 890 newborns discharged from ICN, 10% suffered from hearing loss in one or both ears, and 2% suffered irreversible bilateral sensorineural hearing losses so severe as to require amplification.

Several limitations of ABR evaluations with a neonatal population have been identified by Stockhard and Westmoreland (1981). A heightened vulnerability of the neonatal wave potentials to certain technical and subject factors should be of concern. Stimulus intensity calibration can be a major source of variability in peak and interpeak latencies. Uncertainty about the conceptual age versus gestational age of the infant may confuse the interpretation, because of the rapid change of maturational levels in auditory transmission time.

Many waveform criteria of auditory evoked potentials are used to identify a hearing-impaired infant and to distinguish peripheral hearing loss from intracranial pathology (Finitzo-Hieber, 1982): the absolute latency of waves I and V, the latency-intensity function, the wave I–V interwave interval, and the amplitude ratio of wave V to wave I. She indicates that accurate infant assessment requires age-specific norms for each of the measurements. These waveforms are first visible in a premature infant at 28–30 weeks *postconception* (or 28–30 weeks gestational age), not postbirth. However, latencies are prolonged and thresholds are elevated when compared with those of a term newborn. The maturation of the auditory brainstem response is not complete until 12–18 months postterm (with term being 38–40 weeks gestational age). Figure 7.6 illustrates the maturation of wave V and wave I over time. Note that the critical time is expressed in *postconception* rather than in time *postbirth*.

Finitzo-Hieber (1982) makes the following recommendations in conducting ABR in premature infants. First, if a premature infant is tested far in advance of discharge, the baby can present with a significant, but transient, impairment that may show partial or complete recovery at the time of dis-

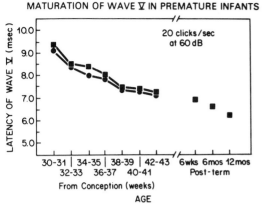

MATURATION OF WAVE V IN PREMATURE INFANTS

20 clicks/sec
at 60 dB

From Conception (weeks)

AGE

MATURATION OF WAVE I IN PREMATURE INFANTS

20 clicks/sec
at 60 dB

● Despland/Galambos
■ Finitzo-Hieber

From Conception (weeks)

AGE

Figure 7.6. Maturation of wave V and wave I over time. (Reproduced with permission from T. Finitzo-Hieber: Auditory brainstem response: its place in infant audiological evaluations. *Seminars in Speech, Language and Hearing* 3:76–87, 1982.)

charge. If ABR is to be effective, assessment should take place near discharge time, when the infant is in an open crib and is not less than 37 weeks of gestational age. Second, a single ABR assessment is not sufficient in premature infants. Both improvement and deterioration in auditory function have been documented on follow-up testing. Therefore, at-risk infants should be monitored with ABR every 3 months in the first year of life.

It should then be questioned if ABR monitoring in itself constitutes adequate follow-up for a child. According to Stein et al. (1983a), otologic, audiologic, and neurologic examinations, as well as postdischarge ABR, are mandatory before any inferences

can be made about hearing loss or neurodevelopmental disorders. The intent of the initial screening procedure will help dictate the appropriate follow-up examinations. A behavioral audiometric evaluation would be necessary to obtain accurate frequency-specific information and to determine the existence or extent of a conductive hearing loss.

Dennis et al. (1984) summarized the ABR evaluations obtained from a group of 200 infants from the NICU, which provide an overview of results to be expected in such a screening program. There were 177 instances of pass (88.5%) and 23 instances of failure (11.5%). Despite diligent efforts to retest all the "failure" babies, 8 of the 23 were lost to follow-up. The remaining 15 "failure" babies were given thorough medical and audiologic evaluation. Ten babies (5% of the original sample of 200 babies) were confirmed to have sensorineural hearing loss, with 3 of the 10 failing the initial ABR screen at 30 dB hearing level (HL) and 7 of the 10 failing the initial screening at 70 dB HL.

Auditory Evoked Response Infant Protocol. A recommended protocol for audiologic screening of newborn infants who are at risk for hearing impairment has recently been published by the American Speech-Language-Hearing Association (Asha, 1989). ASHA recommends that all newborns at risk for hearing impairment be screened with ABR audiometry prior to discharge from the hospital. Should the infant be discharged without the ABR screening, the parent or caretaker should be informed that audiologic evaluation is important for the infant.

The acoustic stimulus for ABR screening should include the frequency band important for speech recognition and may consist of clicks, tone pips, or tone bursts. The pass criterion for ABR infant screening is a response from both ears at intensity levels of 40 dB nHL (normal hearing level) or less. The ASHA recommendations point out that it is important for the parents, caretakers, and those who provide primary health care to understand that "pass" on ABR screening does not rule out development of hearing impairment in infancy or early childhood. Infants who "pass" the ABR screen should receive audiologic follow-up as necessary for medical evaluation and management and/or developmental evaluation. Infants whose responses meet the "pass" criterion and who are at risk for progressive hearing impairment should receive audiologic monitoring on a periodic basis probably throughout the preschool years.

Infants who do not demonstrate responses at intensity levels of 40 dB nHL or less in both ears should enter the audiologic evaluation, follow-up, and management system. In fact, early habilitation is believed to be so important to the development of hearing-impaired infants that continued efforts to confirm electrophysiologic estimates of peripheral sensitivity may coincide with ongoing habilitation. Infants who demonstrate responses at 40 dB nHL or less from only one ear should receive audiologic monitoring until either (a) both ears meet the pass criterion, or (b) stable unilateral hearing loss is confirmed and follow-up and management are initiated. It is important to note that the ASHA recommendations include a statement that the electrophysiologic test results (ABR) be confirmed by behavioral techniques as soon as possible.

A flow diagram of the ASHA audiologic screening program for newborn infants at risk for hearing impairment is presented in Figure 7.7. The total infant hearing screening program is described as a three-part effort: (1) parent/caregiver education to ensure that they understand the relationship between hearing, speech, and language development and that they receive information to enhance their ability to observe and monitor normal developmental milestones; (2) the ABR audiologic hearing screening protocol described above; and (3) evaluation, follow-up, and management systems to ensure that the identified hearing-impaired infant receives immediate habitation action.

Crib-o-gram. An ingenious automated system for detecting hearing loss in newborns was devised by F. Blair Simmons at the Stanford University School of Medicine in 1974 (Simmons and Russ, 1974; Simmons, 1976; Jones and Simmons, 1977). The technique, known as the Crib-o-gram, uses a motion-sensitive transducer placed under the crib mattress in the ICN or between the crib and frame in the well-baby nursery (WBN). The transducer is capable of detecting virtually any motor activity from the infant stranger than an eye-blink or facial grimace, including respiration.

The Crib-o-gram is a timed self-cycling system that turns on and shuts off automatically following each complete stimulus presentation and response measurement interval. The Crib-o-gram is a microprocessor-based unit that performs the test and scores and interprets the results.

The baby's state is monitored automatically by measuring crib movement for 10–15 seconds before and 6 seconds after each test sound presentation. The test sound presentation is delivered from an earphone placed in the bassinette (2000–4000-Hz band-pass noise stimulus). The auditory test stimulus is presented 20 or more times over a 7–24 hour period. Responses in the form of baby movement (or lack of responses) are noted by the microprocessor and are analyzed until a statistically valid decision can be made by the unit regarding whether the baby passed or failed the hearing screening. The Stanford group used the Crib-o-gram to establish an incidence of 1:1000 of deafness in the WBN and of 1:52 in the ICN (Simmons, 1982).

McFarland et al. (1980), using the Crib-o-gram, found a sensitivity rate of 91% of the WBN and 82% in the ICN, while specificity for the WBN was 92% and 79% for the ICN. Many of the ICN babies are less responsive to external stimuli, and rescreening is necessary for some 20% of the ICN babies screened.

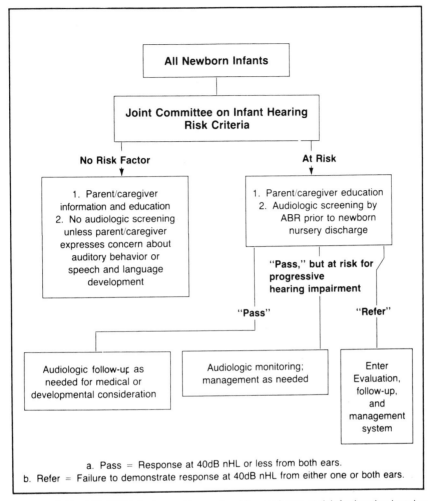

Figure 7.7. ASHA 1989 ABR infant screening protocol for newborns at risk for hearing impairment.

Durieux-Smith et al. (1985) compared the Crib-o-gram as a screening test in NICU infants by using ABR as the standard threshold estimation method. They reported that approximately one third of babies with normal ABR thresholds failed Crib-o-gram screening, raising serious question about the validity of the Crib-o-gram technique. In this study, two Crib-o-gram tests were administered to 280 babies within 48 hours, resulting in poor test-retest reliability scores. The correct identification of hearing loss by the Crib-o-gram increased with severity, so that this technique was able to identify moderately severe hearing loss in full-term and older babies. Wright and

Rybak (1983) also reported a high incidence of false positive results with ICU babies with normal ABR auditory findings.

Auditory Response Cradle. The auditory response cradle was developed in England as a fully automatic, microprocessor-controlled, newborn screening device. The system consists of a "cradle" with head and body support that is capable of monitoring four measures of infant behavioral response following auditory stimulation. Trunk and limb movements are monitored by a pressure-sensitive mattress; the head-jerk component of the startle reflex is monitored by a transducer, embedded in the foam of a headrest, that is pivoted on low-friction bearings to detect head-turn reactions; infant respiratory pattern is sensed by a transducer, fitted in a plastic belt, that is placed around the upper abdomen of the baby.

A high-pass noise of 85 dB sound pressure level (SPL) (bandwidth from 2600 to 4500 Hz) is used as the test stimulus and presented through close-coupled ear probes fitted with tips similar to those used for acoustic impedance testing. The auditory stimulus is presented to the infant under test on a number of occasions, and resulting motor and respiratory responses are detected and stored by the microprocessor. Equal numbers of no-sound "control" trials enable calculation of the probability that the sound responses are genuine and not spontaneous events. When the microprocessor determines that the probability of response exceeds 97%, the baby is considered to have normal-hearing responses and to have passed. The average test time takes 2–10 minutes.

Over 5000 babies have been evaluated with the auditory response cradle (Bhattacharya et al., 1980). To date, infants with severe hearing loss as well as infants with middle ear dysfunction diagnosed as serous otitis media have been identified with this hearing screening technique (Bennett, 1979, 1980; Bennett and Lawrence, 1980).

Identification and Follow-up in Infant Screening. The effectiveness of any screening program is only as good as the subsequent follow-up program (McFarland et al., 1980). If experienced audiologists are unavailable or if parents have difficulty gaining access to audiologic assistance, hearing-impaired babies may not receive the necessary follow-up and intervention. The philosophical question remains, who is responsible for follow-up—the parents or the institution? Who should bear the financial burden of further evaluation, the parents or the institution, when the baby is called back for additional testing?

Individuals involved in infant screening must also be concerned about the ever-present possibility of progressive sensorineural hearing loss. When high-risk babies pass the initial screening test and are later determined to have hearing loss, the question always remains, did the screening test miss this baby or did the hearing loss occur after the hearing screening was applied (Simmons, 1980a)? Simmons argues that genetic delayed-onset hearing losses are probably very rare and that nearly all, if not all, sensorineural hearing losses in very young children occur before they are discharged from the newborn nursery.

An interesting point can be made by examining the reported age of *detection* of hearing loss against the age of *confirmation* of hearing loss. Bergstrom (1984) called the situation disgraceful in a referral clinic in which hearing loss in a severely to profoundly deaf child is initially suspected, on the average, at age 10 months, the loss is detected at age 21 months, and training and amplification are first begun at 27 months of age. In 1977, Jones and Simmons published a table showing that the age of suspicion of deafness with 24 infants screened with the Crib-o-gram was approximately 42 days; age of confirmation of hearing loss in these infants was nearly 13 months. Statistics based on behavioral infant screening performed at Colorado General Hospital between 1972 and 1976 indicate that the average time between *confirmation* of hearing loss and the beginning of *habilitation* procedures in these youngsters was 6.5 months. It should be noted that these data preceded the use of auditory evoked response as a technique to validate hearing loss in infants.

Shah et al. (1978) reviewed 200 questionnaires completed by parents of hearing-impaired youngsters in Toronto. Nearly half of the parents reported that they experienced difficulties and prolonged delays in reaching a firm diagnosis of hearing impairment in their children. Although the mean age of suspicion of hearing loss was 16 months of age, the average additional delay until audiologic assessment was completed was 11.5 months, with a range between 0 and 60 months! The parents viewed the chief obstacles as the primary care physician's unwillingness to accept the parent's opinions, the failure of these physicians to perform simple hearing screening tests, and, finally, the reluctance of the physicians to arrange for referral of the child for audiologic evaluation. The detection of the child's hearing problem was found to depend on the astuteness and insistence of the parents as well as the alertness of the physician.

More recently, Simmons (1980b) reviewed the records of 42 babies whose average age of first hearing aid purchase was 22 months. While this statistic alone is not surprising, 83% of these babies were suspects for deafness before they were discharged from the newborn nursery, and 43% of those who were not newborn suspects failed their initial hearing test by 11 months of age. Simmons' review of the referral processes and professional judgments is worthwhile reading for all clinicians faced with decision-making responsibilities. His data indicate that the problem is generally not in the audiologist's diagnosis but in such hearing losses escaping the notice of parents and physicians. Although many of the babies had other medical problems manifested in delayed development of motor skills and moderate-to-severe visual impairments, ABR testing was conducted in only a few of the babies.

The pattern of delays between the recommendation and the fitting of a hearing aid seemed to be threefold: (1) referral back to the physician for ear examinations and medical clearances, then long, silent intervals without action; (2) babies with multiple physical and developmental problems in which hearing was only part of the total concern of the parents; and (3) parental disbelief or avoidance of the fact that their child had an important hearing loss.

Since the intent of an infant hearing screening program is to identify and habilitate deaf children as early as possible, programs must build in strict time schedules for action following the identification of an infant suspected to have hearing loss. Simmons recommends that any child failing a hearing screen be retested at least once within 2 weeks. A child then suspected of hearing loss should be referred for a formal hearing evaluation, not more than 2 weeks hence, and a final opinion on hearing status should be forthcoming within 6 weeks of the initial hearing screen. A thorough medical examination, impedance audiometry and, if question still exists about the hearing, an ABR evaluation are a necessity. Even under this rigid time regimen, the typical child who is suspect at birth and rescreened at 7 months, when behavioral responses are more obvious, will still perhaps require 4 additional months before habilitation is in full swing.

A committee from the Never Too Young project of Arizona organized and distributed a questionnaire to parents of congenitally hearing-impaired children to probe for information regarding the identification and intervention processes that the parents had experienced, as well as to inquire regarding the children's birth and medical histories. The findings revealed a number of important facts that have important relevance to our goal of the early identification of deafness in infants (Elssmann et al., 1987):

- Approximately one half of the babies with congenital deafness would not have been detected by the 1982 high-risk register factors;

- Approximately one third of the babies with congenital hearing loss had spent time in a NICU;

- Advice given by managing physicians in response to parental concern (of good and poor value) had significant influence on the early identification (or lack thereof) of their child's hearing loss;

- The average age of identification of deafness in this group of surveyed children was 19 months regardless of whether the infant was high-risk for hearing loss or not;

- Audiologists were estimated to have contributed, on the average, to a delay of as much as 6 months between identification of the hearing loss and the initial hearing aid fitting;

- Finally, the hearing loss of babies born between 1960 and 1969 was identified at approximately 19 months of age, while babies born later than 1982 were identified to have hearing loss at about 15 months of age.

Stein et al. (1989) compared patterns of initial identification and habilitation between a group of 88 hearing-impaired infants studied between 1980 and 1983 and a comparable group of 107 hearing-impaired infants identified between 1983 and 1988. Their findings include:

- Only one third of hearing-impaired infants spent time in the NICU;

- Of the seven high-risk deafness factors identified by the 1982 Joint Committee on Infant Hearing, meningitis was the leading cause of deafness in children less than 5 years of age, while fewer instances on very low birthweight seemed related to deafness;

- The 1980–1982 hearing-impaired babies were enrolled in habilitation programs at 18 months (ICU infants) and 22 months (WBN babies), which is not much different from the 1983–1986 data of 20 months (ICU babies) and 19 months (WBN babies). Although the ages at diagnosis of 12 months in the earlier study and 13 months in the later study for ICU infants is significantly earlier than for the WBN graduates, any potential advantage that might result from earlier diagnosis is apparently lost because of delays in habilitation program enrollment. The Stein et al., study concludes that even at this current level of activity with early identification programs using the high-risk registry program, the number of hearing-

impaired infants diagnosed and enrolled in therapy by the optimum 6 months of age as recommended by the Joint Committee on Infant Hearing 1982 Statement is disappointingly low.

James Jerger of Baylor School of Medicine relates that the clinical audiologist can make two mistakes when counseling parents of an infant suspected to have hearing loss; one of the mistakes, however, has considerably more serious consequences than the other mistake. The *lesser* of the two mistakes (the false positive) is for the audiologist to decide that the infant is deaf and subsequently to determine that the infant has normal hearing. An embarrassing mistake to be sure, but probably every experienced clinician has fallen prey to this error, but the final outcome of normal hearing is a great relief to all involved with the infant.

The more serious mistake, however, is devastating to the infant in question. In this grave error (the false negative) the clinician informs the parent that their baby has normal hearing when, in fact, the infant has severe-to-profound hearing loss. In this situation, the parent assumes with confidence that the baby hears normally, but by the time the mistake is identified, maximum habilitation may never be achieved.

Armed with knowledge about the potential for these two mistakes in infant-hearing assessment, the audiologist must practice extreme care in pronouncing an infant to have normal hearing. When in doubt, it behooves the clinician to assume the infant has a hearing problem until proved otherwise. The audiologist is still the best professional to serve as an advocate for the child and to be the one whose ultimate responsibility is to provide the maximum in support for the infant under evaluation.

Issues in the Early Identification of Hearing Loss. A comprehensive discussion of numerous issues related to a hospital infant hearing screening program was published by Alberti et al. (1985) based on their experiences with more than 8000 live births between the years 1981 and 1983. They point out that it is difficult and prohibitively expensive to test every infant by ABR. The current high-risk register has some limitation, in that many hearing-impaired infants will not manifest any classical register factor (Riko et al., 1985). One consideration is to test all babies in the ICU where these infants are at greatly increased risk, comprising about 5% of all live births, and where a yield of hearing loss incidence of 2% or more may be identified. The ICU infant group includes many of the babies who would be under the high-risk registry for deafness, especially those infants with low birthweight and asphyxia. On the other hand, to attempt to screen all ICU infants for hearing would include some babies who are not at risk for hearing loss and yet exclude those infants with minor (but important) defects of the head and neck or with a family history of childhood hearing loss. The Alberti group screening for hearing a random sampling of non-ICU infants and found a significant number of hearing loss cases, which suggests that it is unsatisfactory to restrict hearing screening just to ICU infants.

A further issue examined was when should the ABR hearing screening test be done and still conform to the Joint Committee recommendation that management of hearing-impaired infants should be instituted by 6 months of age. The Alberti study concluded from careful examination of its infant screening records that there is great advantage to be gained by deferring the ABR test until about 4 months of age. The reasons for this delay include: (*a*) hearing tests must be performed immediately prior to the initiation of habilitation, so even if predischarge ABR was conducted, subsequent hearing tests would have to be accomplished anyway; (*b*) by waiting until 4 months of age the likelihood of identifying progressive or adventitious hearing loss increases; (*c*) the infant is stronger and healthier, thereby creating less confounding of test results by sequelae of se-

vere neonatal illness and normal maturational effect; (*d*) time is provided whereby logistic ease of test scheduling and case selection can be done on an outpatient basis; and (*e*) the scope and propriety of intervention and habilation during the first 3 months of life are questionable.

On the other hand, there is no doubt that in favor of predischarge ABR screening is the fact that the infant is available, because in the current United States health system, once the infant is discharged there is no assurance that follow-up testing can be scheduled and successfully accomplished. Indeed, with the quick discharge system followed in most hospitals, it is often impossible to perform the hearing screening test before the baby and mother go home. The greatest weakness of most infant hearing screening programs is the inability to comply with follow-up programs after the infant has left the hospital. Alberti et al. (1985) agree that it is probably better to have a predischarge ABR screen than no hearing test at all.

GOALS AND METHOD USED IN TESTING PRE-SCHOOLERS 2–4 YEARS OLD

Goals. The period of 2–4 years gives us real problems in identification of hearing loss. These children are usually seen at well-baby clinics or at doctors' offices. Although Head Start programs are making many children available, there are large numbers who are not seen for health visits unless special efforts are made to reach them. Nursery schools, play schools, and child care centers are prime locations for hearing screening programs.

At this age we look primarily for medically remediable hearing losses, on the assumption that the more severely handicapping losses will have been found by 2 years. The chief pathology we are looking for is otitis media—the disease that can result at this age in subtle auditory disorders or permanent middle ear damage. The disorders that should be screened for at this age include middle ear pathologies, viral diseases, and sensorineural hearing loss. The tests that are adequate to identify these disorders are hearing screening, acoustic immittance testing, audiometry, and/or otoscopic examination.

Method. Numerous efforts have been made to develop effective screening methods for the preschool child. The problems arise from the definition of screening as "rapid, simple measurements applied to large numbers of children." Any test that requires a voluntary response from 2–3 year olds will be neither rapid nor simple. The 2–3 year olds can be negativistic, apprehensive, or "eager beavers"—all attitudes that hardly make for easy testing.

The ideal program would utilize both pure tone and acoustic immittance testing. Various studies have shown that immittance testing will identify 90–95% of all the significant ear pathologies in children. The pure tone screening test may identify 50% of the ear pathologies (Melnick et al., 1964). The pure tone preschool screening test is described below:

- *Pure Tone Screening Test*
  a. Play-conditioning procedure for testing the 3 and 4 year old child:
     (1) Have available a peg board, a ring tower, plain blocks, or other simple toys that are motivating to young children.
     (2) With headphones on your ears, take a block (or peg) and hold it up to one ear as if listening. Make believe you hear a sound, say "I hear it," and put the block on the table.
     (3) Put the phones on the child's ear and hold his or her hand with the block up to the child's ear.
     (4) Present a 50 dB tone at 1000 Hz and guide the child's hand to build the block tower. Repeat once or twice and then see if he or she can do it alone. If he or she can, go on.
     (5) Decrease the hearing level to 20 dB and repeat the test. If the child responds, go on to the other fre-

quencies (2000 and 4000 Hz) and repeat the procedure. Praise him or her for each correct response. After each presentation, place another block in the child's hand.
     (6) Switch to the opposite ear and repeat the test starting at 4000 Hz, then to 2000 Hz and 1000 Hz.

- *Criterion for Referral.* Failure to respond to 20 dB HL at any frequency and/or failure on impedance screening evaluation is criterion for referral.

Weber (1987) described a portable visual reinforcement audiometry (VRA) system that has been used extensively in a statewide program to screen infants, toddlers, and preschoolers at risk for hearing loss in rural Colorado. The statistics from the community-wide screenings between 1977 and 1986 demonstrate the effectiveness of the VRA technique. Of the nearly 25,000 children tested during the 9-year period of the report, nearly one half were less than 2 years of age. Sixteen percent of all children screened were referred for medical consultation, and 30 of the children were found to have significant sensorineural hearing loss.

SCREENING FOR COMMUNICATIVE DISORDERS IN THE 2–4 YEAR OLD

Screening for communicative disorder (i.e., hearing, speech and language) in the 2–4 year old may be done in local preschool programs, Head Start programs, child care centers, or primary care physician's offices. The close relationship of auditory development in the young child with evolving speech and language skills makes it possible for screening procedures to identify those children who are significantly delayed in developmental milestones to be referred for more complete evaluation. Because the foundations of language are fully established in normal children between 38 and 40 months of age, sufficient language milestones should be accessible prior to 36 months of age to permit screening at an early age. And significant delay in language development may provide the clue of suspicion for the presence of hearing loss.

Physicians who treat children are in a key position to identify language and hearing delay at the earliest possible age. Routine use of developmental screening tests by pediatricians occurs infrequently (Smith, 1978). Screening tests are customarily used when pediatricians already suspect a problem. Thus, the screening test is not being used for its intended purpose of separating from the larger population those children who are at increased risk for the disorder. Instead, the screen is being used as a post hoc confirmation of a problem. The test most frequently used for screening young children in pediatric offices is the Denver Developmental Screening Test (DDST) (Frankenburg and Dodds, 1967). A recent study compared results of performances on the language sector of the DDST with results of speech and language evaluations. With the DDST, 47% of children with delayed expressive language were not identified, thereby rendering it an insensitive screen for language disorders (Borowitz and Glascoe, 1986).

A majority of pediatricians judge a child's developmental level by parental recall of milestones or through observations during the routine physical examination. It has been shown that pediatricians' informal appraisals of children's mental abilities are inaccurate, with overestimation of abilities occurring most often (Bierman et al., 1964). Furthermore, no significant correlation exists between the pediatrician's confidence in making appraisals and the accuracy of their appraisals. The extent of their pediatric experience likewise does not increase their accuracy.

The problem of pediatricians' overestimating children's mental abilities through informal appraisals suggests that fewer children are referred for diagnostic testing than are actually developmentally delayed. A survey of Colorado pediatricians and family practitioners who provide general medical care to children younger than 3 years of age was conducted by Walker et al. (1989).

The 429 physicians who responded to the survey refer children in this age range to speech/language pathologists at rates varying from 0.3% to 0.6%. These figures are strikingly small when compared with prevalence estimates. Leske (1981) reported that 2–3% of 3 year old children are language-impaired. This figure does not include language delay due to causes such as mental retardation, cerebral palsy, or deafness. Routine screening of young children is paramount if language and hearing problems are to be identified early, accurately, and consistently.

Although the present state of screening for communicative disorders in the young child is not sophisticated, screening tools are available that, if applied at appropriate ages, would constitute an adequate screening program. A protocol utilizing such tools has been developed through the Robert Wood Johnson Foundation project in Colorado (Walker et al., 1989; Northern et al., 1989). For 4 years the staff of the project screened more than 800 children under 36 months of age for speech, language, and hearing. The screening was conducted in the offices of primary care physicians, health maintenance organizations, neighborhood health clinics, and university health clinics. During the course of the project the team determined that the brief screening protocol could be effectively incorporated into a busy office schedule (Fig. 7.8).

Before the screening was initiated, the Colorado project assessed the current state of speech, language, and hearing screening in the office of the primary physician. In a response to a questionnaire, 484 primary care physicians who manage the medical care of children under age 3 years indicated that they screened language skills with a wide variety of methods. Most of the physicians reported informal screening of language through patient history (parental report) and listening to and observing the child.

The protocol described in Figure 7.6 has been in use for more than 3 years in a

GUIDELINES FOR HEARING AND LANGUAGE SCREENING
OF YOUNG CHILDREN IN PHYSICIANS' OFFICES
HEARING SCREENING

AGE RANGE OF TEST	RECOMMENDED AGES TO TEST	SCREENING TEST	APPROPRIATE RESPONSE	RULES OUT	MANAGEMENT REFERRAL
Any age after birth	Neonatal period	Review child's history for these high risk factors for deafness: Asphyxia or anoxia Bacterial Meningitis Congenital perinatal infections Defects of head or neck Elevated bilirubin Family history of childhood deafness Gram birthweight less than 1500g.	No high risk factors in history	Most congenital hearing losses	If any factor is positive, refer for audiological testing
1-4 months	1-2 months	Loud horn 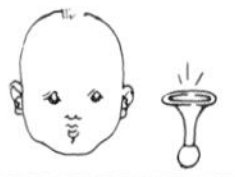	Eye Blink or Startle	Severe to profound loss	For failed screening tests, rescreen in 2 weeks
4-36 months	6-9 months and after each middle ear effusion	1. Soft noisemakers (Bell, squeeze toys, rattles, or keys) 2. Loud horn 3. Tympanometry for children 7 months and older	See chart on back for age appropriate response Eye blink or startle Normal tympanogram	Moderate to severe loss Effusion	If rescreen is failed, refer for audiological testing
36 months and older	4 - 5 years	Pure-tone audiometry* screen at 20 dBHL at 1000, 2000, 4000 Hz	Finger Raising 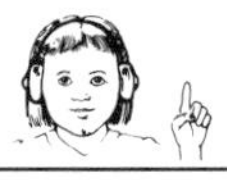	Mild loss and greater	

LANGUAGE SCREENING

AGE RANGE OF TEST	RECOMMENDED AGES TO TEST	SCREENING TEST	APPROPRIATE RESPONSE	RULES OUT	MANAGEMENT REFERRAL
0 - 36 months	13 - 36 months Best Age Range 24 - 30 months	Early Language Milestone Scale (ELM)	Pass Test at appropriate age level	Significant Language Delay	For failed screenin tests, rescreen in 1 - 2 weeks If rescreen is failed, refer for audiological and language testing

ADDITIONAL GUIDELINES FOR FOLLOWING CHILDREN
WITH EAR DISEASE

CRITERIA FOR ADDITIONAL FOLLOW-UP	MANAGEMENT		
	HEARING	LANGUAGE	MEDICAL
3 episodes of otitis media in 3-6 months or Persistent middle ear effusion for 3 months or more §	Refer for audiological testing regardless of age	Under 3 yrs: Screen every 6 mos. with ELM	Consider other medical management to interrupt cycle of disease

Figure 7.8. Guidelines for hearing and language screening of young children in physician offices. *Play conditioning may facilitate testing the younger children in the 3–5 age range. §Tympanometry is useful to document the duration of middle ear effusion.

number of offices of Colorado primary care physicians. In many office situations, the screening procedures are conducted by allied health personnel or office assistants. The screening test battery includes the Early Language Milestone (ELM) scale (Coplan et al., 1982), hearing screening with noisemakers, and tympanometry. This screening package has been developed specifically for children between birth and 3 years of age.

Hearing Screening. Between the ages of 4 and 16 months of age, the baby with normal hearing goes through an orderly auditory maturation process described previously and shown in Figure 7.4. During this age period, behavioral responses to quiet auditory noisemakers are seen as localization, i.e., head-turns for the visual observation of the noisemakers. The tester presents a quiet auditory stimulus, below or above the infant, but well out of the infant's sight. A normal response is for the baby to search out the source of the sound visually to either side in the early months or to turn the head briskly toward the sound source as the auditory response matures. The absence of this auditory localization response constitutes a failed screening test and raises the question of a hearing deficit. Although this procedure typically rules out moderate-to-severe hearing loss, experienced examiners with quiet noisemakers can often identify unilateral or bilateral mild hearing loss due to middle ear effusion.

The hearing screening should be done in a sound-treated room in which noise and visual distraction are at a minimum. Failure of a child to localize properly to an auditory signal does not indicate that the child did not hear it. The absence of a response may be due to lack of interest in the sound, delayed auditory maturation, or mental and/or physical impairment. The use of noisemakers, in accordance with expected auditory maturation responses, is intended to be a screening technique only. Additional evaluation by an experienced audiologist is recommended for any child who repeatedly fails to produce appropriate auditory-orienting responses.

Children with a mental age of 36 months are often able to comply with traditional pure tone hearing tests. Techniques of play conditioning may facilitate hearing testing in children between 3 and 4 years of age. Hearing screening is recommended for all children at about the age of 4 years or prior to their entering preschool. Hearing screening is performed, as recommended by the ASHA (1985), with pure tones of 1000, 2000, and 4000 Hz at 20 dB HL in each ear, with a finger-raising response by the child as each tone is heard. Failure of the hearing screening test occurs when any one of the tones in either ear is not heard. This technique may identify even mild hearing loss in one or both ears. Children who fail the hearing screening test should be rescreened within 2 weeks. If the rescreen is also failed, the child should be referred to an audiologist for further hearing evaluation with VRA techniques.

Tympanometry. Auditory evaluation of a child cannot be considered complete without inclusion of tympanometry. Tympanometry is an objective method of determining the status of the middle ear space and tympanic membrane compliance. It is particularly useful in identifying the presence of middle ear effusion or documenting the duration and number of episodes of otitis media. Tympanometry can detect the presence of middle ear pathology in some young children who are able to hear well enough to pass the behavioral auditory noisemaker screening. The usefulness of tympanometry cannot be overstated. Primary care physicians who routinely use tympanometry often comment that their diagnostic accuracy with otoscopy is greatly enhanced. Tympanometry in infants less than 7 months of age is *not* recommended in screening because of high false negative rates.

Language Screening. We use the Early Language Milestone scale (ELM).

The ELM is a well-normed language-screening instrument designed to be a rapid means of evaluating language development of children under 3 years of age. The test addresses both receptive and expressive language through parent report and direct testing of the child. The administration time of the ELM is 1–4 minutes. Each child's ELM profile is scored as "pass" or "fail."

Following 2 years of our experience administering the ELM in physicians' offices, an overall failure rate of 8% was noted. Children who failed an initial ELM screening, as well as a randomly selected sample of children who passed the ELM screening, were subsequently evaluated with a more sophisticated language test, the Sequenced Inventory of Communication Development (SICD). Based on an analysis of this evaluation procedure, it was determined that the best age range for ELM administration is between 24 and 30 months of age. Because the ELM is quickly and easily administered and because of improvement in the accuracy of parental report during a second ELM screen, it is recommended that children who fail to pass the ELM at their appropriate age level should be rescreened with the ELM within 1–2 weeks. If the ELM rescreen is also failed, referral to a speech/language pathologist is recommended. All children with language delay should also be referred for a hearing test to rule out the possibility of hearing impairment as a cause of language problems.

Following Children with Middle Ear Effusion. Physicians must be sensitive to the identification of communication disorders in children with recurrent middle ear effusion. The criteria presented for additional follow-up implicate those children with three episodes of otitis media within a 3 to 6 month period and those children who present with persistent middle ear effusion of 3 months or longer. It is important for physicians to maintain written notations of each episode of middle ear effusion, from the initial diagnosis to the complete resolu-

tion of the problem. Children identified by these criteria should be: (1) referred for audiologic evaluation, regardless of age; (2) screened with a formal, standardized language development assessment tool, such as the ELM, every 6 months to ensure adequate language appropriate for age level; and (3) some means other than continued medical treatment management to interrupt the cycle of the middle ear disease.

Home Language Stimulation. Screening without follow-up is of no benefit to the child. Providers of health care must assume the responsibility for arranging definitive diagnostic evaluations for suspect patients and for providing for remediation when appropriate and possible.

Children who exhibit mild language delay on the screening test may be enrolled in a home language enrichment program. Materials may be recommended for the parents that can be used in the home to enhance the child's speech and language. It is generally accepted that working with parents and instituting a home-based, moderately structured program can produce impressive short- and long-term gains for children.

SCREENING FOR OTITIS MEDIA

Controversies exist regarding the need, purpose, and technique of screening for middle ear disease and hearing loss in children. Middle ear disease generally refers to otitis media, one of the most common diseases of childhood. Identification, treatment, and management of otitis media spreads across the territories of numerous professional groups and thus has important economic and health care implications in society. A special national workshop was held during 1985 during which experts in pediatrics, infectious disease, otolaryngology, epidemiology, audiology, and biostatistics gathered to assess the current status of screening for otitis media in infants and children (Bluestone et al., 1986).

A principal problem that accompanies all cases of otitis media is hearing loss. Although usually mild in degree, the hearing loss may be the basis of an adverse effect upon the development of speech, language, and cognition of young children. (See Chapter 1 for a complete discussion of the developmental and educational aspects of otitis media.) Undoubtedly, many variables influence the outcome of otitis media upon the development of any young child. The potential seriousness of the consequences of unidentified and, therefore, untreated asymptomatic otitis media is too important to overlook. The sequela of otitis media with effusion that is of most concern to audiologists and educators is the suspected association between frequency occurrences of otitis media during early childhood and impaired speech and language development. Whether this association is valid has certainly been questioned by some researchers. Many believe that the overwhelming majority of cases of otitis media sooner or later subside spontaneously without lasting physical or developmental consequences. Nonetheless, although research continues, most speech-language specialists and audiologists believe that to wait for a definitive answer while doing nothing is an untenable position.

Because the hearing loss associated with otitis media is often episodic and mild, numerous issues concerning screening for middle ear disease exist. It is well-established that traditional pure tone hearing screening testing alone may miss as many as 70% of ears with pathologic findings (Melnick et al., 1964), and accordingly tympanometry has become a critical component of mass hearing screening programs. It must be admitted that mass screening with tympanometry may indeed produce overreferrals, i.e., children referred from screening programs to physicians who have found them to have normal middle ears on examination. But such findings are to be expected in light of the fact that otitis media with effusion is fluctuant and recurrent and that there is great seasonal variation in the presence and absence of the disorder. Immittance audiometry, especially tympa-

nometry, is an effective screening tool, although there seems to be disagreement about its precise role in various screening strategies. Tympanometry is easy to use, objective, efficient, acceptable to the screening population, inexpensive, and accurate in identifying those children with significant negative middle ear pressure and effusion. Whether or not the child will experience serious consequences if the otitis media disorder is left untreated is probably not a simple and easy question, since so many other variables have influence on the final outcome measures.

According to Bess and McConnell (1981), at least 16 states incorporate immittance as part of their recommended identification procedures. Consistent use of immittance screening is also evident in local educational agencies, day care centers, Head Start programs, well-baby clinics, and private primary care medical offices. Although there is no clear-cut resolution to the many questions that surround the immittance screening for middle ear disease and mild hearing loss controversy, the fact is that the technique has been a positive addition to hearing screening programs. To be sure, there is need for comprehensive, well-controlled research concerning the differential and cumulative effects of otitis media with effusion and mild conductive hearing loss.

In a report of the Fourth International Research Conference on Otitis Media (Lim, 1989), concern was expressed for the accurate identification of otitis media in those patients who are prelingual, patients without obvious symptoms, well babies, symptomatic infants and children, and at-risk groups. Recognizing the controversy regarding universal mass screening for otitis media, this report recommends that the real goals of screening should be the identification of the 10% of cases of otitis media that are truly chronic. Emphasis in screening should be directed toward settings in which early recognition may forestall educational sequela (as in infants) and those in which recognition of the problem by any other means is unlikely (such as under-served populations).

Although the International Otitis Media Report (Lim, 1989) endorses the ASHA Guidelines for Identification Audiometry (Asha, 1985) specific protocol, several additional suggestions are made that warrant careful consideration. A recommendation is offered to conduct hearing and middle ear screening (immittance screening) only during the initial year of school entry and 1 year later. This strategy will make screening more cost-effective and will survey children at the ages most likely to have unrecognized middle ear effusion. Screening of children 7 years of age or older is not likely to identify new cases of children with significant hearing loss.

The hearing and middle ear screening is suggested to be done at least biannually, preferably early in the school year and near the end of the school year. This is recommended for two reasons: (1) children with effusion early in the fall are more likely to have chronic, persistent effusion over the summer months; and (2) screening during the winter months is likely to identify cases associated with upper respiratory tract infections.

The International Otitis Media Report indicates that *bilateral* middle ear problem is the key condition being sought by pure tone and immittance screening and is grounds for an *immediate alerting letter* to parents with a recommendation for assessment by the family's primary care physician at the earliest opportunity. A child with a *unilateral* middle ear screening failure, by pure tone and immittance testing, should be rescreened at the next routine time. Two successive unilateral failures should result in an alerting letter to the parents. All children who fail, whether unilaterally or bilaterally, should be rescreened at every routine biannual screening examination.

HEARING SCREENING IN SCHOOL PROGRAMS

At school age the primary goal is to keep the child functioning adequately in the classroom, which means that it is necessary to identify the milder hearing loss caused by middle ear effusion. In the majority of school situations it is impossible to screen at levels lower than 20 dB HL because of the presence of ambient noise. Thus, the traditional pure tone screening tests must be supplemented by other tests such as acoustic immittance or acoustic reflectometry if educationally handicapping hearing losses are to be identified.

Pure Tone Screening Test. School hearing screening has a long and honorable history. As early as 1924 a group of dedicated otolaryngologists utilized and reported a new instrument for the testing and the hearing of school children (McFarlan, 1927). The instrument was developed for the Western Electric Company. The Western Electric 4-A audiometer was a phonograph, connected to an assembly of 30 earphones, that would simultaneously present well-calibrated speech signals to the earphones. In the Western Electric Fading Numbers test, numbers were spoken by both a man's and a woman's voice, starting at 33 dB and ending at 9 dB (re: normal threshold). The reason for the change to pure tone testing was that the gross speech signals used in the Western Electric test did not identify children with high-frequency losses.

Individual Pure Tone Sweep Test. In 1961 the Conference on Identification Audiometry of the American Speech and Hearing Association issued a monograph providing guidelines for school screening (Darley, 1961). It recommended individual pure tone screening as the most accurate procedure but started that group screening tests were less costly and could be used where cost is a factor. The Conference on Identification Audiometry recommended that four frequencies be tested: 1000, 2000, 4000, and 6000 Hz; 500 Hz was to be omitted because testing environments often produce too-high ambient noise levels.

Melnick et al. (1964) conducted a study, which utilized the Conference's recommendations, and found that the use of 6000 Hz as a test frequency produced too many failures. The variable interactions between earphones and children's ear canals at 6000 Hz make this test frequency a poor choice for inclusion in a school screening program.

A second set of Guidelines for Identification Audiometry was published by the ASHA in 1975. The Guidelines recommended a manually administered, individual, pure tone, air conduction hearing screening procedure with test frequencies of 1000, 2000, and 4000 Hz. The screening intensity level was 20 dB HL (re: ANSI 1969) at 1000 and 2000 Hz and 25 dB HL at 4000 Hz. It was recommended to screen at 20 dB HL at all three test frequencies, but if the 4000 Hz presentation was not heard, the intensity output was increased to 25 dB HL. Failure of the child to respond at the recommended screening level at any frequency in either ear was to be considered as failure of the screening test. All children who are "failures" were to be rescreened, preferably within the same testing session during which they failed, but definitely within 1 week.

The following referral priority scheme for audiologic evaluation was recommended in the 1975 Guidelines for those children who fail the screening and rescreening procedures:

1. Binaural hearing loss in both ears at all frequencies;
2. Binaural hearing loss at 1000 and 2000 Hz only;
3. Binaural hearing loss at 1000 or 2000 Hz only;
4. Monaural hearing loss at all frequencies;
5. Monaural hearing loss at 1000 and 2000 Hz;
6. Binaural or monaural hearing loss at 4000 Hz only.

The ASHA Guidelines for Identification Audiometry were designed with the basic assumption that hearing screening is often conducted in the relatively poor acoustic environments of schools and offices. Although the Guidelines detail specific procedures and protocols for screening hearing in children, it is pointed out that identification audiometry is only *one* part of a hearing conservation program. A well-planned program must go beyond initial hearing screening with consideration of rescreening, threshold audiometry, referral for audiologic and medical evaluations, education and counseling for parents and teachers, as well as commitment to follow-up procedure to ensure that adequate steps have been taken to alleviate or manage the hearing problem identified in each screening failure. Obviously, without concurrent follow-up programs, identification of hearing loss in children is a meaningless effort.

Recommended Hearing Screening Guidelines. The ASHA Guidelines for Identification Audiometry (1985) focus on children of third grade or younger, pointing out that these children are most at risk for hearing problems leading to educational, psychologic, and social problems. The pure tone screening procedure should be part of a program that includes acoustic immittance screening for identification of children with middle ear disorders. Individualized, manual, pure tone screening at 20 dB HL (re: ANSI-1969) should be conducted for each ear of every child. Recommended test frequencies include 1000, 2000, and 4000 Hz when the program is conducted in conjunction with acoustic immittance screening. If acoustic immittance is not part of the screening program, the test frequency of 500 Hz should be added, provided the ambient noise level does not exceed acceptable levels. Frequencies of 3000 and 6000 Hz should *not* be included in the pure tone hearing screening protocol (Table 7.11).

The failure criterion is failure of the child to respond to the recommended screening levels at any test frequency in either ear. All failures should be rescreened during the same session in which they failed or within a 2 week period of the initial screen. Failures on rescreening should be referred for audiologic evaluation by an audiologist with additional referrals as appropriate, based

Table 7.11.
ASHA 1985 Recommended Guidelines for Pure Tone Hearing Screening

Test Frequencies	Intensity Level	Pass-Fail Criteria
1000-2000-4000 Hz (with acoustic immittance) 500-1000-2000-4000 Hz (without acoustic immittance)	20 dB HL	Failure to respond at any test presentation in either ear

on the audiologist's findings. The ASHA Guidelines warn that the word "fail" should be avoided in reporting screening results to parents because of the negative connotation of the word. It must be remembered that many causes exist for "failing" hearing screening tests, and confirmation of the presence of hearing loss cannot be assumed until the audiometric evaluation is completed. Table 7.12 identifies a number of considerations that must be taken into account during any school hearing and immittance screening program.

A qualified audiologist should conduct or supervise the identification audiometry program, although nonprofessional support personnel may be used for the screening testing after appropriate training. The recommendations for audiologic and medical evaluations should be based on local realities and on the availability of referral sources.

The paperwork associated with a hearing screening program can be massive. Test forms, calibration data, student records, etc. must be carefully considered and planned prior to the testing sessions. The language used in notices sent to parents and referral physicians about screening or rescreening results should avoid diagnostic conclusions and alarming predictions. Remember that the hearing impairment is not confirmed until the stage of the audiometric evaluation has been completed. The Guidelines recommend speaking directly with the parents and child about test results, if possible, rather than written notices. Some parents will become overly concerned,

others will show little or no concern, and still others would like to cooperate but fear the potential expense that might be involved. If parents believe that their child can "hear," despite the results of the hearing screening, special tact and persuasion will be required to convince them that a problem truly exists. Because of its negative connotation, the word "fail" should be avoided in reporting hearing screening results. The reporting aspect of the identification audiometry program will require more time and thought than initially is anticipated. Detail concerning the operation of a school hearing screening program has recently been described by Feldman et al. (1981).

Rosenberg and Swogger-Rosenberg (1982) present an interesting discussion and review of the status of hearing screening procedures in each state of our country. They have compiled a list or, as they describe it, "a chaotic myriad of standards, regulations, guidelines, techniques and recommendations" that they gathered by survey. They noted that most states did have a hearing screening program of some sort but that the extraordinary range of screening techniques and policies is a sad commentary upon our ability to sell a health program in which we believe so strongly.

ACOUSTIC REFLECTOMETRY

A device known as the acoustic otoscope has been introduced as a simple, noninvasive screening instrument for identifying the presence of middle ear fluid in children (Fig. 7.9). Initially described by Teele and Teele (1984), the acoustic otoscope was designed to overcome the disadvantages of acoustic immittance measurement. The acoustic otoscope requires no hermetic seal at the ear canal and is effective even when the child is crying or when the ear canal is partially obscured with cerumen.

The acoustic otoscope generates a 100 msec multifrequency sweep between 20,000 and 4,500 Hz at 80 dB SPL. The pickup microphone measures the amplitude of the re-

Table 7.12.
Pitfalls to Avoid in Hearing Screening and Immittance Screening[a]

Hearing Screening Pitfalls

Child observing dials. This should be avoided at all times, because children will respond to the visual cues. The most appropriate position to seat the child is at an oblique angle, so the tester and audiometer are out of the child's peripheral vision.

Examiner giving visual cues (facial expression, eye or head movements, etc.).

Incorrect adjustment of the head band and earphone placement. Care must be taken to place the earphones carefully over the ears so that the protective screen mesh of the earphone diaphragm is directly over the entrance of the external auditory canal. Misplacement of the earphone by only 1 inch can cause as great as a 30–35 dB threshold shift.

Vague instructions.

Noise in the test area.

Overlong test sessions. The screening should require only 3–5 minutes. If a child requires significantly more time than this, the routine screening should be discontinued, and a short rest taken. If the child continues to be difficult to test, play conditioning should be used.

Too long or too short a presentation of the test tone. The test stimulus should be presented for 1–2 seconds. If the stimulus is for a shorter or longer time than this, inaccurate responses may be obtained.

Immittance Screening Pitfalls

Clogged probe and probe tip. The probe and probe tips must be kept free from earwax.

Probe tip too large or too small. Each ear canal is different and may require a different-sized probe tip. Utilization of the correct size for each child will avoid possible errors.

Head movement, swallowing, or eye-blinks. The child should be kept still during testing, as a sudden abnormal movement during testing may be interpreted as a reflex.

Probe tip against ear canal wall. The probe tip must be inserted directly into the ear canal, and when the canal is not straight, the tip must be kept away from the canal wall.

Debris in ear canal. The ear canal should be inspected before testing to ensure that it is clear.

[a]From R. J. Roeser and J. L. Northern: Screening for hearing loss and middle ear disorders. In R. J. Roeser and M. P. Downs (eds.): *Auditory Disorders in School Children*, ed. 2. New York, Thieme-Stratton, 1988, with permission.

flected probe tone from the plane of the tympanic membrane. The instrument

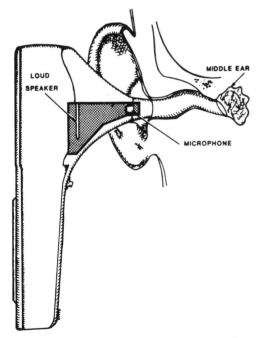

Figure 7.9.   Cross-section diagram of the acoustic re-flectometer (also known as the acoustic otoscope).

works on quarter-wavelength theory, so that the reflected wave completely cancels the principle wave in the external ear canal at a distance of one-quarter wavelength from the tympanic membrane. Thus, the reflected sound is inversely proportional to the total sound; a greater reflection produces a reduced amplitude suggestive of middle ear effusion.

To conduct the test, the examiner simply "aims" the speculum of the acoustic otoscope into the child's ear canal and presses the activator button. The instrument is positioned until the highest level of reflectometry is noted on a vertical display. Vertical display readings of 0–2 represent a normal middle ear; readings of 3–4 represent possible middle ear effusion; and readings greater than 5 indicate the presence of middle ear fluid.

Teele and Teele (1984) reported results from nearly 260 children examined with the acoustic otoscope. Their acoustic otoscope reflectivity sensitivity scores were 94% and 99% with specificity scores of 79% and 83%. These investigators concluded that acoustic reflectometry adds considerably to the screening tools currently available for identifying children with middle ear effusion. Lampe et al. (1985) compared results from acoustic reflectometry with tympanocentesis or myringotomy in 75 patients between 6 months and 13 years of age. They found a highly significant relationship between ears with middle ear effusion and reflectivity values of 5 or greater and ears with no middle ear effusion and reflectivity values of 4 or less. With a reflectivity reading of 5 or greater, the acoustic otoscope correctly identified nearly 87% of ears with middle ear effuson, and with a reading of 4 or less, it correctly identified 70% of ears without effusion. These authors found the reflectometry technique to be a valuable adjunct to current diagnostic tools because it is objective, rapid, and reliable irrespective of age, crying, cerumen, or lack of cooperation from the child.

A less positive report on the reflectometer was published by Buhrer et al. (1985), who evaluated 60 children with the acoustic reflectometer, pure tones, immittance, and otologic evaluation. They found reflectometry to be the least sensitive and least specific of the screening procedures. Their study differed from previous studies in that they used the acoustic otoscope in a general otologic clinic situation—not just for identifying the presence or absence of middle ear fluid. Buhrer et al. concluded that when the acoustic otoscope is used as intended, i.e., as a supplement to pneumatic otoscopy in the diagnosis of middle ear effusion, the test can be beneficial and can save clinical time.

Holmes et al. (1989) compared acoustic reflectometry with tympanometry in pediatric middle ear screening in 357 children. They found high positive sensitivity rates (correct identification of children with middle ear effusion) but low specificity rates (children failing tympanometry) with use of the acoustic otoscope. Unfortunately, the Holmes et al. study did not have medical confirmation of the presence or absence of pathology in the children.

A thorough evaluation of the acoustic otoscope in children was reported by Schwartz and Schwartz (1987) from a cohort of 511 ears of 256 children seen in a private practice pediatric office. The ages of the children ranged from 2 months to 14 years. Schwartz and Schwartz applied decision-making analyses and established receiver operating characteristic curves in a large sample of 160 children to illustrate the effects of various cutoff criteria on true and false positive rates for reflectometry and tympanometry. For example, consistent with the manufacturer's suggestion, the cutoff criterion of 5 provides a sensitivity rate of 88% and a specificity rate of 83%. They noted that the length measurement provided by the acoustic otoscope has no clinical usefulness. Schwartz and Schwartz concluded that the acoustic otoscope complements traditional methods for detecting middle ear fluid in otherwise asymptomatic children. They caution, however, that the acoustic otoscope should not be used as a technique to diagnose general pathologies of the ear.

The acoustic reflectometer has received considerable attention regarding its potential as a screening device for otitis media. It should be noted that the device requires little training or skill in its use, but given the diverse range of results, considerable caution must be used in interpretation, since no single value may be used as a threshold for the presence or absence of effusion. Further research and technologic development are necessary to establish the role of acoustic reflectometry in the screening and clinical practice.

IMMITTANCE SCREENING

The evaluation of children in hearing screening programs has changed considerably with the use of audiometry. The immittance technique is well-suited to use with children, since it requires little cooperation, provides objective results, and is quick and easy to administer. However, considerable controversy has arisen about the use of immittance measurements in school screening programs. Brooks (1969, 1973, 1975) has long and often advocated the use of acoustic immittance measurement as a supplement to the standard pure tone hearing screening test in school populations. A large number of studies have been conducted to compare the efficacy of immittance screening in the identification of hearing problems in children. A comprehensive review of the status of this topic was published by Brooks in 1980.

The debate about the role of immittance screening was summarized in two points of view by Bess (1980) and Northern (1980b). Much of the discussion presented below has been taken from these two reports.

The goal of a hearing screening program is to identify those individuals who probably have some hearing problem from those individuals who probably do not have a hearing problem. Children who "fail" the screening tests may or may not have ear problems and are thus "tagged" for additional testing to determine the cause of screening failure. Virtually every state has an active hearing screening program, and for nearly 40 years hearing screening has proven to be one of the most acceptable screening procedures in a multitude of health detection programs. Unfortunately, traditional pure tone techniques for screening hearing fail to identify numerous persons who have mild hearing loss often due to the presence of middle ear disease.

The single "bright light" in the history of auditory screening has been the development of acoustic immittance measurements. It is only natural that the vast numbers of persons responsible for hearing screening programs utilize the best testing techniques to identify children with hearing disorders. The immittance technique is capable of yielding more accurate screening results in the identification of middle ear disease than is possible with otoscopy or pure tone audiometry—a firm fact substantiated in numerous studies.

Professionals active in hearing screening are well aware of the inadequacies of pure tone screening audiometry and thus welcome the opportunity to supplement their test protocol with immittance screening. The use of immittance in conjunction with pure tone hearing testing increases the overall accuracy of the screening program, reduces the number of children who must be retested prior to referral, and, in fact, increases assurance that children who are referred for additional workup have legitimate otologic problems.

Opponents to the use of immittance in mass screening raise legitimate concern that the technique will identify asymptomatic persons who have fluctuant otitis media with effusion for which specific treatment may be inadvisable. Although the otitis media with middle ear effusion may resolve spontaneously in many individuals, undetected and untreated middle ear effusions may, indeed, create serious otologic complications, speech, language, and/or educational problems. Medical complications from otitis media include sensorineural hearing loss, ossicular fixation through adhesions, tympanic membrane perforations and/or retraction pockets, cholesteatoma, ossicular necrosis, mastoiditis, and even meningitis. Although specific treatment may not be in order for every person with middle ear effusion, certainly accurate identification of such persons is desirable and easily within our technical means.

As shown by Cooper et al. (1975) and Queen et al. (1981), immittance screening is economically the most cost-effective technique for sampling asymptomatic children to identify those children who have middle ear problems. Immittance screening is not intended to be a diagnostic procedure; nor is isolated immittance screening advocated without support from audiometry and/or otoscopic examination. Not only immittance screening will identify those persons who have otitis media with effusion, but the technique is also sensitive to all the complications or sequelae of otitis media.

Immittance Validity. Much discussion has been published questioning the validity of immittance screening. Validity is determined by examining the sensitivity and specificity of a screening technique. *Sensitivity* is defined as accuracy in identifying persons who have the target condition. *Specificity* is the accuracy of the technique in identifying nondiseased persons. Knowledgeable professionals cannot deny the high sensitivity of immittance screening in correctly identifying persons with low sensitivity of pure tone screening. For example, statistics have shown that pure tone screening missed 259 of 1651 tympanic membrane perforations (17%) and failed to identify 33 of 60 (55%) cholesteatomas (Northern, 1977a). However, the major criticism of immittance screening relates to its low specificity, i.e., the false identification of persons who do not have middle ear disease.

Admittedly the monumental number of articles published about immittance screening provides little conclusive data for establishing validity credentials. To determine validity of a screening technique, one screening procedure is used as a criterion measure against which to compare other screening tests. Otoscopy is most often accepted as the criterion test against which to compare screening, in spite of the fact that the accuracy of otoscopy varies tremendously as a function of the person behind the otoscope (Paradise et al., 1976; Roeser et al., 1977). Otoscopy is so subjective it can be argued that immittance should be the criterion procedure because of its objectivity and test-retest reliability. Generally, the use of otoscopy as the criterion produces higher sensitivity agreement, since fewer subjects "fail" otoscopy, while many subjects may "fail" screening.

Paradise and Smith (1979) analyzed 14 published studies of immittance screening in preschool children and found that only 2 studies provided ample data from which to calculate validity. In the two cited studies (Paradise et al., 1976; Roeser et al., 1977), immittance sensitivity with otoscopy as the criterion measure was 94% and 97%, respectively, while specificity was 42% and

61%, respectively. The amount of pathology in the sample population affects the sensitivity rate, since it is easy to obtain high agreement between immittance and otoscopy when many normal subjects are examined. The low specificity rates of immittance audiometry are most often due to the use of too-rigid failure criteria for peaked negative pressure curves. Adherence to middle ear pressure failure criteria of -200 mm H_2O should do much to alleviate the overreferral and low specificity problem.

Of course, the ultimate validation technique for middle ear effusion is myringotomy. The studies reported by Orchik et al. (1978a, 1978b) with immittance and myringotomy in 218 ears have shown that the combined use of tympanometry and acoustic reflex measurement showed a statistically significant correlation with the presence of middle ear fluid. Their studies, as well as the report by Paradise et al. (1976), show the correlation between "flat" impedance curves and the presence of effusion proven by myringotomy to be 82–90% accurate. This high correlation between "flat" impedance curves and absent acoustic reflexes speaks highly for referral and medical evaluation of such children.

Additional research of this sort is important if we hope to establish the positive and negative attributes of immittance as a screening test. The importance of the sensitivity-specificity relationship, with various combinations of immittance measures used in a number of childhood populations, cannot be overemphasized. Our goal should be to establish a cutoff that can identify most children with disease but does not result in overreferral. Although abnormal tympanograms appear to be associated with a diseased ear, normal tympanograms do not necessarily imply a nondiseased ear.

Recognizing that many screening programs were already in operation and that others were soon to be implemented, procedural guidelines and criteria to be used in the screening of preschool and school-age children have been developed. The Nash-

Table 7.13.
Nashville Task Force Classifications and Criteria[a]

Classification	Initial Screen	Retest	Subject Outcome
I	Acoustic reflex present and tympanogram normal	Not required	Cleared
II	Acoustic reflex absent and/or tympanogram abnormal	Acoustic reflex absent and/or tympanogram abnormal	Referred
III	Acoustic reflex absent and/or tympanogram abnormal	Acoustic reflex present and tympanogram normal	At risk; recheck at later date

[a]From E. R. Harford et al.: *Impedance Screening for Middle Ear Disease in Children.* New York, Grune & Stratton, 1978, p. 6.

ville Task Force (Harford et al., 1978) hoped that the data collected from screening programs already in existence would be obtained in a uniform and systematic manner and that such data could be used to refine future guidelines. Toward this end, the classification scheme shown in Table 7.13 was developed for various screening results. Failure on the initial screening test is determined by an absent acoustic reflex at 1000 Hz (presented at 105 dB HL in the contralateral mode) or by an abnormal tympanogram. An abnormal tympanogram is defined as one that is either flat or rounded, having no discernable peak, or one that has a negative pressure equivalent to or greater than −200 mm H_2O. It was recommended that any child who failed the initial screening be retested in 4–6 weeks. Classification 1 is represented by a pass on the initial screening, whereas classifications 2 and 3 are for those children who fail the initial test. As denoted by classification 2, referral is made to an appropriate health care provider if the child fails the retest. A child who passes the retest, as designated by classification 3, is categorized as "at risk," and a close monitoring program is recommended.

An alternative set of screening guidelines was developed by the American Speech and Hearing Association (1978). In these guidelines, not only was the need to identify middle ear disease based on medical considerations, but much emphasis was also placed on the possible educational, social, and psychologic sequelae. Although the procedural considerations for both sets of recommen-

dations are remarkably similar, the American Speech and Hearing Association guidelines differ from the Nashville Task Force recommendations in two significant ways. First, the American Speech and Hearing Association guidelines refrain from making any value judgments pertaining to the need for mass screening. That is, they neither recommend nor oppose immittance screening on a routine basis for the detection of middle ear disorders in children. Rather, procedural guidelines are merely outlined for those who wish to implement a screening program. Second, the referral criteria of the American Speech and Hearing Association guidelines differ from the Nashville Task Force recommendations. The middle ear screening criteria advocated by the American Speech and Hearing Association are summarized in Table 7.14. Although somewhat more detail is provided, the "pass" and "risk" classifications do not differ significantly from the Nashville Task Force scheme. The "fail" classification, however, is considerably different, in that a failure in the initial screen results in an immediate referral. Recall that the Nashville Task Force recommended a retest in 4–6 weeks following a fail on the initial screen.

Lucker (1980) reported results of a screening project in which the American Speech and Hearing Association guidelines were followed and pass/fail criteria were applied after a single test session. A pilot project so conducted yielded a large number of failures, many of whom were not found to have middle ear disorders when examined by their physicians within 2

Table 7.14.
American Speech and Language Association Guidelines and Middle Ear Screening Criteria[a]

Classification	Screening Pass/Fail Criteria Results of Initial Screen	Disposition
1. Pass	Middle ear pressure normal or mildly positive/negative and acoustic reflex (AR) present	Cleared; no return
2. At risk	Middle ear pressure abnormal (and acoustic reflex present) or Acoustic reflex absent (and middle ear pressure normal or mildly positive/negative)	Retest in 3-5 weeks (a) if tympanometry and AR fall into Classification 1: PASS; (b) If tympanometry or AR remain in Classification 2: Fail and refer
3. Fail	Middle ear pressure abnormal and Acoustic reflex absent	Refer

[a]American Speech-Language-Hearing Association: Guidelines for acoustic immittance screening of middle-ear function. *Asha* 21:283-288, 1979.

weeks from the date of referral. Lucker was able to reduce the number of failures in the immittance screening program by altering the guideline pass/fail criteria by retesting all the children in the "fail" category 1–2 weeks following the initial screening prior to referral.

Queen et al. (1981) reported results of an immittance screening project conducted in the Kansas City, Missouri, Public School District involving nearly 20,000 elementary students. Although they attempted to utilize the American Speech and Hearing Association guidelines, they soon found need to delete the acoustic reflex from the test procedure except in "borderline" cases, i.e., -200 mm H_2O middle ear pressure. They also combined the recommended AT RISK and FAIL categories into a simple REFERRAL category for retesting at a later date. They report that their initial retest rate was 17%, compared with a 25% rate reported by Lucker (1980). They finally identified 6.2% of their total elementary population for further audiologic evaluation.

Roush and Tait (1985) examined 75 3 and 4 year old children with pure tone and acoustic immittance measures. Their results confirmed that pure tone audiometry was not effective as a means to identify otologic abnormalities and that the 1979 Guidelines for Acoustic Immittance Screening are likely to result in an excessive number of false positive medical referrals.

Guidelines for Screening for Hearing Impairment and Middle Ear Disorders were published by ASHA in 1990. This revised set of guidelines incorporates the 1985 Guidelines for Identification Audiometry with a new protocol for identifying persons with potentially medically significant ear disorders that have been undetected or untreated. This new immittance protocol is written to incorporate standard terminology for aural acoustic immittance measurements, as well as to acknowledge improved technologic advances in instrumentation.

To avoid the excessive overreferral rates that characterized earlier screening protocols based solely on tympanometry and acoustic reflex measurement, the 1990 screening protocol includes four sources of data for each child: (*1*) history of recent occurrence of otalgia (ear pain) or otorrhea (ear discharge) is cause for immediate medical referral; (*2*) visual inspection of structural defects of the ear, head, and neck, ear canal abnormalities, or eardrum abnormalities that may require medical referral; (*3*) identification audiometry in accordance with the 1985 manual pure tone screening protocol; and (*4*) acoustic immittance measurements. This screening protocol is summarized in Table 7.15 and Figure 7.10.

The current state of affairs in immittance screening programs is that we now have three significant sets of guidelines for those school clinicians who wish to include immittance measurements as part of the hearing

Table 7.15.
Referral Criteria, ASHA (1990)

I. History
  A. Otalgia
  B. Otorrhea
II. Visual Inspection of the Ear
  A. Structural defect of the ear, head, or neck
  B. Ear canal abnormalities
    1. Blood or effusion
    2. Occlusion
    3. Inflammation
    4. Excessive cerumen, tumor, foreign material
  C. Eardrum abnormalities
    1. Abnormal color
    2. Bulging eardrum
    3. Fluid line or bubbles
    4. Perforation
    5. Retraction
III. Identification Audiometry—Fail air conduction screening at 20 dB HL at 1, 2, or 4 kHz in either ear (ASHA, 1985; these criteria may require alteration for various clinical settings and populations).
IV. Tympanometry
  A. Flat tympanogram and equivalent ear canal volume (Vec) outside normal range
  B. Low static admittance (Peak Y) on two successive occurrences in a 4–6 week interval
  C. Abnormally wide tympanometric width (TW) on two successive occurrences in a 4–6 week interval

screening program. There is still an urgent need, however, for carefully planned and rigorously controlled scientific screening projects to clarify further the benefits and limitations of immittance screening. Further, there is need to gather additional data on the natural history, medical management, and educational complications of middle ear effusions.

AUDITORY SCREENING OF THE MENTALLY DELAYED

Standards for institutions serving the mentally retarded as set forth by the Accreditation Council for Facilities for the Mentally Retarded provide operational guidelines for audiology services. In reference to audiometric screening, the standards state that all new residents, children under 10 at annual intervals, other residents at regular intervals, and any resident referred shall be screened. In addition, many facilities provide outpatient evaluation and services including audiometric screening. As a result, audiologists in such facilities are finding themselves faced with great numbers of retarded, of all ages and functioning levels, for audiometric screening.

Comprehensive audiologic assessment implies pure tone thresholds, speech audiometry, and any other significant diagnostic information obtainable. However, when large number of mentally retarded are involved, the need for a more efficient method of screening becomes evident. A variety of conditioning techniques, evoked response audiometry, special diagnostic procedures, and other auditory assessment techniques have been suggested; although these may be reliable clinical tools, the technical problems of applying them to rapid mass screening have not been resolved. Subjective approaches that employ behavioral observation alone give limited information and no indication of cause of hearing loss.

We have developed a screening procedure for the retarded that is based on behavioral observation as a function of mental age (Downs, 1970) and acoustic immittance audiometry (Lamb and Norris, 1970; Northern, 1971a, 1978c, 1980d). Our screening technique is designed for use with the severely and profoundly retarded and other patients who would be classified as difficult to test. It is not proposed as a substitute for pure tone screening when pure tone results are obtainable within the limitations of a screening program. Rather, it is designed to use when traditional clinical assessment techniques are not applicable.

The subject is seated or held in the sound suite facing one speaker. Initially the stimulus is presented through the opposite speaker so that if the subject localizes he or she must make an overt lateralization, which is very obvious, to seek the sound from the speaker furthest away. If he or she localizes, as soon as his or her head is turned toward the speaker, the examiner quickly switches the signal to the other side. Speech is primarily used as the sound

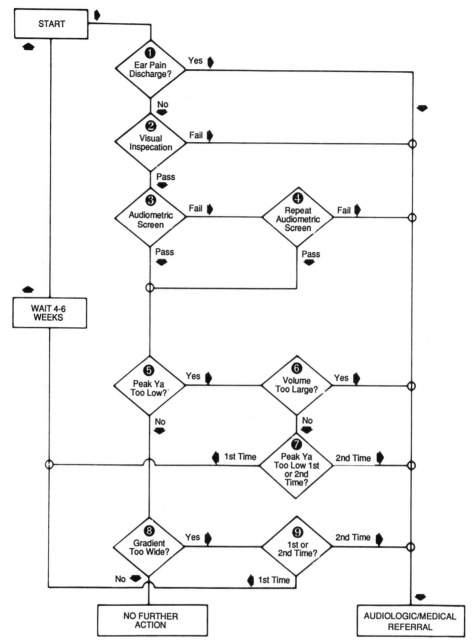

Figure 7.10. Flow chart for determination of the need for audiological/medical referral incorporating case history, visual inspection, pure tone audiometry, and tympanometry. The flow chart represents the logic used to determine the need for referral but does not indicate the order of test procedures to be followed. Each *numbered box* is discussed in the text.

stimulus, but a variety of other stimuli can be employed. It is sometimes necessary to change the stimuli during testing to pure tones, warble tones, white noise, or complex noise.

Observations are made by an audiologist and, if possible, trained observers. Response categories include: (*1*) responses that indicate awareness such as eye opening, quieting, assuming a listening attitude, smiling, laughing, cessation of activity; (*2*) localization responses, which are the overt learned responses that take the place of generalized body movements as the child matures; (*3*) startle responses, which are the involuntary reflexive responses that are expected 65 to 85 dB above threshold and include eye-blink, orientation reflex, tonic neck reflex, Moro reflex; and (*4*) no response.

- Auditory Screening of Mentally Delayed Children
  (1) An ascending approach should be employed in an attempt to obtain response from the person at levels of 45 dB HL or better. Awareness, or preferably localization by 45 dB HL, constitutes passing the observational portion of the screening.
  (2) If no response is obtained by 45 dB, ascend in 10 dB steps in an attempt to elicit a response. It is necessary to vary the time between presentations in an attempt to catch the person off guard. If the person shows awareness or localizes by 65 dB HL and a startle can be elicited, it may be concluded that he or she either has grossly normal hearing or a mild-to-moderate hearing loss.

(3) Even when a subject shows awareness and/or localization at levels below 45 dB, an attempt is made to elicit a startle. If no startle is obtainable, the person fails screening and probably has a hearing loss. Even as the examiner attempts to elicit a startle at high intensity levels, it is important to continue to watch for awareness and/or localization responses. Responses at these levels will provide inferences about auditory sensitivity.

(4) The final step in the screening procedure is immittance audiometry. Tympanograms and acoustic reflexes, if possible, are obtained bilaterally. The objective measurements obtained with the immittance audiometer not only rule out or establish conductive problems but also serve as an objective means of examining the more difficult-to-test students.

Operant conditioning techniques as described in Chapter 5 may also be used as hearing screening methods for the mentally retarded.

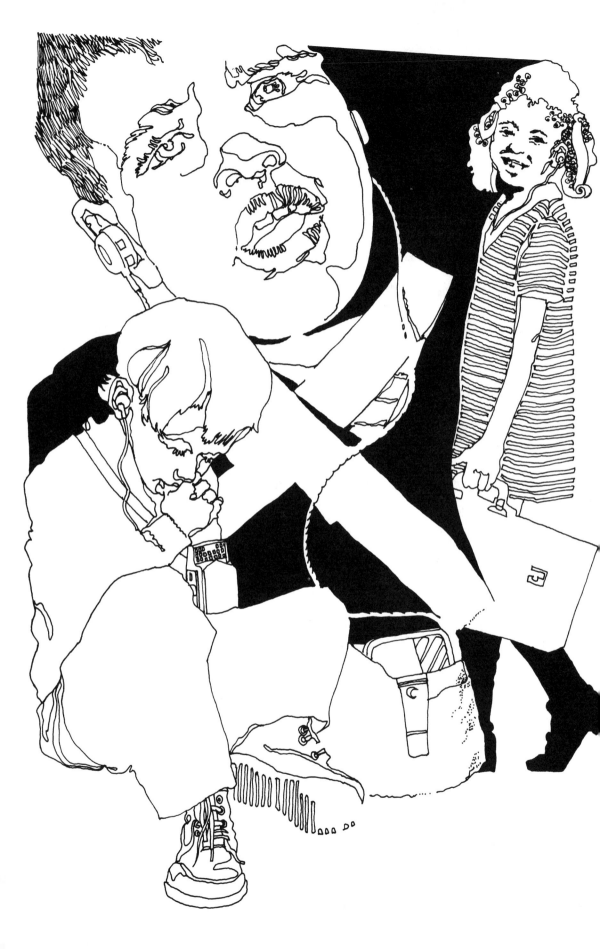

CHAPTER 8

Amplification for Hearing-Impaired Children

HEARING AIDS FOR CHILDREN

There is little doubt that the single most important invention to help the hearing-handicapped child is the amplifying hearing aid. There is an old adage, "as we hear, so shall we speak," and it is this very close relationship between hearing, speech, and language that is so important to the deaf child. New technology has been developed to help the deaf child learn to speak, including voice pitch indicators, speech timing equipment, vowel indicators, voice/non-voice meters, speech spectrum displays, and visible speech machines. None of these devices, however, is more fundamental to the hearing-impaired child's education and ability to learn speech than the properly fitted hearing aid.

The task of selecting and fitting hearing aids for a child is not to be taken lightly. Selection and fitting of hearing aids for the hearing-impaired or deaf child must not be undertaken by the inexperienced clinician or the nonprofessionally trained individual. The procedure involved in the process of selecting hearing aids for a child involves many people including the otolaryngologist, the pediatrician, the audiologist/dispenser, the speech/language pathologist, the teacher of the deaf, and other auxiliary professionals, such as the public health or school nurse and the social worker. These individuals must work together more closely, in a coordinated effort, to ensure that the hearing-impaired child obtains maximal benefit from amplification.

The audiologist is clearly the individual to coordinate and guide the hearing aid se-

lection procedure. The audiologist is able to identify the nature and degree of the child's hearing loss, which may in itself be a challenging task. The audiologist ensures that proper medical clearance is obtained prior to the hearing aid selection procedure. The audiologist is able to evaluate the performance of various hearing aids on the child, make an earmold impression, and select and dispense the hearing aids to obtain the best amplification available for the child's hearing loss. As part of this process, the audiologist counsels the parents about the new hearing aids and their care and use and arranges for therapy for the child and special training if necessary. Finally, the audiologist is able to devote the necessary time to follow up the progress of the patient and to maintain an ever-vigilant eye to be sure the hearing aids are in top operating condition. The audiologist must be careful not to use the hearing aids as a device to test a youngster's hearing, as it is no substitute for an accurate, knowledgeable hearing assessment. Do not confuse the situation by mixing the audiometric evaluation with the hearing aid evaluation.

Although acoustic immittance (impedance) measurements have long been recommended for routine inclusion in every hearing evaluation, only in the past few years have clinicians recognized the importance of acoustic immittance measurements in hearing aid management. Acoustic immittance testing should precede *every* hearing aid evaluation session. Rubin (1976) cited the importance of immittance measurements with hearing-impaired children because of the high incidence of middle ear pathology. She reported that 50% of the hearing-impaired toddlers and babies in the Lexington Infant Center had cases of middle ear effusion during a 1 year period. Thorough discussions of immittance measurements and their utilization in hearing aid clinical practice may be found in materials published by Northern (1978a) and McCandless and Keith (1980).

Clinical hearing aid evaluations with children should include ample consideration for therapy. Time for thorough preparation is involved in the preselection hearing aid workup for the hearing-impaired child. Nearly as much time may then be necessary to select the proper hearing aid and earmold. Additional telephone calls and letters may be necessary to appropriate agencies to obtain financial assistance for the purchase of the aid. Electroacoustic analysis of the hearing aids is important to confirm optimal operation of the hearing instrument. But the time consumed by these procedures is only fleeting seconds, when compared with the long-term therapy and follow-up programs that the child will need through the remainder of the school years.

Tremendous technologic advances in the hearing aid have been made over the past three decades. Only a few years ago, hearing aids were heavy, cumbersome units with large, unsightly battery requirements. The electronic hearing aid became a reality in the 1930s; the vacuum tube became part of the system in the 1940s; transistors permitted the hearing aid to be a much smaller unit in the 1950s. Today, tiny "solid state" electronic devices have reduced the instrument and its power source to a practical size and weight. Developments in the microphone component of the hearing aid have extended both ends of the frequency reproduction range. Microphones are now available that are truly directional—amplifying only sounds that are immediately in front of the hearing aid and at the same time attenuating sounds emitted from the sides or back of the listener.

The operation of the hearing aid has been likened to a miniature high-fidelity set made up of a group of tiny components that picks up sound wave vibrations from the air and converts them into electrical signals. Actually, modern hearing aids are much more than just ultraminiature electroacoustic amplifiers. They are sophisticated personal signal processing systems comprising not only the hearing instrument itself but also a technically elaborate acoustic coupling system that plays a significant role in processing and modification of the acoustic signal, as well as conducting the signal to the tympanic membrane (Ely, 1981). Although the major amplification, signal limiting, and complex controlling functions are achieved within the hearing aid itself, spectral shaping takes place not only in the hearing aid but also in the acoustic coupling system, which includes the earmold, earhook, and tubing.

Most hearing aids operate through three basic components as shown in Figure 8.1. Sound from the environment enters the hearing aid through a *microphone*, which changes the acoustic (sound) signals into electrical signals. The electrical signal is enhanced, or increased in intensity, through an *amplifier*. The amplified electrical signal is then passed through the *receiver*, which changes the signal back into amplified acoustic sound. The amplified acoustic sound is delivered into the user's ear canal through some type of earmold. The hearing aid system is powered by a small battery.

The continued development of digital-based hearing aids will likely have a significant impact on personal amplification. We can expect major changes in the physical hardware and appearance of hearing aids, accompanied by computerized evaluation techniques to ensure improved fitting protocols. Advanced signal processing technology will, it is hoped, improve aided performance. These new hearing aids will utilize programmable settings and adjustments, so that very specific prescriptive fittings can be applied to each individual hearing loss and audiometric configuration. Each hearing aid will literally be as adjustable as the wide variety of settings and mod-

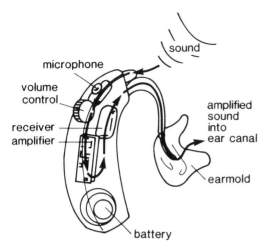

microphone

volume
control

receiver

amplifier

sound

amplified
sound
into
ear canal

earmold

battery

Figure 8.1. Components of a contemporary behind-the-ear hearing aid.

els now offered by each manufacturer. Although this new technology will be developed initially for adult users, the long-term benefit to hearing-impaired children will be most valuable.

A large number of textbooks concerning all aspects of hearing aids are now available to the interested reader. Readers interested in more information about hearing aids are referred to Pollack (1988), Hodgson (1986), Skinner (1988), or Sandlin (1988, 1990).

Persons working with children who use hearing aids are familiar with the wide variety of occurrences and bizarre experiences that can render the hearing aid inoperable. Zink (1972) reported results from a 2 year longitudinal electroacoustic hearing aid program of analysis of aids worn by children. He warned that just because a child wears his or her hearing aid faithfully, the assumption cannot be made that the aid is functioning adequately. In the evaluation of 92 hearing aids in use by children, only 55% were found to be acceptable. Zink recommends that each amplification unit in regular use receive regular longitudinal electroacoustic analysis. Potts and Greenwood (1983) described a daily hearing aid monitoring program, the results of which created a significant decrease in the incidence of hearing aid malfunction in their school.

The program was based on a detailed visual-auditory inspection (Table 8.1) and routine electroacoustic analysis. These authors commented that the increased emphasis on hearing aid performance appeared to promote other improvements in the child's utilization of amplification.

The regulations of the recent Education for All Handicapped Children Act of 1975 (Public Law 94-142) state that each public agency shall ensure that hearing aids worn by hearing-impaired students in school are functioning properly (*Federal Register*, August 23, 1977, 121a.303). Bendet (1980) reported a successful public school hearing aid maintenance program carried out by the teachers of the hearing-impaired students. Woodford (1987) published results of a survey indicating that the majority of speech/language pathologists lack the basic knowledge and skills necessary to provide help with amplification to aided hearing-impaired students.

Food and Drug Administration regulations were put into effect in August 1977 for the protection of potential hearing aid consumers. These regulations include the following rules related to hearing aids for children:

- Before purchase of a hearing aid, an individual with a hearing loss must have a medical evaluation of the hearing loss by a physician (preferably a physician specializing in diseases of the ear) within 6 months preceding the sale of the aid.

- Adult patients, under carefully defined circumstances, can sign a waiver of the medical clearance requirements. However, there is no waiver option of persons under 18 years of age. The physician who examines the child must provide a written statement that the patient's hearing loss has been medically evaluated.

- In addition to seeing a physician for a medical evaluation, a child with a hearing loss should be directed to an audiologist for evaluation and rehabilitation, since hearing loss may cause problems in lan-

Table 8.1.
Total Looking/Listening Check for Hearing Aids[a]

Remove aid from child, noting "as worn" volume setting.

Component	Looking	Listening (use sounds /a/ /u/ /i/ /ʃ/ /s/)
Earmold	Opening clear? Cracks, rough areas?	
Battery	Read voltage (replace at 1.1 or below)—Compartment clean?	
Case	Cracks? Separating?	Press case gently—Interruption in amplification?
Microphone	Clean? Visible damage?	
Dials	Clean? Easily rotated?	Rotate—Reasonable gain variation: Static?
Switches	Clean? Easy to move?	Turn on and off—Static?
Cord (body aid)	Cracked? Frayed? Connection plugs clean?	Run fingers down cord—Interruption in amplification? Connections tight?
Tubing (ear-level aid)	Cracks? Good connection to mold and aid? Moisture? Debris?	Cover opening of earmold and turn to maximum gain—Feedback?
Receiver (body aid)	Cracks? Firmly attached to earmold snap ring?	Distortion? Static? Reduced gain? Substitute spare receiver and recheck.
Oscillator (bone aid)	Cracks? Plug clean? Attached well to band?	Listen with oscillator on mastoid, ears plugged to block air-conducted sound.
Variable Controls	Proper SSPL[b], frequency response, gain setting?	5 speech sounds clearly amplified? Gain sounds normal for this aid?
Distortion		Clear quality?
Feedback	Recheck receiver snap, tubing, earmold.	Turn to maximum gain to check—External feedback? Internal?

Replace aid and check fit of the earmold to the child's ear.

[a]From P. Potts and J. Greenwood: Hearing aid monitoring. *Language, Speech and Hearing Services in Schools* 14:163, 1983.
[b]SSPL, saturated sound pressure level.

guage development and the educational and social growth of a child.

Basic to the concept of hearing aid recommendations is a realistic understanding of what the aid can do for the patient. No hearing aid will enable a hard-of-hearing youngster to perform normally in *all* situations. The primary reason for recommending the use of personal amplification is to enable the child to communicate better with a hearing aid than without it. Such improvement may be possible in only a few select conditions for a child, but he or she will ultimately learn, with good teaching, to utilize the aid to its maximal benefit. In the words of Mark Ross (1969). "merely because one can 'get along' without a hearing aid is *not* an adequate reason to discourage its use."

Curran (1982) described four basic factors for successful hearing aid fittings that may be applied to children: (*1*) He identified the importance of the case history and basic hearing evaluation to confirm the patient's hearing status and qualify his or her candidacy for amplification. (*2*) The method for selection of the hearing aid is often a function of the experience of the audiologist. Although no specific method provides exact, precise information regarding the correct amount of gain, output, or frequency response, final selection may be influenced by ergonomic characteristics such as motor skills of the child, cosmetic considerations, manipulation of trimmer controls, availability of options, and, of course, cost. (*3*) The third important factor is to use instruments that have a wide range of adjustable trimmers such as a saturated sound pressure level (SSPL) reduction control, a low-cut tone control of at least 15 dB at 500 Hz, a gain trimmer, a high-frequency roll-off trimmer, and compression adjustments. The wide range of adjustments is especially valuable in children's fittings because of the questionable hearing threshold measurements and the fact that the patient's listening skills will change over time after the hearing aids are fitted. (*4*) The fourth factor to consider is modifications to the hearing aid coupling system. All parts of the coupling system, including the earmold, tubing, and earhook, are under direct control of the dispenser of the hearing aid. Small, almost imperceptible changes in the physical dimensions of the earmold and associated "plumbing" system can produce significant auditory changes in the response of the hearing aid system.

The selection of children's hearing aids requires some special consideration. The hearing aid must have maximum performance flexibility, so that a significant range of adjustments and modifications can be made without the need to purchase new hearing aids as the child's needs develop. Telecoil circuitry may be included to allow the hearing aid to accept sound conveyed by magnetic signals as picked up from a telephone receiver or other special assistive listening aids. The telecoil microphone picks up magnetic signals while not amplifying background noise. Some hearing aids have a special microphone-telecoil two-position switch to change from the normal microphone use to the special telecoil microphone when compatible telephone receivers are being used. Children's hearing aids should always have the capability for direct audio input (DAI), which allows for direct connection of the hearing aid to a telephone receiver, radio, television, movie projector, stereo, or other assistive listening system. Common wisdom requires that a child's hearing aid be exceedingly durable, and of course, consideration should be given to a protection plan for extended warranty, loss, or damage.

Young children have not developed a "listening strategy," and it is important to re-emphasize that the hearing aid evaluation in children is a continuing process. Other factors to be considered require the best possible amplified signal with good quality and clear sound. This *must* be checked electroacoustically and with real-ear measurements by the audiologist/dispenser for *every* hearing aid on *every* child at *every* clinic visit. Townsend and Olsen (1982) reported that only 69% of new hearing aid instruments they evaluated met the manufac-

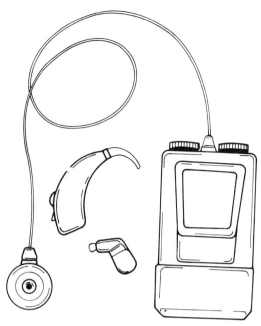

Figure 8.2. The three basic types of hearing aids are shown: a body-worn instrument, an all-in-the-ear hearing aid, and a behind-the-ear hearing aid.

turer's specifications, which stresses the need for electroacoustic analysis with all new hearing aids.

TYPES OF HEARING AIDS

Body-Type Hearing Aids. The on-the-body model of hearing aids has a relatively large microphone, amplifier, and power supply enclosed in a case attached to the clothing, placed in a pocket, or carried in a harness around the chest (Fig. 8.2). An external receiver attaches directly to the earmold and is driven by power supplied through a thin flexible wire from the instrument case. Body-type hearing aids usually provide greater gain and power output than ear-level instruments. Since the microphone and receiver are separated by considerable distance, the probability of acoustic feedback (or squeal) from amplified sound that leaks out around the earmold and "feeds back" into the microphone of the hearing aid is reduced.

Body-type hearing aids are now less often recommended for children because of current improvements in ear-level hearing aids. In spite of their size, bulk, and cord, body aids can be firmly carried by young children in garment-type carrier harnesses. The body aid is more durable and less likely to be broken than ear-level instruments. The external controls are easier to adjust, although this often creates problems with children who play with the aids or inadvertently turn the hearing aid volume down or shut it off. Body-type hearing aids may be recommended for children too often, with not enough consideration given to ear-level instruments. We reserve the fitting of body-type hearing aids to children with congenital anomalies of the pinna and ear canal, children with multiple handicaps in addition to hearing loss, and other special situations where ear-level hearing aids cannot be used.

Ear-Level Hearing Aids. Ear-level instruments include behind-the-ear models, eyeglass models, or all-in-the-ear (ITE) aids, and the new all-in-the-ear-canal aids (ITC). The ITE and ITC instruments fit directly into the ear canal. They have no external wires or tubes and are very lightweight. They are generally used for patients of all degrees of hearing loss, from mild to severe. The ITE and ITC instruments may be used with children and adults (Fig. 8.2).

The behind-the-ear model hearing aid has all its components housed in one curved case that fits neatly behind the pinna and rests against the mastoid surface. A short plastic tube connects the earmold to the hearing aid case. Ear-level hearing aids are nearly as powerful as body-type aids and deliver up to 70 dB full-on gain and 125–130 dB SSPL. Since the microphone and receiver are in the same case and in very close proximity to the earmold, increased opportunity exists for acoustic feedback.

Ear-level hearing aids (behind-the-ear, ITE, and ITC) have been the most popular type of amplification instrument since the 1960s. This type of aid is less conspicuous than the body hearing aid; it does not amplify clothing noise, since it is worn on the

head; and most importantly, from the audiologist's point of view, hearing reception is at a more natural position on the head. Our success with ear-level hearing aids with children has been very good, and we tend to recommend this type of aid whenever possible. We have fit ear-level instruments on youngsters as young as 2 years of age with little problem.

The eyeglass type of hearing aid was quite popular when it first appeared on the commercial market in the late 1950s. The eyeglass unit is essentially the same aid as the behind-the-ear type, except that the plastic case that enclosed the components is part of the eyeglass temple piece. These units have become less popular in recent years, and we seldom recommend eyeglass aids for children. The major problem is that when repairs are necessary on either the eyeglass set or the hearing aid, both units are lost to the child while service is performed.

As children grow older they become more concerned about the cosmetic appearance of their hearing aid. As they reach those trying "teen" years, they often demand smaller, less visible, ear-level (or especially ITC) hearing aids, and we make this recommendation when possible. Better to underfit the patient with a hearing aid that will be willingly used daily, than to force the use of an unwanted hearing aid that will not be worn.

Bone Conduction Hearing Aids. Bone conduction hearing aids are used in selected children with significant conductive hearing loss who cannot use, for whatever reason, an air conduction hearing aid. The bone conduction hearing aid has a vibratory flat surface that rests on the mastoid and transduces sound waves into vibrotactile sensation, thereby stimulating the cochlear cells via the bone conduction auditory pathway. Bone conduction hearing aids are not commonly used today except in infants and young children with maximum conductive hearing loss due to congenital anomalies such as severe microtia of the pinnae and/or atresia of the external ear canal. We have placed bone conduction hearing aids on infants as young as one month of age. Soft material can be used to pad the headband for a small child or infant if necessary. The bone oscillator can be used any place on the infant's skull, including the mastoid area behind the ear, or the forehead, or at the back or top of the skull when the infant is placed stomach-down.

Everyone involved should understand that the bone conduction hearing aid fitting is not permanent. Chances are quite good that the cause of the conductive-type hearing problem will ultimately be alleviated through surgical intervention. Successful surgical treatment will, it is hoped, permit the fitting of a traditional air conduction ear-level hearing aid.

CROS Hearing Aid. Harford and Barry (1965) of Northwestern University fitted 20 persons who had severe unilateral hearing loss with a special instrument that utilized a microphone on the side of the head with the bad ear and transmitted sound electrically as picked up by this microphone to the good ear through an open-type earmold. They named this special instrument CROS, for "contralateral routing of signals." This simple procedure opened up many new applications of amplification for hearing-impaired persons.

The basic premise of this amplification system is to improve hearing by eliminating the "head shadow effect." This arrangement, of placing the microphone beside the patient's poorer ear and feeding the amplified sound to the better ear, prevents the head from blocking sounds directed to the bad side from reaching the better ear. The most common arrangement for this apparatus is shown in Figure 8.3. Some patients who do not wear glasses use a wire or a thin plastic tube draped around the back of their head, often under their hair, to connect the microphone to their good ear or to use an FM wireless set. The open-type earpiece is an essential part of the CROS system, since the good ear when left unoccluded allows normal reception of sound directed to the better ear.

The use of an open-type earmold or the use of a tube without an earmold enhances speech discrimination for persons with high-frequency hearing loss. The success of the open canal fitting is due to a reduction in gain and maximal power output, so that even very loud sounds in the low-frequency spectrum do not produce discomfort to the patient.

The success of the CROS aid was immediate. Some 10 versions of the CROS principle have now been incorporated into various designs and applications (Rintelmann et al., 1970). The most common variant of the CROS aid is termed the BiCROS system (Fig. 8.3). The BiCROS consists of two microphones—one above each ear—that send electrical signals to a single amplifier. The output from the amplifier goes to a single receiver that delivers sound to the better ear through a conventional earmold. Matkin and Thomas (1972) verified that children benefit from CROS hearing aids. They report the need for careful consideration of CROS aids in youngsters with unilateral hearing loss only or in new hearing aid users in their teenage years.

Extended-Frequency Hearing Aids. Conventional hearing aids attempt to provide optimal amplification for the speech frequency range between 200 and 5000 Hz. For years, however, attempts have been made to produce amplification systems that can provide supplemental speech cues for the profoundly hearing-impaired.

In recent years, special amplification systems have been developed to enable hearing-impaired children with residual hearing in the low frequencies to use amplification. These special hearing aids provide greater low-frequency acoustic stimulation than does the conventional hearing aid. Initial evaluations of these amplification systems by their proponents were reported to be favorable, but later studies have produced conflicting results.

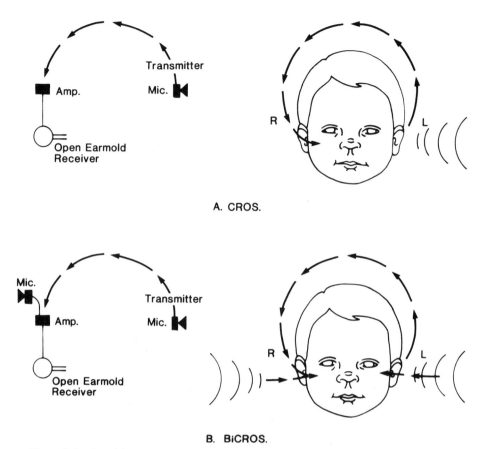

A. CROS.

B. BiCROS.

Figure 8.3.   Special use hearing aid systems. **A.** CROS hearing aid. **B.** BiCROS hearing aid.

Berlin (1982) described hearing loss in which hearing is poor in the standard audiometric ranges but nearly normal at frequencies between 8,000 and 15,000 Hz. In his report, Berlin described the development of an upward-shifting translating hearing aid that has a frequency response extending well beyond 10,000 Hz. Candidates for his special translating hearing aid are difficult to diagnose. They typically have unusually good speech and sensitivity to environmental sounds in the presence of poor speech perception and severe pure tone hearing losses with unusually good speech-detection thresholds. Their audiograms suggest severe-to-profound deafness, poor speech understanding, and good speech production. Many of these patients reject standard hearing aids and often function well without them.

HEARING AID SELECTION

In the words of Ross and Tomassetti (1980), "for most hearing-impaired children, the early and appropriate selection and use of amplification is the single most important habilitation tool available to us." In their excellent material on hearing selection for preverbal hearing-impaired children, Ross and Tomassetti emphasize the need for hearing aid preselection procedures including analyzing the electroacoustic characteristics of various aids and examining features of the hearing aids to eliminate consideration of those aids that are not appropriate, to provide the child with maximum auditory information consistent with his or her hearing loss. Their key word in the hearing aid selection is "flexibility," since initial information concerning the childs residual hearing may be limited; and since the audiologist-dispenser has some control over the response of the hearing aid itself through earmold and tube considerations, the selected aid must have adjustable output and frequency response systems (Ross and Tomassetti, 1980).

Ross and Tomassetti summarize their thoughts about hearing aid fittings in children by stating that the goal for most children is properly used and adjusted binaural hearing aids, preferably at ear level. They base hearing aid selection on the viewpoint that all initial electroacoustic recommendations are tentative and may need to be altered in time and that, foremost, children's hearing aid selection and fitting must be considered an ongoing process that is part of a complete habilitation program. Matkin (1981) writes that the focus of routine audiologic monitoring of amplification must include not only the child's auditory status and the function of the hearing aids but also the function of the auditory training system (in school) and the parent's participation in the habilitation program.

Wherever possible an ear-level type is the aid of choice for a child. For some very active children of age 3 or so, the parents may not be able to maintain an ear-level aid. On the other hand, a well-behaved 2½ year old may be given consideration for an ear-level aid. We have, however, on numerous occasions, fitted a small ear-level hearing aid on young infants as soon as a diagnosis of hearing loss is strongly suspected or confirmed. Parents should be warned that the hearing aids may end up flushed down a toilet, chewed up by the family dog, thrown out of a window, or used as a pacifier. The parents must be willing to handle the problems of the ear-level aid. They will then assume the responsibility of seeing that it is cared for and protected against loss and/or damage.

The selection of a specific hearing aid for a hearing-impaired child challenges the skills of even the most experienced audiologists. When a child has both receptive and expressive speech and language, the selec-

tion of a hearing aid is certainly easier. It is the nonverbal child who poses problems, since this youngster is not capable of communicating with the audiologist about the quality of various hearing aids. Appropriate selection of the frequency response and output characteristics must be carefully considered in fitting amplification to children. A number of techniques, both behavioral and electroacoustic, have evolved as a means to select the optimal hearing aid for each patient. None of the methods provides exact, precise information that is valid for *every* hearing aid fitting, but each procedure provides direction about the appropriate range of performance that the hearing aid must encompass. Often, more than one hearing aid instrument will meet the appropriate gain and output requirements, and selection is then based on other considerations, such as hearing aid size, durability, cosmetics, ease of use, cost, and availability of service and insurance (Matkin, 1986).

It is common wisdom to select a hearing aid that has a broad range of adjustable controls that can provide flexibility for changing the response of the hearing aid as necessary. As more data are accumulated and the accuracy of test results improves as the child grows older and matures, changes in the hearing aid system will undoubtedly be necessary. Routine hearing aid assessment and alteration for all children using amplification is an important part of the process, and the audiologist must be prepared to make hearing aid response changes as often as necessary. We do not advocate any specific procedure because no single technique fits all circumstances for all children. The audiologist must be prepared and willing to utilize the technique that provides the most useful information in a reasonable time period.

Preselection. The preselection procedure begins with consideration of the type of hearing aids to be utilized. Body-type hearing aids are now less often recommended for children because of technologic improvements in ear-level hearing aids, especially in terms of adjustment, flexibility, and amount of power. Ear-level aids are lightweight, have no external wires or tubes, do not amplify clothing noise, and, most importantly, provide hearing reception at the natural position of the head. Ear-level hearing aids are the general choice for most children, with the exception of the multiply-handicapped child with poor head control that may lead to persistent feedback problems when ear-level aids are utilized.

ITE hearing instruments have not been widely used with children according to a survey reported by Curran (1985). Although tremendous strides have been made in the technology of ITE hearing aids, their major limitations for children involve their inability to provide direct audio input (DAI) and weak telecoil response. These limitations prohibit the use of personal FM systems and assistive listening devices with the child's hearing aid. Until the addition of DAI and improved telecoil response in ITE hearing aids, it seems likely that ITE hearing aids will be recommended only for children with mild hearing losses. The problem of a child outgrowing the ITE hearing aid is actually easily solved by simple recasing of the instrument as often as necessary.

Binaural Hearing Aids. Although considerable controversy concerning the merits of binaural versus monaural amplification has existed over the years, the critical need for optimal hearing by children demands binaural hearing aids. Our policy is that *all children should be fitted with binaural hearing aids whenever possible* to maximize auditory potential. The fitting of binaural amplification with all hearing-impaired children should prevail unless contraindication (such as total deafness in one ear) is determined. A binaural hearing aid system consists of two complete hearing aids worn simultaneously—one in each ear.

Certainly, common wisdom prevails that two ears are better than one, and thus two hearing aids must be better than one hearing aid. However, professionals have long debated the empirical evidence to prove this point. Obviously, the binaural hearing system is twice as expensive as a single, monaural system. However, hearing-impaired adults often state their preference for the binaural system, and although the audiologist can often successfully add a second hearing aid to a monaural hearing aid user, the reverse is never true. That is, the audiologist can never talk a binaural hearing aid user into changing to a monaural hearing aid. In spite of the expense, there is obviously something about using a binaural hearing system that makes better listening for hearing-impaired users.

Mueller and Hawkins (1990) present an up-to-date review of the advantages of binaural hearing aid systems. They describe three main advantages for binaural hearing aids to include *binaural summation, elimination of head shadow, and binaural squelch.* These three factors work together to improve speech recognition for the hearing-impaired binaural amplification user:

• *Binaural Summation.* When a sound is presented binaurally, it is perceived louder than if the same sound is presented monaurally. Hawkins et al. (1987) demonstrated that persons with bilateral sensorineural hearing loss have 6–10 dB of binaural summation. This loudness summation has significant benefit to hearing-impaired amplification users, since they can have equivalent perceived loudness at lower volume control settings, thus reducing potential feedback problems and prolonging battery life.

• *Elimination of Head Shadow.* Head shadow occurs when an individual is wearing a single hearing aid, and speech is presented from the nonaided side. Head shadow can attenuate the speech signal 6–12 dB as sound "bends" around the head to reach the hearing aid on the opposite ear. Thus, the binaurally hearing-impaired patient who is unfortunately wearing only one hearing aid is constantly attempting to manipulate the hearing aid to be on the side of the speech signal. This situation adds increased stress to the monaural hearing aid user who is often in a situation where it is not easy to continually turn the hearing aid towards the signal of interest, as might be encountered in theater seats, a dinner party, the automobile, etc. According to Mueller and Hawkins (1990), in a worse case scenario, the monaural hearing aid user may lose as much as 10–18 dB less gain than the binaural hearing aid wearer in the same situation because of the head shadow effect.

- *Binaural Squelch.* Binaural squelch is the term applied to the reported ability of the auditory system to diminish noise or reverberation more efficiently when input is received from two ears rather than one ear. The immediate effect of this phenomenon is to increase speech recognition in noise for the binaural hearing aid user. This single advantage of binaural hearing aid use is the main reason that audiologists justify encouraging their patients to use two hearing aids rather than one hearing aid.

Other advantages attributed to binaural hearing aids include increased auditory localization abilities, improved sound quality (fidelity), spatial balance, and ease of listening. These factors are often difficult, if not impossible, to demonstrate in sound-treated test chambers where testing is often accomplished in the presence of a particularly quiet background. Experienced binaural hearing aid users are quick to endorse the wearing of two hearing aids rather than one hearing aid and generally accept the increased financial consequence as a well-invested expenditure. Ear-level binaural hearing aids are especially advantageous, since the microphones are at the level of the ears, separated by the head, resulting in improved time-intensity parameters of the acoustic signal.

Children may be unable to make judgments regarding monaural versus binaural hearing aid use, and the decision falls to someone else. The traditional hearing aid evaluation procedures using functional gain measurements at threshold levels are hard-

pressed to show superior performance of binaural hearing aids over a monaural hearing aid. However, as audiologists gain first-hand experience in dispensing, fitting, and managing patients with hearing aids, the advantage in speech recognition in noise created by binaural hearing aids as reported by hearing-impaired patients is providing cumulative evidence for the superiority of listening with two ears rather than one ear.

The easiest persons to fit with binaural hearing aids are those children with bilateral, symmetrical hearing loss. However, asymmetrical hearing loss should not be a contraindication to binaural amplification, although the audiologist is challenged to attempt to balance out the two hearing aids until aided symmetry is achieved. The use of computerized real-ear probe microphone-aided measurements from each ear canal can be used to achieve symmetry in a binaural hearing aid fitting for a child with asymmetrical bilateral hearing loss.

An intriguing research project conducted by Silman et al. (1984) studied auditory deprivation in monaural and binaural aided adult subjects. The auditory performance of the subjects prior to the use of hearing aids was compared to their auditory performance after 4–5 years of hearing aid use to determine whether the unaided ear would show effects of auditory deprivation. The most revealing finding was that the speech recognition scores remained stable in both ears of the binaurally fitted patients, while the unaided scores of the monaurally fitted patients showed a significant reduction, apparently the result of auditory deprivation. This study has important implications that urge the binaural fitting of all children who need hearing aids.

In light of the evidence that binaural amplification results in improved speech recognition skills, especially in the presence of background noise, which is undoubtedly an important feature for hearing-impaired children, we continue to be astounded by the reluctance of audiologists to commit to this concept. Recent statements by Rintlemann and Bess (1988) that "in young children a recommendation of binaural amplification should be made with extreme caution" and "amplification (in children) should be periodically alternated between ears when feasible" show a lack of understanding regarding the importance of binaural hearing for the education and social development of a young hearing-impaired child.

Frequency Response of Hearing Aids.

Early in the history of hearing aid fitting a controversy arose between the "selective" frequency response proponents and those preferring a "flat," more uniform response curve. The controversy soon became rather one-sided, with the selective fitting proponents enjoying the recognition and acceptance of the majority. The selective method was based upon the patient's audiogram and provided amplification only where most needed. Amplification was restricted to the frequency areas in which the user still had residual hearing to be reached.

However, in 1946 (Davis et al., 1946), reports of the Harvard Study began to question the advantage of selective fitting. The Harvard group conclusions were very emphatic that selective fitting was of no value and that a uniform response would almost invariably yield as good, if not better, speech discrimination response. "For every subject the best performance could be obtained by using either the flat response system or the high pass 6 dB per octave tilt."

There has been a reevaluation of the importance of low-frequency hearing aid amplification, suggesting that the relative intensity level of the low-frequency band is critical. Danaher and Pickett (1975) and Franklin (1988) clearly demonstrated that when a low-frequency sound is presented at high-intensity levels, a type of masking is produced that reduces the person's ability to detect sounds in the higher frequency regions. This effect is termed "upward spread of masking" and occurs in normal-hearing persons and most persons with sensorineural loss. When amplified with a low-frequency emphasis aid, moderate levels of environmental noise may be sufficiently intense to produce spread of masking, making speech intelligibility frustratingly difficult for the hearing-impaired listener.

The audiologist's task, then, is to discover an acoustic system that will provide the patient with all of the acoustic cues necessary to achieve maximum use of his or her residual hearing for daily real-world communication while minimizing the degradation of signal through "upward spread of masking" in most (preferably all) listening situations. This task is, of course, confounded when the patient is very young, nonverbal or noncooperative!

Hearing Aid Output.

Hearing aids should not be selected because of their power output—also known as saturated sound pressure level (SSPL)—alone. After all, every hearing aid has a volume control that can be adjusted within the limits of the hearing aid. The output range of the hearing aid fixes the minimum-to-maximum decibel levels of the receiver when sound enters the microphone. Typically, the audiologist adjusts the hearing aid output control so that sound that comes out of the receiver into the user's ear canal is limited below the level of discomfort. Various electronic circuits are used in hearing aids to automatically suppress loud sound picked up by the hearing aid. The maximum power output of the hearing aid describes the decibel level of the greatest possible intensity that a hearing aid is capable of producing through amplification. Although one would not purposefully choose a hearing aid with inadequate output, a common error is to "overfit" with too much power. Seewald et al. (1985) pointed out that the selection of real-ear SSPL is a compromise. The SSPL must be high enough to provide adequate amplification without exceeding the saturation level frequently, yet the SSPL must not exceed the child's loudness discomfort level.

Clinicians must be aware that hearing aid specifications are reported relative to a 2 cc hard-walled cavity. A hearing aid coupled to a child's ear canal will enclose a cavity that is considerably less than 2 cc, resulting in increased sound pressure levels (SPLs) at the tympanic membrane. Children with small ear canal volumes may actually receive considerably more amplification than indicated by the hearing aid technical specification sheet; i.e., an instrument with an SSPL of 130 dB as measured in a 2.0 cc coupler may be capable of creating 142 dB SPL when coupled to an ear having a 0.5 cc space between the tip of the earmold and the eardrum.

Gain. Hearing aid gain is defined as the amount of amplification measured in decibels. The gain of each hearing aid must be considered by the audiologist in selecting personal amplification for a hearing-impaired child. In general terms, we attempt to assure optimal audibility of the speech spectrum between 750 and 3000 Hz while avoiding overamplification of low-frequency sound energy found in background noise. Gain adjustment may be accomplished to a limited degree through the tone controls (or gain adjustments) of the hearing aid. Modification of the "earmold plumbing" can also effect gain in specific regions of the frequency spectrum.

The selection of appropriate gain in children's hearing aids is an especially difficult task, as often the youngsters cannot verbalize their perceptions of the amplified sound quality. Thus, we use a number of "prescriptive formulae" to determine target gain requirements relative to the patient's auditory thresholds. There are different prescriptive rules to be used with various types of hearing loss and the personal preference and experience of the audiologist. Curran (1988) states that none of the prescriptive rules provide a precise prediction of appropriate hearing aid performance, but rather since each rule varies by formula and methodology, there is little to suggest that one prescriptive technique is intrinsically superior to another. Davis and Mueller (1987) and McCandless (1988) provide

good discussions and overviews of each of the prescriptive rules described below.

- Half-Gain Rule. The half-gain rule of Lybarger is the simplest and most widely used prescriptive fitting technique. The threshold hearing loss values at test frequencies between 250 and 4000 Hz are divided by 2, with the result taken as the desired gain for the hearing aid.

- Berger Rule. This prescriptive fitting formula is very similar to the half-gain rule, except that the speech frequency around 2000 Hz is particularly amplified.

- POGO Rule. POGO (prescription of gain/output), described initially by McCandless, is based on the half-gain rule but provides additional amplification reduction in the low frequencies. A POGO II rule has also been described with a special correction factor for hearing losses greater than 65 dB hearing level (HL).

- One-Third Gain Rule. This prescriptive fitting rule described by Libby uses less amplification gain than the other methods and is thus especially useful with mild hearing impairment.

- NAL Rule. This method, developed at the National Acoustic Laboratories in Sydney, Australia, attempts to amplify all the frequency bands of speech to equal loudness.

Although these formulae can be calculated manually for each hearing aid patient to determine target gain values, the computerized probe-microphone real-ear instruments usually include a feature that permits the audiologist to select any of the fitting rules and then the computer instantly calculates the gain values for each frequency and displays the target fitting result on the video screen.

HEARING AID FITTING METHODS

Hearing aid fittings in children may be accomplished through a number of different techniques. The steps of the various procedures do have some elements in common, such as preselection of the hearing aid(s), determination of frequency response, gain and output characteristics, and acoustic and/or electronic adjustments and modifications, and every fitting should incorporate some procedure to verify or validate the final fitting. All aspects of the pediatric audiometric test battery are utilized to obtain as much information as possible regarding the child's hearing impairment.

Parents of young children must understand that the hearing aid fitting process is an ongoing activity to be analyzed and reconsidered at each clinic visit. As more audiometric information is obtained, and careful observation of the child's behavior and development is noted with the hearing aids in place, the audiologist may decide to modify or adjust the hearing aids when necessary. Computerized probe-microphone real-ear measurements, when available, should be checked at each clinic visit as a means of monitoring the performance of the child's hearing aids as they are worn. Permanent hard copy of these real-ear measurements will permit comparative evaluation of the hearing aids' performance from visit to visit. Probe-microphone real-ear measurements may be utilized to identify malfunctioning hearing aids that need repair or adjustment, particularly in children who are too young or unsophisticated to voice complaint. In addition, Jerger (1987) reminds us of the importance of using a speech-based evaluation measure in hearing aid fitting protocols.

Traditionally, the most common procedure for selecting and fitting hearing aids in children is the functional gain method described below. Increasing in popularity at this time is the computerized probe-microphone real-ear technique. We also describe briefly the new amplified speech spectrum method, as well as physiologic evaluation techniques utilizing the auditory brainstem evoked response (ABR) and the acoustic reflex. It is certainly possible that audiologists may use more than one of the described procedures in each pediatric hearing aid fitting session.

Especially important in working with hearing-impaired children and their hearing aids is the concept of a "target" fitting. The target fitting is the audiologist's best prediction for final optimal amplification, taking into account the patient's audiometric configuration, the hearing aid frequency response, and its gain and output characteristics. It is often possible, once the target fitting has been ascertained, to modify or adjust the hearing aids to come as close as possible to the desired (predicted) amplified configuration. A number of prescription rules have been developed to help audiologists in their determination of the hearing aid gain. These prescriptive rules are briefly described under hearing aid gain.

Functional Gain. Functional gain is the difference between *unaided* and *aided* minimal response levels. The purpose of functional gain measurements is to compare unaided and aided responses under identical conditions. The young child is typically seated on the parent's lap between two sound field speakers. Through visual response audiometry, minimal response levels are obtained for speech signals and narrow bands of noise, 250–8000 Hz, without the hearing aids. Then with the hearing aids in place on the child and the gain controls set at preselected levels, minimal response levels are again obtained for speech and narrow bands of noise. The difference between the aided and unaided minimal response levels is the functional gain. If the functional is different from the target gain, appropriate adjustments should be made. A major disadvantage with functional gain procedures is that the sound field audiogram reflects performance only at minimal response or threshold levels, and thus there is no assurance that the child will receive meaningful perception of speech at intensities sufficiently above threshold. Rines et al. (1984) suggest that minimal response levels in sound field underestimate functional gain when unaided hearing levels are near normal limits.

"Reasonable" levels can be estimated in relation to the degree of hearing loss. An approximation of what should be expected is as follows:

Degree of Loss	Reasonable Level of Awareness
100 dB HL +	45–55 dB HL
75–100 dB HL average	25–50 dB HL
50–75 dB HL	15–30 dB HL
25–50 dB HL	0–15 dB HL

A greater gain can be tolerated by the child with a conductive or mixed loss than by one with a sensorineural loss. For example, a child with a conductive loss of 60 dB HL average can easily tolerate a gain that brings his or her awareness level to 20 dB HL or even less. But a sensorineural loss of that degree will not allow the child to tolerate receiving such thresholds; a 25–30 dB HL may be the best that can be expected. It is probably not realistic to expect normal or near-normal thresholds of awareness in children. They will not wear an aid giving those levels, despite all our ambitions to bring them to normal levels.

Uses for functional gain measurements include comparing the performance of hearing aids with different internal settings, obtaining information regarding various types of earmolds, monitoring stability of the young child's amplification system over time, and demonstrating improvement in unaided versus aided conditions. However, since functional gain measurements are typically made in 5 dB intervals, smaller differences due to hearing aid adjustment may not be noticeable with functional gain measurements. Humes and Kirn (1990) report increased test-retest variability related to functional gain measurements.

Infants and 2–3 Year Olds. Subjective evaluation of infants and small children can be conducted while the youngster is wearing both hearing aids. The child should be given various levels of gross speech through a loudspeaker. Thresholds of

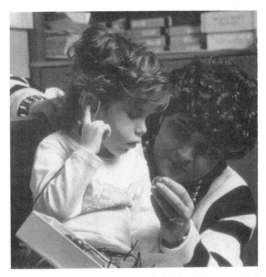

Figure 8.4. Hearing-impaired children have special needs and require additional attention to obtain maximum benefit from their hearing aids.

should be obtained, plus observations of reactions to louder levels.

The child 2 or 3 years and older who can be play-conditioned or taught hand-raising responses to sounds can be given a satisfactory hearing aid evaluation (Fig. 8.4). The principle of such an evaluation is to compare the unaided audiogram and the speech awareness levels with similar measures using hearing aids. The initial choice of which hearing aids to try may be made on the basis of the principles listed in Table 8.2.

It may be necessary to schedule more than one testing session for the 2 or 3 year old. The child's tolerance for testing has a limited time span, and it is fruitless to try to extend it. Some bright 2 or 2½ year olds are able to learn play-conditioning techniques for speech or pure tones and sustain their interest for very short periods of time. A 2 year old may surprise you by learning play-conditioning long enough to give a speech awareness level or a threshold at one frequency during short periods of time. Two or three frequencies are sufficient to place the loss: 500 and 2000 Hz, or 500, 1000, and 2000 Hz. This is the major frequency range of hearing aid amplification.

Table 8.2.
Synopsis of Standard Hearing Aid Specifications

SSPL	Curve (minimum range recorded 200—5000 Hz)
SSPL (maximum)	dB (+ 0 dB tolerance)
High frequency—average SSPL 90	dB (average of 1000, 1600, 2500 Hz outputs) ± 4 dB tolerance
Full-on gain	Curve (60 dB input, 50 dB for automatic gain control aids)
High frequency—average full-on gain	dB (average of 1000, 1600, 2500 Hz gain) ± 5 dB tolerance
Reference test position	17 dB below high-frequency SSPL 90. Input 60 dB
Reference test position automatic gain control aids	Maximum gain; input 50 dB
Reference test gain	dB (average of 1000, 1600, 2500 Hz at reference test position)
Frequency response at reference test position	Curve (input 60 dB, 200–5000 Hz)
	Low band (below 2000 Hz + 4 dB tolerance)
	High band (above 2000 Hz + 6 dB tolerance)
ANSI[a] frequency range	Hz (average of 1000, 1600, 2500 Hz minus 20 dB)
Total harmonic distortion 500, 800, and 1600 Hz	(Reference test position, input 70 dB, at each frequency)

[a]ANSI, American National Standards Institute.

Given a threshold audiogram, plus observed tolerance limits obtained from observation or acoustic reflexes, the following is a suggested functional gain procedure for hearing aid selection. On each hearing aid selected for trial, obtain the five measures listed below. (The approximate volume setting can be estimated from the hearing aid analysis charts in relation to the midpoint of the dynamic range).

1. Using gross speech, obtain a speech awareness level through play-conditioning techniques or hand-raising. The simple word "now" is as good a speech signal as any.
2. Using warbled pure tones, obtain an aided free-field audiogram on each aid. Use intermediate frequencies in addition to the standard frequencies (750, 1500, 3000 Hz) if possible.
3. Test the tolerance limits of the hearing aid on the child by raising the speech level gradually until the child evidences discomfort.
4. Evaluate the hearing aids first on the basis of the best speech awareness in relation to tolerance levels.
5. The next evaluation of the hearing aids should be made on the basis of the aided pure tone thresholds. The threshold at 2000 Hz is the most critical, and the

hearing aid showing the best threshold there should be given preference. The contour of the audiogram should be fairly even, without high peaks at any frequencies.

This procedure should allow a selection of one or two acceptable aids that can be recommended. If there is any question, a trial of the finally selected aids can be suggested. During the trials, observations of the child's performance with each aid can be made by parents, teachers, or clinicians. From these observations the ultimate selection can be made.

Verbal Child 3–16 Years Old. When receptive language is present in the child, speech recognition testing can be accomplished with hearing aids; when, in addition, there is expressive language present, finer word recognition tests such as Pediatric Speech Intelligibility (PSI) test described in Chapter 5 are applicable (S. Jerger et al., 1985).

A minimum of two and a maximum of three hearing aids should be selected for trial. In the descriptions of testing at the various age levels that follow, there will be overlapping in the ages at which children can perform the tests. The variable factors are the degree of hearing loss, the level of language skills, and the intellectual function of the child. A mentally retarded child of 9, for example, may have to be handled like a 3 year old. Previous audiometric testing should have determined the level of testing that can be used on each child.

Age 3–5 Years. A hearing-handicapped child of this age may require special motivational techniques, even for speech reception testing. Therefore, toys or pictures of objects should be used to sustain interest in the test. The steps that can be followed are:

1. Set the volume of each aid in accordance with your best estimate of necessary gain. A hearing aid should never be tested at full volume, as some distortion may occur at high output levels.
2. Obtain a speech reception threshold (SRT) by using the toys suggested in Chapter 5 or the picture tests described. Work as fast as possible, foregoing the standard three-out-of-six-words criterion for threshold. Select as threshold the last word repeated on a descending threshold starting at 40 dB and proceeding rapidly downward in 5 dB steps. Express pleasure or clap your hands at each response. Record the level.
3. Starting at 40 dB, sweep upward in 5 dB steps, giving a "buh-buh" at each step. Observe carefully the first sign of discomfort the child shows, such as wincing or putting a hand to the ear, or grimacing, or even attempting to take off the hearing aid. Record this level as the tolerance threshold.
4. Use as criteria for selection the combination of the best SRT and highest tolerance level, giving more weight to the tolerance level. No hearing aid with a tolerance level under 65 dB should be chosen, nor a hearing aid with an SRT higher than 25 dB. These general criteria can be set because the child of this age who has receptive language is likely to have a mild-to-moderate hearing loss.

Age 6–10 Years. The cooperative child at this age can be given more sophisticated audiology tests. Follow the procedures listed below:

1. Set each hearing aid at an appropriate gain level between one-half and two-thirds volume.
2. Obtain a SRT by using 8–10 children's spondees. Start at 40 dB HL and descend in 5 dB steps, giving one word at each level. Bracket the threshold level with no more than three words around threshold. Keep the child's interest by smiling with pleasure and give praise at each correct response.
3. Give a half list of PBK discrimination words at 40 dB HL, maintaining attention with praise. The 40 dB level is selected because the goal for the child should be to hear normal conversational speech. The PSI test is an excellent alternative to the PBK list. Verbal children of this age most likely have moderate to moderately severe losses at worst and should be expected to understand normal conversational speech with an aid. The vocalized responses may not be clear enough on any words to be correct, but you should set up a mental criterion of what is probably correct, even if the child cannot pronounce it correctly. A consistent criterion will produce meaningful results. Another useful criterion is the latency of the responses. One hearing aid may provide the child with a signal that permits immediate response; another hearing aid may produce hesitation on each word. This observation should be noted.
4. To establish the aided discomfort threshold, start at 40 dB HL with spondee words, and ascend in 5 dB steps. Watch for the first sign or discomfort. If the child has sufficient understanding, he or she can be instructed to tell you when it becomes too loud. In this case, make three presentations of the ascending levels and record the average level of the three discomfort responses.
5. Use as criterion for final selection of the aid, the combination of the best word

discrimination score, the best SRT, and the highest tolerance level. Speech understanding should be given the greatest weight, tolerance level follows closely, and SRT is of least importance.

Age 10–16 Years. Depending on the language level and capacity of the child, standard or slightly modified adult techniques can be used at this age range. The procedure is:

1. Turn each aid to a most comfortable loudness gain setting. Speaking normally at a distance of 3 or 4 feet, ask the child, "Do you like it this loud?" or "Is it better this loud?" Often the child will indicate a quite definite preference for one particular volume setting.
2. Obtain a SRT. Standard SRT technique can be used but should be shortened in the case of poor attention span.
3. Give a half list of phonetically-balanced (PB) words (or PBK words) at 40 dB HL or perform the PSI procedure to establish a performance-intensity function with each hearing aid under consideration.
4. Instruct the child to tell you when your voice becomes "too loud," and give spondees in 5 dB ascending steps from 40 dB HL. Repeat 3 times and take the average of the response levels.
5. Use as criteria for the final selection the best discrimination score, the highest tolerance level, and the best SRT, in that level of importance. At this age the child may voice a preference for one aid over the other. If it is not the aid that performed the best, determine on what basis the choice has been made. If it is on size, shape, or color, try to point out better features of the hearing aid that performed best. Assure the child that he or she will hear the best with the selected aids.

One should always keep in mind the audiologist's adage: "The best hearing aids are the ones that are worn." The pediatric hearing aid evaluation procedure is nearly al-ways an ongoing process, and parents must be aware that changes will probably be made in the hearing aid fitting as more accurate and detailed information is determined regarding the child's hearing loss, development, social-educational needs and circumstances, etc. Occasionally, the audiologist should be prepared to accept a temporary compromise hearing aid fitting to maintain the child's and parents' interest and cooperation, knowing full well that modifications to the hearing aids or finer acoustic tuning can be accomplished at a near-future appointment time.

Probe-Microphone Real-Ear Measurements. Computerized probe-microphone real-ear hearing aid analysis offers an important opportunity to evaluate hearing aid fittings with children (Fig. 8.5). This technique utilizes a soft silicone tube that is inserted into the ear canal with the hearing aid and earmold in place. The amplified sound in the ear canal is picked up by a probe microphone through the silicone tube and is subjected to signal processing by a special purpose computer and presented on a visual display or printout. It is now possible for the audiologist to know precisely the aided frequency response and amplified signal intensity in the child's ear canal. For many years it has been necessary to estimate ear canal sound pressure at each frequency by interpolating data obtained from a 2 cc cavity and utilizing correction factors as a mathematical means to determine real-ear specifications.

The major advantage of the computerized probe-microphone real-ear measuring device is that the entire amplification system is evaluated so the effects of tubing, earmold, filters, and so forth can be acknowledged. Physiologic differences among children, such as the length, diameter, and the shape of the ear canal, which are extremely important considerations in fitting hearing aids with children, are taken into account in probe-microphone real-ear measurements. Computerized probe-microphone real-ear measurements provide

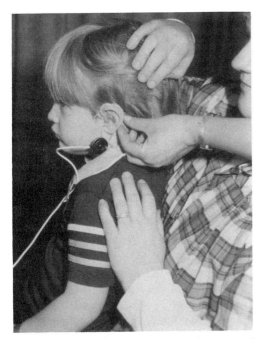

Figure 8.5. Computerized probe-microphone real-ear measurements provide electroacoustic information while the hearing aid is being worn. This technique has proven to be especially valuable with children's hearing aid fittings and evaluations.

quick, objective data regarding insertion gain, in situ response, and relative gain, as well as the telemagnetic response of the hearing aid. The measurements may be read in 1 dB intervals; every acoustic modification or electroacoustic adjustment made with the hearing aids will be clearly noted. This information is valuable during the hearing aid selection, fitting verification, and postfitting management of the hearing-impaired child. Most real-ear measurement equipment also includes a "listening" system, through high-fidelity lightweight earphones, so that the amplified sound can be heard easily by the child's parents, who thereby gain full appreciation of exactly how their youngster's hearing aids amplify environmental and speech sounds.

An important aspect of this revolutionary new equipment is the ability to plot visually on the video screen a target amplified hearing aid response. The hearing aid fitter is able to use any method of gain prediction (i.e., the half-gain rule, POGO, and so forth) to achieve the best amplified responses for each child. Then, acoustic measurements performed in the ear with probe microphone systems can provide information regarding the total effect of the hearing aids, earmold plumbing, and sound field effects with minimal patient cooperation (Libby, 1982). It is important to note that probe-microphone measurements in infant ear canals have documented that the fundamental resonance frequency of the external ear decreases from approximately 6000 Hz at birth to the adult resonance value of 2700 Hz by the second year of age (Kruger, 1987). This information is of value in selecting appropriate hearing aid frequency characteristics in babies.

Comparison of the real-ear response with the target amplification response permits manipulation of the acoustic coupling system with predictable effects on the frequency range to be modified. Earmold venting may be used to suppress low-frequency output and reduce tolerance problems by limiting amplified output. Acoustic dampers (filters) may be used as midfrequency controls to smooth out the amplified frequency response between 1000 and 3000 Hz. An acoustic horn may be used to extend the amplified high-frequency response to improve speech intelligibility. Following each acoustic modification it is a simple matter to verify the result of manipulation.

A recommended procedure for probe-microphone real-ear hearing aid fittings in hearing-impaired infants and children is as follows:

- Examine the child with an otoscope to be sure ear canals are clear.

- Situate infant or child in parent's lap approximately 1 meter from loudspeaker.

- Set marker on silicone probe tube at 5 mm longer than earmold canal.

- Insert probe into child's open ear canal with marker at tragus so that marker is observable.

- Measure "open" real-ear unaided response (REUR) to obtain insertion gain curve.

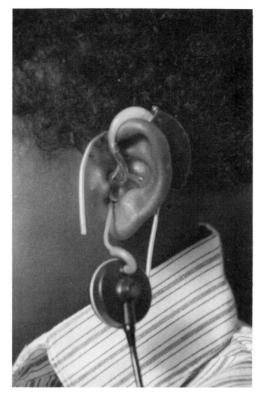

Figure 8.6. Close-up view of computerized probe-microphone system in place on a hearing-impaired child's ear.

- Enter threshold data or threshold estimate into computer program.

- Select fitting formula to obtain target goal at each frequency to be achieved with "ideal" amplification.

- Place hearing aid and earmold in infant or child's ear; silicone probe-microphone is placed in ear canal under earmold with marker at same initial tragus location.

- Measure real-ear insertion response (REIR) and compare to target insertion gain response.

- Make acoustic modifications as necessary to achieve "ideal" amplification response, and remeasure real-ear aided response.

- Measure *in situ* real-ear response (REAR), if desired, to monitor overall SPL of amplification system in the infant or child's ear canal;

- Print out results.

Computerized probe-microphone real-ear measurements have numerous distinct advantages over functional gain measurements as a method of assessing hearing aid performance, especially with hearing-impaired children. These advantages include: (*1*) elimination of dependency on the behavioral threshold responses; (*2*) electroacoustic information across the entire frequency range of interest rather than only octave or half-octave intervals; (*3*) no contamination of aided threshold measures by internal hearing aid and/or room noise—a significant problem with functional gain measurements when hearing thresholds are in the normal or near-normal range; and (*4*) considerable savings in time and efficiency, with improved accuracy and reliability in the electroacoustic analysis of the hearing aid under evaluation (Fig. 8.6).

The use of this technology in fitting hearing aids and managing amplification with hearing-impaired children should have widespread application. The real-ear response in no way can be construed to represent what the child hears, which requires cerebral integration. Probe-microphone evaluation gives audiologists confidence in their selection and fitting of hearing aids for this difficult-to-test population. We currently use the probe-microphone real-ear system with all of our pediatric hearing aid patients.

It is not uncommon for the audiologist to realize very different amplification results from patients with similar audiograms and similar speech discrimination abilities who are fitted with precisely the same hearing aid. Consideration of probe-microphone real-ear measurements will help the audiologist understand the reasons for these different results in similar patients. Real-ear measurements can provide information to modify the acoustic coupling system to resolve hearing aid problems and permit in-office modifications.

Numerous broad clinical applications of probe-microphone real-ear measurements will undoubtedly be developed during the next few years. To be sure, all facts and data concerning the critical factors of successful hearing aid fittings are not yet available. Although we can now control the shape, smoothness, and bandwidth of the amplified frequency response, we still do not know the "best" way to determine precise insertion gain necessary to achieve optimal speech intelligibility.

Amplified Speech Spectrum Method.
A hearing aid selection procedure introduced by Gengel et al. (1971) assumes that a positive correlation exists between aided speech discrimination performance and the area of speech spectrum received with amplification. Thus, the goal of hearing aid selection is to utilize a hearing aid that amplifies, at a comfortable gain setting, as much of the speech spectrum as possible. Bands of noise corresponding to the intensity of corresponding segments in normal conversational speech are used to compute average speech spectrum levels for octaves over the standard frequency range. Gengel and colleagues computed approximate average speech levels for bands of noise centered at five test frequencies, when the overall SPL of the spectrum was 70 dB SPL, to be 60 dB at 250 Hz, 61 dB at 500 Hz, 58 dB at 1000 Hz, 54 dB at 2000 Hz, and 46 dB at 4000 Hz.

The protocol of this procedure is to establish aided thresholds (functional gain) with these selected narrow bands of noise when the hearing aid is set at a comfortable listening level. To estimate the average levels above threshold at which the child receives the speech spectrum at conversational level, the aided threshold SPLs are subtracted from the average speech spectrum levels. The difference values in decibels represent the approximate sensation level at which each frequency band of speech will be perceived during normal conversation. Gengel and colleagues suggested that the hearing aid of choice is the unit that amplifies the widest possible speech spectrum 10–20 dB above the aided threshold. The authors proposed this procedure for evalu-

ating and selecting hearing aids for children with severe-to-profound hearing loss. Schwartz and Larson (1977) confirmed the value of this procedure with severely hearing-impaired children.

The publications of Ross and Seewald (1988) and Seewald and Ross (1988) have continued to develop this suprathreshold approach to selection of hearing aids for hearing-impaired children. Their procedure has been to determine amplification target levels by using estimates of the average levels associated with the long-term speech spectrum relative to the child's unaided sound field detection levels. Although some controversy exists among researchers as to the exact intensity levels representative of frequency segments within the long-term speech frequency spectrum (Olsen et al., 1987), the overall concept is to provide children with an amplified speech signal that is audible throughout the broadest frequency range possible. In general, the desired sensation level of the amplified speech decreases in an accelerated nonlinear function with increasing hearing loss. Although older children can be assessed with this technique through behavioral sound field measures, probe microphone measurements provide information regarding the real-ear frequency characteristics quickly and easily in the child's ear canal.

Hawkins (1987) described a similar procedure using computerized probe-microphone real-ear measures and behavioral techniques in which the child's auditory detection levels were determined in sound field. Then, an unoccluded frequency-specific stimulus was presented with the probe microphone in the child's ear canal (REUR) at the level at which threshold was obtained and ear canal SPLs of the stimulus were recorded. With the probe tube in the same position, the hearing aid was fitted and REARs were determined with the input stimuli presented at levels determined by the long-term speech spectrum. By comparing the real-ear unoccluded response (REUR) at threshold levels with the REAR produced with the speech spectrum level input, an estimate can be made of the sensation level at each frequency of the amplified long-term speech spectrum.

In general, the principles behind the selection of hearing aids for children are no different from hearing aid characteristics used by adults. Libby (1982) has summarized these considerations as follows: (1) select an amplification system with a smooth frequency response and no sharp peaks; (2) plan to compensate for the 10–15 dB insertion loss at 2700 Hz created by the occluding earmold; (3) ensure a wide-frequency bandwidth to ensure greater fidelity for speech and music; (4) preserve an appropriate balance between high-frequency amplification for speech recognition and low-frequency energy for intelligibility and sound quality; and (5) the output of the hearing aid should not exceed the patient's loudness discomfort level.

Aided Auditory Brainstem Evoked Response. Numerous authors have suggested using ABR measurements for hearing aid evaluation in young children because patient participation is not necessary. However, questions have been raised about the accuracy of ABR hearing aid measurements, as well as genuine concerns about the lengthy time and high expense of the procedure. Another major limiting factor is that the ABR technique does not provide specific frequency information.

In reviewing literature on aided ABR procedures, there is no agreed-on evaluation technique. Mahoney (1985) proposed the following protocol: (1) At 50 dB SPL, begin the aided ABR with a high-gain hearing aid, and if there is no response, increase the click stimulus; (2) following an aided ABR recording, increase the gain until wave V latency and amplitude stabilize; and (3) establish a latency-intensity function at varying frequency and compression settings. Kiessling (1982) utilized aided ABR amplitude-intensity information to determine appropriate hearing aid settings. He offered a mathematical technique for opti-

mal hearing aid fitting from unaided earphone-stimulated ABR intensity amplitude curves. The computation includes the intensity in decibels of the stimulus and the amplitude of the ABR wave V in nanovolts. The hearing aid components calculated are average gain in decibels, dynamic range in decibels, compression factor, and type of compression. The steepness of the ABR intensity-amplitude curve dictates the amount of compression that is needed.

Cox and Metz (1980) suggested that the gain of the hearing aid be adjusted to the level where additional increases in gain no longer produce further decreases in ABR wave V latency. They reported that the accuracy rate of hearing aid prescription by ABR may be as much as 75% of the accuracy rate of traditional hearing aid fitting procedures. The authors concluded that accuracy is associated with the configuration of the hearing loss, with greater accuracy for flat and precipitous losses than for gradually sloping losses. They also believe that clicks, in addition to tone pips, yield greater accuracy in hearing aid fittings. An extensive discussion of hearing aid assessment and ABR has been published recently by Seitz and Kisiel (1990).

Acoustic Reflex Method. McCandless and Miller (1972) described a technique for establishing hearing aid gain by use of acoustic reflex thresholds as measured with an immittance meter. With this procedure, the patient is fitted with a hearing aid to one ear and an immittance probe tip placed in the contralateral ear. Using constant sound pressure input of average environmental sounds or conversational speech, the gain control of the hearing aid is slowly raised until the acoustic reflex is barely observed in the contralateral ear. A gain setting is accomplished by adjusting the controls just below this level, which will be safely under the patient's loudness discomfort level. This technique appears to determine a gain level that provides a maximum intelligibility for speech (Rappaport and Tait, 1976). In persons with significant hearing loss, behavioral and acoustic reflex estimates of functional gains were found to be in good agreement (Rines et al., 1984). Ross and Tomassetti (1980) suggested that the SSPL of the hearing aid should not exceed the SPL that elicits an aided stapedial reflex. They described a real-ear 2 cc coupler correction factor to be added to the acoustic reflex threshold for a particular frequency. For example, if at 2000 Hz the coupler overestimates the frequency response by 10 dB and the acoustic reflex sound field threshold is 125 dB, then the coupler maximum output at 2000 Hz should not exceed 135 dB.

Unfortunately, the acoustic reflex is often absent in severe-to-profound sensorineural hearing loss. In addition, acoustic reflexes may be absent due to unilateral or bilateral middle ear effusion, a common finding in young children. Hall and Ruth (1986) reported that the acoustic reflex technique is probably useful in only 40–50% of the average pediatric population undergoing hearing aid evaluation.

HEARING AID COUPLING AND MODIFICATIONS

Today's audiologist-dispenser must be especially cognizant of the methods of hearing aid response modification technology. Level and spectral modifications can be implemented to produce a uniform effect over the entire spectrum or to selectively effect frequency ranges of the overall spectrum. Modifications to the hearing aid response can be influenced by a number of factors including the microphone location, frequency response adjustments, the earhook and tubing length, diameter, configuration and filter characteristics, the earmold shape and size, the seal or openness of the earmold (which can strongly influence low-frequency amplification), and the ear canal space between the tip of the earmold and the tympanic membrane. The clinical side of the evaluation reminds us that even when the above considerations have been accurately worked out for maximum benefit in amplification, changes in the impedance

of the tympanic membrane and middle ear due to pathology may render the "best fitting" somewhat less than desired. All of these considerations must be second nature to the audiologist-dispenser who works with hearing-impaired children.

The acoustic coupling of the hearing aid refers to the "plumbing" of the system, i.e., all of the external components that convey sound from the hearing aid itself into the ear canal of the user. With behind-the-ear hearing aids the acoustic coupling refers to the earmold, tubing, and earhook. Audiologists now understand the importance of the acoustic coupling in modifying the performance of the hearing aid. Inadequate acoustic coupling efforts can essentially ruin the performance of even the best of hearing aids. In recent years, the skill involved in successful hearing aid fitting often is a direct result of the care and consideration given to the acoustic modifications provided by the earmold and the associated connections to the hearing aid. Curran (1988) points out that the relevant literature over the past 15 years is replete with examples of how alterations in electroacoustic performance occur as a result of particular forms of earmold modification and with examples of changes in listener performance that appear to be related to changes in earmold modification.

Dalsgaard and Dyrlund-Jensen (1976) used a probe microphone in the ear canal to measure the natural acoustic resonance that in adult ears occurs at approximately 2700 Hz with a natural amplification of nearly 17 dB. Thus, nature has provided us with a natural amplifier, because of the size and shape of the ear canal, that actually helps amplify the frequency spectrum of speech. Unfortunately, when an earmold is placed into the ear canal, the acoustic properties of the system is disrupted, the natural ear canal resonance is altered in frequency range, and the natural amplification is typically diminished. This creates the often-heard response from first-time hearing aid users, "The sound just doesn't sound natural to me." The presence of the earmold in the ear canal creates an obstruction, or occlusion, which tends to keep natural sound out of the ear canal, an effect that we term *"insertion loss."*

The work of Dalsgaard and Jensen (1976) led to the acknowledgment that the standardized 2 cc hard-walled cavity electroacoustic measurements supplied for each hearing aid by the manufacturer were substantially altered when the hearing aid was coupled to an earmold and placed into an ear canal. In general, the 2 cc coupler response of the hearing aid and earmold overestimates gain between 2000 and 4000 Hz by 12–18 dB and underestimates gain below 1500 Hz by 5–7 dB when compared with real-ear insertion gain measurements. Thus, real-ear measurements differ considerably from the physical cavity measurements, making it impossible to predict accurately the acoustical performance of a hearing aid when it is attached to a coupling system and inserted into a hearing-impaired patient's ear canal.

The earmold itself is an essential feature of the hearing aid system. It provides support for the hearing aid on or in the patient's external ear, while directing the sound into the ear canal, and, if properly fitted, prevents acoustic feedback. Since even minor variations in the fitting and configuration of the earmold can alter the electroacoustic parameters of the hearing aid, it is important to evaluate each hearing aid with the earmold that is to be used with it. This may require two or more sessions for fitting hearing aids on children: one session during which the earmold impression is obtained, and an additional session after the permanent custom earmold has been fabricated. It is particularly difficult to conduct hearing aid evaluations with children using stock earmolds, since the stock earmolds often do not fit well in the child's ear canals and most certainly do not represent how the hearing aid will perform when the child has his or her own earmold. The pinna continues to grow in size, and the concha changes shape, until the child reaches the age of about 9 years. Thus, earmolds and

custom ITE hearing aids should routinely be reevaluated and remade every 3–6 months during the child's early years, and once a year after age 5 to ensure satisfactory fit.

The earmold may be crafted in many ways (with open vents, various tubing, filters, and so on) to enhance the hearing aid. The material of the earmold is relatively insignificant in terms of general acoustics. The most important factor about the earmold is that acoustic feedback must be prevented if the child is to obtain maximum benefit from the hearing aid.

Through developments in subminiature transducers and electronics, the physical performance of hearing aids has been vastly improved, and problems previously associated with the earmold and acoustic coupling are now sufficiently understood so that a smooth frequency response of the hearing aid, as perceived by the user, can be individually tailored in a highly predictable manner (Killion, 1982). One of the most important electroacoustic characteristics of a hearing aid is the absence of "peaks and valleys" in the frequency response curve.

The development of transducers with wideband capabilities, and the "stepped diameter" approach to the conventional acoustic coupling system, which can be extended to the earmold to improve the high-frequency response of the aid, have had tremendous impact on the fidelity of amplification (Fig. 8.5). Libby (1982) described various earmold and tubing construction to influence the electroacoustic frequency response of the hearing aid system in a predictable fashion. Venting the earmold is an effective technique to influence low-frequency responses below 1000 Hz, which in effect reduces the patient's total SPL exposure significantly (by as much as 20 dB at some frequencies). Damping is a useful technique to smooth the frequency range between 1000 and 3000 Hz, and the acoustic horn or stepped-diameter approach to the acoustic coupling system often extends the frequency response beyond 3000 Hz. Construction of the earmold becomes increas-

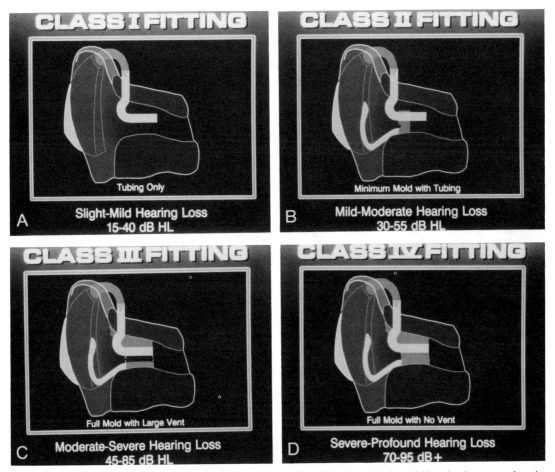

Figure 8.7. Sullivan classification system for acoustic coupling of hearing aids for mild hearing loss to profound hearing loss.

ingly important to preserve the high-frequency response of the hearing aid. To meet these needs, a one-piece, tapered, internally stepped bore horn can be used effectively to conserve high-frequency components of amplified sound, which are so important to hearing-impaired children in the learning of speech and auditory discrimination.

Acoustic Coupling Classification System. Sullivan (1985) developed an acoustic coupling-based classification system for hearing aid fitting. The Sullivan classification system takes into consideration a number of important acoustic coupling variables including whether the system is essentially parallel or in series, transmission loss of the hearing aid-earmold system, venting, the hermetic seal of the earmold, the residual ear canal volume between the earmold bore and the tympanic membrane, and the in situ gain and output. Sullivan's classification system also takes into consideration the effects of pinna diffraction and the resonances of the ear, concha, and ear canal. The Sullivan classification system organizes the acoustic coupling components into four general classes, ranging from mild hearing losses with open ear canal fittings to profound hearing loss requiring tight, full earmold coupling (Fig. 8.7).

Class I Acoustic Couplings. Class I acoustic coupling is the most open-canal type fitting, used frequently with mild hearing impairment or high-frequency hearing loss. This type of fitting permits the amplification of the instrument to be augmented by the direct transmission of unamplified sounds through the open ear canal. Examples of class I fittings include tube fittings, soundfield or CROS open earmolds, and shell earmolds with no ear canal occlusion.

Class II Acoustic Couplings. The class II fitting utilizes a minimal earmold and is used with mild-to-moderate hearing impairments. Class II fittings include acoustic modifier earmolds with various venting systems. The class II fitting is essentially a parallel fitting with a slight high-frequency acoustic transmission loss. A minimal acoustic vent system is used with no hermetic seal on the earmold and moderate ear canal volume. The class II in situ gain is 20–35 dB with an in situ output of 80–100 dB SPL.

Class III Acoustic Couplings. Class III acoustic couplings utilize closed earmold fittings with vents of sufficiently small size to preclude acoustic feedback. In class III fittings the external ear effects are displaced if the hearing aid is of the behind-the-ear type. Class III ITE hearing aid fittings retain pinna diffraction with no usable concha or ear canal resonance. The class III hearing aid coupling system is characterized as a closed earmold with adequate hermetic seal. The in situ gain is 30–55 dB, and the in situ output is 95–115 dB SPL.

Class IV Acoustic Couplings. Class IV acoustic coupling fittings are applied to patients with severe and profound hearing loss. These patients generally require the tightest earmold hermetic seal, which, of course, creates the greatest magnitude of direct acoustic transmission loss. The class IV closed earmold system requires a tightly fitted earmold with no vents and deep canal insertion to obtain an in situ gain of 50–75 dB and to accomplish an in situ output of 110–135 dB SPL. Sullivan (1985) suggests that probe-tube microphone real-ear measurements may be accomplished by pre-drilling a 1.5-mm hole in the earmold, which is then sealed with a removal plug. The plug may be removed when future probe-microphone real-ear measurements are desired.

EAR CANAL PHYSICAL VOLUME AND HEARING AIDS

Clinicians are aware, of course, that hearing aid technical specifications are reported in decibels relative to a 2.0 cc coupler. The hearing aid specifications relative to a 2.0 cc cavity are altered significantly when the hearing aid is coupled tightly to an ear canal that is less than 2.0 cc in volume. In fact, each time the cavity volume is reduced by one half, sound pressure is increased by 6 dB. It can be expected that hearing aid sound pressures measured in a 2.0 cc cavity will be delivered to an adult 1.0 cc canal with 6 dB more intensity than that shown on the standard hearing aid frequency response curve (Cole, 1975). Infants with ear canal volumes of approximately 0.5 cc may actually receive as much as 12 dB more amplification than that shown on the hearing aid technical specification sheet. That is, an instrument with an SSPL 90 of 130 dB, as measured in a 2.0 cc coupler, becomes capable of delivering 142 dB SPL when coupled to an ear having a 0.5 cc space between the tip of the earmold and the eardrum (Fig. 8.8).

Jirsa and Norris (1978) examined changes in hearing aid performance characteristics, which resulted from a reduction in coupler volume from 2.0 cc to 1.0 cc and 0.5 cc, in an effort to determine the differences that might exist between cavity size and SPL. Results showed that as volume was reduced, the SPL developed inside the cavity increased. In addition, Jirsa and Norris examined the relationship between threshold improvement and acoustic gain, aided and unaided speech reception thresholds, and ear canal volume, in eight hearing-impaired children. Acoustic gain as meas-

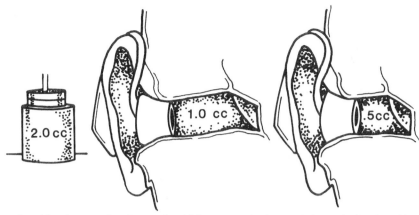

Figure 8.8. Consideration must be given to the child's ear canal volume relative to the hearing aid specifications obtained on a 2 cc coupler. Children's small ear canals may lead to overamplification.

ured via the threshold improvement procedure was compared with that measured in the standard 2.0 cc and the experimental 1.0 cc and 0.5 cc couplers. Results showed that functional threshold improvement always exceeded the 2.0 cc coupler acoustic gain measure. The results reported by these investigators again suggest that it is important to consider the increase in SPL that will occur in real ears when determining appropriate acoustic gain and maximum power output (SSPL 90) requirements from electroacoustic data. Failure to account for these differences may result in overamplification and cause the child either to reject the aid or to reduce the hearing aid gain to allow for a more comfortable listening level (Schwartz and Larson, 1977).

Bragg (1977) reported that the most common problem in hearing aid fitting is "overamplification." Clinicians who select hearing aids based on 2.0 cc coupler measurements must be aware, therefore, that overamplification may result from coupling an aid and a full earmold to an ear having a volume of less than 2.0 cc. According to Sachs and Burkhard (1972), the 2.0 cc coupler underestimates aided SPL relative to the human ear canal by as much as 15 dB in the higher frequencies. The acoustic immittance meter can provide important information if the physical volume test (PVT) is conducted to estimate ear canal volume prior to selection of the hearing aid. In addition, it is important to measure the overall SPL in the child's ear canal with computerized probe-microphone real-ear-aided response (REAR) to verify actual "in situ" amplification levels.

CAN HEARING AIDS DAMAGE HEARING?

Clinicians often worry that powerful hearing aids fitted to children may cause additional hearing damage due to overamplification. In fact, case studies have been published over the years that show that the use of a hearing aid may cause temporary and permanent threshold shift, resulting in further hearing loss.

Kasten and Braunlin (1970) presented a case study in which they could create deterioration in patient's hearing through the use of a hearing aid. Their patient was a 10 year old girl with bilateral, moderate sensorineural hearing loss. She wore a body-type hearing aid satisfactorily in one ear for 14 months and then began to complain that the aid was not helping as much as it did previously. An audiometric evaluation showed marked worsening of the hearing in the aided ear and no change in the hearing of the unaided ear. Kasten and Braunlin alternated the hearing aid between ears and were able to show temporary deterioration in the aided ear, regardless of which ear wore the hearing aid.

Two patients exhibiting temporary increases in sensorineural hearing loss following hearing aid use were reported by Heffernan and Simons (1979). The use of different hearing aids with decreased power output did not cause temporary threshold shifts. Based on their experiences, Heffernan and Simons offer specific follow-up routine to include: (1) check of performance with the new hearing aid within 30 days of purchase, (2) electroacoustic analysis of the new aid within 30 days of purchase, (3) monthly appointments thereafter to monitor hearing thresholds until the hearing levels have stabilized for at least 3 months of continual hearing aid use, (4) reevaluation at least every 3 months for the next calendar year, and (5) annual otologic and audiologic evaluations as long as the aid is worn.

Rojskjaer (1960) reported an evaluation of 390 cases of all types of hearing loss treated with hearing aids for 5 years or more. He found 9 cases with additional hearing loss in the aided ear. No cases were noted where hearing deteriorated in nonaided ears. Naunton (1957) reviewed charts of 120 patients selected from a population of 1480. He compared thresholds from the nonaided ear with the aided ear of these patients and concluded that changes in hearing as a result of hearing aid use are statistically and clinically nonsignificant.

Macrae and Farrant (1965) evaluated changes in the aided and unaided ears of 87 children and concluded that (a) individuals with sensorineural hearing loss should be fitted with limited maximal power output hearing aids, (b) frequent audiologic follow-up of aided children should be required, (c) children should alternate use of the aid in each ear whenever practical, and (d) users should be cautioned about wearing hearing aids in high ambient noise environments. Macrae (1968a, 1968b) found temporary threshold shift in the aided ears of children with sensorineural deafness following use of powerful hearing aids. He measured the hearing levels of four children from a school for the deaf on Friday afternoon after the youngsters had worn their hearing aids all week. He then kept the aids and deprived the children of amplification for 66 hours, until the following Monday morning. Hearing levels in all four children showed improvement on Monday morning but again deteriorated after 4 hours of hearing aid use.

Jerger and Lewis (1975) described an incident of progressive hearing loss in a young patient attributed to excessive sound pressure from a high-power hearing aid. These authors suggest caution in fitting high-power hearing aids binaurally in children. Reilly et al. (1981) examined the effects of hearing aid use on progressive hearing loss in children. Careful examination of the role of amplification and the time period of progressive hearing loss "probably" implicated the hearing aid in 11% and "questionably" implicated the hearing in an additional 20% of the patients. These authors warn that it is unwise to conclude that hearing aid use is the cause of hearing deterioration without considering all other plausible factors. Details of several experimental investigations regarding the use of amplification and its effect on residual hearing have been summarized by Rintelmann and Bess (1988). Humes and Bess (1981) published a tutorial on the potential deterioration in hearing as a result of hearing aid use, based on studies of temporary threshold shift induced by overamplification.

The evidence for powerful hearing aids causing threshold changes in the aided ear certainly seems to us to suggest this unfortunate circumstance as a possibility to be considered by clinicians. Further developments will hopefully assist in identifying children, in advance, who might suffer trauma from hearing aid use. There is much we still do not know about some basic psychophysical facts related to hearing loss and hearing aid use. Many patients with profound hearing loss have no loudness discomfort at any level, while other patients, with seemingly similar hearing loss, have loudness tolerance problems so severe that they cannot tolerate any type of amplification.

Darbyshire (1976) and Titche et al. (1977) examined large groups of children with hearing aids for signs of possible effects of amplification on auditory sensitivity. The conclusion that hearing aids have no damaging effects on the hearing sensitivity of children was reported in each study.

A comprehensive review of the literature by Mills (1975) provides the most logical conclusions available. In general, he states, "the results of all studies indicate that habitual use of a hearing aid is not associated with additional deterioration of hearing in a large majority of persons tested. In some subjects, however, decreases in auditory sensitivity are observed." However, Mills questions whether the additional hearing losses are due to genetic or to disease-related factors, or whether they are due to the chronic temporary threshold shifts of 5–20 dB reported on many hard-of-hearing adults who use powerful hearing aids. Auditory threshold shifts of 5–20 dB may be a small cost for the many benefits of a hearing aid.

We wholeheartedly support the recommendations of Ross and Lerman (1967) to alleviate or lessen the possibility of inadvertent traumatic hearing loss related to overamplification:

1. Additional hearing loss is most likely related to use of extremely high levels of maximal power output that exceed 130 dB SSPL; hearing aid recommendations for children with sensorineural hearing loss should include only hearing aids with less than 130 dB SSPL.
2. Although we recognize that traumatic hearing loss may be related to hearing aid use, the incidence seems quite small, and our concern is by no means to be interpreted as contradictory to amplification. In fact, we believe that denying a child a hearing aid during the critical language years may only be saving his or her hearing for no good purpose. If the

aid is fitted too late, it will not help anyway.
3. Frequent follow-up audiometric and hearing aid evaluation is an absolute must for all children with sensorineural hearing loss who wear hearing aids. We reevaluate our aided children twice a year.

AMPLIFICATION IN THE CLASSROOM

One of the most important aspects of amplification is its use in the school or educational setting. Important technologic advancements have occurred in the past few years that make amplification in the classroom an essential component in the education of hearing-impaired children. Excellent reviews of classroom amplification have been written by Freeman et al. (1980), Bess and Logan (1984), and Bess and Sinclair (1985).

The acoustic environment in which hearing-impaired students do their learning typically has high noise levels and poor acoustic reverberation conditions. Olsen (1981) and Finitzo-Hieber (1982) have shown that classroom acoustics are an important consideration that can be deleterious to the hearing-impaired student. The three critical factors are the level of noise in the classroom, the level of speech or the desired signal, and the amount of room acoustic reverberation. To be sure, certain architectural improvements can be made in school rooms to help reduce unwanted noise and limit reverberation (May and Brackett, 1984), but in these days of mainstreaming it is unlikely that all classrooms can be modified to meet the needs of the hearing-impaired student. Sanders (1965) reported the mean noise values of normal school-occupied classrooms to be 55–65 dBA or as high as 69 dBA, while Bess and McConnell (1981) indicate that the highest acceptable noise level in classrooms used by hearing-impaired children is 30–35 dBA.

Hearing aid users complain about the difficulty of understanding speech in the presence of background noise. In fact, Walden et al. (1984) showed that the noise in the environment is the most significant factor limiting benefit from the use of personal amplification. The challenge of helping hearing-impaired children who wear hearing aids in the typical noisy classroom situation creates serious problems for the teacher and the educational audiologist.

The personal hearing aid is, of course, the most common means of providing schoolroom amplification. The major drawback to the personal unit is its dependence on close distance to the speaker to achieve a high signal-to-noise effect. Unfortunately, this is difficult to control in the typical classroom, and as the teacher moves away from the child wearing a personal hearing aid, the increase in distance contributes quickly to the demise of signal amplification for the hearing-impaired child. When faced with a weak sound signal, the hearing aid user must turn up the gain of the unit, which also increases the background noise, creating unavoidable masking effects.

These problems led to the development of radio frequency transmission units (FM) with wireless microphones. FM amplification represents the best means of combating poor classroom acoustics. The wireless microphone is worn by the teacher, which strengthens and stabilizes the reception of the speaker's voice while simultaneously minimizing the effect of background sounds. External receivers may be coupled to the personal earmolds worn by the hearing-impaired child. The student receivers can be adjusted to make them adaptable to a wide range of individual needs.

Even more recently, a number of newer techniques permit the "dovetailing" of the personal hearing aid to the FM system (Bess and Logan, 1984). The coupling of the FM system to the personal hearing aid can be accomplished by several techniques including electrical, induction, or acoustical. The advantages to an FM radio transmission through a wireless microphone attached close to the mouth of the speaker, sending high-fidelity signals to the personal hearing aid of the hearing-impaired child

(who may be as far as 200 meters (650 feet) away) are obvious.

Hawkins (1984) states that the optimum classroom amplification system using the personal FM system concept would consist of (a) a directional microphone as close as possible to the teacher's mouth, (b) a FM receiver coupled via direct input to binaural hearing aids on each hearing-impaired child, and (c) switch positions on the hearing aids, allowing for choice of hearing aids only, FM reception only, or FM plus hearing aid microphones. Hawkins showed that the advantage of the FM system over hearing aids alone is substantial, equivalent to a 12–18 dB improvement in signal-to-noise ratio even when the child is in an optimal classroom position. For the child with less than optimal classroom position, the FM advantage over hearing aids alone would even be greater.

The application of the FM personal hearing aid system is much broader than just schoolroom use. These systems are practical for at-home use, learning sports activities, driver's education, and large group theater or auditorium activities. The FM system is no longer a "special instrument" consideration but is an important part of every hearing-impaired child's daily life.

TACTILE SENSORY AIDS

Interest in tactile sensory aids for the hearing-impaired has been a long-time research activity, although wide acceptance and utilization of these devices have not occurred. Levitt (1988) reviewed the issues underlying the development of tactile sensory aids and pointed out that the current interest in cochlear implants has stimulated new research in alternatives to traditional amplification instruments. Amid concern for the surgical intervention and finality of cochlear implants, many have questioned whether hearing-impaired persons could do just as well with a technologically advanced, noninvasive sensory aid.

Tactile aids change auditory signals into either vibratory or electrical patterns on the skin. The vibrotactile approach presents a vibration to the skin through a bone conduction vibrator, a small solenoid, or other mechanical transducer. The electrotactile approach presents the acoustical signal through the skin via a tiny electrical current. As Roeser (1985) described it, "the goal of a tactile communication system is to extract relevant information from the acoustic signal and to present it to the individual as a means of supplementing or replacing the auditory reception of speech as the ultimate challenge." These devices are also used to teach and reinforce speech production.

Vibrotactile devices have been preferred over the electrotactile instruments due to the availability of vibrators and difficulties of applying electrical current to the skin. Vibrotactile devices, however, have generally poor frequency response and have high-power requirements, and users have difficulties in background noise environments. Sachs et al. (1980) compared vibrotactile and electrotactile devices and showed that the vibrotactile instruments were more efficient in transmitting lower frequencies, while the electrotactile devices were more efficient with higher frequency signals. According to Levitt (1988), new technologic advances, combined with ongoing research on cochlear implants, have resulted in the development of new tactile aids that include spectral or vocoder-type displays in which the spectrum of the encoded sound is represented with a one- or two-dimensional array of stimulators, as well as speech-processing tactile devices in which specific features of the speech signal are displayed.

Research reports into the effect of tactile aids on speech reception and speech production are encouraging. At the simplest levels, with only modest training, children are helped at the syllable level in recognizing supersegmental features of speech, such as rhythm, number of syllables, contrasting voiced/unvoiced sounds, nasal versus oral production, and stop continuants (Franklin, 1988). Goldstein and Stark (1976) analyzed consonant-vowel syllables of four profoundly deaf children using tactile, visual, and nonspeech displays. They found significant increase in consonant-vowel production in both tactile and visual groups, while the control group demonstrated no significant change. Oller et al. (1980) reported improvement in pronunciation of fricative and nasal consonants with tactile aid use. Friel-Patti and Roeser (1985) reported increased vocalization and sign language communication in deaf children with use of the vibrotactile aid and decreased vocalization and sign language without use of the tactile aid. Boothroyd's continued research with tactile transformation of voice as a supplement to speech reading has recently been published (1988).

COCHLEAR IMPLANTS FOR CHILDREN

One of the most dramatic and exciting developments in hearing and deafness has been the cochlear implant. Over the past 20 years, the idea of restoring hearing to profoundly deaf patients by artificially stimulating the sensory system has progressed from a futuristic possibility to reality. The cochlear implant is a surgically inserted device that delivers electrical stimulation within the inner ear. A cochlear implant relies on the fact that many auditory nerve fibers remain viable in patients with cochlear-type deafness. The surviving neurons of the eighth nerve can be stimulated to excitation by applying external electric currents of the proper strength, duration, and orientation, resulting in actively propagating neural impulses. These evoked electrical neural potentials arrive at the temporal lobes of the cortex just like the normal neural impulses generated by acoustic signals that intact cochlear hair cells transduce. The brain interprets these artificial potentials as sound (Loeb, 1985).

Several paradigms have been developed into various types of cochlear implants to create direct stimulation of the eighth nerve. Sophisticated single-channel and multichannel devices have been manufactured in the United States, Australia, and Europe and have undergone considerable animal and human research. Each device has a microphone for picking up external sounds and an elaborate microelectronic processor for converting the sound into electrical signals and sending them to the tiny electrode array that is surgically implanted into the cochlea as shown in Figure 8.9. Only carefully selected patients can benefit from cochlear implants, in particular, those deafened individuals who have defective sensory elements (hair cells) in the cochlea with surviving, intact fibers of the auditory (VIII) nerve. Basically, the cochlear implant replaces the defective hair cells of the inner ear with an array of stimulation electrodes (Shallop and Mecklenburg, 1988).

Loeb (1985) described the operation of the cochlear implant in a *Scientific American* article:

The loudness of the sound perceived depends roughly on the number of nerve fibers activated and their rates of firing. Both variables are functions of the amplitude of the stimulus current. The pitch is related to the place on the basilar membrane from which those nerve fibers once derived their acoustic input, in agreement with the place-pitch theory. In principle, with enough independent channels of stimulation, each controlling the activity of a small, local subset of the auditory nerve fibers, one could recreate the normal neural response to acoustic stimuli of any spectral composition. The brain would then process that information in its usual manner and the subject would "hear" the "sounds".

Cochlear implants have been used with adult deaf patients since the mid-1970s. All of the initial cochlear implants in the United States used the 3M/House single-channel device. It was generally agreed that while the early 3M/House single-channel device could not actually reproduce speech sounds to the patient, the implant could provide important and useful sound cues to aid in speechreading and in the identification of environmental sounds. It was not until 1982 that federal investigational device exemption was granted for the 3M/House single-channel device to be implanted into profoundly deaf children. By 1986, more than

200 children, between the ages of 2 and 17 years, received the 3M/House single-channel cochlear implant (Berliner et al., 1985).

The use of cochlear implants in children raises a number of special questions regarding potential problems related to the long-term effects of the implant in the child's body. In addition, many clinicians questioned results from surgically implanted amplification devices that did not appear significantly better than results obtained with traditional hearing aids. Finally, what about new, improved technology that would be available in future cochlear implant devices that may or may not be exchangeable for the child's original implant? And yet, it was agreed among professionals that maximum benefit afforded by these surgically implanted devices, if successful, would be most valuable to young deaf children in their quest to learn speech and develop social communication skills.

Subsequent advances in technology (*a*) led to the development of more sophisticated multichannel cochlear implants that enabled adult users to recognize more environmental sounds, (*b*) provided more speechreading enhancement, and (*c*) enabled users to understand limited open speech materials than were provided by single-channel implants (Gantz et al., 1988). Based on the success of the Cochlear Nucleus 22-channel cochlear implant with adults and on the introduction of a new, smaller, receiver and stimulator, the federal government granted investigational device exception to Cochlear Corporation to begin carefully controlled studies with profoundly deaf children. Because of the concern and need for thorough evaluations of child candidates for cochlear implants, only approved implant centers with an active children's cochlear implant team composed of an otologist, audiologist, speech/language pathologist, psychologist, deaf educator, and pediatrician can perform the surgery and carry out the extensive post-surgical auditory training.

The Cochlear Nucleus group began their children's project by implanting the mul-

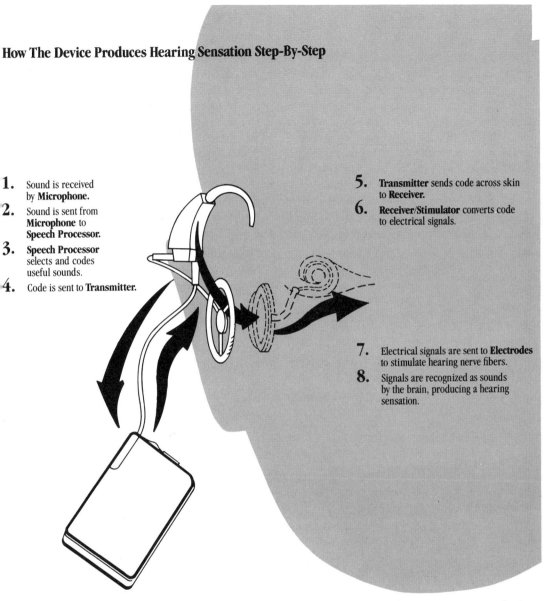

How The Device Produces Hearing Sensation Step-By-Step

1. Sound is received by **Microphone.**

2. Sound is sent from **Microphone** to **Speech Processor.**

3. **Speech Processor** selects and codes useful sounds.

4. Code is sent to **Transmitter.**

5. **Transmitter** sends code across skin to **Receiver.**

6. **Receiver/Stimulator** converts code to electrical signals.

7. Electrical signals are sent to **Electrodes** to stimulate hearing nerve fibers.

8. Signals are recognized as sounds by the brain, producing a hearing sensation.

Figure 8.9. Diagrammatic representation of the operation of the cochlear implant. (Photograph provided by Cochlear Corporation, Englewood, Colorado.)

tichannel device in two groups of children. One group consisted of postlingually deafened children between the ages of 10 and 17 years, while the second group included prelingually deaf children from 2 to 9 years of age (Mecklenburg, 1987). As of January 1990, 263 profoundly deaf children have been implanted in the United States under the approved protocol for the Cochlear Nucleus 22-channel device (Staller et al.,

1991). The preliminary results have been very promising. All the children in the study respond to electrical stimulation and are able to detect sound at normal conversational intensities across the speech frequency range. This result is astonishing, considering the fact that all the children included in the study had profound, bilateral sensorineural deafness from birth or at a very early age. Nearly half of the study group had a deafness etiology of meningitis, while in the other half of the sample group the cause of deafness was unknown.

A tiny audio receiver is implanted in the temporal bone behind the pinna, and a special wire electrode array with 22 separate channels is surgically inserted into the cochlea. After about 1 month for healing, the patient is fitted with the system's external parts: a microphone and a transmitter that are connected by wires to a computerized speech processor worn in a shoulder pouch, in a pocket, or on a belt. A microphone within a behind-the-ear case picks up sounds and relays them to the speech processor, which is postsurgically set by an audiologist to transmit those sounds that will help the patient interpret speech (Fig. 8.8).

The implanted device is capable of delivering biphasic stimulus current pulses between any pair of electrodes or between any one electrode and the remaining common electrodes. This system requires postsurgical programming that permits individual electrodes to be "tuned" to fit the specific hearing loss pattern of the patient. This programming is conducted through audiologic behavioral hearing responses from the newly implanted patient. An advantage of this system is that if any changes in hearing occur over time, the speech processor and electrodes can be reprogrammed as many times as needed with no disturbance to the implant or the patient. Typically, the audiologist is the cochlear implant team member responsible for programming the implant device to the individual child's needs.

Extensive training using visual and/or tactile stimuli is necessary to teach the young deaf child to give reliable, time-locked behavioral responses to discrete electrical stimulation of the electrodes. Special programming concepts are taught to each young child prior to implant placement, so that the child can respond to electrode threshold levels, establish loudness comfort levels across frequency, comprehend loudness concepts to determine effective electrical dynamic range, and loudness scaling to assess loudness growth relative

to electrical current levels (Fig. 8.10). Prior to the initiation of the children's implant study program, concern was expressed by professionals that deaf children could not be taught to respond to such subtle differences in the acoustic stimuli necessary to program the multichannel cochlear implant. It is to the merit of the skilled audiologists involved in these early children's implant programs that techniques were successfully developed, even with the youngest of deaf children, to measure the various psychophysical parameters to permit accurate programming of the cochlear implant.

Selection of Children for Cochlear Implants. A multidisciplinary colloquium composed of experts in the fields of audiology, hearing science, medicine, psychology, linguistics, statistics, speech/language pathology, and deaf education met in 1986 to discuss the ramifications of cochlear implants for deaf children (Mecklenburg, 1986). One of the critical issues discussed was the minimum patient selection criteria. The recommended minimal criteria for patient selection that should be applied to every child being considered for cochlear implantation is shown in Table 8.3. Only children with profound or total, bilateral sensorineural deafness should be considered for a cochlear implant with a minimum age of 2 years. This age constraint was imposed not for technical surgical considerations but rather to permit time to establish the diagnosis of deafness, with full audiologic information and hearing aid performance evaluation.

The colloquium proceedings recommended that only deaf children with normal intelligence be considered for cochlear implants during the initial years. To perform cochlear implants on children with less than normal intelligence would certainly confound the child's prognosis with the implant and create difficulties in interpreting the child's subsequent development. By the same logic, it was suggested that deaf children with additional handicaps, such as autism and significant learning disabilities that might adversely affect their success with a

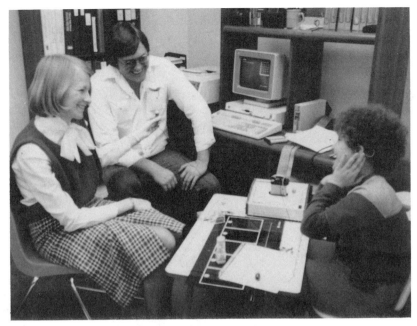

Figure 8.10. An audiologist programs a child's cochlear implant. (Photograph provided by Jon Shallop, Ph.D., Denver Ear Institute.)

cochlear implant, not be implanted. Another important consideration in selecting child implant patients is evidence of strong family support exemplified by an understanding of the problems that may be associated with the implant device. It is necessary that the immediate family of the child have appropriate expectations and a strong commitment to the responsibilities of postimplant auditory training with their child.

A final important consideration is the auditory development of the hearing-impaired

child prior to selection as a cochlear implant candidate. Before the decision is made to implant the child, the colloquium proceedings recommended that the entire implant team reach consensus that satisfactory progress in auditory development is *not* being made, despite "effective training and appropriately fitted hearing aids." Since the recognition of satisfactory progress in auditory development may be difficult to ascertain in a deaf infant or young child, two guidelines were offered to describe *lack of auditory development:*

- Little or no ability to discriminate spectral information of the segmental aspects of speech after at least 1 year of effective auditory training and appropriately fitted hearing aids; or

- Inadequate progress in verbal language skill according to preselected criteria after at least 1 year of effective auditory training and appropriately fitted hearing aids.

Table 8.3.
Minimum Required Conditions for Selection of Children for Cochlear Implants[a]

Minimum 2 years of age
Bilateral, profound or total, sensorineural deafness
Completion of all preevaluation procedures
IQ at least within normal limits
No additional handicaps (such as autism or significant learning disabilities) that might adversely affect potential success with implant
Strong evidence of family support
Team decision that satisfactory progress in auditory development is not being made despite effective training and appropriately fitted hearing aids

[a]From J. L. Northern: Selection of children for cochlear implantation. *Seminars in Hearing* 7:4, p. 342, 1986.

Suggested Hierarchy for Potential Success with Cochlear Implants. Because

Table 8.4.
Potential for Success Hierarchy for Children with Cochlear Implants[a]

Group	Onset of Profound, Bilateral Deafness[b]	Duration of Deprivation[b]	Type of Educational Training
I	Acquired after 4 years	Short-term	Oral-auditory
IIa	Acquired before 4 years	Short-term, implanted before age 5 years	Oral-auditory
IIb	Acquired before 4 years	Long-term	Oral-auditory
IIIa	Acquired after 4 years	Long-term	Total communication
IIIb	Acquired before 4 years	Short-term	Total communication
IVa	Congenital[c]	Short-term	Oral-auditory
IVb	Congenital	Short-term	Total communication
V	Acquired before 4 years	Long-term, implanted after age 5 years	Total communication
VI	Congenital	Long-term	Total communication

[a]From J. L. Northern: Selection of children for cochlear implantation. *Seminars in Hearing* 7:4, p. 344, 1986.
[b]Acquired, short-term: 6–24 months. Congenital, short-term: Before 5 years of age.
[c]See text for explanation.

deaf children are not a homogeneous population and because numerous variables associated with each child may influence the potential success of a cochlear implant, the colloquium members developed a classification system to identify a general hierarchy of potential success with cochlear implants as shown in Table 8.4. This classification system was based largely on previous experiences with deaf children implant recipients and on knowledge of cochlear implant results in children as reported by Berliner et al. (1985) and Eisenberg et al. (1986).

The hierarchy suggested for potential success with cochlear implants in children, as shown in Table 8.4, includes six categories. The categories represent a progression of success levels, with group I representing the children with the most potential for success and group VI representing the children with the least potential for success. Previous experience had established that a child's success with a cochlear implant depends on the age of deafness onset, the duration of auditory deprivation due to deafness, and the type of educational training the child has been given since the onset of the deafness. In general, children with acquired deafness are better candidates for cochlear implants than children with congenital deafness; children who have been deaf for only a short time do better with cochlear implants than children who have been deafened for some extended length of time; and deaf children who have had auditory-oral educational training are more

likely to achieve success with a cochlear implant than deaf children in total communication (manual) educational settings. These classification systems serve as guidelines for surgeons and audiologists in assessing children as potential candidates for cochlear implants and assume that the child has met all the minimum requirements for patient selection. This classification system is useful in counseling parents and educators about the relative potential for a child's success with a cochlear implant.

The future for cochlear implants in children is especially bright, and technology is continually improving in terms of better speech-processing paradigms and hardware design. At this point in time, those hearing-impaired children who can benefit from well-fit hearing aids are far better off than those children who must rely on cochlear implants for auditory input. It is likely that as more experience is gained with today's cochlear implants, future applications will be attempted with individuals who have severe sensorineural loss and will not be limited to only those with profound, total deafness.

FAMILY MANAGEMENT

The importance of parental involvement in the habilitation process of their hearing-impaired children is absolutely crucial to the child's success with amplification. Unfortunately, there are no specific guidelines that can always be followed when dealing with parents. Just like the children, each child's parents are unique and have individual backgrounds, attitudes, and needs that must be dealt with on a very personal basis. The audiologist may be well-advised to plan on spending at least as much time talking with parents as working with the child. Often the parents develop a special relationship with the audiologist, as it is the audiologist who probably confirmed the presence of hearing loss in the child. It would be worthwhile for the reader to review the discussion of parent management in Chapter 5, Clinical Audiologic Testing, as most of the same principles involved in discussing the child's handicapping hearing loss also apply to helping the parents accept their role in working with the amplification device worn by their child.

The prognosis for the hearing-handicapped child to obtain maximum benefit from amplification has a direct relation to the level of support provided by the immediate family. Evidence of strong family support can actually be noted with empirical observation by the audiologist and are not just based on subjective intuition. Family behavior can be observed over time and modified when necessary through careful and appropriate counseling. Behaviors to be noted that may have influence over the child's use of amplification include:

- Family accepts and understands child's hearing loss.

- Family shows responsibility for scheduling and keeping all medical and educational appointments on behalf of the child.

- Family is knowledgeable about the etiology of and the prognosis for the child's hearing loss.

- Family communicates well with the child by encouraging conversation under all circumstances.

- Family has appropriate expectations about the amplification devices utilized by the child.

- Family displays high interest and motivational levels in child-related activities.

- Family spends ample, constructive time with the child.

- Family has genuine concern for child's educational and physical development.

In Luterman's book, *Counseling Parents of Hearing-Impaired Children* (1979), he describes different approaches for the audiologist to use in order for parents to cope with their child's special needs. Luterman emphasizes that the parents, not the professional, must make the decisions regarding their child's habilitation because they must accept and take the ultimate responsibility. Certainly, parents must accept and understand the need for amplification before hearing aids can be successfully placed and utilized by the hearing-impaired youngster.

Once hearing aids have been recommended and selected, it is important for the parents to observe the child's aided and unaided responses in a sound field situation to see for themselves that their child benefits from using personal amplification. Once convinced of the need and benefits provided by amplification, the parents will likely not be embarrassed or apologetic about the hearing aids. The parents must understand that although personal amplification is absolutely necessary for the development of their child, it may require extensive auditory therapy before these newly amplified sounds will be meaningful to the child. The parents should also be made aware of the number of important assistive listening devices that are available to help the hearing-impaired child gain maximum benefit and relate effectively with daily communication and listening tasks.

The audiologist's role in parental management of their child's personal amplification and assistive listening devices has a great deal to do with the ultimate successful acceptance and utilization of these hearing instruments. That role should include education, guidance, and counseling, since the parents' attitude regarding amplification may be the single most important factor in successful hearing aid use by the hearing-impaired child.

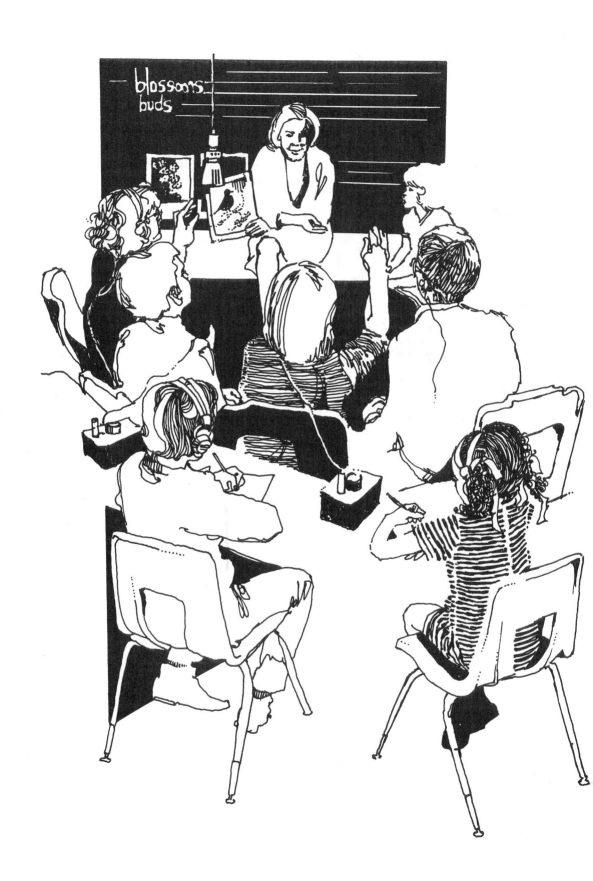

CHAPTER 9

Education of Hearing-Impaired Children

AUDIOLOGY AND EDUCATION OF THE HEARING-IMPAIRED CHILD

One of the first issues to be clarified in this chapter is that of terminology and definition. Our definition of "hearing-impaired" children includes all those children with hearing loss who are handicapped to such an extent that some form of special education is required. Obviously, this broad definition includes those we traditionally define as "deaf." The Conference of Executives of American Schools for the Deaf defines "the deaf" as having a hearing loss of 70 dB hearing level (HL) or greater in their better ear, while the "hard-of-hearing" student has a loss of 35–69 dB HL in the better hearing ear. Amon (1981) defines "deaf" as a hearing impairment so severe that a child experiences difficulty in processing linguistic information through hearing, with or without amplification. Although it is easy to speak in general terms about the education of deaf and/or hard-of-hearing students, the point must be made that these groups are by no means homogeneous, and there is no single educational "method," "system," or "approach" that is uniformly applicable to all members of each group.

Of all the information published throughout the years in previous editions of this textbook, this chapter, "Education of Hearing-Impaired Children," elicits more controversial commentary from our colleagues than any other chapter. But such is the nature of this topic, and it is unlikely that the information presented below will satisfy all readers. Our goal is to acquaint speech-language-hearing students with the single most important aspect of management of the child with hearing impairment—achieving the maximum potential of the child through education.

The audiologist is often hard-pressed to maintain the distinction between being an expert in hearing and being an advocate for the hearing-impaired child. When the audiologist expresses an objective statement within the field of hearing measurement, the facts are based on solid data. However, when the audiologist expresses a viewpoint or an opinion advocating a chosen position on questions of general policy not directly related to audiology, the stated opinion may be rather tenuous. In the area of education for hearing-impaired children, it certainly behooves the audiologist to know as much as possible about all avenues, methodologies, techniques, and systems for teaching this special population. It is obligatory that the audiologist who specializes in pediatric hearing evaluation also be knowledgeable and well-informed on the current status of education for hearing-impaired children.

The educational audiologist may prove to be the appropriate intermediary trained in deafness education and management with special emphasis in audiologic aspects of hearing-impaired children. As defined by the Educational Audiology Association, an educational audiologist is a specialist who ensures that all aspects of children's hearing and learning are maximized in order that their educational and real-life capabilities can be met. The educational audiologist is the person responsible for the child with hearing difficulties. In many instances, the role could be one of the case manager. The educational audiologist is qualified in the overall ramifications of sound, hearing, hearing loss, hearing aids, auditory perception (including central auditory abilities), and their impact on learning and life. The educational audiologist is responsible for identification, diagnosis, assessment, amplification programming, aural rehabilitation programming (and training when feasible), and central auditory programming. In addition, this professional is responsible for the selection of classrooms, training of supportive personnel, parent training and support, specialist coordination, listening training, hearing conservation programming, supervision of specialized testing, otologic referral, and ongoing evaluations of the child's classroom and educational functioning.

The audiologist is the professional best able to manage the complete hearing care of a child who experiences hearing loss of any degree (Flexer, 1990). Even a "mild" hearing loss can sabotage the development of academic competencies, and there is a growing population of school children with mild-moderate hearing loss. Unfortunately, there are far too few audiologists employed in educational settings (approximately 700 nationally), with an average ratio of 1 audiologist for every 12,000 children (Blair et al., 1989)!

Ross and Calvert (1977) recommend a minimum ratio of 1 audiologist to every 75 hearing-impaired children in school programs, in addition to necessary equipment and supportive personnel, to effectively exploit the residual hearing of the children. Excellent materials on the audiologist's role in the school setting are available, written by Bess and McConnell (1981) and Ross (1982).

In this book we have described objective measures that have been fairly adequately standardized, and we have also outlined subjective assessments that lend themselves to some measurable degree of judgment. Here we are under a fair amount of control. However, in the field of directing hearing-impaired children into educational channels, the audiologist becomes an advocate of a cause. Many audiologists do not have knowledge of all training methods and

what they can do, nor do they have an understanding of all the variables that will affect the child's functioning in a given training method. To rectify these inadequacies, we point out that the audiologist, in addition to personal empirical testing, must seek the judgments of various physicians, educators, psychologists, sociologists, and others. With these people the clinician must evolve a decision concerning the direction of management of the child—one that is flexible enough to change with the further accumulation of information.

Certainly there is a need for a variety of experts in the field of deafness. The difficulty comes from the fact that few "experts" have the important ingredient of objectiveness when it comes to evaluating the field of deaf education. The professional groups who know most about this area are the teachers themselves or program administrators. Yet these people are limited in number and isolated from new parents of a deaf child.

It is our philosophy that the audiologist can become an "advocate without a cause" in the field of educational management for the child. The audiologist should not be biased in the direction of any training method or philosophy and should consider only what will best ensure the child's maximal ultimate development. In this book we try to give the audiologist the tools to arrive at a working construct concerning the direction of management for a child.

In another sense, however, the audiologist can espouse advocacy for principle or cause alone. This is in the sense of fighting for the child's right to be given a chance to show what he or she can do, despite contrary evidence. We would be something less than human if we failed to let hope play a part in judgments of multiple-handicapped children. We also would be less than human if we failed to glow with satisfaction when a child who was scheduled for institutionalizing becomes trainable with hearing aids and hearing therapy, upon our insistence, or when an infant who was thought to be incapable of developing useful auditory perceptions becomes in every way a hearing person with adequate speech and language abilities.

Among the fundamental rights that we as surrogates for children should demand from society is a child's right to achieve his or her maximal potential communication abilities. We should demand of society that special provision be made to help the hearing-impaired child override the disability and become as "normal" as individual limitations will allow. The world-famous child psychologist, A. L. Gesell (1956), said: "The . . . aim should not be to convert the deaf child into a somewhat fictitious version of a normal hearing child, but into a well-adjusted nonhearing child who is completely managing the limitations of his [or her] sensory deficit." An excellent description of the current state of affairs in the field of education of hearing-impaired learners was written by Ferguson et al. (1988).

GOALS OF EDUCATION FOR THE HEARING-IMPAIRED

Obviously, there are many goals to be achieved in educating hearing-impaired and deaf children, but we have chosen to highlight only the four goals that we believe to be most important. Our goals, presented in order of importance, include achievement of adequate language skills, establishment of sound mental health, intelligible speech, and easy communication with peers. These goals by no means are to be interpreted as limiting the range of objectives that one might have for the hard-of-hearing and deaf child. However, other goals that we might enumerate—high employability, job satisfaction, enrichment of life—all depend on the success of achieving our four goals as described below.

Language. The importance of language cannot be denied. Language comes so easily to normal hearing children and is a giant stone wall for children with significant hearing impairment. Educators of hearing-impaired students realize the long-term commitment and years of diligent work needed to establish communicative competence based on adequate linguistic abilities. The process of developing language competency is very difficult for the child who has significant hearing impairment, and all children who are prelingually deaf will experience serious difficulties and delays in acquiring language skills. The hearing-impaired child with limited language skills will have additional difficulties in subjects other than language studies, since each new step in education requires mastery of the previous steps. It is the role of the school or program to create an environment for learning that maximizes the language acquisition process of deaf children.

Reading ability is highly correlated with language skills, so many hearing-impaired students also have difficulty in becoming proficient readers. The ability to express or comprehend language in written form is closely allied with the ability to express and comprehend language through face-to-face spoken communication. Our deaf education programs have not been very successful in assisting the majority of hearing-impaired students to achieve age-level reading skills (Ferguson et al., 1988).

Osberger and Hesketh (1988) describe the language difficulties experienced by hearing-impaired and deaf children in terms of language form (syntax), content (semantics) and function (pragmatics). According to these authors, hearing-impaired children may have only minor difficulties in acquiring the basic rules of English, compared with the profoundly deaf child who has a great deal of difficulty in syntax acquisition because of his or her dependence on learning language through the visual modality. Language content, as reflected by word knowledge, is commonly limited and delayed even in children with mild hearing losses. Hearing-impaired children have a restricted knowledge of synonyms and special difficulties in recognizing relationships between words. In terms of language function, Osberger and Hesketh suggest that hearing-impaired children must be taught directly the rules that govern conversations, such as turn-taking and topic negotiation.

For many years we have been misled into placing oral speech as the primary goals for deaf children, never realizing that the enrichment of their lives may be sacrificed for the simple ability to mouth words. What words? And in what relationships and context? Our primary goal in education of the hearing-impaired child is to develop linguistic abilities and ensure communication development by whatever means possible. Then, as a secondary goal, we should aim to develop intelligible oral expression of that language—a skill that itself depends upon the acquisition of a high degree of language competence.

An important question that has been debated for years centers around whether combining signing with spoken language contributes to or interferes with the development of spoken language. Geers et al. (1984) attempted to answer this question by testing a nationwide sample of 327 congenital, profoundly deaf children from 13 oral/aural programs and 15 total communication programs, through their own tool, the Grammatical Analysis of Elicited Language–Simple Sentence Level (GAEL-S). The GAEL-S measures production of selected English language structures in a standardized manner, so that each child's "spontaneous" language sample is evoked in precisely the same manner (Moog and Geers, 1979). In their study, Geers et al. examined their data separately for four different response modes: the oral productions of the oral/aural children, the oral productions of the total communication children, the manual productions of the total communication children, and the combined productions of the total communication children. The results showed that the percentage correct scores for the oral productions of the total communication children were substantially below scores for their manual productions and below scores of the oral/aural children in all grammatical categories sampled on the GAEL-S. It was reported

that most of the children in the total communication programs tested in this study did not simultaneously talk and sign, and their signed productions were far superior to their spoken productions. Thus, based on this study, the children in total communication programs did not develop competence with selected simple sentence structures at a rate faster than those children trained in the oral/aural programs. The authors also point out that both groups of children showed relatively poor performance in language production, and urged that more emphasis on systematic instruction in English be included in all training programs regardless of the mode of communication.

Sound Mental Health. The most effective learning takes place in the context of warm, nurturant relationships within the family. This is particularly important for the very young child during the critical years for language development. Whatever type of educational program a child is receiving, the parents should be given close emotional support and guidance in their management of the child's problems. The results should be the development of the child's self-confidence, high self-esteem, and the ability to relate well to people in the environment.

The warm relationship between parents and child can be fostered by helpful, supportive communications from physician and educational personnel. The initial phase of reporting the child's deafness to the parents is crucial to the parents' attitude toward the problem (see Chapter 5). Time should be allowed for the parents to air their feelings and their sorrow over having an "imperfect" child. Grief must be expressed if acceptance of the handicap is to come. These natural feelings should be shared with empathy and understanding. The physician and the audiologist can create the kind of atmosphere out of which nurturant attitudes can grow.

Together with the physician and audiologist the parents can be guided to an educational program for their child that will allow the continuation of a good parent nurturing. As Schlesinger (1973) pointed out: "Early parent-child communication is a traumatic issue between hearing parents and their deaf children. Although the hearing parents talk to and in front of the child, they can only guess at the level of understanding." Frustration results, for both parents and child. Thus it is important that an educational program be chosen that minimizes this frustration. It should be noted that such problems are minimized in the relationships of deaf parents to their deaf children. Denton et al. (1974) stated: "Deaf parents, as they communicate to and in front of the child, can test the child's understanding more easily. The child . . . can learn the symbols, the signs the parents use, and learn to understand and reproduce them more easily." It is estimated that about 10% of all congenitally deaf children are born to deaf parents.

Intelligible Speech. Certainly an important goal in the education of deaf children is intelligible speech. However, we caution against placing this skill too high in the hierarchy of educational goals. Intelligible speech without good language skills is an exercise in futility; intelligible speech in an emotionally disordered mind is a useless function. Articulate speech is greatly to be desired, but a program producing excellence only in this skill and not in language or emotional stability cannot be highly rated. Clear oral speech is greatly to be desired, but should not become the mainstay of the child's educational efforts. So-called "deaf speech" is characterized by a signiificantly higher fundamental frequency, a slower speaking rate than found in normal-hearing persons, and typical increased voice intensity with abnormally large amplitude fluctuations.

Oral production of speech for the deaf child is a problem that stems from inadequate control at nearly all levels of production (Osberger and Hesketh, 1988). In addition, there is a systematic relationship between the degree of hearing impairment and the intelligibility of the child's speech so that the greater the hearing loss, the more unintelligible the child's speech is likely to be. Although exceptions to this rule do exist, for whatever unknown reasons, we all have seen children in our clinics with profound hearing loss and exceptionally clear oral speech.

Increased awareness of the precise parameters of the speech of deaf individuals has accompanied the development of the cochlear implant (see Chapter 8). In general, the immediate effect of the cochlear implant is that the patient has an increased ability to monitor and adjust vocal output, and an increased clarity of oral speech. Even with the best of personal amplification or a cochlear implant, the deafened child is destined to spend long hours in speech therapy. It is to be remembered, however, that the goal of clear oral speech is secondary to our goal of developing a strong language base, so that when the deaf child speaks, something of value will have been spoken.

The problem is not so much the development of better teachers and of greater skills, although these are desirable, as to put into effect that which we already know. The deaf child learns primarily through vision, so we must make the imperceptible become perceptible. When we instill in deaf children the desire to communicate and provide the necessary language skills to do so, teaching speech will become a far easier task.

The family, particularly the parents, are the most important part of the child's support system. But families need assistance in understanding the problems of deafness and in learning those skills that will, in turn, be of benefit to the hearing-impaired child. The family must be inherently involved in all decisions regarding their child and must believe positively about the child's potential. Many parents of deaf children complain that their concerns and desires were not given consideration when their child was beginning special education programs. It is essential that parents be committed to, and trained in the use of, whichever communication system is used by their child. Behind many successful deaf children will be found devoted and concerned parents.

For any child, handicapped or not, a positive self-concept is crucial. Emotional stability and maturity are often problem areas for children who are deaf. When a child has low self-esteem, has tendencies to be withdrawn, or exhibits inappropriate behaviors, strategies must be established to improve the child's emotional well-being. Both the home and the school environment should be evaluated, and everyone concerned must be flexible to make the necessary adjustments for the good of the child. The goal of sound mental health is essential to any successful achievement that can be desired for the hearing-impaired child.

Communication with Peers. Humans have a special need for communication, and happiness and satisfaction go hand-in-hand with the ease by which we transmit and receive information. It is too often the case that without careful guidance and intervention, the deaf child can become isolated from family and friends. Interaction with peers is an important part of normal development, and it is critical that deaf children be able to communicate freely and easily with children of their own age range. Peer relationships serve as models for appropriate behavior and self-identity. It is recommended that deaf children be exposed to role-models who are also deaf, as recognition of deafness in others provides a sense of belonging rather than of pure isolation in a world of hearing people.

Children have cultural needs. Culture is knowledge that gives individuals a shared understanding of the world of accepted behaviors and values. Culture enables us to know what is expected and anticipated and permits individuals to gauge their place within the group. Differing cultural standards, when not recognized, can interfere with the learning process in the classroom and in the home. Recently, there has been a strong movement among deaf adults to rec-

ognize their unique needs and their accommodation to the world around them as *deaf culture.*

It may be difficult for the uninitiated to appreciate the fact that communication can be secured in milieus other than the one we understand and consider natural—the normal-hearing world. The deaf have developed a full-fledged native minority language, American Sign Language (ASL), which is easily learned by normal-hearing people. ASL is widely used for peer communication among the deaf, enabling them to communicate quickly and effectively under a wide range of daily situations. Over the past 15 years, total communication (which includes speechreading and various forms of manual communication) has become the educational approach of choice for most programs for deaf children (Jordan et al., 1979). These programs have typically included some form of manually coded English to maximize early exposure to language through an unimpaired modality (vision). The acquisition of ASL has been shown, through many studies, to be comparable to the acquisition of spoken English in normal-hearing children in terms of semantic relations, pronouns, and various morphologic markers (Geers et al., 1984).

The deaf child, who most of the time has two hearing parents, may experience rejection through dislike, pity, and misunderstanding from the hearing world. It is thus not surprising that the deaf child of deaf parents seems to be much happier and better adjusted than the deaf child of hearing parents. Many deaf children have social problems that complicate their language disability. Accordingly, the frustrated deaf child is noted to show outbursts of anger and rage throughout the school years. In schools for the hearing-impaired with hearing teachers, deaf children may develop strong emotional ties and loyalties to each other, which leads them to the exclusive and excluded community of the deaf as adults.

Schwartz (1987) states that no method for teaching hearing-impaired children can completely make up for a lack of communication at home. In a classic comment, Schwartz says that "staunch advocates of Oralism, of Total Communication, and of Cued Speech, alternately inspire and terrify parents with various tales of triumph and tragedy." Obviously, success in communication for the hearing-impaired child will be enhanced when the particular methodology used at home is also used at school. Cornett (1985) indicates that fewer than 2% of hearing parents of profoundly deaf children enrolled in signing programs actually become competent themselves in manual communication. Hearing parents, according to Cornett, tend to learn a few signs and do reasonably well in communicating until the child starts to school. As the child's signing sophistication increases, communication with the parents may become more and more limited. It is important that when parents make a choice and commitment to communication that the choice be made for the benefit of the entire family and not just for one parent to be able to talk to the hearing-impaired youngster.

The degree to which hearing-impaired children of hearing-impaired parents demonstrate an advantage in their acquisition of signed and spoken English over hearing-impaired children of hearing parents was studied by Geers and Schick (1988). Their results indicated that by ages 7 and 8, the hearing-impaired children of hearing-impaired parents demonstrated a significant linguistic advantage in both spoken and signed English over hearing-impaired children of normal-hearing parents. The hearing-impaired children of hearing-impaired parents appeared better able to utilize a language training program to produce linguistic structures of English in both manual and oral modes than the hearing-impaired children of hearing parents.

We strongly believe that it is unfair to force a child into a peer relationship where the hearing handicap is such a detriment that the child cannot compete nor be fully accepted. The hearing-impaired child must be in an environment where communication can be accomplished successfully, without stress or censure. Since the child has a strong vested interest in placement decisions, the child's opinions and preferences whenever possible should be given ample consideration. The real world of normal-hearing, fast-talking adults and children is a difficult environment for the deaf child to understand and overcome without achieving some means of easy communication.

FEDERAL LEGISLATIVE ACTS

The passage of the Education for All Handicapped Children Act of 1975 (otherwise known as Public Law 94-142) represents a landmark in federal recognition of their responsibility to provide funding for the costs of special education that will ensure a basic minimum level of program quality for handicapped children and their parents. The law assures the right of all children to be educated in the school districts in which they live.

The basic purposes of the law are to ensure that every handicapped child in the country will be able to receive a free, appropriate public education. The education is to be free—at no charge to the child or parents, appropriately designed to fit the special needs of the child and public—i.e., the state education department has the legal responsibility to provide appropriate educational services under public auspices at public expense. The basic goals of this legislation broaden the options available to educate deaf students, recognizes the diverse needs of individual children, and supports the need for early identification and diagnosis.

The specific provisions of the law include: (*1*) a free, appropriate public education for all handicapped children; (*2*) the identification, location, and evaluation of all handicapped children; (*3*) the preparation and implementation of an individualized education plan (IEP) for each involved child; (*4*) assurance of education in the least restrictive environment; (*5*) procedural safeguards for parents—"due process"; (*6*) maintenance of rights for children placed by the state in private schools; (*7*) in-service training; and (*8*) related services (including some health-related services). Although the 1970s will be remembered for this encompassing law, the economic conditions of the 1980s may create serious challenges for the enactment and fulfillment of the law's provisions. The "education of all handicapped children" is a multibillion dollar per year undertaking for which most of the funding has been allocated to the state and local communities (Palfrey, 1980).

Davila and Brill (1976) point out that the law itself is not a panacea, nor will it automatically improve services and education for deaf students. The small numbers of the deaf require grouping deaf children with other deaf children in day programs or residential school settings. The law does not mean that "least restrictive environment" and "maximal integration" are synonymous. Considering the ultimate objective of producing well-educated, socially adjusted and responsible adults, the "least restrictive environment" is not necessarily the one that is closest to home or has the maximum integration in schools.

In many ways, the law was enacted before answers were ready concerning meeting the educational mandates. Many questions still exist regarding identification, evaluation, and education of hearing-impaired and deaf children. One of the major tenets, which has received mixed reviews, relates to the placement of children in the "least restrictive environment." Although "mainstreamed children" have experienced some of the obvious benefits of association with age-similar peers, they have also experienced isolation and rejection within the classroom. Bess and McConnell (1981) summarize the factors associated with a higher degree of success in mainstream programs to include the onset of hearing loss after oral language has been established, middle- or upper-income-family background, and an ability to speak intelligibly.

Conway (1979) points out that mainstreaming is, indeed, becoming a reality for a high percentage of hearing-impaired students. Success in mainstreaming, however, is dependent upon careful selection of appropriate students. Thompson and Thompson (1981) warn that educators must be wary of getting caught up in a group movement that may not reflect the needs of an individual child and, in fact, may actually be detrimental to the achievement of that child's goals. They state that decisions about school placement should necessarily be made on the basis of the availability of continued professional support by qualified persons after the placement has been made.

Excellent discussions of the implications of Public Law 94-142 for hearing-impaired and deaf children have been published by Bess and McConnell (1981) and Amon (1981). Amon points out that in the past, it could be assumed that as a school hired certified teachers of the hearing-handicapped and provided room, materials, and equipment for the hearing-handicapped children, the school's educational and legal mandate had been fulfilled. But, she continues, *no one system, method or program can meet all the needs of hearing-handicapped children.*

The United States Supreme Court reached its first decision involving the Education for All Handicapped Children Act in 1982. Although in this specific suit, the Rowley case, the Court found that a young deaf student did not require a sign language interpreter in school, it affirmed the right of all handicapped children to receive personalized instruction and the supportive services they need to benefit from their IEP. In addition, the Court upheld the basics of the law that parents are to share in the planning and development of their child's IEP and that if the parents are not satisfied, they can appeal through the due process of law.

Schildroth (1988) reports a definite shift in the educational placement of hearing-impaired students over the 10 year period since implementation of Public Law 94-142.

A significant decrease in the number of hearing-impaired children receiving special education services is attributed to the departure from the secondary schools of the large number of hearing-impaired students born during the 1964–1965 maternal rubella epidemic. With a drop of enrollment of deaf students from special day schools and residential schools, the number of hearing-impaired students enrolled in local school districts has increased 16% in just the past few years. However, a new concern is emerging based on the fact that an increasing number of local school districts report having only one or two hearing-impaired students in their schools. In fact, more than 52% of the 8428 schools reporting data to the 1985–1986 Annual Survey of Hearing-Impaired Children and Youth enrolled only *one* hearing-impaired student.

The proliferation of local schools enrolling hearing-impaired students has resulted in a dispersion of these children away from the special schools in which they were grouped together, usually at one location. These circumstances should be cause for concern regarding special staffing and support services not available in many local schools, as well as future educational implications for these isolated hearing-impaired students. The communication and socialization limits resulting from this "isolation and dispersion" may have serious effects on the hearing-impaired student's development, especially in emotional and behavioral areas. If the preference for local school placement of hearing-impaired students continues, the ability of the local educational structure to cope with these changes will undoubtedly affect the lives of the hearing-impaired students, for better or worse, including their preparation for postsecondary education. The profound effect of a serious hearing impairment on the communication and academic achievement of deaf children is not fully realized by some school officials, boards of education, and lawmakers.

During 1986, Congress enacted Public Law 99-457, known as the Education of the Handicapped Act Amendments. The Amendments reauthorize the Education of the Handicapped Act (PL 94-142) and include a rigorous national agenda pertaining to more and better services to young special-needs children and their families (Sass-Lehrer and Bodner-Johnson, 1989). This legislation requires states receiving federal funds to extend the benefits of a "free appropriate public education to children ages 3 through 5 years." Specifically, these amendments expanded Public Law 94-142 to include handicapped infants from birth to age 2 years as well as preschool children. The new amendments challenge professionals in the field of deaf education to reexamine basic assumptions and develop a new range of services for this population, as well as incorporate and develop the role of families who have children with hearing impairments. This new federal funding presents an opportunity for innovative programs, research and development in early intervention programs, and cooperative working relationships between related-service professionals outside the discipline of deafness. States receiving federal funds must provide full services to this younger special-needs population by 1991.

CURRENT STATUS OF EDUCATION OF THE DEAF

The blue ribbon Commission on Education of the Deaf published a comprehensive report on the current status of education of the deaf in the United States in 1988. The report, entitled *Toward Equality: Education of the Deaf*, stated the primary and inescapable conclusion that the present status of education for persons who are deaf is "unacceptably unsatisfactory". The report points out that we have had available the knowledge to improve the situation significantly, although our good intentions alone have not been sufficient. Granted that it will be an expensive effort to improve the current situation, we really cannot afford not to remediate existing problems in order to minimize the need for remediation in the future. The report places emphasis on action and prevention rather than reaction and remediation to enhance the well-being of the deaf, their families and in fact, all of us.

The Commission was the first national body to consider the status of education of the deaf since the Babbidge Committee met in 1965. The Babbidge report stated that "the American people have no reason to be satisfied with their limited success in educating deaf children and preparing them for full participation in our society." The Babbidge report cited the underlying cause of this poor result as a failure to launch an aggressive assault on the basic problems of language learning by the deaf and on lack of progress in the development of improved systematic and adequate programs for educating the deaf at all grade and age levels.

The 1988 Commission believed that significant strides in educating persons who are deaf had been made during the intervening years since the Babbidge report but that actual implementation of many initiatives had been inadequate. The Commission's report to the President and the Congress of the United States includes 52 recommendations dealing with all aspects of deafness and education, including prevention and early identification, elementary and secondary education issues, parents' rights, the federal postsecondary education programs, research, evaluation, and outreach efforts, utilization of new technologies, and professional standards and training. *Toward Equality: Education of the Deaf* is aimed at federal government agencies who are in position to expend funds and establish the deaf as a priority to increase their present status quo situation. The document is an important contribution to guide those professionals dealing with education issues and deaf children and is recommended reading for the audiologist.

Since the initial contributions of early deaf educators such as Abbé de L'Epée, Thomas Hopkins Gallaudet, and Alexander Graham Bell, education of the deaf is thought by some to be exactly where it was 150 years ago. However, innovations in

teaching, sophistication in psychology and linguistics, and improvements in personal and classroom amplification systems should stimulate the educational establishment to improve the educational level and skills of the deaf and hearing-impaired students.

Where are today's deaf students? Each year the April issue of *The American Annals of the Deaf* is devoted to a directory of information concerning all deaf education programs in the United States. The 1988 Directory issue indicated that 45,000 deaf children were enrolled in 881 schools and special education classes. Only 7763 of these pupils were located in public and private residential schools. Day classes and day school programs, public and private, accounted for 22,515 deaf students.

Traditionally, residential schools are aligned with manual-type communication in their education system, while private day schools are auditory/oral in nature. Such dichotomy, however, is no longer so specific. More than 95% of the students in special schools were reported to use sign language, compared with 76% of the integrated students in the local schools. This discrepancy may, at least in part, be attributed to the fact that the special schools enrolled a higher percentage of the more seriously hearing-impaired students than did the local schools. It may also be due to the greater availability in the special schools of teachers able to sign (Schildroth, 1988). Another meaningful statistic from the Annual Survey reports that of the total enrollment of hearing-impaired students in 1987, 5115 students are totally mainstreamed, while an additional 6792 students are reported to be partially mainstreamed.

PROBLEMS IN TEACHING THE DEAF

All educators would agree that the most vital aspect of any child's intellectual development is language. Upon the child's successful handling of language skills hinges progress in school and in life. The ability to communicate thoughts, wants, and needs to others and, in turn, the understanding of thoughts and feelings of others depend on crucial language skills.

The deaf child's problem is that hearing plays a vital role in language development to build concepts and clarify them. The deaf child lacks this valuable input channel and accordingly throughout life has trouble developing and clarifying concepts. The entire process is slowed down and becomes laborious.

Language and concept developments clearly proceed hand-in-hand with communication. For the hearing child, the early states of communication are primarily via speech and hearing and may be categorized into five components:

- Reception: Sensory data are fed into the brain via the senses.

- Symbols: Words, signs, gestures that are used in *reception*.

- Encoding: Meaningful arrangement of symbols.

- Transmission: Meaningful sending of encoded material to someone else.

- Decoding: The receiver's mind now utilizes the message and extracts meaning from it.

For smooth, free-flowing communication, all five components must be operating efficiently. There must be a sufficient number of symbols to represent the message (vocabulary). There must be sufficient skill to encode the symbols (grammar). There must be sufficient mechanisms for transmission, such as speech and writing. The process of decoding involves understanding the vocabulary and grammar that form the very basis of the most important factor, the substance or content of the message itself. Incomplete communication and frustration result from a breakdown anywhere along the line.

So the educator of the deaf faces the problem with every deaf child. The child is stuck at the very first element of the communication process. The deaf child's mind is deprived of the rich sensory data supplied normally through the auditory mechanism, and depends only on a meager supply of symbols to use for labeling, categorizing, and storing. New symbols are difficult to come by. The deaf child functions on the concrete level of mental operations, and thus, abstract operations are most difficult because they are performed with words—the very commodity of which the deaf child never has enough. Abstract operations demand precise encoding and decoding and mastery of "word" concepts. Deaf children seldom attain sufficient language skills to master abstract operations even after arduous effort.

The usual process of trial and error learning—or teaching for that matter—is seriously hampered for the deaf child. The deaf child cannot hear errors of vocabulary or grammar. Attempts to correct the deaf child's errors are chancy undertakings. Because of the often indistinct transmissions (speech), the listener cannot be certain that the child made an error in the use of words or grammar or whether the listener just did not understand the spoken phrase. Suppose the listener thinks an error was, indeed, committed; imagine the task of trying to correct the error. Or suppose an error was committed, but the listener is unsure and, because of the problems in trying to correct the error situation, is content to deduce an answer and let the error go. Thus, the child's error is reinforced and will surely be perpetuated.

One is never really sure what the hearing-impaired child is thinking because of difficulties in communication. Consider this example relayed to us by a teacher of the deaf. In her classroom of hard-of-hearing preschoolers, when some object would drop accidentally on the floor with a loud noise, the concept was conveyed to the children by the teacher who quickly held her hands over her ears and showed exaggerated facial expression of disdain. The children could see that the situation clearly and quickly followed example, with similar behavior each time an object was dropped. A few days later following this lesson, a pencil was dropped on a soft carpet accidentally. As expected, the preschoolers clapped their hands over their ears and made exaggerated faces! To what were they reacting? Surely not "noise" as the teacher thought she was teaching a few days previously. And so every concept must be carefully considered by the deaf educator from the eyes and mind of the hearing-impaired child.

Today, the problems of teaching the deaf are further complicated by the fact that a greater proportion of our deaf young people were born deaf, or lost their hearing before the acquisition of language, than was the case 25 years ago. In fact, today, with medical achievements creating more control over the various etiologies of deafness, the communication dilemma is even more of a problem, for there are fewer adventitiously deaf children, who might have some language acquisition prior to their deafness, entering our deaf education programs. Today's hearing-impaired child is usually congenitally deaf (at least, prelinguistic) and exhibits many more difficulties and frustration in meeting language needs and speech skills than the child who may have lost hearing after the critical language age of 2 years. Further, many of today's deaf children, if born 20 years ago, might not have lived to enter school. Today they live, often exhibiting multiple handicaps and creating very special problems for the educator of the deaf to solve. Northcott (1981) indicates that 91% of all hearing-impaired children have two normal-hearing parents, 6% have one normal-hearing parent, while 3% have two deaf parents.

Individualized Educational Program.
One of the key factors in successful mainstreaming is the guarantee that hearing-impaired students will not be "dumped and forgotten" into the regular classroom. This proviso is covered by the requirement in Public Law 94-142 for all handicapped children to receive personalized instruction and supportive services they need to benefit from an IEP. The IEP is confirmation for hearing-impaired children that a more ob-

jective and scientific educational decision-making process will be followed. Withrow (1981) believes that with the use of IEPs, educators can no longer rely on biases and preconceived ideas of what is "best" for the hearing-impaired child.

The term IEP means a written statement for each handicapped child developed in any meeting by a representative of the local educational agency or an intermediate educational unit who shall be qualified to provide, or supervise the provision of, specially designed instruction to meet the unique needs of handicapped children, the teacher, the parents or guardian of such child, and, wherever appropriate, such child, which statement shall include (a) a statement of the present level of educational performance of such child, (b) a statement of annual goals including short-term instructional objectives, (c) a statement of the specific educational services to be provided to such child, and the extent to which such child will be able to participate in regular educational programs, (d) the projected date for initiation and anticipated duration of such services, and appropriate objective criteria and evaluation procedures and schedules for determining, on at least an annual basis, whether instructional objectives are being achieved.

Flexer (1990) points out that it is the school audiologist's role to actively integrate hearing services into the overall educational program of the hearing-impaired child in a manner consistent with the philosophy, goals, and objectives of the child's IEP. If the provision of hearing services or auditory pieces of equipment is not mentioned in the IEP, there is no assurance that the child's hearing needs will be met. When the audiologist is included as an IEP team member and a signatory of the IEP, there is greater probability that the hearing needs will be noted, understood, and appropriately managed.

No one is more important to the success of today's mainstreamed hearing-impaired student than are well-informed and assertive parents who can become intimately involved in their child's mainstreamed program on a regular basis as an IEP team member. Hearing-impaired children must have strong advocates if they are to be educated successfully in public schools. Most regular teachers, special educators, and administrators receive little training in the effects of hearing loss. Moreover, administrators are responsible for a wide variety of students and programs under their jurisdiction. Their problem is to stretch inadequate resources to cover many programs; they cannot serve as effective advocates for individual or small groups of children, much as they might like to be able to (Davis, 1988).

Data regarding the psychoeducational status of children with mild and moderate hearing loss are scarce. In spite of this limited data base, audiologists and speech/language pathologists often counsel parent regarding the possible deleterious effects of hearing loss and must help establish IEPs to enhance communication with these children and thus enrich their academic achievement. A project conducted by the University of Iowa (Davis et al., 1986) attempted to evaluate the psychoeducational performance of 40 hearing-impaired children to study the effects of degree of hearing loss, age, and other factors on the intellectual, social, academic, and language behavior. Their data did not predict the hearing-impaired children's language or educational performance on the basis of the degree of hearing impairment alone. Although some of the children evaluated in this study were performing exceptionally well, as a group the children fell into three major categories of significant delay: verbal skills, academic achievement, and social development. Some of these deficits did not manifest themselves until the child was in school for several years. The differences exhibited by the hearing-impaired children on the personality inventories suggest that these children are more likely to show aggressive tendencies, to express physical complaints, and to show significant behavior difficulties, especially social problems involving isolation and adjustment to school. It must be pointed out, however, that the individual results of this study confirmed the heterogeneity of hearing-impaired children and that the effects of hearing loss vary from child to child. The study did conclude that children with any degree of hearing loss appear to be at risk for delayed development of verbal skills and reduced academic achievement.

An informal article was written by Simmons (1988) concerning the parent's role in developing the child's individualized educational program. He points out that if parents expect to have a meaningful role in developing the mainstreamed child's IEP, a responsibility exists for the parents to be well-informed and knowledgeable about the needs of hearing-impaired children. This article offers a number of suggestions for parents to review during the regular IEP meetings with the school staff members.

DEAFNESS AND VISUAL ACUITY

The concern for visual acuity in deaf children cannot be overemphasized. Given the importance of good vision to persons with hearing loss, the *American Annals of the Deaf* devoted a recent issue detailing the relationship between deafness and vision (Johnson and Caccamise, 1981). It was recommended that (*a*) an indepth ophthalmologic examination be done routinely for every child with hearing loss, (*b*) reassessment of visual and auditory function be conducted periodically for all persons with severe-to-profound hearing losses, and (*c*) information be provided for hearing-impaired persons, parents, and professionals concerning the importance of visual assessment and visual hygiene for persons with hearing loss.

Clinicians should be well-acquainted with the symptoms of *retinitis pigmentosa*, which are not uncommon in deaf individuals. Retinitis pigmentosa is generally characterized by an initial loss of night vision followed by loss of peripheral field vision. These symptoms are usually initially noted during the teenage years.

Retinitis pigmentosa is defined as a disorder associated with a group of diseases that are frequently hereditary, marked by progressive loss of retinal response (as elicited by the electroretinogram), retinal atrophy, attenuation of the retinal vessels, and clumping of the pigment, with contraction of the field of vision. Retinitis pigmentosa may be transmitted as a dominant, recessive, or X-linked trait.

The combination of retinitis pigmentosa and deafness is known as Usher's syndrome. Vernon (1969, 1976) noted that Usher's syndrome is currently the leading cause of deafblindness. The incidence of Usher's syndrome among the congenitally deaf is approximately 3–6%, while its occurrence in the general population is 3/100,000. The concern for identification of Usher's syndrome in the congenitally deaf child is very important, because the child will need extensive special education, counseling, social-emotional support, and vocational consideration. Although most hearing loss associated with retinitis pigmentosa is severe-to-profound in degree, some moderate sensorineural hearing loss patients have been reported. The hearing loss may also be progressive and may start at the same time as the visual degeneration.

Hicks and Hicks (1981) presented a five-stage program for dealing with deaf youngsters with symptoms of retinitis pigmentosa. Stage I is an *awareness period* between the ages of 6 and 12 years and consists of a comprehensive diagnosis and explanation of the disease to the child and parents. Stage II involves *general counseling* including genetic counseling and educational and career planning. Stage III is the *general planning and community resource identification* stage during which the child is established with an appropriate resource agency that can assume primary responsibility for case management. By this period, the deaf patient has probably suffered considerable loss of vision. Stage IV consists of the *specific planning and adjustment counseling* stage and deals with the middle adult years and stresses. Finally, Stage V,

the *adjustment stage*, deals with the later adult years when the Usher's syndrome has rendered the deaf client a complete loss of usable vision. This is an extremely important article to acquaint the uninitiated with the real severity of this problem.

EDUCATIONAL PROGNOSIS FOR HEARING-IMPAIRED CHILDREN

Deafness Management Quotient. Downs (1974) proposed the deafness management quotient (DMQ) formula to predict whether a hearing-impaired child could be successful in an oral educational program or whether he or she required the supplementary visual information of a total communication program. The proposed formula consists of weighted scales that take into account many aspects of the child and his or her environment. Table 9.1 shows the DMQ, weighted on a 100-point scale, with a suggested score of 81 or better to qualify for an auditory/oral program.

Luterman and Chasin (1981) applied the DMQ to 31 severely hearing-impaired children who had attended a preschool nursery program and were now 6–13 years of age. They reported that those children with high DMQs were found to be in mainstreamed classes, while those children with low DMQs were indeed in total communication programs. The children with high DMQ scores were deemed superior in their use of hearing, language and speech and were more oral. Luterman and Chasin stated that the DMQ is a viable sorting device for distinguishing auditory/verbal children from those requiring total communication. They suggested the addition of a measure of the child's use and acceptance of amplification as being more important than the pure tone average.

The Spoken Language Predictor (SLP) was devised by Geers and Moog (1987) in an effort to improve on the concept of the DMQ by (*a*) selecting factors that better reflect a hearing-impaired child's potential for acquiring spoken language, (*b*) specifying more precisely the procedures for assigning

Table 9.1.
Suggested Scale for Deafness Management Quotient (DMQ)—Total: 100 Points

Residual hearing: 30 points possible
   0 = no true hearing
  10 = 250–500 < 100 dB
  20 = 250–500–1000 < 100 dB
  30 = 2000 < 100 dB

                              } Add 10 points for conductive element to hearing loss

Central intactness: 30 points possible
   0 = diagnosis of brain damage
  10 = known history of events conducive to birth defects
  20 = perceptual dysfunction
  30 = intact central processing
Intellectual factors: 20 points possible
   0 = MR[a] < 85 IQ
  10 = average 85–100 IQ
  20 = above average: > 100 IQ
Family constellation: 10 points possible
   0 = no support
  10 = completely supportive and understanding
Socioeconomic: 10 points possible
   0 = substandard
  10 = completely adequate
Auditory program leading to oral: 81–100 points
Total communicative program: 0–80 points

[a]MR, mental retardation.

weights to the factors, and (*c*) providing an option for a diagnostic category for those children for whom intensive instruction and periodic reevaluations will be required.

Five factors were selected in the SLP that were judged to contribute significantly to a child's success in *oral instruction* and that could be reliably estimated in clinical evaluations of hearing-impaired children as young as *3 years of age*. The five factors are (*1*) hearing capacity, (*2*) language competence, (*3*) nonverbal intelligence, (*4*) family support, and (*5*) speech communication attitude. The score sheet that is used to assign points to each factor is presented in Table 9.2. Geers and Moog describe in detail all of the tests used in each category to determine the point rating awarded to the hearing-impaired child in terms of educational recommendations. The SLP scale was validated in a sample of students at the Central Institute for the Deaf who were between 11 and 16 years of age. Each child's hearing, language, intelligence, family support, and communication attitude were obtained from test results and clinician ratings in their file that had been obtained between the ages of 3 and 5 years during their initial evaluation

for school placement. The results suggest that children with a SLP score of 80–100 points have excellent potential for acquiring spoken language and should be enrolled in programs emphasizing oral communication. Children with SLP scores of 0–55 are not likely to develop communicative competence with spoken language even with intensive oral instruction. These children should be referred to programs emphasizing instruction in using manual signs.

Geers and Moog indicate that the SLP index is intended to assist the responsible clinician in placement of the young hearing-impaired child in the appropriate education program. Careful and continuous reassessment of the SLP factors must be conducted to monitor the advisability of switching educational emphasis to a manual program, if the SLP drops below 60, or to reassignment to a speech-emphasis educational program when the SLP increases to 80 or above.

Obviously, many factors are involved in attempting to predict the educational outcome for hearing-impaired and deaf children. The concept of the indices described above may be too simple for such a complex problem, but the guidelines offered

Table 9.2.
Spoken Language Predictor (SLP) Index Score Sheet for Assigning SLP Point Values to Each of the Five Predictor Factors and the Educational Recommendation for Each Range of the SLP Index[a]

Factor	Score Type	Points							Point Value
		0	5	10	15	20	25	30	
Hearing[b]	Speech reception capability Aided	No pattern perception		Pattern perception		Some word recognition		Consistent word recognition 70–100	
	Articulation Index (AI)	0–20		21–48		49–69	81–100		
Language	Percentile rank	0–10	11–20	21–40	41–60	61–80	81–100		
Nonverbal intelligence	IQ	70	71–85	86–100	101–115	115			
Family support	Rating	No support	Minimal support	Adequate support	Above-average support				
Speech communication attitude	Rating	Poor	Fair	Good					
								Total SLP Index[c]	

[a]From A. Geers and J. Moog: Predicting spoken language acquisition of profoundly hearing-impaired children. *Journal of Speech and Hearing Disorders* 52:86, 1987.
[b]Select one hearing measurement or speech reception.
[c]Educational recommendations:
SLP = 80–100: Speech emphasis
SLP = 60–75: Provisional speech instruction
SLP = 0–55: Sign language emphasis

can tune the audiologist into those important variables that are necessary for successful educational outcomes.

METHODOLOGIES

Many claims have been made for success of education of the deaf. Many claims, however, are from teachers of the deaf who have a personal belief in their own teaching techniques. Most claims, furthermore, are testimonials supported by a demonstration from one or two deaf children who have performed exceedingly well under the advocated, or advertised, method. During this past decade, more and better research efforts have been conducted to evaluate various methodologies used to teach deaf children. It still appears, however, that *no single methodology works for all deaf children*. In this section we will limit our discussion to the oral, manual, and total communications philosophies of deaf education and a few of the most significant variations of these three major categories. Although virtually volumes of material have been written on the methodologies in education of the deaf, we can provide only a basic, and necessarily shallow, synopsis in these pages.

Auditory/Oral Method. We have chosen to use the nomenclature described by Musselman et al. (1988). The term *auditory/oral* is used to describe programs that use spoken language alone for communication and teaching. The descriptor *manual communication* is used to refer to programs that incorporate signs and/or fingerspelling. The term *total communication* is used to describe the simultaneous use of speech and signs with fingerspelling.

In terms of preschool hearing-impaired children, recent educational trends are similar to trends noted in older hearing-impaired children. There has been, in recent years, a definite shift from the use of auditory/oral to total communication methods, a decrease in the age of intervention, an increase in the number of hearing-impaired children who are integrated (mainstreamed) with normal-hearing peers, and an increased emphasis on parental involvement (Musselman et al., 1988). Contrary to expectations, there were no widespread and consistent interactions between degree of hearing loss and communication mode or between intelligence and communication mode.

Although an enormous amount of research effort has been expended to determine the "best" communication mode for hearing-impaired children, the overall results have been inconsistent. Studies favoring auditory/oral programs have been published, and studies favoring total communication systems may be cited. Obviously a number of factors, which may or may not be interrelated, influence the results as well as the interpretation of the results among these many studies.

An interesting study of 139 preschool children with severe-to-profound hearing loss from Ontario, Canada attempted to investigate the relationship of several background and educational variables with the linguistic, academic, and social aspects of the children over a 4-year period (Musselman et al., 1988). Despite their careful analysis, they concluded that unequivocal statements about the value of particular approaches or the consequences of not following one approach or another were unwarranted. They did state strongly, however, that no approach succeeded in reversing the devastating effects on language of severe-to-profound hearing impairment. As they tracked the children's movement among programs, it was found that auditory/oral programs and IEPs were the programs of choice, whereas the children in total communication programs and group education programs tended to do less well.

Musselman et al. (1988) noted that language itself is not a unitary ability but consists of a number of skills that respond differently to different interventions. In particular, it is necessary to distinguish among spoken language, receptive language, and mother-child communication. In spite of the placement factors that operated in their study, these researchers found that children in total communication programs scored higher on measures of receptive language and mother-child communication, whereas children in auditory/oral programs had better spoken language.

Silverman and Lane (1970) report that 85% of children enrolled in schools for the deaf are instructed by the oral method, at least in their early years. The fundamental assumption is that every deaf child should be given an opportunity to communicate by speech. Advocates of this method indicate that an employer is more inclined to hire a deaf person to whom he or she can give oral instructions over an equally capable deaf person to whom the employer must communicate in gestures and writing. Proponents of this approach believe that orally trained children do very well in life and that training in speech and lipreading permits an earlier adjustment to a world in which speech is the chief means of communication.

According to McConnell and Liff (1975), children who become good listeners also use vision as necessary to become good lipreaders. Since the two events do not happen simultaneously, it is necessary to establish the acoustic channel as the primary input channel if at all possible. The use of the visual channel then seems to come naturally as needed. Conversely, if the visual channel is established first as the main source of the child's perceptions and information, the use of hearing does not come naturally but only laboriously and slowly and with much intensive training.

Essentially three methods of auditory/oral education for deaf children are in use in the United States today. The traditional approach is to use them in the order described below. All three methods have the commonality that they essentially depend on training lipreading and audition and wholly exclude the use of any natural signs or gestures. The main aim of the auditory/oral system is to make the deaf youngster a part of the hearing society through good speechreading and lipreading.

At times it is difficult to separate these auditory/oral education approaches, and some eclectic programs choose to utilize the best from all three methods. It would seem that the children who do best in such programs are those with good residual hearing and good listening skills.

The first and primary oral method may be termed *pure oralism* or *auditory stimulation*. It was developed in America at the Clarke School for the Deaf during the late 19th century. All sign language is discouraged, and the child is exposed to sounds and spoken language at every opportunity. The child is fitted with hearing aids and every excuse for auditory stimulation is utilized. In theory, the deaf youngster is to "hear" everything that a youngster with normal hearing might be exposed to, only the auditory stimulation must be conducted with more deliberate action and intensity than usual circumstances might dictate. The method starts with visual attention to lipreading and includes isolated sound elements, sound combinations, words, and finally speech. Much of the work is done at home, and if a nearby preschool for the hearing handicapped is not available, a home-study course is offered by the John Tracy Clinic in Los Angeles.

When auditory stimulation alone or lipreading is not sufficient to initiate satisfactory speech and language development, a second oral method known as the *multisensory/syllable unit method* is called into use. It is essentially the same as the pure oral procedure with lipreading, except that reading and writing of orthographic forms of English are included. Sight and touch are utilized as well as sound. This system is probably the most widely used oral method.

Everything in the deaf child's environment is labeled, and his or her attention is drawn to the relation between the written form and the object, as well as the relation between the written form and the spoken word. The teacher may use the motokinesthetic approach to learning speech, where the child mimics speech production by feeling the teacher's face and reproducing the same breathing and vibration effects.

The third oral method is called the *language association-element method* or *"natural language" method*. It was proposed and developed by the long time principal of the Lexington School for the Deaf in New York City, Mildred Groht, who believed that the deaf child should learn to speak through activity. This type of program is developed around activities, and teachers continually talk to the deaf children and encourage them to ask questions with speech. Activities are supplemented with specialized instruction in lipreading and speech.

According to Luterman (1976), the auditory/oral approach presupposes that lipreading or visual awareness of the face need not be taught; rather, the impaired auditory modality must be trained while allowing the child to use visual information as he or she needs it. This approach differs from the multisensory (visual/oral) system in which no formal work is attempted in lipreading, nor is the child's attention deliberately directed toward the speaker's face. While all agree that auditory training is an important part of the auditory/oral and the visual/oral program, the visual/oral proponents view auditory training as a supplement to vision.

Arguments against the aural/verbal methods cite several objections to the approach. In general, the complaints are against lipreading itself and the fact that the oral method depends too heavily on lipreading as the primary mode of reception. Lipreading is ambiguous because (*a*) many sounds and words look alike on the lips (homophonous words such as mat, pan, and bat); (*b*) many sounds are not visible because they are made in the back of the throat, such as k, g, ng; and (*c*) many people do not speak clearly and distinctly and speaking styles vary tremendously. Lipreading is an art mastered by very few. Those who have the talent do very well and serve as demonstration students. Lipreading depends on good language skills, acute vision, good lighting, and exposure of the

lips and is limited by distance between speakers. Lipreading is less useful in dimly lit environments, within groups of talkers, or for speaker-audience formats.

A well-recognized variant of the oral method is the so-called "unisensory" or "aural approach" to education of the deaf (Pollack, 1971). Rupp (1971) cites the features of an auditory emphasis program: (*a*) audition is the most suitable perceptual modality by which a child learns speech and language; (*b*) it develops the impaired-hearing modality to its fullest by focusing attention on audition; (*c*) the unisensory approach has applicability to the very young child; and (*d*) normalcy of environmental contacts at all levels is necessary for success of the method. The unisensory approach is dependent on very early identification, early parental guidance, early amplification, and total exposure to normal language stimulation. The unisensory approach to deaf education has numerous advocates and is practiced throughout the United States. Pollack (1982) published a most informative "how to" article dealing with early amplification and auditory/verbal training of hearing-impaired infants.

Eric Greenway (1964), well-known British educator of the deaf, indicted oralism with the following comments:

> [F]or almost a century we have witnessed the great oral experiment. . . . In theory it is ideal and there are essential virtues in its principles. In many respects it has been a courageous attempt to bring the deaf into the world of the hearing by simulation of the normal means of communication. But an honest appraisal of the results shows plainly that it has not met with the overall success that teachers hope for or that the deaf themselves desire and demand. . . . It cannot be denied that there have been some outstanding successes with an exclusive oral system, but for the majority it fails because it is unable to provide the fullest and most congenial means of communication.

A classic study initiated at the University of Minnesota in 1969 and terminated in 1975 (Weiss et al., 1975) intensively evaluated children in seven well-known programs for the deaf and hard-of-hearing during these years. The programs provided a diverse representation of approaches to deaf education, ranging from auditory/oral to visual/oral. One of the findings regarding children who were integrated into mainstream education was that these children had had better hearing acuity and superior articulation prior to integration. It seemed conclusively evident that children do not speak better because of integration but are integrated because they speak better.

Other measures in the 6-year Minnesota study compared relative communication efficiency between modes of training. Children were found to receive communication most efficiently when stimuli were presented simultaneously through speech and signs. Next were simultaneous speech and fingerspelling, followed by speechreading and sound. The least efficient means was sound alone. In the area of expressive speech, the better articulation scores were made by the better-hearing students. The type of training seemed not to affect articulation scores; rather, skill in articulation related purely to the emphasis on auditory training and articulation given by a program.

Clearly the auditory/oral method is not for every deaf child. For example, we know that some deaf children have no measurable hearing for one reason or another. Temporal bone studies from children with profound deafness have been reported with total absence of the cochlear structures or eighth nerve fibers (Fig. 9.1). Amplification, or traditional hearing aids, can provide no substantive benefit except possible tactual cues. Some of these children, however, with appropriate diagnosis and evaluation, may be candidates for cochlear implantation (see Chapter 8).

Visual/Oral Methods. *American Sign Language.* It is said by many, including the vast majority of deaf adults, that the sign language is the common, natural language of the deaf. The signs have concrete meanings. Words can be spelled on the fingers to connect the signs into sentences.

According to Ridgeway (1969), "the sign language with deaf children is part mime; it is beautiful to watch, highly expressive and receptive."

L'Abbé de L'Epée, a French priest, undertook the education of two deaf sisters in the year 1750. Fingerspelling had been used earlier to teach language to the deaf in France, but to it L'Epée added a "natural language of gestures." He established a school to teach the deaf in Paris in 1860 and was later succeeded by his equally famous pupil, L'Abbé Sicard.

In 1815 an American named Thomas Hopkins Gallaudet, a minister from Hartford, Connecticut, met a young deaf neighbor girl, Alice Cogswell. Gallaudet was deeply taken by Alice's plight of mutism and the fact that she had no place to go to school. He sought support from families of other deaf children and ultimately went to Europe to study methods of teaching the deaf. He visited London and was refused access to Watson's Asylum, where secret and expensive educational methods were jealously guarded. However, he met L'Abbé Sicard and was invited to Paris to learn L'Epée's system of sign language. From this warm welcome in France, he returned to America with a young deaf teacher, Laurent Clerc, and established the first school for the deaf in the United States in 1817, the American School for the Deaf in Hartford. The school was replicated throughout the United States, and L'Epée's sign language was fused with the natural gestures used in America and became the basis for our present day sign language.

Years later, Thomas Hopkins Gallaudet, enjoying the success of establishing schools for the deaf across the United States, was still not satisfied. As an old man he passed his vision of visions on to his son, Edward Miner Gallaudet, and his dream was realized with the establishment of Gallaudet College in 1864, the world's first college of the deaf, in Washington, D.C. The establishment of the National Technical Institute for the Deaf, associated with Rochester In-

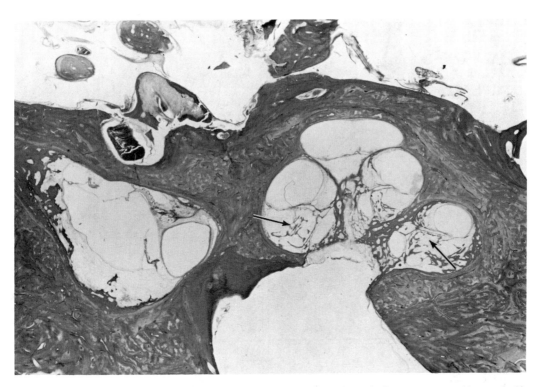

Figure 9.1. Midmodiolar section from the temporal bone of a patient whose deafness was caused by meningitis. Note the partial ossification that has taken place in the scala vestibuli portion of the cochlea (*arrows*) and the lack of eighth nerve fibers and spiral ganglia. This patient had no measurable hearing. The absence of essential sensory and neural structures makes amplification with a hearing aid useless. (Courtesy of I. Sando, M.D., University of Colorado Medical Center.)

stitute of Technology in New York, was the second full college program for the deaf—more than 100 years following the dedication of Gallaudet College.

The language of signs has been subjected to systematic analysis by several investigators including Tervoort (1964) and Bornstein (1973, 1978, 1979). Their conclusion is that sign language is an independent language that is not just a translation of oral language. Natural gestures and fingerspelling depend on situational understanding; when a sign has a tendency to become repeated and understood by more than one person the sign is "formalized" and no longer a natural gesture. The manual alphabet and samples of sign language from David Watson's book, *Talk with Your Hands* (1964), are shown in Figures 9.2 and 9.3.

Louie Fant, one of the finest interpreters for the deaf in the United States, and author of the book, *Say It with Hands* (1964), points out the importance of facial expression as one communicates with the sign language. The face, in fact, carries much of the meaning and many of the subtleties needed to enrich the communication. The limitations of sign language are also recognized and acknowledged by the experts. It is limited in scope and expressive power when compared with oral language. The sign language is bound to the concrete and limited in expression of abstractions, metaphor, irony, and humor.

The standardization of ASL or "Ameslan" has been enhanced by two important developments: the valuable contribution of Stokoe's *Dictionary of American Sign Language* and the establishment of a National Registry of Interpreters for the Deaf

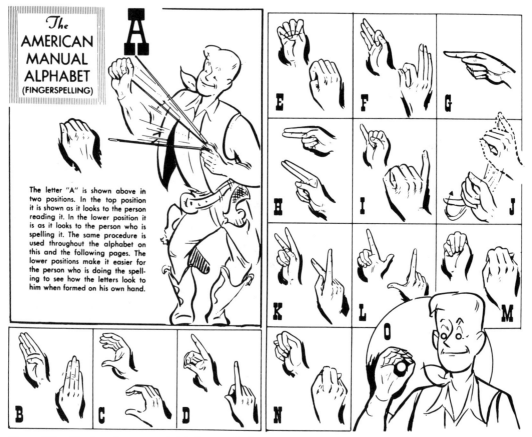

Figure 9.2. The American manual alphabet used in fingerspelling. (Reproduced with permission from D. O. Watson: *Talk with Your Hands*. Winneconne, Wisconsin, 1964, pp. 185–189.)

(RID), with three levels of certification according to interpreting skill based on standardized tests administered by expert hearing and deaf interpreters.

The manualists define the role of an educational program as that of providing an education to the deaf child that is equitable to the education of a hearing child. A manualist questions the implementation of speechreading and lipreading into the curriculum to the diminution of the three R's and submits that language skills are paramount to speech both educationally and socially.

Garretson (1963), a respected deaf educator and long-time advocate of the use of fingerspelling and signs in spite of the fact that he was brought up in the oral tradition, cites the following factors as assets for the manual method:

- Denying a child the right to use his [or her] hands along with speech and lipreading creates anxiety and emotional stress on the pupil.

- With the use of fingerspelling, signs, and speech, there is no doubt as to what is being communicated.

- Signs on the hands are considerably larger and clearer than lip movements.

- Fingerspelling and signs do not discriminate against anyone, and all have equal opportunity to participate and learn from classroom activities.

Garretson concluded that during the past 75 years of education of the deaf, signs and fingerspelling had never been made compulsory for the student, while speechreading and lipreading are usually taught in spe-

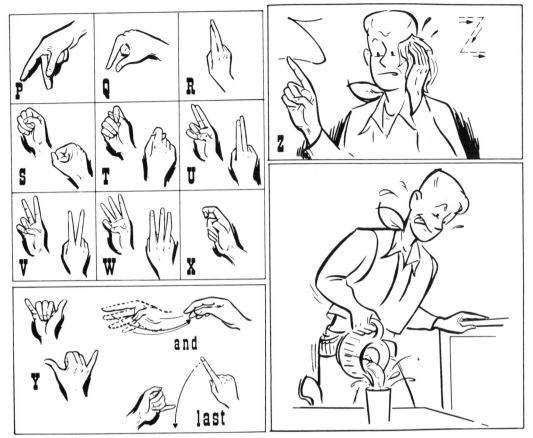

Figure 9.2–*Continued*

cial sessions in schools for the deaf. That the manual system has persisted among deaf adults and is the preferred method of communication by the majority of the deaf speaks for the value of the manual system.

Mention should be made of two early variants of the manual system known as the *combined method* and the *simultaneous method*. The combined method utilizes speech, speechreading, hearing aids, and fingerspelling. The simultaneous method is essentially the same as the combined method with the addition of the language of signs.

One of the major drawbacks to Ameslan is that its syntax is not conducive to the development of acceptable English. With the Ameslan system it is difficult to express pronouns; verb tense is indicated by context, signs follow each other according to

convenience and not necessarily accepted English order; and what is acceptable for communication is the *general concept*, not the *specific intent*.

Rochester Method. The New York state deaf residential school staff questioned the educational validity of signed English. They noted that deaf children, who had been taught in the oral method during elementary school years and then introduced to Ameslan still were not acquiring educationally acceptable English. There arose subsequently the Rochester method, which is the simultaneous use of speech and fingerspelling—a sort of "writing in air" technique superimposed on normal speech. This technique is also known as "visible speech" because the teacher is able to face the class and synchronize what is said and

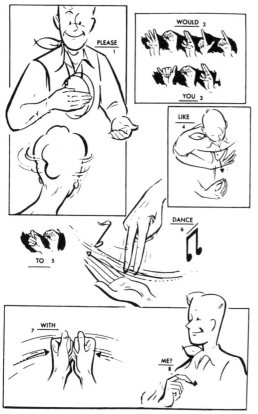

Figure 9.3. Signs and fingerspelling used in the sentence, "Please, would you like to dance with me?" (Reproduced with permission from D. O. Watson: *Talk with Your Hands.* Winneconne, Wisconsin, 1964, p. 220.)

shown on the lips with a more visible form of English as spelled on the hands.

The more visible approach of the Rochester method is the best supplement to an otherwise oral method, because it is a pure, visible, English medium. It represents a multisensory visible oral-plus approach to language development. This method is said to continuously emphasize the traditional oral approach, supplemented by simultaneous and very visible fingerspelling.

Total Communication. Comparatively recently, in terms of deaf education tradition, a philosophy termed total communication has arisen. The proponents of total communication recognized the educational advantages of visible speech, yet they also noted certain difficulties. The manual dexterity of the preschool child limits his or her ability to fingerspell quickly, and the child's limited attention span makes it difficult to attend intensely on "flying fingers and fleeting flexible faces" for an all day instruction session. Total communication is a philosophy requiring the incorporation of appropriate aural, manual, and oral modes of communication in order to ensure effective communication with and among hearing-impaired persons (Brill, 1976).

Total communication, as it is stressed by its advocates, is a *philosophy* and not simply another method for teaching deaf children. The basic premise is to use every and all means to communicate with deaf children from infancy to school age. No particular method or system is to be omitted or stressed. The student is exposed to natural gestures, Ameslan, fingerspelling, facial expression, body English, all accompanied simultaneously with speech heard through hearing aids. The idea is to use any means that works to convey vocabulary, language, and idea concepts between the deaf child and everyone to whom he is exposed. The important concept is to provide an easy, free, two-way communication means between the deaf child and his or her family, teacher, and schoolmates. In some environments and educational facilities, total communication is practiced continually with all pupils throughout their school years.

Opponents of total communication complain that if a teacher of the deaf really favors one method over another, the teacher will unwittingly move the students in the direction of that approach under the guise of teaching total communication. Some educators believe that it is not possible to evaluate the effectiveness of any one approach while using all the approaches at the same time. These arguments, however, seem to miss the main concept of total communication, which says that it is paramount to communicate without regard for which "method" is really doing it. The total communication approach has been criticized because it is too much of a shotgun approach to education of the deaf. Critics argue that the overstimulation of the deaf child is actually detrimental to communication.

For years, the approach to deaf education was to start all children in an oral-type program for their early years of school. At some point in time, second or third grade or age 7 or 8, the child would be evaluated with regard to educational progress and the oral method. As long as the child was progressing well, the oral/verbal approach would be continued. If the child was not doing well, consideration would be given for transfer into a manually oriented class. For most children, this timing of selecting their educational method so long after the critical years of language and speech development makes education prognosis very poor.

Total communication is an important concept in behalf of the deaf child and should add years of head start toward formal education. The concept of total communication has caught on and spread quickly in the United States. The progress, thus far, is encouraging, and the change in attitude from stressing a particular "method" to overall concern for the deaf child's needs to be immersed in two-way communication may turn out to be the most significant change in deaf education for over 100 years.

An interesting survey was conducted by Matkin and Matkin (1985) of parents whose hearing-impaired children had initially been enrolled in an aural/oral program for a minimum of 2 years and then subsequently enrolled in a total communication class in a day school setting for at least 2 years. The parents were asked a series of questions concerning the social, emotional, and educational growth of their child, as well as the impact of the change in school communication system upon their speech, speechreading, and hearing aid use. The study found a significant positive correlation between parents' overall perception as to the benefits of total communication and their perception of their children's educational and emotional growth. In addition, the parents did not perceive the use of total communication as adversely affecting speechreading, speech production, or hearing aid use.

OTHER SIGN SYSTEMS

During the past few years, several manual sign systems have been developed as improvements to Ameslan, since their design is such that they represent English. These sign systems are described here to orient readers to the basic philosophies, approaches, nomenclature, and differences, since these approaches have been developed to overcome apparent inadequacies of the ASL or Ameslan. The other sign systems have as their premise that Ameslan, with linguistically generated variations, can be the visual equivalent of spoken English. Furthermore, they share the idea that if this type of system is introduced to the deaf child at a very early age, the language skills, total experiences, mental health, and communicative abilities will be improved over our traditional approaches.

The sign systems discussed below have several principles in common as described by Cokely and Gawlik (1973). The basic premise is that deaf children need a visual symbol system to develop their language competency to its fullest potential. They assume that the more syntactically correct the symbols, the more it will aid in development of language in the deaf child. Apparently, all argue that although the American Sign Language is an adequate communication tool, its syntax is such that it is not necessarily related to the grammatical structure of English. Finally, with exception of "cued speech," each believes that a visual symbol system can be developed to incorporate basic Ameslan signs with modifications that encourage the use of meaning through context that is consistent with the form of spoken English.

Obviously, these sign systems are in a state of flux and transition. Incongruities and contradictions may be seen within the systems. To judge the systems today would be imprudent and unfair, and decision, as of yet with few data, must be based on personal intuition. The advent of the systems reflects dissatisfaction with the ASL as a basic language instructional tool. Final judgment must be reserved until the results can be examined objectively.

Cued Speech. Cued speech is a method of communication developed by R. Orin Cornett for the hard-of-hearing in which 8 hand configurations and 4 hand placements are used to supplement the visible manifestations of natural speech. Cued speech was hailed in 1967 as a possible answer to the oralism versus manualism controversy. The 12 cues described above are used around the chin, cheek, and neck, drawing attention to the speaker's face and lips. The cued speech system provides a visible phonetic analog of speech in the form of lip movements supplemented by hand cues with both vowel and consonant cues.

According to Cornett (1985), most users of the auditory-only and multisensory approaches do not introduce the written language until there is sufficient foundation in the basic oral skills to permit mutually supportive use of oral communication and written language. He believes that cued speech offers specific advantages for supportive use in oral programs. The greatest advantage of cued speech is that it facilitates the acquisition of the vocabulary and the syllabic-phonemic-rhythmic patterns of the spoken language without interrupting the natural process of communication to interpolate the written form.

Cornett argues that another advantage to cued speech is that it meets the objections of total communication and other manual-language advocates and that early communication through exclusively oral methods is insufficient to meet the psychosocial needs of the child. Cued speech forces the use of information on the lips by the hearing-impaired child without subjecting the child to the confusion of lipreading. Finally, Cornett states, cued speech is self-limiting, in that the child with speech does not use cues to hearing persons and ignores the cues he or she does not need.

Actually, the cues are not intelligible without proper mouth motions. Because "cueing" is completely dependent upon spo-

ken language and lipreading, it satisfies the oralist's demand that emphasis be placed on learning to communicate with those who do not know sign language.

Seeing Essential English. Seeing Essential English (SEE$_1$), a sign system originated by David Anthony in 1962 and developed in Southern California, uses modifications of Ameslan to resemble English. SEE$_1$ is intended for use by all age groups and now has as its basis an impressive two-volume manual that includes an introduction to the system, how it is used, grammar and syntax guidelines, and over 5000 vocabulary entries (Anthony et al., 1971). The SEE$_1$ system has the largest vocabulary of any of the new systems.

SEE$_1$ signs represent word forms or word parts such as roots, prefixes, or suffixes. The signs are used in combinations to form any desired word. To reflect English syntax, SEE$_1$ emphasizes complete English word order. Verb tense is clearly indicated and irregular verb forms have signed representation. In general, English words are represented by the traditional American sign word plus a suffix and/or prefix. English compound words are often made up of elements different from the single sign element often used in Ameslan. As a result, SEE$_1$ words often do not closely resemble the original source sign in Ameslan. SEE$_1$ is similar enough to Ameslan that ASL users can almost read it in context but may not be able to identify specific SEE$_1$ signs without previous exposure or explanation.

Signing Exact English. Signing Exact English (SEE$_2$) was a sign system developed in 1972 by a group of former members of the Seeing Essential English group headed by Dr. Gerilee Gustasan. It is perhaps unfortunate that the new group did not select another name for their system that did not mimic Anthony's SEE$_1$ system. Cokely and Gawlik (1973) use the notations SEE$_1$ and SEE$_2$ to differentiate the two systems. According to Bornstein (1973), the reasons leading to the development of

Signing Exact English is that SEE$_1$ utilized too many signs that were too distant from Ameslan, that it was too radical in its use of the root word, and that was too complex for the needs of parents and teachers. Accordingly, SEE$_2$ uses signs that represent words rather than roots, as well as basic affixes as needed. SEE$_2$ has a vocabulary of some 2800 words published in booklet form.

SEE$_2$ is also intended to be used by young children. It is readily apparent, then, that a situation can develop whereby parents and children who interact with persons trained in another system will use different signs for the same word. According to calculations reported in Bornstein (1973), 61% of the SEE$_2$ vocabulary is based on traditional Ameslan signs, 18% is based on modified Ameslan signs, and 21% consists of entirely new signs. When SEE$_2$ signs were compared with SEE$_1$ signs, some 80% of the traditional sign group were identical in both systems. Bornstein et al. (1980) and Bornstein and Saulnier (1981) conclude that difficulties created by these sign word differences are relatively minor.

VERBOTONAL METHOD

In about 1952, Professor Petar Guberina from the University of Zagreb, Yugoslavia, began developing a method to improve foreign language teaching through emphasis on the spoken rhythm of the language to be learned. He later applied his theory and methods to teaching deaf children and adults—still with emphasis on the rhythm of spoken language and on speech perception and production as an interacting loop system.

According to Craig and Craig (1972), the verbotonal approach is characterized by (*a*) emphasis on low frequencies (below 500 Hz) and on vibratory clues in perception of spoken language patterns; (*b*) matching of special amplification devices known as SUVAG to the deaf person's optimum "field of hearing"; (*c*) use of body movements to assist both in production and perception of speech; (*d*) emphasis on acoustic memory

for language patterns aided by body movements and by articulatory movements from the production of speech; (*e*) providing speech and language work in active "play"-type situations, so that much longer periods of concentrated work on spoken language are possible; and (*f*) emphasis on language in meaningful context of "situations."

Guberina's concept is based on his theory that the low frequencies of spoken language do not mask the high spoken frequencies. He believes that amplifications of auditory clues, below 500 Hz, to include rhythmic patterns and the sound fundamentals, can actually help the deaf person to perceive the higher speech frequencies. In an additional effort to reach the low-frequency residual hearing of profoundly deaf children, the verbotonal approach includes the use of vibrators, or bone oscillators, to provide vibratory cues in the perception of language rhythms and sound patterns. Body movements are an important part of the technique and lipreading is taught only incidentally.

Asp (1985) reports that in the University of Tennessee verbotonal preschool program, between 65% and 75% of the hearing-impaired children (average hearing loss of 90 dB HL in the better ear) have been successfully integrated into regular public school classrooms.

The goal of verbotonal therapy is to help hearing-impaired children develop good oral communication skills that will allow them to freely interact with normal-hearing people. A review of a number of studies of international verbotonal programs summarized by Guberina and Asp (1981) concludes that these programs have been "extremely successful in integrating the deaf children who began therapy at 2 or 3 years of age . . . and that these children can continue in therapy beyond the first grade suggest[s] that the children who are integrated are not the exception—they are the rule."

MAINSTREAMING

Mainstreaming is one of the single most important issues in education of deaf children to appear in the past few decades. By formal definition, mainstreaming is "an educational programming option for handicapped youth which provides support to the handicapped student(s) and his teacher(s) while he pursues all or a majority of his education within a regular school program with nonhandicapped students." In short, mainstreaming is the current term for the practice that used to be known as "integration" of the hearing-impaired student into regular classrooms with hearing children. Mainstreaming is a procedure that is already well-established in the United States and is the crest of a fast-moving wave in education circles. The real push for mainstreaming has been the stimulation provided by the "least restrictive" portion of the new federal law known as the Education for All Handicapped Children Act of 1975. Excellent materials on mainstreaming hearing-impaired youngsters have been published by Northcott (1979) and Hoversten and Fornby (1988).

The organization of educational programs for hearing-impaired students is undergoing considerable change in many states. The change is from serving only a few students, mainly in residential schools, toward serving many deaf students in local community programs with a system that provides a variety of educational opportunities to the hearing-handicapped child and his or her parents (Macklin, 1976). Northcott (1973) clearly stated, however, that partial or full-time integration for hearing-impaired students into regular classes is not a realistic goal for every child; nor is the policy of self-containment from kindergarten through grade 12 suitable for all hearing-impaired children.

Bricker (1978) suggests that integration is a means of eliminating the deleterious effects of segregation and the stigma often attached to the "handicapped" student. Normal children are thus exposed to the handicapped child with positive and enlightened responses toward the integrated person. Of course, it is also possible that a negative response to the integrated child, or handicap-

ping condition, is also possible, with devastating results to the integrated child.

Birch (1976) indicates that mainstreaming deaf children is to be done only after thorough preparation, with sensitivity to the needs of all parties and with careful monitoring and support. He states that degree and onset of hearing loss are not the primary factors in selecting children for mainstreaming. Regular classroom teachers are very accepting of hearing-impaired pupils and are willing to design programs for complete or partial mainstreaming, depending on the child's capabilities, requirements, and the school's resources. Mainstreaming has been tried for years, and its success is the reason for its continued survival and growth.

In one mainstreaming program described by Holcomb and Corbett (1975), the deaf child is put into a class with hearing children only when a tutor-interpreter is available to translate everything said in the classroom into sign language and fingerspelling. The tutor-interpreter is a trained teacher of the deaf so that the teacher aide function is utilized constantly to help the hearing-impaired student. The tutor helps the deaf child to keep up with the rest of the class and grasp fully what is going on at all times. Acceptance of such a program in the regular school is enhanced by teaching all normal-hearing students and classroom teachers elements of sign language and fingerspelling.

Special consideration must be given when hearing aids are worn by the hearing-impaired child mainstreamed into the regular classroom without regard for the acoustic characteristics of the normal school room. Poor signal-to-noise ratios produce detrimental effects on speech discrimination and understanding by the hearing-impaired student using amplification aids. A study of this problem in the Detroit metropolitan area indicated that hearing-impaired children with malfunctioning hearing aids studying in regular classrooms suffered a high scholastic failure rate (Robinson and Sterling, 1980). Mussen

(1981) has prepared an excellent chapter to aid speech/language clinicians and teachers with one or more hearing-impaired children in their regular classrooms in special techniques to enhance listening and auditory training skills of the handicapped youngsters.

Madell (1984) and the staff at the New York League for the Hard of Hearing published a monograph based on their years of experience in helping hearing-impaired children succeed in mainstreamed educational settings. Their monograph, *Mainstreaming the School-Aged Hearing-Impaired Child*, offers excellent practical information to help any audiologist meet the challenge of assisting an auditory-handicapped child in a regular school setting, as well as suggestions to adapt the school environment to achieve optimal opportunities for the integrated children as well as the normal-hearing students.

Brackett and Maxon (1986) published a useful listing of services for hearing-impaired mainstreamed children that might be provided by the educational audiologist in the public school setting:

1. Comprehensive audiological and amplification evaluation
   a. Unaided: pure-tone air and bone conduction thresholds
   b. Unaided: speech reception and speech discrimination
   c. Electroacoustic impedance measures
   d. Aided (aids and FM): sound field warbletone thresholds
   e. Aided (aids and FM): sound field speech measures
   f. Electroacoustic analysis of hearing aids and FM system
   g. Thorough report from evaluator
2. Comprehensive communication evaluation
   a. Preferred receptive mode: auditory only, visual only, auditory-visual combined
   b. Comprehension of spoken language: vocabulary level, sentence level, connected discourse
   c. Production of spoken language: vocabulary level, sentence level, connected discourse
   d. Speech intelligibility
   e. Written language
   f. Annual reevaluation
3. Educational evaluation

   a. Skill differentiation within subtests important
   b. Test presentation and format to be considered during interpretation of results
   c. Annual reevaluation
4. Psychosocial evaluation
   a. Performance subtests used as an estimate of potential
   b. Verbal subtests measure language ability
   c. Triennial reevaluation
5. Classroom observation
   a. Child/teacher interaction
   b. Child/child interaction
   c. Child participation
   d. Classroom modifications
   e. Learning strategies
   f. Use of FM systems
   g. Analysis of noise sources
   h. Visual distractions
   i. Use of classroom aide/interpreter
6. Audiological management
   a. Improving classroom acoustics
   b. Recommending and using FM systems
   c. Daily troubleshooting of personal aids and FM system
   d. Assessing use of FM system within various settings
   e. Monitoring of middle ear problems with appropriate referrals
7. Speech-language management
   a. Focus on deficit areas which impact on academic performance and social interaction
   b. Coordination with other support personnel and classroom teacher
8. Educational management
   a. Favorable seating
   b. Buddy system
   c. Notetaker
   d. Discussion of hearing impairment/amplification
   e. Improving classroom presentation: characteristics of teacher's speech paraphrasing of content directing classroom discussion using visual aids
   f. Improving the use of classroom amplification
   g. Improving classroom flexibility
   h. Discussing teacher's expectations
   i. Facilitating teacher/tutor exchange
9. Preview/review tutoring
   a. Academic vocabulary
   b. Academic content
10. Classroom aide/interpreter
11. Psycho/social management
    a. Adolescent group, including career information
    b. Parent support group
    c. Extra-curricular social activities

12. Parent involvement
   a. Home support
   b. Program planning
   c. Regular contact with school personnel
13. In-service training
   a. Staff: whole school once per year
        direct service personnel twice per year
        individual as needed
   b. Peers: once per year
14. Alternative educational placement
   a. Full mainstreaming
   b. Partial mainstreaming
   c. Social mainstreaming
   d. Self-contained class in regular school

A thought-provoking essay questioning the quality of a mainstreamed education for prelingually deaf children was written recently by Brill (1975), a veteran of 25 years as the Superintendent of the California School for the Deaf in Riverside. He worries that we are in an era of simplistic solutions to complex programs. Until a few years ago many deaf children were postlingually deafened as a result of some childhood illness. However, today's deaf children are most *prelingually* deaf and present different educational problems.

Brill points out that the deaf child learns best when in a small class composed of children who are about the same age and educational level. It is likely that a limited geographical area will contain only a small number of deaf children of about the same age and educational level. Mainstreaming philosophy requiring the right to an education in the least restrictive or most typical school setting possible has held, first, that every child is generally best placed in a regular classroom; second, that he or she is best placed in a special class by being provided special supportive services while still in local school; and third, that only as a last resort should he or she be separated physically from all of the so-called typical children in his or her educational placement.

Brill cautions that the integration of deaf children in a special class with the hearing children in a school is sometimes only a token integration. The deaf child with a tremendous communication handicap is not best placed in a regular classroom. The teacher in the regular classroom does not have the competencies to meet the child's special needs. The prelingually deaf child is almost never appropriately placed in a regular classroom. The policy of placing the child with less severe hearing loss in integrated programs while the profoundly deaf child attends a specialized deaf school eliminates destructive conclusions or comparisons of academic or social achievements.

In view of the current social climate, mainstreaming is here to stay. Ferguson et al. (1988) cautions that care must be exercised so that professionals and parents do not perceive mainstreaming as "the only way to go." These respected educators of the deaf believe that special schools including residential schools should remain a part of our educational system for hearing-handicapped children. Ling (1975) likens the deaf education controversy to cyclic sunspot activity. It has flared up on numerous occasions in the past and abates only when the protagonists realize that there is no one method or mixture of methods that can possibly meet all the needs of hearing-impaired children and their parents.

PARENT TRAINING

For perhaps too many years, attention of professionals has been devoted solely to the hard-of-hearing or deaf child, and little consideration has been given to the parents. We believe that the parents of the deaf child may be the key to one of the most significant factors in the deaf youngster's development. Fortunately, during the past few years, parent-oriented habilitation programs for children with hearing impairment have emerged. The importance of families of hearing-impaired children and the role they play in the development of the handicapped child is the subject of an excellent textbook by Schuyler and Rushmer (1987).

Horton (1975) summarized the objectives of parent training programs into categories:

• To teach parents to optimize the auditory environment for their child;

- To teach parents how to talk with their child;

- To teach parents strategies of behavior management;

- To familiarize parents with the principles, stages and sequence of normal development, including language development, and apply this frame to reference in stimulating their child;

- To supply effective support to aid parents in coping with their feelings about their child, and to reduce the stresses that a handicapped child places on the integrity of the family.

The major emphasis of parent training includes emotional support for the parents by helping them recognize, realize, accept, and understand the implications of their child's hearing problem. This increased awareness should help reduce anxiety and worry often expressed by parents of handicapped children. Education for the parents is important so that they might fully understand the nature of their child's hearing loss with realistic ramifications of the educational future for their youngster. The parent is taught to understand child growth and development as well as the need for communication skills, social contact, and emotional expression. A clear reference source such as Caplar's *The First Twelve Months of Life* (1973) is especially valuable to parents, and we have been successful in recommending *Learning Games for the First Three Years* (Sparling and Lewis, 1979).

Parents must be involved in the choice of the communication system the family wishes to use with the hearing-handicapped child. The choice between communication systems is secondary to the desirability of the parents being in ageement, enthusiastic, and committed to the system of their choice. Professionals can provide guidance, exposure, and background to the parents, but the final choice should be made with full cooperation and agreement with the parents. Imposing the use of signs on parents who lack confidence in their ability to inter-

act with the child is a common cause of failure. If the parents choose to use signs, the entire family must develop fluency with this means of communication.

Another project in parent training is to teach the parents how to utilize and adapt daily activities of the home as experiential teaching events for the preschool child. Hopefully, the result is a stimulating home environment for the hearing-impaired child, where auditory, speech, and language development is a daily, ongoing, and natural activity for the youngster. Some programs have a model home completely furnished and operational with kitchen, bathroom, bedroom, playroom, etc. The home is stocked with typical utensils and furnishings. Parents spend time with the parent-training supervisor to learn how to develop a repertoire of experiences and activities to stimulate interaction with their children. Video tape is used extensively to observe parent-child interaction with immediate feedback to the parents in order to increase their abilities with their children.

A number of practical publications are now available to help the professional deal with parents of hearing-impaired children, including Stewart (1978), Stream and Stream (1978), Luterman (1979), and Mitchell (1981). A study course for parents has been published as a two-part guide, *Talk To Me* (Alpiner et al., 1977).

Major cities and most large clinic programs have parent-centered projects underway, and it would appear that the deaf child will be the ultimate beneficiary of the support and education aimed at his or her parents during the initial stages of discovery of the hearing loss. Meadow and Trybus (1979), in a review of emotional problems of the deaf, report three family variables of importance to a deaf child's mental health: (*a*) degree of parental overprotectiveness, (*b*) development of unrealistic expectations for the child's progress, and (*c*) effectiveness of parent-child communication.

An important study that examined the attitudes and stress of hearing families with a profoundly deaf preschool child was published by Greenberg (1975). The author studied 28 families that were equally divided into those using oral and simultaneous communication and then further divided into these groups into subdivisions based on communicative ability (high versus low). Mothers completed questionnaires and interviews on stress concerns, parent attitudes, and their child's developmental level. Results showed few differences between simultaneous and oral families. However, comparison of the four subgroups indicated that those with high-competence simultaneous communication skills had more positive attitude and less stress than highly competent oral communication families. Studies such as that conducted by Greenberg suggest the need for additional research on key variables in the deaf child's life, such as the family, which undoubtedly have significant impact.

SUMMARY

Dr. Julia Davis of the University of Iowa discussed utilization of audition in the edu-

cation of the hearing-impaired child (Davis et al., 1981). They describe the population of hearing-impaired children as "vastly heterogeneous" and correctly points out that the best use of the residual hearing in each child will require different procedures and emphasis. In summary, as Davis states, "we really must stop arguing over whether children use the auditory system *alone* or in conjunction with visual or tactual information during educational endeavors. If the energy spent in futile attempts to convince each other of the supremacy of one educational method over another had been spent in devising ways to maximize reception through *all* modalities, including hearing, it is unlikely that the educational achievement levels of hearing-impaired children would be as low as they are today."

CONCLUSION

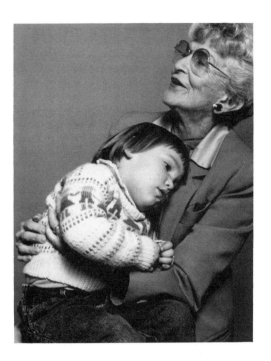

FUTURE DIRECTIONS IN PEDIATRIC AUDIOLOGY

Pediatric audiology came quietly into being in the early 1940s, spurred by dedicated educators of the deaf who studied the auditory behaviors of normal children. These educators were Lord and Lady Ewing in England. They combined the use of gross noisemakers with their own sophisticated skills of observation, developing those simple techniques into an art.

And what an art! A case can still be made that the highest form of pediatric audiology is a known sound stimulus in the hand of a zealous, practiced, observer, pointed at an infant's ear. Many thousands of hearing-impaired individuals are getting on with more successful lives as a result of having been identified early in life by such techniques. But there are not enough of those fortunate ones. In this book we find the full 20th century response to the need for a pediatric audiology that utilizes a state-of-the-art technology to ensure that *all* children will have available to them the identification of their problems at the earliest possible moment.

For the goal is *all*! Not just the children with parents who can afford testing and monitoring. Not just those who happen to fall into a category that places them *at risk* for deafness. Not just the ones that happen to be in the right place at the right time to be screened. But *all children*! They are all entitled to be touched by the screening hand of modern technology. There is too much at stake to miss any.

Not only those severe and profound losses so devastating to speech and language but even the mildest losses with their sequelae in delayed expressive language must be identified early enough to allow interventions that will lessen their problems.

The development of cochlear implants make it even more critical that losses be identified early. We can now envision a world where a deaf baby can be implanted at birth and, with the plasticity of the young brain, can utilize the implant code to become a functional hearing person.

The field of preventive medicine gives us an analog: It has been said that "medicine is unique among the sciences in that it strives incessantly to defeat the object of its own invention." This object, of course, is disease—and there is a parallel in audiology. Since our beginnings in the mid-1940s, we have measured, described, researched, cataloged, analyzed, and synthesized the entity of hearing loss exhaustively—and now, having defined it, we must busy ourselves with preventing the devastation of its effects on children. In such terms preventive audiology becomes a viable endeavor—a discipline devoted to preventing the effects of ear disease on the individual who suffers from it. Such prevention can only be accomplished by early detection of the condition and by proper provision for remedial therapy and education.

Marion P. Downs (1990)

Appendix of Hearing Disorders

A synopsis of various syndromes associated with congenital deafness is presented in this appendix of hearing disorders. The material is a summary of information we believe is pertinent to the clinician. The information is by no means intended to be exhaustive or even complete; our intent is to provide a concise, clear, and informative reference regarding special patients who have an inordinately high risk for impairment of their hearing. We recognize that children with symptoms that are variants from our generalized information about each disorder will be seen and that readers will immediately wish to revise our summary. So be it; our intent is to provide only an orientation or a guide to clinicians who might come into contact with children who demonstrate these disorders and to instill a desire to learn more about the disease.

General References. Some students may wish to consult more general reference sources for detailed accounts of syndromes included in this section of the book or to pursue information on syndromes not included here. Such general references cover much more than individual articles and may touch on many aspects of the disorders not covered in our necessarily scant summaries. Accordingly, such a list is given below, which we have found to be immeasurably useful in our review of birth defects associated with hearing loss.

Bergsma D (ed): *Birth Defects Compendium*, ed 2. New York: Alan R Liss, 1979.

Bess F: *Childhood Deafness: Causation, Assessment and Management*. New York: Grune & Stratton, 1977.

Fraser GR: *The Causes of Profound Deafness in Childhood*. Baltimore: Johns Hopkins University Press, 1976.

Hemenway WG, Bergstrom L: Symposium on congenital deafness. *Otolaryngol Clin. North Am.* 4: 1971.

Jung JH: *Genetic Syndromes in Communication Disorders*. Boston: Little, Brown, 1989.

Konigsmark BW, Gorlin RJ: *Genetic and Metabolic Deafness*. Philadelphia: WB Saunders, 1976.

Lindsay JR: Profound childhood deafness. *Ann Otol Rhinol Laryngol* 82 (suppl 5): 1973.

Salmon MA: *Developmental Defects and Syndromes*. Aylesbury, England: HM & M Publishers Ltd, 1978.

Siegel-Sadewitz V, Shprintzen R: The relationship of communication disorders to syndrome identification. *J Speech Hear Disord* 47:338, 1982.

Smith DW: *Recognizable Patterns of Human Malformation*. Philadelphia: WB Saunders, 1970.

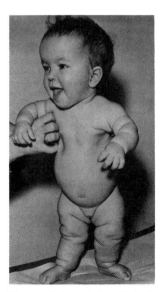

Figure A.1. Achondroplasia. (Reproduced with permission from T. H. Shepard and B. Graham: The congenitally malformed: achondroplastic dwarfism: diagnosis and management. *Northwest Medicine* 66:451–456, 1967).

Absence of the Tibia

(Robert's Syndrome)

Skeletal disorder; recessive trait; characterized by congenital absence of one or both tibias (lower legs), shortened, malformed fibulas, and severe, congenital sensorineural hearing loss (Pashayan et al., 1971).

Achondroplasia

(Chondrodystrophia Fetalis)

A congenital skeletal anomaly characterized by slow growth of cartilage, retarded endochondrial ossification, and almost normal periosteal bone formation (Fig. A.1). As a result, those affected are very short in stature with dispro-portionately short limbs, large heads with prominent foreheads, depressed nasal bridge, and "button" nose. Mentality is usually normal, but retardation may appear secondary to hydrocephalus and increased cranial pressure. Deafness may be present. Respiratory, pulmonary, and other complications increase with age. Diagnosis may be suspected by clinical examination but is confirmed by radiographic evaluation.

This is a hereditary dominant disorder; however, over 80% of cases are due to fresh mutation, with both parents being normal. Incidence increases with increasing parental age.

Both conductive and/or sensorineural loss may be present. Middle ear anomalies include fusion of ossicles to surrounding bony structures as well as dense thick trabeculae without islands of cartilage in the endochondrial and periosteal bone. Associated anomalies of the inner ear include deformed cochlea and thickened intercochlear partitions. Incidence of serous otitis high.

General treatment consists of genetic counseling and surgical treatment as indicated (Cohen, 1967; Langer et al., 1967; Langer, 1968).

Acoustic Neuroma

(See Von Recklinghausen's Neurofibromatosis)

Acrocephalosyndactyly

(See Apert's Syndrome)

Albers-Schönberg Disease of Osteopetrosis

(Chalk Bone Disease; Ivory Bone Disease; Marble Bone Disease)

Craniofacial and skeletal disorder; recessive form associated with deafness. Brittle but paradoxically sclerotic thickened bones. Head may be somewhat enlarged; retarded growth in one third of cases. Visual loss noted in about 80% of cases, which may lead to blindness. Mental retardation in 20% of cases; facial palsy, unilateral or bilateral, in 10%. Little detailed audiometric data available, but 25–50% of patients are reported to have moderate, progressive sensorineural or conductive hearing loss (Johnston et al., 1968; Jones and Mulcahy, 1968; Myers and Stool, 1969).

Albinism with Blue Irides

(Oculocutaneous Albinism)

Integumentary and pigmentary disorder; dominant; scalp hair white, fine, and silky, sometimes with patches of pigmentation. Fair skin. Possible heterochromia of iris. Severe sensorineural congenital deafness (Tietz, 1963; Reed et al., 1967).

Alport's Syndrome

(Hereditary Nephritis with Nerve Deafness)

Renal disorder associated with deafness and ocular anomalies. Characteristics include autosomal dominant inheritance with men being more severely affected than

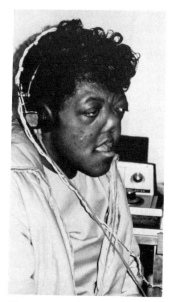

Figure A.2. Apert's syndrome.

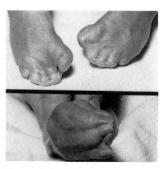

Figure A.3. Apert's syndrome.

women, progressive nephritis with uremia, ocular lens abnormalities such as cataracts, and progressive sensorineural hearing loss. Hearing loss occurs in 40–60% of cases; ocular defects in 15%. Hearing impairment is typically mild to severe, high frequency, usually bilaterally symmetrical, and may occur alone or in combination with the renal disease. Hearing loss is more frequent and tends to be more severe in men. Age of onset of hearing impairment is in preadolescence (Bergstrom et al., 1973; Rintelmann, 1976; Johnsson and Arenberg, 1981).

Amyloidosis, Nephritis, and Urticaria

(Muckle-Wells Syndrome)

Dominant. Onset in teens of recurrent urticaria (vascular reaction of skin with elevated patches and itching) with malaise and chills with onset of recurrent limb and joint pain. Amyloidosis (starchy-like substance in the blood) precedes nephropathy and renal failure. Progression of hearing loss parallels progression of renal failure, resulting in severe hearing impairment by third or fourth decade of life. Endocrine and metabolic disorder with progressive sensorineural hearing loss of late onset.

Apert's Syndrome

(Acrocephalosyndactyly)

Skeletal and associated skull malformations that include craniofacial dysostosis, syndactyly, brachiocephaly, hypertelorism, bilateral ptosis, saddle nose, high arched palate, ankylosis of joints, spinal bifida, and mental retardation (Figs. A.2 and A.3). Syndactyly (fusion of fingers and toes) is complete on both hands and feet. Hearing loss common. Characteristic "tower skull," with flat forehead.

Most reported cases appear sporadic. When reproduction is possible, the disorder is apparently of autosomal dominant transmission. There also appears to be a high mutation rate related to increasing parent age. Manifestation present at birth. Risk of occurrence is 1 in 160,000.

Audiometric findings usually show flat conductive loss. However, a sensorineural component is suspected in some cases. Surgical explorations have revealed congenital stapedial footplate fixation, abnormal patency of cochlear aqueduct, and enlarged internal auditory meatus. Impedance audiometry shows manifestations of conductive hearing loss with low compliance and absent acoustic reflexes (Bergstrom et al., 1972; Lindsay et al., 1975).

Atopic Dermatitis

Recessive. Congenital moderate nonprogressive sensorineural hearing loss that may not be detected until school years. About age 10, affected persons develop lichenified, skin eruptions especially on forearms, hands, elbows, and trunk and arms. Very rare. Integumentary and pigmentary disorder with congenital sensorineural hearing loss (Konigsmark et al., 1968, 1970).

Brevicollis

(See Klippel-Feil Syndrome)

Cardioauditory Syndrome

(See Jervell and Lange-Nielsen Syndrome)

Cerebral Palsy

Recessive or sporadic trait; 1 of 330 babies is born with cerebral palsy. Paralysis due to a lesion of the brain, usually suffered at birth, and characterized by uncontrollable motor spasms. Cerebral palsy involves paralysis, weakness, incoordination, or other abnormality of motor function due to pathology of the motor control centers of the brain. Damage to the brain may occur during embryonic, fetal, or early infantile life. Essentially nonprogressive, clinical symptoms of the disorder include spasticity (40%), athetosis (40%), ataxia (10%), or combinations of these basic motor dysfunctions. Mental deficiency and convulsive disorders are common. Feeding problems, retarded growth, eye difficulties such as strabismus and nystagmus, developmental delay, orthopedic problems, communication disorders, and educational problems often are evidenced in varying degrees. Damage to the brain may occur during embryonic, fetal, or early infantile life and may result from an antecedent disorder such as trauma, metabolic disorder of infection, destructive intercranial cerebral processes, and/or developmental defects of the brain. Location of the lesion may be in cerebral cortex, basal ganglia, or other sites in the pyramidal system or extrapyramidal system; coexistent involvement in both systems is observed. Less frequently, cerebellar damage may be evident. Patients may have mild-to-moderate sensorineural hearing loss, typically more severe in high frequencies.

Cervico-oculoacoustic Dysplasia

(See Klippel-Feil Syndrome)

Cleft Palate and/or Lip

High incidence of recurrent middle ear effusion episodes. Approximately 35–50% of cleft palate babies have associated anomalies (Fig. A.4).

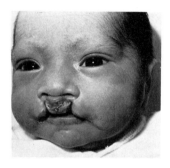

Figure A.4. Bilateral cleft palate and lip.

See Chapter 3 for additional information (Bzoch, 1979).

Cleidocranial Dysostosis

(Cleidocranial Dysplasia; Osteodental Dysplasia)

A general disorder of skeleton due to retarded ossification of membranous and cartilagi-

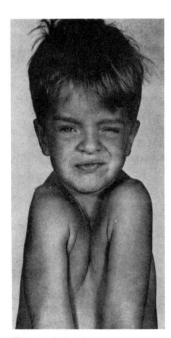

Figure A.5. Cleidocranial dysostosis. (Reproduced with permission from I. S. Jaffee: Congenital shoulder-neck-auditory anomalies. *Laryngoscope* 58:2119–2139, 1968).

nous precursors of bone characterized by congenital absence of clavicles, softness of skull, and irregular ossification of bones (Fig. A.5). In addition, shortness of stature, narrow drooping shoulders, widely spaced eyes, irregular or absent teeth, and high arched palate or submucous cleft have been noted. Concentric narrowing of external auditory canals. Mental development is usually normal. Chromosome analyses show normal karyotypes. Autosomal dominant with high percentage and wide variability in expression. About one third of the cases appear to be sporadic. Occasionally, progressive deafness is reported. May be conductive or sensorineural due to retarded bone ossification.

Cockayne's Syndrome

Recessive. Generally rare with about 30 cases described in the literature. Dwarfism, mental retardation, retinal atrophy, and motor disturbances. Progressive disorder. Appearance normal at birth. Growth and development normal through first year. During the second year, growth falls below normal range and mental-motor development becomes abnormal. Minimal diagnostic characteristics include dwarfism, retinal degeneration, microcephaly, cataracts, neurologic impairment including progressive mental retardation, sun-sensitive skin, thickening of the skull bones, disproportionately long extremities with large hands and feet, eye disorder, and progressive sensorineural hearing loss of later onset, usually of moderate-to-severe degree. Prognosis is poor with severe blindness and deafness. Hearing aid is possible; however, mental retardation precludes much suc-

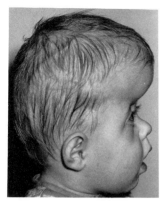

Figure A.6. Crouzon's syndrome.

cess (Riggs and Seibert, 1972; Shemen et al., 1984).

Cornelia de Lange Syndrome

Polygenetic-multifactorial syndrome characterized by severe-to-profound mental and growth retardation, hirsutism, microcephaly, confluent eyebrows often accompanied by anomalies of the external ear, including low-set auricles and small external auditory canals. Usually, full-term infants although small at birth. Severely malformed upper limbs; may have missing toes or fingers and possible webbing between toes. Cardiac defects are common; possible cleft palate accompanied by neonatal feeding and respiratory difficulties. Speech and language problems are severe, and hearing loss attributed to conductive, sensorineural, and mixed etiologies has been reported. Prognosis is poor with diminished life expectancy (Silver, 1964; Moore, 1970; Fraser and Cambell, 1978).

Craniofacial Dysostosis

(See Crouzon's Syndrome)

Crouzon's Syndrome

(Craniofacial Dysostosis)

Abnormally shaped head characterized by a central prominence in the frontal region, a peculiar nose resembling a beak, and marked bilateral exophthalmos caused by premature closure of cranial sutures (Fig. A.6). Shape of the skull depends on which sutures are involved. Mentality may be low but usually is not unless there is brain damage secondary to increased intracranial pressure. Bifid uvula and cleft palate may be present. Autosomal dominant with variable expression. Approximately one fourth of reported cases arise as fresh mutations. Detected at birth or during first year. Ears may be low set. About one third of cases have nonprogressive conductive hearing impairment. May have mixed-type deafness. Middle ear manifestations include deformed stapes with bony fusion of promontory, ankylosis of malleus to outer wall of the epitympanum, distortion and narrowing of middle ear space, absence of the tympanic membrane, and perhaps bilateral atresia. Stenosis or atresia of external canal common. Early surgical intervention is usually recommended to prevent damage to the brain and eyes. Genetic counseling is recommended (Dodge et al., 1959; Vulliamy and Normandale, 1966; Baldwin, 1968).

Cryptophthalmus

Eye disorder. Recessive. Adherent eyelids that hide the eyes, often accompanied by external ear malformations. In its most severe form, unilateral or, more often, bilateral extension of skin of the forehead completely covers

eye or eyes to the cheeks. In less severe form, the upper or lower eyelid may be absent. Syndactyly of fingers and/or toes may be present. Laryngeal atresia has been reported. Cleft lip and palate are not uncommon. Hearing loss is of mixed type, with atresia of external auditory canals (Fraser, 1962; Ide and Wollschlaeger, 1969).

Cytomegalovirus Disease

Intrauterine perinatal viral infection or postnatal viral infection, usually transmitted in utero, that may cause hearing loss and other serious central nervous system disorders. See Chapters 3 and 7 for additional information.

Diastrophic Dwarfism

Craniofacial disorder. Recessive trait. Marked shortness of stature, characteristic hand deformity with short fingers, and severe bilateral clubfoot. The auricles show cystic swellings in infancy that later develop into cauliflower-like deformities that may calcify. There is 25% incidence of cleft palate. Congenital sensorineural hearing loss (Langer, 1965).

Down's Syndrome

(Trisomy 21 Syndrome; Mongolism)

Syndrome (Fig. A.7) is the result of a chromosomal abnormality, either as a 21 trisomy, translocation trisomy (Fig. A.8, *A* and *B*), or mosaicism. High incidence of occurrence— 1 in 770 live births—with approximately 5000 new Down's

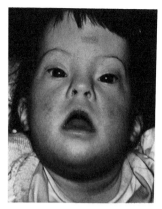

Figure A.7. Down's syndrome.

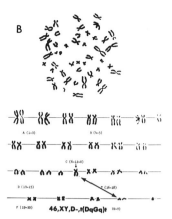

Figure A.8B. Karyotype of Down's syndrome (note translocation). (Courtesy of A. Robinson, M.D., Cytogenetics Laboratory, University of Colorado Medical Center, Denver, Colorado.)

births each year in the United States. Clinical findings include a list of 50 features with varying penetrance. Mental retardation is almost universal. Characteristic personality that is warm, friendly, and affectionate. Common diagnostic features include flattened facial features, oblique palpebral fissures, flat occiput, short limbs, short broad hands, short fingers (especially the fifth finger), depressed nasal bridge, congenital hearing defects, absent moro reflex in infancy, mouth breathing, dental abnormalities, and mental retarda-

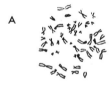

DOWN'S SYNDROME

47,XY,21+

Figure A.8A. Karyotype of Down's syndrome (note extra 21st chromosome). (Courtesy of A. Robinson, M.D., Cytogenetics Laboratory, University of Colorado Medical Center, Denver, Colorado.)

tion. Ear symptoms in Down's syndrome include small pinnae, narrow external ear canals, abnormal ear configuration, and a strong tendency for repeated bouts of otitis media. Incidence of hearing loss is very high with implications of sensorineural, conductive, and mixed hearing problems. Anomalies of middle ear ossicles have been reported. Risk of occurrence increases with age of mother: 1 in 1200 at age 25, but increasing to 1 in 100 for a 40 year old. Can be identified in early pregnancy with amniocentesis. See Chapter 3 for additional information.

Duane's Syndrome

(Cervico-oculoacoustic Dysplasia)

Eye disorder. Recessive. Congenital paralysis of the sixth cranial nerve (abducens palsy) with retracted bulb and severe congenital sensorineural and/or conductive deafness. Striking appearance because head seems to sit directly on trunk. The abducens paralysis prevents external rotation of eyes, may be unilateral or bi-

lateral; occasional cleft palate. Various ear anomalies have been described, including periauricular tags, malformation, atresia or absence of external ear canal, abnormal ossicles, etc. Congenital and nonprogressive (Kirkham, 1969; Singh et al, 1969; Cross and Pfaffenbach, 1972; Stark and Borton, 1973).

Dyschondrosteosis

(See Madelung's Deformity)

Ectodermal Dysplasia

(Ectrosyndactyly, Ectodermal Dysplasia, and Cleft Palate Syndrome; Lobster-Claw Syndrome)

Integumentary and pigmentary disorder sometimes accompanied by congenital progressive sensorineural and/or conductive hearing loss. Depressed vestibular function. Abnormality of middle and inner ears has been described. Syndrome seems to have dominant transmission with poor penetrance and variable expressivity. Peculiar lobster-claw deformity of hands and feet, nasolacrimal obstruction and cleft lippalate. Microcephaly and/or mental retardation present in about 20% of cases (Preus and Fraser, 1973; Robinson et al., 1973; Pashayan et al., 1974).

Engelmann's Syndrome

(Craniodiaphyseal Dysplasia; Diaphyseal Dysplasia)

Skeletal disorder; dominant and/or recessive transmission. Radiologically, this syndrome is characterized by bilateral fusiform enlargement of the diaphyses of the long bones. Skull base may be sclerotic. Deafness is universal and may appear as progressive sensorineural mixed or conductive in nature (Nelson and Scott, 1969; Sparkes and Graham, 1972).

Fanconi's Anemia Syndrome

(Infantile and/or Adolescent Renal Tubular Acidosis)

A syndrome of many causes, some of which are inherited, yet often unidentified. Exposure to toxic agents directly precedes most acquired cases. The clinical manifestations are dependent upon the causes of the syndrome. All aspects of the disorder reflect impaired renal tubular transport. Growth retardation common. In the infantile form, high-frequency sensorineural deafness is noted in infancy; in adolescent form, slowly progressive sensorineural deafness noted during teen years (McDonough, 1970; Walker, 1971).

Fehr's Corneal Dystrophy

(Harboyan Syndrome)

Eye disorder. Recessive. Age of detectability is usually between 5 and 9 years. Congenital corneal dystrophy with slow progression leading to blindness at age 40. Progressive sensorineural deafness of delayed onset (Maumenee, 1960; Harboyan et al., 1971).

Fetal Alcohol Syndrome

Neuroectoderm syndrome that includes a combination of low birthweight, failure to thrive, and mental retardation seen in children of women who abuse alcohol during pregnancy. Occurrence is between 1:500 and 1:1000 births. Full or partial expression of congenital malformations is associated with prenatal and postnatal growth deficiencies, central nervous system dysfunctions, and anomalies of the skeletal system and internal organs. Characterized by a variety of craniofacial disorders traditionally associated with hearing disorders, such as micrognathia, cleft palate, and abnormal pinnae. Frequently includes congenital abnormalities of the heart and eyes. Church and Gerkin (1987) noted hearing disorders in 13 of 14 children affected by fetal alcohol syndrome. Of the 14 study children, 13 had significant recurrent otitis media histories, including 4 with sensorineural hearing loss. Speech and language disorders have been described by Sparks (1984).

Fragile X Syndrome

Fragile X syndrome is an inherited abnormality of the X chromosome that causes disabilities ranging from varying degrees of learning problems to mental retardation. Features commonly associated with the syndrome include: severe language delay, behavior problems, autism or autistic-like behaviors (including poor eye contact and hand-flapping), macroorchidism, large prominent ears, hyperactivity, delayed motor development, and poor sensory skills. Hearing loss has seldom been associated with fragile X syndrome. Fragile X

syndrome affects approximately 1 in 1000 persons.

Most children affected with fragile X syndrome will have some form of speech or language delay. Because they do not speak in short phrases until 2½ years of age, these children should have routine auditory evaluation. The speech of fragile X children has been described as compulsive, narrative, and perseverative. Fragile X speech has been described as "cluttered" and "mumbled" with poor topic maintenance; frequent tangential comments may occur. Syntax is usually appropriate for mental age; a high receptive vocabulary score is usually seen, although auditory memory and processing skills are weak (Paul et al., 1984; Wolf-Schein et al., 1987).

Friedrich's Ataxia

Nervous system disorder. Recessive. Progressive spinocerebellar ataxia appearing between the ages of 7 and 18 years. Nystagmus, optic atrophy, oculomotor paralysis, retinitis pigmentosa, cataracts, cardiac complications and organic psychologic problems. Progressive sensorineural deafness of late onset that may be mild or severe, possibly progressive, symmetrical or asymmetrical with better hearing in the middle frequencies (Sylvester, 1958, 1972; Shanon et al., 1981).

Goiter, Stippled Epiphysis, and High Protein-Bound Iodine

Endocrine-metabolic disorder. Congenital metabolic defect associated with thyroid overactivity, congenital profound sensorineural deafness, birdlike facies, pigeon breast,

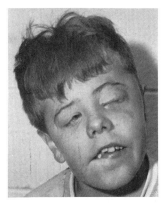

Figure A.9. Goldenhar's syndrome.

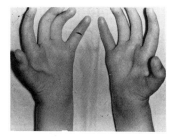

Figure A.10. Hand-hearing syndrome.

and winged scapulae. Goiter appears in early infancy. Congenital sensorineural hearing loss (Refetoff et al., 1967).

Goldenhar's Syndrome

(Oculoauriculovertebral Dysplasia)

Eye, oral, and musculoskeletal anomalies (Fig. A.9). Eye abnormalities include cleft or upper lid, epibulbar dermoids, extraocular muscle defects, and antimongoloid obliquity. Auricular abnormalities include auricular appendices, unilateral posteriorly placed ear, unilateral microtia, atresia of external auditory meatus (40%), and blind-ended fistulas. Oral abnormalities include unilateral facial hypoplasia of ramus and condyle, high arched palate, and open bite. Musculoskeletal abnormalities such as hemivertebrae and clubfoot. Congenital heart disease. Mental retardation not common. Etiology unknown but may not be hereditary. Most cases are sporadic. Possibly secondary to vascular abnormality during embryologic development of first and second arches. Conductive hearing loss present in 40–50% of reported cases as a result of atresia of external auditory canals (Sugar, 1966; Berkman and Feingold, 1968).

Hallgren's Syndrome

Eye disorder. Recessive. Congenital sensorineural hearing loss. Retinitis pigmentosa, progressive ataxia, and mental retardation in 25% of cases. Some patients show later psychosis; 90% have profound deafness (Hallgren, 1959).

Hand-Hearing Syndrome

(Hand Muscle Wasting and Sensorineural Deafness)

Dominant inheritance. Patients manifest familial congenital bilateral or unilateral sensorineural hearing loss of varying degrees. A congenital hand abnormality is seen in both normal hearing and deaf patients (Fig. A.10). Congenital contractures of the digits and wasting of finger muscles. No pain and no other deficits (Stewart and Bergstrom, 1971).

Hemifacial Microsomia

Craniofacial disorder with unknown etiology. Abnormalities are unilateral and include ear aplasia and hypoplasia with various pinna malformations. Preauricular tags are present in nearly all cases. External ear canals may be absent or present with the opening covered with skin. Other characteristics include eye abnormalities, lower palpebral fissure in the affected side, microphthalmia, cysts, iris, and choroid colobomas and strabismus, hypoplastic facial muscles, malocclusion (90%), and hypoplasia of the maxilla and mandible (95%). May have unilateral conductive hearing loss.

Hereditary Hyperphosphatasia

(See Paget's Disease)

Herrmann's Syndrome

(Photomyelonus, Diabetes Mellitus, Nephropathy, and Sensorineural Deafness)

Nervous system disorder; dominant inheritance. Photomyoclonic and grand mal epilepsy. Later course of syndrome includes personality changes leading to severe dementia, slurring of speech, progressive hemiparesis, and mild ataxia, renal disease, and diabetes. Age of detectability is third or fourth decade. Progressive sensorineural hearing loss of late origin (Herrmann et al., 1964).

Hurler's Syndrome-Hunter's Syndrome

(Mucopolysaccharidosis I and II)

Hurler's is thought to be autosomal recessive, and Hunter's is X-linked recessive

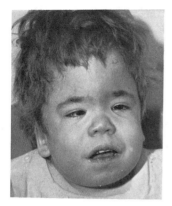

Figure A.11. Hurler's syndrome.

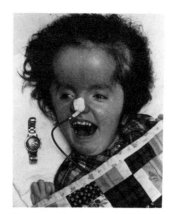

Figure A.13. Hydrocephalus.

fluid in and around the brain (Fig. A.13). May be congenital or acquired; typically detected at birth or within first 3 months of life. Mental retardation if not treated. Risk of occurrence is 1 in 2000. Accompanied by enlargement of the head, prominence of the brain, mental deterioration, and convulsions. With successful shunt treatment 80% of children reach 5 years of age, and 80% of survivors are normal or educable. No data available regarding hearing impairment, although Walker et al. (1987) discuss auditory evoked brainstem response measurement in neonatal hydrocephalus. (Shulman, 1973).

(Fig. A.11 and A.12). Although the two disorders are clinically identical, Hunter's is generally less severe and affects only males. Hurler's can affect both sexes. In contrast to patients with Hurler's syndrome, patients with Hunter's syndrome usually do not show gross evidence of corneal clouding. Patients have normal appearance at birth, but during early months of life there is onset of progressive abnormal traits. Often described as an "inborn error of metabolism." Diagnostic features include growth failure, marked mental retardation, progressive coarsening of facial features, chronic nasal discharge, joint stiffness, and biochemical evidence of intracellular storage and acid mu-

copolysaccharides. Death usually occurs before 10 years of age in patients with Hurler's syndrome, while patients with Hunter's syndrome in mild form may survive until adulthood, or those with severe type may die before puberty. Auditory symptoms have not been satisfactorily described according to Konigsmark and Gorlin (1976). They describe most patients with Hurler's syndrome as having some degree of progressive deafness. Hunter's syndrome has been accompanied by deafness in about half the cases, although the loss is usually not severe and most likely mixed sensorineural and conductive in nature. Otolaryngologic manifestations include upper and lower respiratory infections, narrow nasal passages, hypertrophied adenoids, mucopurulent rhinorrhea, and noisy breathing. Affected individuals are prone to eustachian tube dysfunction and middle ear effusions (Keleman, 1966; Leroy and Crocker, 1966; Hayes et al., 1980).

Hyperprolinemia I and II

A biochemical phenotype. No proven association with clinical disease, although identified frequently in pedigrees containing renal disease or convulsive disorders. Recessive disorder. Metabolic problem. Hearing loss has been described as sensorineural in some individuals affected with type I disease (Schafer et al., 1962).

Hyperuricemia

Endocrine-metabolic problem. Dominant transmission with variable expressivity. Slowly progressive ataxia beginning in second decade. Renal insufficiency. Cardiopathy, myopathy and gout have been noted in some patients. Progressive sensorineural hearing loss of late onset, usually high frequency in nature; may progress to total hearing loss with vestibular abnormalities (Rosenberg et al., 1970).

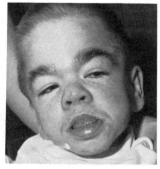

Figure A.12. Hunter's syndrome.

Hydrocephalus

A condition characterized by abnormal accumulation of

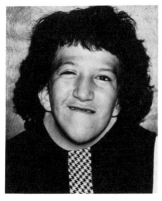

Figure A.14. Klippel-Feil syndrome with right facial paralysis.

Jervell and Lange-Nielsen Syndrome

(Cardioauditory Syndrome; Surdocardiac Syndrome)

Cardiovascular disorder affects 0.3% of congenitally deaf persons. Autosomal recessive trait. Consanguinity is common. Profound congenital bilateral sensorineural deafness accompanied by electrocardiographic abnormalities, fainting attacks, and, occasionally, sudden unexplained death in childhood. Death usually occurs between 3 and 14 years of age in over half the cases of cardiac problems. Hearing loss is usually symmetrical. Often erroneously diagnosed as a seizure disorder and thus improperly treated (Jervell and Lange-Nielsen, 1957; Friedmann et al., 1966; Wahl and Dick, 1980).

Keratopachyderma and Digital Constrictions

Integumentary disorder, dominant trait. Hyperkeratosis involving the palms, soles, knees, and elbows. Ringlike furrows developing on fingers and toes. Mild-to-severe congenital sensorineural deafness, mainly for frequencies above 4000 Hz, which may be slowly progressive. May include renal disease (Bitici, 1975).

Klippel-Feil Syndrome

(Brevicollis; Cervico-oculoacoustic Dysplasia; Wildervanck's Syndrome)

Craniofacial disorder (Fig. A.14) of debatable etiology, probably due to faulty mesodermal differentiation at about the second month of gestation. Involves fusion of some or all cervical vertebrae and is characterized by a short neck with limited mobility, which gives the impression that the head sits on the shoulders. Diagnostic criteria include involvement of ear, eye, and neck. Other malformations may occur such as clubfoot and cleft palate. Associated neurologic disturbances. Debatable etiology. If familial, autosomal dominance with poor penetrance and variable expression. Faulty segmentation of mesodermal somites in utero, defects in maternal intestinal tract, and environmental factors have been suggested. Summary of syndrome characteristics includes multifactorial inheritance, fusion of cervical vertebrae, abducens nerve palsy, occasional cleft palate, torticollis, and severe sensorineural or conductive hearing loss. May range from mild conductive to profound sensorineural. Ear deformities occur in one third of cases; temporal bone and roentgenogram findings include narrow to absent external auditory meatus and/or middle ear space, deformed ossicles, narrow oval window niche, underdevelopment of cochlea and vestibular structures (electronystagmograms abnormal), absence of semicircular canals, and absence of eighth cranial nerve. Central nervous system involvement is also frequently described and may contribute to audiologic findings. This syndrome is much more common in females (McLay and Maran, 1969; Stark and Borton, 1973; Windle-Taylor et al., 1981; Miyamoto et al., 1983).

Knuckle Pads and Leukonychia

Dominant. Callous-like thickening over dorsal aspects of interphalangeal joints of fingers and toes first observed in infancy and early childhood. Progressive whitening of finger and toenails (leukonychia). Integumentary-pigmentary disorder; congenital sensorineural or conductive hearing loss. Hearing loss usually noted in infancy or early childhood. Cochlear involvement of mixed mild-to-moderate degree (Bart and Pumphrey, 1967).

Laurence-Moon-Biedl-Bardet Syndromes

Eye disorder with progressive sensorineural hearing loss of recessive inheritance. Patients with the Laurence-Moon syndrome have retinitis pigmentosa, mental retardation, hypogenitalism, and spastic paraplegia. Patients with Biedl-Bardet syndrome show obesity and retinitis pigmentosa in association with polydactyly, hypogonadism and mental retardation (Weinstein et al., 1969; Konigsmark and Gorlin, 1976).

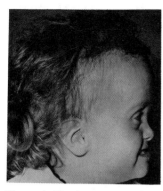

Figure A.15. Long arm 18 deletion syndrome. (Reproduced with permission from D. Bergsma: *Birth Defects Compendium*, ed. 2, National Foundation-March of Dimes. New York: Alan R. Liss, 1979.)

Leri-Weill Disease

(See Madelung's Deformity)

Lobster-Claw Syndrome

(See Ectodermal Dysplasia)

Long Arm 18 Deletion Syndrome

Abnormalities include mental retardation, microcephaly, short stature, hearing impairment with malformations of

PARTIAL DELETION OF 18 LONG ARM

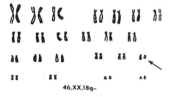

46,XX,18q-

Figure A.16. Karyotype of partial deletion of long arm of 18th chromosome. (Courtesy of A. Robinson, M.D., Cytogenetics Laboratory, University of Colorado Medical Center, Denver, Colorado.)

auricles and external auditory canals, retinal changes, facial peculiarities, and a high count of whorls on the fingers (Fig. A.15). Congenital heart disease, horseshoe kidney, cryptorchidism, spinal defects, and foot abnormalities have also been described. Genetic imbalance syndrome involving partial deletion of the long arm of the 18th chromosome (Fig. A.16). If translocation is responsible for deletion, transmission to children is possible. Conductive hearing loss associated with external and middle ear anomalies most frequently reported. Temporal bone study has shown collapsed Reissner's membrane in all turns of the cochlea, rolled and retracted tectorial membrane, and hypoplastic cochlear aqueduct (Smith, 1962; Kos et al., 1966; Bergstrom et al., 1974).

Madelung's Deformity

(Dyschondrosteosis; Leri-Weill Disease)

Craniofacial-skeletal disorder. Dominant. Characterized by deformity of the distal radius and ulna bones and mild dwarfism. Congenital bilateral conductive loss with abnormal ossicles and narrow external auditory canals (Nassif and Harboyan, 1970).

Malformed Low-Set Ears Syndrome

Craniofacial disorder with unilateral or bilateral, mild-to-severe, conductive hearing loss associated with malformed low-set ears (usually bilateral). Conductive loss usually worse in the most affected external ear. May be accompanied by mental retar-

dation in 50% of cases (Mengel et al., 1969).

Marfan's Syndrome

Craniofacial-skeletal disorder of dominant inheritance. Characteristic symptoms include arachnodactyly, scoliosis, joint hypermobility, dislocated lenses, and cardiac anomalies. Deafness associated with Marfan's syndrome is rare (Konigsmark and Gorlin, 1976).

Measles

A highly contagious viral infection involving the respiratory tract. The skin becomes covered with red papules that appear behind the ears and on the face before spreading rapidly down the trunk and onto the arms and legs. Measles may be complicated by bacterial pneumonia, otitis media, and a demyelinating encephalitis. According to Bergstrom (1984), measles may cause hearing loss as a result of invasion of the inner ear via the blood stream or central nervous system or through purulent labyrinthitis secondary to suppurative otitis media.

Meningitis

Infection or inflammation of the meningeal membrane surrounding the brain and spinal cord. May be a complication of otitis media. Etiology is varied and may be due to bacteria, virus, or fungi. Symptoms include stiff neck, headache, high fever, nausea, vomiting, and sometimes coma. Approximately 40% of children with deafness due to meningitis have at least one other major handicapping condition. Recovery of auditory function

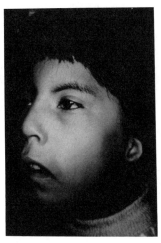

Figure A.17. Möbius' syndrome.

following meningitic deafness has been documented in numerous reports. Fairly common cause of sudden, severe-to-profound sensorineural deafness (8–16%) that is usually bilateral but may occasionally be unilateral. See Chapter 3 for more information (Vernon, 1967; Roeser et al., 1975; Keane et al., 1979; Finitzo-Hieber et al., 1981b).

Möbius' Syndrome

(Facial Dysplagia)

Dominant. Craniofacial nervous system disorder (Fig. A.17). Bilateral congenital facial paralysis, due to paralysis of cranial nerves VI and VII, severe but incomplete, with varying degrees of ophthalmoplegia, external ear malformations, micrognathia. Hands, feet, or digits may be missing; tongue paralysis and mental retardation may be present. Middle ear anomalies may be associated, as well as aberrant facial nerve. Congenital sensorineural and/or conductive hearing loss (Kahane, 1979).

Mohr's Syndrome

(Oral-Facial-Digital II; OFD II)

Deformities of face, mouth, and fingers transmitted as recessive trait. Characterized by cleft lip and lobulated tongue, broad nasal root, hypoplasia of the mandible, polydactyly, and syndactyly. Oral deformities may cause speech problems and conductive hearing loss associated with malformed ossicles (Rimoin and Edgerton, 1967).

Mongolism

(See Down's Syndrome)

Muckle-Wells Syndrome

(See Amyloidosis, Nephritis, and Urticaria)

Multiple Lentigines Syndrome

(LEOPARD Syndrome)

Integumentary-pigmentary disorder. Dominant trait. Freckly, dark brown, small spots concentrated on the neck and upper trunk. The term LEOPARD syndrome is an acronym derived from *len*tigines, *e*lectrocardiographic defects, *o*cular hypertelorism, *p*ulmonary stenosis, *a*bnormalities of genitalia, *r*etardation of growth, and sensorineural *d*eafness in 15% of cases. Hearing loss is usually detected in childhood (Gorlin et al., 1969; Voron et al., 1976).

Mucopoly saccharidosis

(See Hurler's Syndrome-Hunter's Syndrome)

Mumps

A contagious viral disease occurring mainly in children. It is acquired by aspiration, with the heaviest inoculation of virus being in the salivary and parotid glands. The incubation period is 18–22 days, with fever and painful inflammation of the involved glands. Symptoms are most pronounced during the first 2 days and subside slowly over the next 4 or 5 days. Classic symptoms involve fever, headache, anorexia, malaise, earache, and enlargement of parotids. Relatively common cause of sudden, total unilateral sensorineural hearing loss. Hearing loss is nearly always permanent. Bilateral total deafness has been reported, but only in rare instances. Exact incidence of hearing loss is difficult to ascertain because of undetected, or undiagnosed, unilateral cases. Deafness may be approximately 5% (Fowler, 1960; Vuori et al., 1962).

Muscular Dystrophy

Recessive or X-linked. Muscle wasting of various types classified by transmission mode, age of onset, damaged muscle set, rate of disease development, associated problems. *Pseudohypertrophic* muscular dystrophy usually begins prior to age 5 years and affects most body muscles including cardiac and pulmonary systems. *Facioscapulohumeral* type affects face, shoulder, and upper arm muscles; slowly progressive with age of onset at 13–14 years. *Limb-girdle* type initially affects muscles of hips and shoulders. *Myotonic* muscular dystrophy associated with diabetes mellitus and cataracts, usually of late onset at age 30–40 or older. Severe infantile muscular dystrophy noted to be accompanied by sloping, sensorineural hearing loss of mild-to-moderate degree. Risk of occurrence is 1 in 100,000; childhood form is usually noted during initial 3 years of life. Extremely rare in females (Black et al., 1971).

Myoclonic Epilepsy

Dominant nervous system disorder with variable expressivity. Seizure disorder characterized by myoclonic movements that include jerking motions involving head, trunk, and limbs. Slowly progressive ataxia. No mental retardation. Progressive sensorineural hearing loss of late onset (May and White, 1968).

Myopia and Congenital Deafness

Recessive transmission. Patients demonstrate a combination of symptoms including myopia, congenital moderate-to-severe, nonprogressive sensorineural hearing loss and, in some cases, low intelligence (Eldridge et al., 1968).

Nephrosis, Urinary Tract Malformations

Sex-linked or recessive transmission. Renal disorder with congenital conductive hearing impairment. Characterized by renal anomalies, nephrosis, digital anomalies, bifurcation of uvula. Congenital moderate-to-severe con-

ductive-type hearing impairment (Winter et al., 1968).

Neurofibromatosis

(See Von Recklinghausen's Neurofibromatosis)

Norrie's Syndrome

(Oculoacousticocerebral Degeneration)

X-linked recessive with progressive eye degeneration leading to total blindness. Approximately one third are severely mental retarded, one third are mildly retarded, and one third are of normal intelligence. Auditory impairment is progressive, of late onset, and usually bilaterally symmetric sensorineural hearing loss in one third of cases (Holmes, 1971).

Oculoacousticocerebral Degeneration

(See Norrie's Syndrome)

Onychodystrophy

Recessive integumentary disorder characterized by rudimentary fingernails and toenails, triphalangeal thumbs with congenital severe sensorineural hearing loss (Goodman et al., 1969).

Optic Atrophy and Diabetes Mellitus

Autosomal recessive with onset in childhood of progressive visual impairment. Diabetes mellitus onset prior to second decade, with childhood

progressive sensorineural hearing loss (Stevens and Macfayden, 1972).

Optic Atrophy and Polyneuropathy

Recessive or X-linked transmission. Symptoms include progressive visual loss with bilateral and symmetric optic atrophy beginning in second decade and leading to rapid deterioration of vision. Polyneuropathy from childhood. Progressive severe sensorineural deafness in childhood that tends to affect high frequencies. Risk of occurrence is 1 in 100,000 or less (Iwashita et al., 1970).

Opticocochleodentate Degeneration

Eye and nervous system disorder. Recessive trait. This fairly rare syndrome is characterized by progressive visual and sensorineural hearing loss and progressive spastic quadriplegia. Vision is normal until about 1 year of age, with total blindness occurring at about age 3 years. Microcephaly, mental deterioration, and speech problems may be evident, with death in later childhood (Konigsmark and Gorlin, 1976).

Osteogenesis Imperfecta

(Van Der Hoeve's Syndrome)

High percentage of infant death, multiple fractures may be present at birth, weak joints, blue sclera, thin and translucent skin, yellowish-brown and easily broken teeth, deafness. Deformities such as kyphoscoliosis and pectus excavation (Fig. A.18),

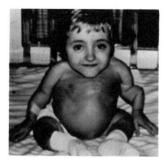

Figure A.18. Osteogenesis imperfecta.

internal hydrocephalus, nerve root compression, cardiovascular lesions, and thin atrophic skin may also occur. Also known as "brittle bone" disease. Etiology is hereditary autosomal dominant, present at birth. Majority of severe cases are sporadic, and because of clinical variability, detection may range from birth through adulthood. Of reported cases, 60% have conductive hearing loss reportedly due to otosclerotic changes, the footplate of the stapes, and the posterior semicircular canal. Temporal bone findings show diminished or immature bone formation in otic capsule and ossicles. Degeneration of stapes crura so no contact is possible between crura and footplate. Sensorineural hearing loss has also been demonstrated in high frequencies. Genetic counseling, magnesium therapy, orthopedic correction. Rate of occurrence is about 2–5 per 100,000 births. Otologic surgery is usually successful. Estimates of hearing loss range between 26% and 60% of cases (Hall and Rohrt, 1968; Bretlau et al., 1970; Quisling et al., 1979; Riedner et al., 1980).

Osteopetrosis

(See Albers-Schönberg Disease)

Otopalatodigital Syndrome

Sex-linked recessive craniofacial-skeletal disorder. Features include cleft palate, stubby clubbed fingers and toes, wide-spaced nasal bridge giving pugilistic facies, low-set and small ears, winged scapulae, downward obliquity of the eyes, and downturned mouth. Mild mental retardation and congenital conductive-type hearing loss due to ossicular abnormalities (Buran and Duvall, 1967).

Paget's Disease (Juvenile)

(Hereditary Hyperphosphatasia)

Recessive skeletal disorder. Juvenile form is characterized by progressive skeletal deformities that become apparent during the second or third year of life. May result in sporadic cranial nerve involvement. Progressive enlargement of head and long bones. Occasional progressive mixed-type hearing disorder due to continued new bone formation at the skull base (Thompson et al., 1969).

Pendred's Syndrome

(Goiter and Profound Deafness)

Recessive endocrine-metabolic disorder. The goiter is usually apparent by age 8 years but may be noted at birth in some cases. Auditory manifestations are variable but usually demonstrate a moderate-to-profound sensorineural hearing loss. Hearing loss is usually detected in the first 2 years of life and is

almost always symmetrical. Risk of occurrence is about 1 in 14,500. Fairly common disorder related to profound deafness (Batsakis and Nishiyama, 1962; Fraser, 1965; Illum et al., 1972).

Piebaldness

Divided into three integumentary-pigmentary syndromes by Konigsmark and Gorlin (1976). (1) Recessive piebaldness and profound congenital sensorineural deafness. Head, hair, upper chest, and both arms show substantial depigmentation. Normal vision with blue irides. (2) X-linked pigmentary abnormalities and congenital sensorineural deafness. Similar pigmentary skin changes as seen in (1) above. Profound deafness. (3) Dominant piebaldism, ataxis, and sensorineural hearing loss. About 80% have ataxia and mental retardation, and 60% have progressive sensorineural deafness (Woolf et al., 1965).

Pierre Robin Sequence

(Cleft Palate, Micrognatha, and Glossoptosis)

Dominant, craniofacial-skeletal disorder. Oral findings include cleft palate, smallness of jaw and chin, and downward displacement or retraction of the tongue. Ears may be low-set. About 20% of cases are associated with mental retardation. Congenital amputations, hip dislocation, sternal anomalies, spina bifida, hydrocephaly, and microcephaly have been reported. A variety of cardiac and middle ear anomalies have been reported. Congenital conductive and/or sensorineural hearing loss. A 10 year

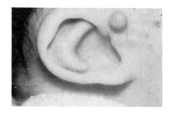

Figure A.19. Preauricular abnormalities.

follow-up study of 55 cases showed high incidence of speech-language-hearing problems. Gould (1989) reports 50% incidence of conductive hearing loss in a sample of 20 Pierre patients with Pierre Robin sequence. Risk of occurrence is 1 in 30,000 (Williams et al., 1981).

Pili Torti

Recessive integumentary disorder. Dry, brittle, flat, twisted hair of scalp, eyebrows and eyelashes accompanied by moderate-to-severe bilateral severe sensorineural hearing loss (Singh and Bresman, 1973).

Preauricular Abnormalities

Includes preauricular pits, preauricular tags (Fig. A.19), and branchial fistulas, which may be multiple and are usually bilateral. Dominant craniofacial disorder often accompanied by conductive hearing loss or sensorineural hearing loss and sometimes by external ear canal atresia, facial paralysis, or mandibular anomalies. Preauricular tag and/or pits usually require no treatment except for cosmetic surgery or excision if draining. See Chapter 3 for more detail. (Melnick et al., 1976; Cremers et al., 1981).

Pyle's Disease

(Craniometaphysial Dysplasia)

Recessive form of craniofacial-skeletal disorder. Expressivity is somewhat variable; facial features include hypertelorism, broad nasal ridge, enlarge paranasal area, and cranial sclerosis. Nystagmus is common. Progressive sensorineural and/or conductive hearing loss (Miller et al., 1969; Gladney and Monteleone, 1970).

Refsum's Syndrome

Recessive eye disorder. Onset in second decade with visual loss, night blindness due to retinitis pigmentosa, progressive ataxia, muscle wasting, obesity, ichthyosis, and polyneuritis. Major clinical symptoms include triad of retinitis pigmentosa, peripheral neuropathy, and cerebellar ataxia. May be related to enzymatic defect. Sensorineural progressive hearing loss (50%) with one side often worse than the other (Fryer et al., 1971; Nance, 1973).

Renal-Genital Syndrome

Recessive disorder. Renal anomalies and internal genital malformations. Malformation of middle ear with low-set auricles and stenotic external canals. Moderate-to-severe conductive hearing loss (Winter et al., 1968; Turner, 1970).

Renal Tubular Acidosis

(Fanconi's Anemia Syndrome)

Richards-Rundle Syndrome

(Ataxia-Hypogonadism Syndrome)

Recessive trait. Nervous system disorder. Includes ataxia, muscle wasting in early childhood. Progressive severe mental retardation, absent deep tendon reflexes with failure to develop secondary sexual characteristics. Early onset of progressive, severe, sensorineural hearing loss; horizontal nystagmus (Richards and Rundle, 1959).

Rubella, Congenital

Rubella embryopathy is a most important prenatally acquired cause of profound childhood deafness. Infants with congenital rubella virus infections have a variety of defects of varying severity depending on the embryonic stage during which the infection occurred. Hearing impairment can result from fetal rubella not only during the first trimester of pregnancy but also in the second and even third trimester (Bordly et al., 1968). Several million persons were affected by the widespread rubella epidemic in the United States during 1963–1965.

Diagnostic features include transient neonatal manifestations of low birthweight, hepatosplenomegaly, purpura, bulging anterior suture, corneal clouding, and jaundice. Anemia, pneumonia, meningitis, and encephalitis may develop. Major associated problems include hearing loss (50%), heart disease (50%), cataract or glaucoma (40%), and psychomotor and mental retardation (40%) (Cooper et al., 1969). A major feature of the rubella embryopathy is a characteristic "salt and pepper" retinal pigmentation, noted in rubella children without cataracts, that does not interfere with visual acuity. Dental abnormalities, microcephaly, and behavioral problems are common in congenital rubella children.

Rubella deafness is commonly sensorineural in nature, often severe to profound in degree. Although sometimes complicated by a conductive component, the typical configuration in rubella deafness tends to be flat or gradually sloping downward from low to high frequencies. Evidence of central auditory deafness due to central nervous system lesion has been reported. Variation in audiometric configuration is common.

The pathology of rubella deafness includes a variety of inner ear abnormalities and middle ear and external ear anomalies. General treatment includes special education considerations as necessary, with possible surgery for cataracts when indicated. Early amplification and auditory training are mandatory when significant hearing loss is determined. See Chapter 8 for additional information (Stuckless, 1980).

Saddle Nose and Myopia

(Marshall Syndrome)

Dominant transmission. Characterized by severe myopia, saddle-nose defect, congenital and/or juvenile cataracts, and congenital progressive sensorineural hearing loss of moderate degree (Ruppert et al., 1970; Zellweger et al., 1974).

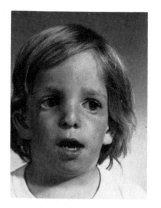

Figure A.20. Treacher Collins syndrome.

Sensory Radicular Neuropathy

Dominant trait, nervous system disorder. Onset in late teens or early adulthood of lightning pains that involve the distal extremities with painless ulcerations of feet. Progressive moderate-to-severe sensorineural hearing loss (Mandell and Smith, 1960; Stanley et al., 1975).

Symphalangism

Dominant skeletal disorder. Stiff fingers and toes due to bony ankylosis of the proximal interphalangeal joints. Congenital conductive hearing loss due to stapes fixation (Spoendlin, 1974).

Syphilis, Congenital

Infectious disease contracted by unborn fetus from infected mother. Sensorineural hearing impairment of slow progressive nature. Pattern of deafness shows variation dependent upon time of onset and rapidity of progression. Youngster may initially

show normal hearing. Typically associated with other sensory defects. See Chapter 3 for additional information (Kerr et al., 1973).

Treacher Collins Syndrome

(Mandibular Dysostosis, First Arch Syndrome)

Major diagnostic features include facial bone abnormalities of structures formed from the first branchial arch including downward sloping palpebral fissures, depressed check bones, deformed pinna, receding chin, and large fishlike mouth with frequent dental abnormalities (Fig. A.20). Atresia of auditory canal, defects of auditory canal and ossicles, and cleft palate are common. Mental deficiency reported in about 5% of cases.

Treacher Collins is a genetic defect leading to multiple congenital anomalies. Autosomal dominant with incomplete penetrance and variable expression. More than half of cases reported are fresh mutations.

The external ears may be small, displaced, or simply nubbins. Atresia of external auditory canal is common. The middle ear is often poorly developed, the tympanic ossicles being absent or deformed. Hypoplasia of the horizontal semicircular canal of the cochlea has been observed, as have branching of nerve to horizontal canal cristae bilaterally and abnormalities of bony and membranous vestibular labyrinth. Deafness generally completely conductive but may be sensorineural.

General treatment includes genetic counseling, surgical repair of ear anomalies, hearing aid if recommended, orthodontic treatment, and speech therapy if indicated

(Fernandez and Ronis, 1964; Frazen et al., 1967; Sando et al., 1968; Lindsay, 1971a, 1971b).

Trisomy 13–15 Syndrome

Major diagnostic features include chromosomal aberration resulting in minimal characteristics of microphthalmia, cleft lip and palate, and polydactyly. A host of other abnormalities may be present, including mental retardation; deafness; broad-nose hypotelorism; microcephaly; heart and/or skin defects; retroflexed thumbs; "rocker-bottom" feet; seizures; and renal, abdominal, and genitalia abnormalities. Those affected frequently suffer with feeding problems, failure to thrive, jitteryness, apneic spells, hypotonia, and jaundice. Meiotic nondisjunction appears to be the cause of the extra chromosome in 13–15 group (Fig. A.21). Trisomy 13 syndrome with 47 chromosomes frequently associated with increased maternal age. Low-set external ears are found in 80%; malformed ears, in 80%; and cleft lip and palate, in 50–80%. Middle ear findings have included deformed stapes, distorted incudostapedial joint posteriorly, and absence of stapedial muscle and tendon. Inner ear abnormalities have included distorted and shortened cochlea, shortened endolymphatic valve, abnormal branch of nerve to posterior semicircular canal crista from posterior cranial fossa, degeneration of organ of Corti, tectorial membrane, stria vascularis, and saccule. Other studies have been normal. Genetic counseling as indicated. Prognosis is poor; 95% die by 3 years (Cohen, 1966; Maniglia et al., 1970; Black et al., 1971; Scherz et al., 1972).

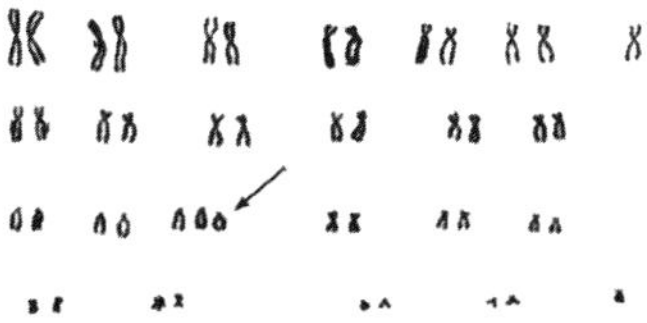

Figure A.21. Trisomy 13–15 (D_1) karyotype. (Courtesy of A. Robinson, M.D., Cytogenetics Laboratory, University of Colorado Medical Center, Denver, Colorado.)

Trisomy 18 Syndrome

Due to chromosomal aberration, features present at birth include being underweight with an undernourished appearance, possible limpness at first soon becoming hypertonic. Microcephaly with triangular shape due to occipital prominence and receding chin. Skin is loose. Flexion of hand with overlapping of index finger over third, "rocker-bottom" feet, short sternum, small pelvis, and agenesis of bones of the extremities. Congenital heart disease, renal abnormalities, cleft lip and palate, deformed ears may also be present. Mental retardation usually profound.

Due to nondisjunction of one chromosome in 17–18 group (Fig. A.22). Advanced maternal age is common. Possibility of recurrence in same family is rare unless translocation is present.

Audiometric testing shows failure to respond to sound. Middle ear anomalies include malformed stapes, deformed incus and malleus, exposed stapedial muscle in the middle ear cavity, absence of stapedial tendon, absence of pyramidal eminence, a split tensor tympanic muscle in separate bony canals, abnormal course of the facial and chorda

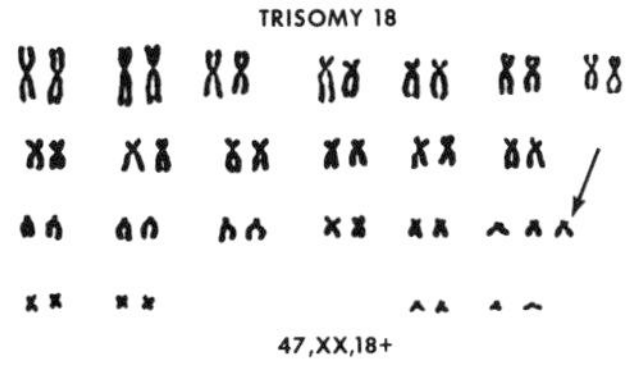

Figure A.22. Trisomy 18 karyotype. (Courtesy of A. Robinson, M.D., Cytogenetics Laboratory, University of Colorado Medical Center, Denver, Colorado.)

tympani nerves, and underdevelopment of facial nerve.

Other anomalies reported include atresia of external canals, decreased spiral ganglion cells, anomalies of cochlea, absence of utriculoendolymphatic valve, and absence of semicircular canals and cristae. Genetic counseling or other treatment as indicated. By 1 year 90% die (Smith, 1962; Kos et al., 1966; Keleman et al., 1968; Chrysostomidou et al., 1971).

Trisomy 21 Syndrome

(See Down's Syndrome)

Turner's Syndrome

(Gonadal Dysgenesis)

Chromosome defect, not inherited. Low hairline, webbing of neck, widely spaced nipples, shieldlike chest, webbing of digits. Chromosomal abnormality recognizable at birth by webbing or loose folds of skin of short neck, swelling of dorsa of hands and feet, deep creases on thickened palms and soles, hypertelorism, epicanthic folds, ptosis of upper lids, elongated "gothic" ears, high arched palate, micrognathia, pinpoint nipples, and enlarged clitoris. Fingernails are hypoplastic and appear small. Later manifestations include shortness of stature, ocular manifestations, hearing impairment, impairment of taste, congenital cardiovascular disease, anomalies of kidneys, and sexual infantilism. It occurs only in females. Mentality may be normal. Mild sensorineural and conductive hearing loss has been reported. Anderson et al. (1969) reported audiometric findings from 79 patients with Turner's syndrome. Of the 79 patients, 64% had sensorineural hearing loss with a bilaterally symmetrical dip in the middle frequency range. An additional 22% showed a conductive or mixed hearing loss. Conductive hearing loss has been attributed to frequent middle ear infections in infancy and early childhood, but congenital hearing loss has also been observed (Stratton, 1965; Anderson et al., 1971).

Usher's Syndrome

Recessive, genetic condition including congenital deafness and progressive loss of vision leading to eventual blindness. The hearing loss is bilateral, moderate to severe, and sensorineural. Patient initially notices difficulty seeing at night during early teens or twenties; narrowing of visual field (tunnel vision); and signs and symptoms of retinitis pigmentosa. May have additional disorders such as mental retardation, vertigo, psychosis, loss of smell, abnormal electroencephalograms, and epilepsy. Prevalence among profoundly deaf children has been estimated to be between 3% and 10%. Early diagnosis is important for provision of appropriate rehabilitation endeavors, genetic counseling, and screening of relatives. Can vary greatly in age of on-

set, severity, and speed of progression.

Vestibular response to caloric testing is generally abnormal; 90% of 177 patients (Hallgren, 1959) had severe bilateral congenital deafness, whereas 10% had moderate (30–70 dB) sensorineural hearing loss, more marked in higher frequencies. In many cases, the deafness is so profound that hearing aid use is not successful; no treatment for retinitis pigmentosa. Most patients are forced to retire by age 30 or 40, because of vision problems and associated disabilities (Kloepfer et al., 1966; McLeod et al., 1971; Hicks and Hicks, 1981).

Van Buchem's Syndrome

(Hyperostosis Corticalis Generalisata)

Recessive craniofacial-skeletal disorder. Generalized osteosclerotic overgrowth of the skeleton. Paralysis of cranial nerve VII and sensorineural deafness are frequent. Onset during puberty demonstrated by narrowing of skull foramina causing cranial nerve paresis with visual and mixed-type hearing loss. Lion-like facial expression with square jaw (Fosmoe et al., 1968).

Van Der Hoeve's Syndrome

(See Osteogenesis Imperfecta)

Von Recklinghausen's Neurofibromatosis

Usually a slowly progressive disease of autosomal dominant inheritance charac-

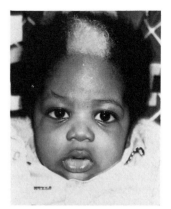

Figure A.23. Waardenburg's syndrome.

terized by café-au-lait spots associated with cutaneous tumors. The tumors may occur in nodules along a peripheral nerve occasionally producing motor or sensory disturbances. Virtually every part of the central nervous system may be affected by the disease process. Cranial nerve signs may be the result of a glioma or neuroma. Optic nerve and acoustic neuromas, particularly in children, are the most frequent cranial nerve tumors. Slow-to-rapid progression of sensorineural hearing loss; prevalence is about 1 in 3000. Congenital skeletal problems may also be associated with this disease. Malignant degeneration of the central nervous system tumors may ultimately cause death. Treatment is genetic counseling and surgery (Nager, 1964; Hitselberger and Hughes, 1968; Young et al., 1970).

Waardenburg's Syndrome

Genetic hearing loss with integumentary system characteristics; inherited as autosomal dominant characteristic with variable penetrance. Major diagnostic features include white forelock (20%) (Fig.

A.23); lateral displacement of medial canthi (95–99%); iris bicolor or heterochromia (45%); prominence of root of nose; hyperplasia of medial portion of eyebrows (50%). Other findings include thin nose with flaring alae nasi, "cupid bow" configuration of lips, prominent mandible, and occasionally cleft palate (5%). All characteristics are not found in each patient. Mental retardation is not typical.

Congenital mild-to-severe sensorineural hearing loss is present in 50% of patients and may be unilateral, bilateral, and/or progressive. Hearing impairment may be evidenced primarily in low and middle frequencies, but profound deafness may also be present. Histopathologic findings include absence of organ of Corti and atrophy of spiral ganglion (Marcus and Valvasori, 1970; Pantke and Cohen, 1971).

Wildervanck's Syndrome

(Otofaciocervical Dysmorphia; Cervico-oculoacoustic Dysplasia)

Multifactorial inheritance. Depressed nasal root, protruding narrow nose, narrow elongated face, flattened maxilla and zygoma, prominent ears, preauricular fistulas, poorly developed neck muscles. Facial asymmetry combines the Klippel-Feil characteristics with retraction of the eyeball, sixth nerve paralysis, and total deafness. Integumentary and pigmentary disorder; congenital sensorineural or mixed-type hearing loss. Female preponderance, 7:75 (Cremers et al., 1984).

References

Abbs JH, Sussman HM: Neurological feature detectors and speech perception: a discussion of theatrical implications. *J Speech Hear Res* 14:23–36, 1971.

Abramovich S, Gregory S, Slemick M, et al: Hearing loss in very low birthweight infants treated with neonatal intensive care. *Arch Dis Child* 54:421, 1979.

Accreditation Council for Facilities for the Mentally Retarded: *Standards for Residential Facilities for the Mentally Retarded.* Chicago: Joint Commission on Accreditation of Hospitals, 1971.

Ahram DM, Nation JE: Preschool language disorders and subsequent language and academic difficulties. *J Commun Dis* 13:159–170, 1980.

Alberti PW, Hyde ML, Riko K, Corbin H, Fitzhardinge PM: Issues in early identification of hearing loss. *Laryngoscope* 95:373–381, 1985.

Alberti PWRM, Kristensen R: The clinical application of impedance audiometry. *Laryngoscope* 80:735–746, 1970.

Alpiner JG, Amon C, Gibson J, et al: *Talk To Me.* Baltimore: Williams & Wilkins, 1977.

Altmann F: Histologic picture of inherited nerve deafness in man and animals. *Arch Otolaryngol* 51:852–890, 1950.

Alvord LS, Doxey GP, Smith DM: Hearing aids worn with tympanic membrane perforations: complications and solutions. *Am J Otol* 10:277–280, 1989.

American Academy of Audiology: *Position Statement on Early Identification of Hearing Loss in Infants and Children.* Houston, TX, 1989.

American Academy of Otolaryngology and American Council of Otolaryngology: Guide for the evaluation of hearing handicap. *JAMA* 241:2055–2059, 1979.

American Academy of Otolaryngology Committee on Hearing and Equilibrium and the American Council of Otolaryngology Committee on the Medical Aspects of Noise: Guide for the evaluation of hearing handicap. *JAMA* 251:19, 2055–2059, 1979.

American Academy of Pediatrics: Policy statement on middle ear disease and language development. *Acad Pediatr News and Comments* 35:9, 1984.

American Academy of Pediatrics: Use and abuse of the Apgar score. *Pediatrics* 78:6, 1148–1149, 1986.

American Academy of Pediatrics, Committee on Children with Handicaps: The physician and the deaf child. *Pediatrics* 51:1100, 1973.

American Academy of Pediatrics, Committee on Environmental Hazards: Noise pollution: neonatal aspects. *Pediatrics* 54:476, 1974.

American Academy of Pediatrics, Joint Committee on Infant Hearing: Position statement 1982. *Pediatrics* 70:496–497, 1982.

American National Standards Institute: *Specifications for Audiometers.* ANSI S36-1969. New York: American National Standards Institute, 1969.

American National Standards Institute/Acoustical Society of America: *Specification of Hearing Aid Characteristics.* ANSI S3, 22-1976. New York: American National Standards Institute, 1976.

American Psychiatric Association: *Diagnostic and Statistical Manual of Mental Disorders,* ed 3. Washington, DC: American Psychiatric Association, 1980.

American Psychiatric Association: *Diagnostic and Statistical Manual of Mental Disorders,* ed 3, revised. Washington, DC: American Psychiatric Association, 1987.

American Speech and Hearing Association: Guidelines for manual pure-tone threshold audiometry. *Asha* 29:297–301, 1978.

American Speech and Hearing Association Task Force: The definition of a hearing handicap. *Asha* 23:293–297, 1981.

American Speech-Language-Hearing Association: Guidelines for acoustic immittance screening of middle-ear function. *Asha* 21:283–288, 1979.

American Speech-Language-Hearing Association: Joint Committee on Infant Hearing position statement. *Asha* 24:1017, 1982.

American Speech-Language-Hearing Association: Position statement on language learning disorders. *Asha* 24:937–944, 1982.

American Speech-Language-Hearing Association: Guidelines for identification audiometry. *Asha* 27(5):49–52, 1985.

American Speech-Language-Hearing Association: *The Short Latency Auditory Evoked Potentials.* Rockville, MD: American Speech-Language-Hearing Association, June 1987.

American Speech-Language-Hearing Association: Audiologic screening of infants who are at risk for hearing impairment. *Asha* 31:89–92, 1989.

American Speech-Language-Hearing Association: Guidelines for screening for hearing impairments and middle ear disorders. *Asha* 32 (suppl 2):17–24, 1990.

Amon C: Meeting state and federal guidelines. In Roeser R, Downs M: *Auditory Disorders in School Children.* New York: Thieme-Stratton, 1981, ch 2.

Anderson H. Filipsson R, Fluur E, et al: Hearing impairment in Turner's syndrome. *Acta Otolaryngol Suppl (Stockh)* 247:1–26, 1969.

Anderson H, Lindsten J, Wedenberg E: Hearing defects in males with sex chromosome anomalies. *Acta Otolaryngol (Stockh)* 72:55–58, 1971.

Anderson SD, Kemp DT: The evoked cochlear mechanical response in laboratory primates. *Arch Otorhinolaryngol* 224:47–54, 1979.

Aniansson G: Methods for assessing high frequency hearing loss in everyday listening situations. *Acta Otolaryngol Suppl (Stockh)* 320:1974.

Anson BJ: *An Atlas of Human Anatomy*, ed 2. Philadelphia: WB Saunders, 1963.

Anson BJ: Developmental anatomy of the ear. In Paparella MM, Shumrick DA: *Otolaryngology, Vol I. Basic Sciences and Related Disciplines.* Philadelphia: WB Saunders, 1973.

Anson BJ, Donaldson JA: *The Surgical Anatomy of the Temporal Bone and Ear.* Philadelphia: WB Saunders, 1967.

Anthony DA, et al: *Seeing Essential English.* Greeley, CO: University of Northern Colorado, 1971.

Apgar V: A proposal for a new method of evaluation of the newborn infant. *Anesth Analg* 32:260, 1953.

Apgar V, James L: Further observations on the newborn scoring system. *Am J Dis Child* 104:419, 1962.

Arey LB: *Developmental Anatomy.* Philadelphia: WB Saunders, 1940.

Armitage SE, Baldwin BA, Vince MA: The fetal sound environment of sheep. *Science* 208:1173–1174, 1980.

Arnst D, Katz J (eds): *Central Auditory Assessment: The SSW Test, Development & Clinical Use.* San Diego: College Hill Press, 1982.

Aslin R, Pisoni D, Jusczyk P: Auditory development and speech perception in infancy. In Haith M, Campos J: *Infancy and the Biology of Development*, Vol II of *Carmichael's Manual of Child Psychology*, ed 4, PH Mussen (ser ed). New York: John Wiley & Sons, 1983.

Asp C: The Verbotonal method for management of young, hearing-impaired children. *Ear Hear* 6:1, 39–42, 1985.

Avery CA, Gates GA, Prihoda TJ: Efficacy of acoustic reflectometry in detecting middle ear effusion. *Ann Otol Rhinol Laryngol* 95:472–476, 1986.

Axelsson A, Fagerberg SE: Auditory function in diabetics. *Acta Otolaryngol (Stockh)* 66:49–64, 1968.

Axelsson A, Jerson T: Noisy toys: a possible source of sensorineural hearing loss. *Pediatrics* 76:4, 574–578, 1985.

Axelsson A, Lewis C: Aspects of delivery of ear, nose and throat care to Montana Indians. *Health Care and the Poor* 89:6, 551–557, 1974.

Babbidge HS: *Education of the Deaf. A Report to the Secretary of Health, Education, and Welfare by his Advisory Committee on the Education of the Deaf.* Publication No. 0-765-119. Washington, DC: Government Printing Office, 1965.

Babson SG: *Diagnosis and Management of the Fetus and Neonate at Risk*, ed 4. St. Louis: CV Mosby, 1980.

Baker DB: Severely handicapped: toward an inclusive definition. *AAESPH Review* 4:52–65, 1979.

Baldwin JI: Dysostosis craniofacialis of Crouzon. *Laryngoscope* 78:1660–1675, 1968.

Balkany TJ: Otologic aspects of Down's syndrome. *Semin Speech Lang Hear* 1:39, 1980.

Balkany TJ, Berman SA, Simmons MA, et al: Middle ear effusion in neonates. *Laryngoscope* 88:398–405, 1978.

Balkany TJ, Mischke RE, Downs MP, et al: Ossicular abnormalities in Down's syndrome. *Otolaryngol Head Neck Surg* 87:372, 1979.

Balkany TJ, Pashley NRT (eds): *Clinical Pediatric Otolaryngology.* St. Louis: CV Mosby, 1986.

Ballenger JJ: *Diseases of the Nose, Throat and Ear*, ed 12. Philadelphia: Lea & Febiger, 1977.

BAM World Markets, Inc., Box 10701 (Dept. BHK), University Park Station, Denver, CO 80210.

Barber HO: Head injury: audiological and vestibular findings. *Ann Otol Rhinol Laryngol* 78:239–252, 1969.

Barden T, Peltzman P: Newborn brain stem auditory evoked responses and perinatal clinical events. *Am J Obstet Gynecol* 136:912–917, 1980.

Bart RS, Pumphrey RE: Knuckle pads, leukonychia and deafness, a dominantly inherited syndrome. *N Engl J Med* 276:202–207, 1967.

Basser LS: Benign paroxysmal vertigo of childhood: a variety of vestibular neuronitis. *Brain* 87:141–152, 1964.

Batsakis JG, Nishiyama RH: Deafness with sporadic goiter: Pendred's syndrome. *Arch Otolaryngol* 76:401–406, 1962.

Bax M: The intimate relationship of health, development and behavior in the young child. In Brown CC: *Infants at Risk: Pediatric Round-Table 5.* New Brunswick, NJ: Johnson & Johnson, 1981, pp 106–113.

Bayley N: The development of motor abilities during the first three years. *Monogr Soc Res Child Dev* 1:1–25, 1935.

Beagley HA, Fisch L: Bio-electric potentials available for electric response audiometry: indications and contra-indications. In Beagley HA: *Audiology and Audiological Medicine.* Oxford: Oxford University Press, 1981, ch 31, vol 2.

Beasley D, Freeman B: Time altered speech as a measure of central auditory processing. In Keith RW (ed): *Central Auditory Dysfunction.* New York: Grune and Stratton, 1977.

Beck HL: Counseling parents of retarded children. *Children* 6:225–230, 1959.

Belzile M, Markle DM: A clinical comparison of monaural and binaural hearing aids worn by patients with conductive or perceptive deafness. *Laryngoscope* 69:1317–1323, 1959.

Bench J, Collyer D, Mentz L, et al: Studies in behavioral audiometry. III. Six-month-old infants. *Audiology* 15:384–394, 1977.

Bench RJ: Sound transmission to the human foetus through the maternal abdominal wall. *J Genet Psychol* 113:85–87, 1968.

Bench RJ: Infant audiometry. *Sound* 4:72–74, 1971.

Bench RJ, Boscak N: Some applications of signal detection theory to paedo-audiology. *Sound* 4:3, 1970.

Bender R, Wig E: Binaural hearing aids for hearing impaired children in elementary schools. *Volta Rev* 64:537–542, 1962.

Bendet R: A public school hearing aid maintenance program. *Volta Rev* 82:149, 1980.

Benham-Dunster RA, Dunster JR: Hearing loss in the developmentally handicapped: a comparison of three audiometric procedures. *J Audit Res* 25:175–190, 1985.

Bennett M: Impedance concepts relating to the acoustic reflex. In Silman S (ed): *The Acoustic Reflex: Ba-*

sic Principles and Clinical Applications, 1984, pp 35–61.

Bennett M, Weatherby L: Multiple probe frequency acoustic reflex measurements. *Scand Audiol* 8:233–239, 1979.

Bennett M, Weatherby L: Newborn acoustic reflexes to noise and pure-tone signals. *J Speech Hear Res* 25:383–387, 1982.

Bennett MJ: Trials with the auditory response cradle; I. Neonatal responses to auditory stimuli. *Br J Audiol* 13:125, 1979.

Bennett MJ: Trials with the auditory cradle; III. Head turns and startles as auditory responses in the neonate. *Br J Audiol* 14:122, 1980.

Bennett MJ, Lawrence RJ: Trials with the auditory response cradle; II. The neonatal respiratory response to an auditory stimulus. *Br J Audiol* 14:1, 1980.

Bentler RA: External ear resonance characteristics in children. *J Speech Hear Disord* 54:264–268, 1989.

Berg FS: *Educational Audiology: Hearing and Speech Management*. New York: Grune and Stratton, 1972, p 2.

Bergsma D (ed): *Birth Defects: Compendium*, ed 2. The National Foundation-March of Dimes. New York: Alan R Liss, 1979.

Bergstrom L: Medical problems and their management. In Roeser R, Downs M: *Auditory Disorders in School Children*. New York: Thieme-Stratton, 1981, ch 6.

Bergstrom L: Congenital Hearing Loss. In Northern JL: *Hearing Disorders*, ed 2. Boston: Little, Brown, 1984, ch 13.

Bergstrom L, Hemenway WG: Otologic problems in submucous cleft palate. *South Med J* 64:1172–1177, 1971.

Bergstrom L, Hemenway WG, Downs MP: A high risk registry to find congenital deafness. *Otolaryngol Clin North Am* 4:369–399, 1971.

Bergstrom L, Jenkins P, Sando I, English GM: Hearing loss in renal disease: clinical and pathological studies. *Ann Otol Rhinol Laryngol* 82:555–577, 1973.

Bergstrom L, Neblett LM, Hemenway WG: Otologic manifestations of acrocephalosyndactyly. *Arch Otolaryngol* 96:117–123, 1972.

Bergstrom L, Stewart J, Kenyon B: External auditory atresia and the deletion chromosome. *Laryngoscope* 84:1905–1917, 1974.

Bergstrom L, Thompson P: Ototoxicity. In Northern JL: *Hearing Disorders*, ed 2. Boston: Little, Brown, 1984, ch 10.

Berkman MD, Feingold M: Oculoauriculovertebral dysplasia (Goldenhar's syndrome). *Oral Surg* 25:408, 1968.

Berko, J, Brown R: Psycholinguistic research methods. In Mussen PH: *Handbook of Research Methods in Child Development*. New York: John Wiley & Sons, 1969, p 531.

Berlin CI: Ultra-audiometric hearing in the hearing impaired and use of upward-shifting translating hearing aids. *Volta Rev* 84:352–363, 1982.

Berlin CI, Catlin FI: *Manual of Standard Pure Tone Threshold Procedure, Programmed Instruction: Tactics for Obtaining Valid Pure Tone Clinical Thresholds*. Baltimore: Johns Hopkins Medical Institutions, 1965.

Berlin CI, Lowe SS: Temporal and dichotic factors in central auditory testing. In Katz J: *Handbook of Clinical Audiology*. Baltimore: Williams & Wilkins, 1972, p 280.

Berlin CI, Lowe-Bell SS, Cullen JK, et al: Dichotic speech perception: an interpretation of right-ear advantage and temporal offset effects. *J Acoust Soc Am* 53:699–709, 1973.

Berlin CI, Lowe-Bell SS, Janetta PJ, et al: Central auditory deficits after temporal lobectomy. *Arch Otolaryngol* 96:4–10, 1972.

Berliner K, House W: Cochlear implants: an overview and bibliography. *Am J Otol* 2:277–282, 1981.

Berliner KI, Eisenberg LS, House WF: The cochlear implant: an auditory prosthesis for the profoundly deaf child. *Ear Hear* (suppl) 6:1–69, 1985.

Berlow SJ, Caldarell DD, Matz GJ, et al: Bacterial meningitis in sensorineural loss: a prospective investigation. *Laryngoscope* 90:1445–1452, 1980.

Berman SA, Balkany TJ, Simmons MA: Otitis media in the neonatal intensive care unit. *Pediatrics* 62:198–202, 1978.

Berry J: Parents of the handicapped as consumers: some thoughts for physicians. *Clin Pediatr* 20:363, 1981.

Bess FH: Impedance screening for children: a need for more research. *Ann Otol Rhinol Laryngol* 89 (suppl 68):228, 1980.

Bess FH, Klee T, Culbertson JL: Identification, assessment and management of children with unilateral sensorineural hearing loss. *Ear Hear* 7:43–51, 1986.

Bess FH, Lewis HD, Cieliczka DJ: Acoustic impedance measurements in cleft-palate children. *J Speech Hear Disord* 40:13–24, 1975.

Bess FH, Logan S: Amplification in the educational setting. In Jerger J (ed): *Pediatric Audiology*. San Diego: College-Hill Press, 1984.

Bess FH, McConnell F: *Audiology, Education, and the Hearing Impaired Child*. St. Louis: CV Mosby, 1981.

Bess FH, Peek B, Chapman J: Further observations on noise levels in infant incubators. *Pediatrics* 63:100, 1979.

Bess FH, Schwartz DM, Redfield NP: Audiometric, impedance and otoscopic findings in children with cleft palates. *Arch Otolaryngol* 102:465–469, 1976.

Bess FH, Sinclair JS: Amplification systems used in education. In Katz J (ed): *Handbook of Clinical Audiology*, ed 3. Baltimore: Williams and Wilkins, 1985, pp 970–985.

Bess FH, Tharpe AM: Unilateral hearing impairment in children. *Pediatrics* 74:206–216, 1984.

Bhattacharya J, Bennett MJ, Tucker SM: Long term follow up of newborns tested with the auditory response cradle. *Arch Dis Child* 59:6, 504–511, 1984.

Beyond "V.D." *Medical World News* 21:56–63, 1980.

Bierman JM, Connor A, Vaage M, et al: Pediatricians' assessments of the intelligence of two-year-olds and their mental test scores. *Pediatrics* 34:680–690, 1964.

Birch JW: Mainstream education for hearing-impaired pupils: issues and interviews. *Am Ann Deaf* 121:69–71, 1976.

Birnholz JC, Benacerraf BR: The development of human fetal hearing. *Science* 22:516–518, 1983.

Bitici OC: Familial hereditary progressive sensorineural hearing loss with keratosis and plantaris. *J Laryngol Otol* 89:1143–1146, 1975.

Black FO, Bergstrom L, Downs MP, et al: *Congenital Deafness: A New Approach to Early Detection Through a High Risk Register.* Boulder, CO: Colorado Associated University Press, 1971a.

Black FO, Sando I, Wagner JA, et al: Middle and inner ear abnormalities, 13–15 (D_1) trisomy. *Arch Otolaryngol* 93:615–619, 1971.

Blager FB: The effect of otitis media on speech and language development. *Semin Speech Lang Hear* 3:313, 1982.

Blair JC, Wilson-Vlotman A, Von Almen P: Educational audiologists: practices, problems, directions, recommendations. *Educ Audiol Monogr* 1:2–14, 1989.

Bland RD: Otitis media in the first six weeks of life: diagnosis, bacteriology and management. *Pediatrics* 49:187–197, 1972.

Blennow G, Svenningsen N, Almquist B: Noise levels in infant incubators (adverse effects?). *Pediatrics* 53:29, 1974.

Bloom L, Lahey M: *Language Development and Language Disorders.* New York: John Wiley & Sons, 1978.

Bluestone CD: Relative value of tonsil and adenoid surgery in preventing otitis media. In Wiet RJ, Coulthard SW: *Otitis Media: Proceedings of the Second National Conference on Otitis Media.* Columbus, OH: Ross Laboratories, 1979, pp 73–78.

Bluestone CD, Beery QC, Paradise J: Audiometry and tympanometry in relation to middle ear effusions in children. *Laryngoscope* 83:594–604, 1973.

Bluestone CD, Fria TJ, Arjona SK, et al: Controversies in screening for middle ear disease and hearing loss in children. *Pediatrics* 77:57–70, 1986.

Bluestone C, Klein J, Paradise J, et al: Workshop on the effects of otitis media on the child. *Pediatrics* 71:639–652, 1983.

Bluestone CD, Klein JO: *Otitis Media in Infants and Children.* Philadelphia: WB Saunders, 1988.

Bluestone CD, Shurin PA: Middle ear disease in children: pathogenesis, diagnosis and management. *Pediatr Clin North Am* 21:379–400, 1974.

Bluestone CD, Stool SE, Scheetz MD (eds): *Pediatric Otolaryngology*, ed 2. Philadelphia: WB Saunders, 1990.

Bocca E, Calearo C: Central hearing processes. In Jerger J: *Modern Developments in Audiology.* New York: Academic Press, 1963, pp 337–370.

Bonfils P, Vziel A, Pujol R: Screening for auditory dysfunction in infants by evoked oto-acoustic emissions. *Otolaryngol Head Neck Surg* 114:887–890, 1988.

Bonvillian JD: Manual systems of communication: some background terms. *Shhh*, April 1989, pp 12–14.

Boothroyd A: *Hearing Impairments in Young Children.* Englewood Cliffs, NJ: Prentice-Hall, 1982.

Boothroyd A: Special issue: auditory and tactile presentation of voice fundamental frequency as a supplement to speech reading. *Ear Hear* 9:6, 1988.

Bordley JE, Brookhouser PE, Hardy J, et al: Prenatal rubella. *Acta Otolaryngol (Stockh)* 66:1, 1968.

Bornstein H: A description of some current sign systems designed to represent English. *Am Ann Deaf* 188:454–463, 1973.

Bornstein H: Signed English: a manual approach to English language development. *J Speech Hear Disord* 3:330–343, 1974.

Bornstein H: Sign language in the education of the deaf. In Schlesinger I, Namir L: *Sign Language of the Deaf: Psychological Linguistics and Social Perspectives.* New York: Academic Press, 1978, pp 333–359.

Bornstein H: Systems of sign. In Bradford L, Hardy W: *Hearing and Hearing Impairment.* New York: Academic Press, 1979, pp 331–361.

Bornstein H, Kannapell BM, Saulnier KI, et al: *Signed English Basic Pre-School Dictionary; Little Red Riding Hood, Goldilocks and the Three Bears, etc.* Washington, DC: Gallaudet College Press, 1972.

Bornstein H, Saulnier K: Signed English: a brief follow-up to the first evaluation. *Am Ann Deaf* 124:69–72, 1981.

Bornstein H, Saulnier K, Hamilton L: Signed English: a first evaluation. *Am Ann Deaf* 125:467–481, 1980.

Borowitz KC, Glascoe FP: Sensitivity of the Denver Developmental Screening Test in speech and language screening. *Pediatrics* 78:1075–1078, 1986.

Borus J: Acoustic impedance measurements with hard of hearing mentally retarded children. *J Ment Defic Res* 16:196–202, 1972.

Bower T: Competent newborns. In Levin R: *Child Alive.* Garden City, NY: Anchor Press/Doubleday, 1975.

Bower TGR: Repetitive processes in child development. *Sci Am* 235:38–47, 1976.

Boyd SF: Hearing loss: its educationally measurable effects on achievement. MS degree thesis. Department of Speech Education, Southern Illinois University, Carbondale, IL, 1974.

Brackbill Y, Adams G, Crowell DH, et al: Arousal level in neonates and preschool children under continuous auditory stimulation. *J Exp Child Psychol* 4:178–188, 1966.

Brackett D, Maxon AB: Service delivery alternatives for the mainstreamed hearing-impaired child. *Language, Speech and Hearing Services in Schools* 17:115–125, 1986.

Brackmann DE: Electric response audiometry in a clinical practice. *Laryngoscope* 87 (suppl 5):1–33, 1977.

Bragg V: Toward a more objective hearing aid fitting procedure. *Hear Instrum* 28:6–9, 1977.

Bredberg G: Cellular pattern and nerve supply of the human organ of Corti. *Acta Otolaryngol Suppl (Stockh)* 236, 1968.

Bretlau P, Jorgensen MB, Johansen H: Osteogenesis imperfecta. Light and electronmicroscopic studies of the stapes. *Acta Otolaryngol (Stockh)* 69:172–184, 1970.

Bricker DD: A rationale for the integration of handicapped and nonhandicapped preschool children. In Guralnich MJ: *Early Intervention and the Integration of Handicapped and Nonhandicapped Children.* Baltimore: University Park Press, 1978.

Bridger WH: Sensory discrimination and habituation in the human neonate. *Am J Psychiatry* 117:991–996, 1961.

Bright KE, Roush J: Hearing and immittance screening. In Lass N, McReynolds L, Northern J, Yoder D (eds): *Handbook of Speech-Language Pathology and Audiology.* Toronto: BC Decker, 1988, pp 1202–1214.

Brill RG: Mainstreaming: format or quality. *Am Ann Deaf* 120:377–381, 1975.

Brill RG: Definition of total communication. *Am Ann Deaf* 121:358, 1976.

Brody JA: Notes on the epidemiology of draining ears and hearing loss in Alaska with comments on future studies and control measures. *Alaska Med* 6:1, 1964.

Brody JA: Overfield T, McAlister R: Draining ears and deafness among Eskimos. *Arch Otolaryngol* 81:29–33, 1965.

Brookhouser PE, Moeller MP: Choosing the appropriate habilitative track for the newly identified hearing-impaired child. *Ann Otol Rhinol Laryngol* 95:1, 51–59, 1986.

Brooks D: An objective method of detecting fluid in the middle ear. *Int Audiol* 7:280–286, 1968.

Brooks D: The use of the electro-acoustic impedance bridge in the assessment of middle ear function. *Int Audiol* 8:563–569, 1969.

Brooks D: Electroacoustic impedance bridge studies on normal ears of children. *J Speech Hear Res* 14:247–253, 1971.

Brooks DN: Hearing screening: a comparative study of an impedance method and pure tone screening. *Scand Audiol* 2:67–76, 1973.

Brooks DN: Middle ear effusion in children with severe hearing loss. *Impedance Newsletters* (American Electromedics, New York) 4:6–7, 1975.

Brooks DN: Impedance in screening. In Jerger J, Northern JL: *Clinical Impedance Audiometry.* Acton, MA: American Electromedics Corp., 1980.

Brooks DN, Wooley H, Kanjilal GC: Hearing loss and middle ear disorders in patients with Down's syndrome (mongolism). *J Ment Defic Res* 16:21–29, 1972.

Bross M, Harper D, Sicz G: Visual effects of auditory deprivation: common intermodal and intramodal factors. *Science* 207:667–668, 1980.

Brown JB, Fryer MP, Morgan LR: Problems in reconstruction of the auricle. *Plast Reconstr Surg* 43:597–604, 1969.

Brown RM Jr, Haigler C, Cooper K: The biomodal perception of speech in infancy. *Science* 218:1138–1141, 1982.

Buran DJ, Duvall AJ: The oto-palato-digital (OPD) syndrome. Arch Otolaryngol 85:394–399, 1967.

Butler K: Language processing: selective attention and mnemonic strategies. In Lasky E, Katz J (eds): *Central Auditory Processing Disorders.* Baltimore: University Park Press, 1983.

Bryan EM, Nicholson E: Congenital syphilis. *Clin Pediatr* 20:81–87, 1981.

Buhrer K, Wall L, Schuster L: The acoustic reflectometer as a screening device: a comparison. *Ear Hear* 6:307–314, 1985.

Butterfield EC: An extended version of modification of sucking with auditory feedback. Working Paper 43. Bureau of Child Research Laboratory, Children's Rehabilitation Unit, University of Kansas Medical Center, Kansas City, KS, 1968.

Byrne B, Willerman L, Ashmore L: Severe and moderate language impairment: evidence for distinctive etiologies. *Behav Genet* 4:333–345, 1974.

Byrne D, Tonisson W: Selecting the gain of hearing aids for persons with sensorineural hearing impairments. *Scand Audiol* 5:51–59, 1976.

Bzoch KR (ed): *Communicative Disorders Related to Cleft Lip and Palate*, ed 2. Boston: Little, Brown, 1979.

Campbell AMG, Clifton F: Adult toxoplasmosis in one family. *Brain* 73:281–290, 1950.

Campbell PH, Wilcox MJ: In *Special Needs Report—A Newsletter from the Akron Medical Center.* Akron, OH, 1986.

Caplar F (ed): *The First Twelve Months of Life: Your Baby's Growth Month by Month.* New York: Grosset & Dunlap, 1973.

Carhart R: Speech reception in relation to pattern of pure tone loss. *J Speech Hear Disord* 11:97–108, 1946.

Carhart R: The usefulness of the binaural hearing aid. *J Speech Hear Disord* 23:41–51, 1958.

Carhart R: Monaural and binaural discrimination against competing sentences. *Int Audiol* 4:5–10, 1965.

Carhart R, Jerger J: Preferred method for clinical determination of pure tone thresholds. *J Speech Hear Disord* 24:330–345, 1959.

Carmen RE, Svihovec D, Gocka EF, et al: Audiometric configuration as a reflection of diabetes. *Am J Otol* 9:327–333, 1988.

Casselbrant ML, Brostoff LM, Cantekin EI, et al: Otitis media with effusion in preschool children. *Laryngoscope* 95:428–436, 1985.

Cavanaugh RM: Pneumatic otoscopy in healthy full-term infants. *Pediatrics* 79:4, 520–523, 1987.

Chalmers D, Stewart I, Silva P, Mulvena A: *Otitis Media with Effusion in Children: The Dunedin Study.* Philadelphia: JB Lippincott, 1989.

Chermak GD, Pederson CM, Bendel RB: Equivalent forms and split-half reliability of the NU-CHIPS administered in noise. *J Speech Hear Disord* 49:196–201, 1984.

Cherry K, Kroger B: Selective auditory attention abilities of learning disabled and normal achieving children. *J Learn Disord* 3:202–250, 1983.

Chiappa KH, Ropper AH: Evoked potentials in clinical medicine. Part I, *N Engl J Med* 306:19, 1140–1150, 1982. Part II, *N Engl J Med* 306:20, 1205–1211, 1982.

Chomsky N: *Aspects of the Theory of Syntax.* Cambridge, Mass: MIT Press, 1966.

Chow K: Numerical estimates of the auditory central nervous system of the rhesus monkey. *J Comp Neurol* 95:159, 1951.

Chrysostomidou DM, Caslaris E, Alexion D, et al: Trisomy 18 in Greece. *Acta Paediatr Scand* 69:591–593, 1971.

Church MW, Gerkin KP: Hearing disorders in children with fetal alcohol syndrome: findings from case reports. *Pediatrics* 82:147–154, 1987.

Clark AD, Richards CJ: Auditory discrimination among economically disadvantaged and nondisadvantaged preschool children. *Except Child* 33:259–262, 1966.

Clark B, Conry R: Hearing impairment in children with low birthweight. *J Audit Res* 18:4, 1978.

Clopton BM, Silverman MS: Plasticity of binaural interactions; II. Critical periods and changes in midline response. *J Neurophysiol* 40(6):1275–1280, 1977.

Clopton BM, Winfield JA: Effect of early exposure to patterned sound on unit activity in rat inferior colliculus. *J Neurophysiol* 39:1081–1089, 1976.

Coats AC: Electrocochleography: recording techniques and clinical applications. *Semin Hear* 7:3, 247–266, 1986.

Cohen BA, Schenk VA, Sweeney DB: Meningitis-related hearing loss evaluated with evoked potentials. *Pediatr Neurol* 4:18–22, 1988.

Cohen D, Sade J: Hearing in secretory otitis media. *Can J Otol* 1:27, 1972.

Cohen ME: Neurological abnormalities in achondroplastic children. *J Pediatr* 71:367, 1967.

Cohen PE: The "D" syndrome. *Am J Dis Child* 111:235, 1966.

Cohen S, Glass DC, Singer JE: Apartment noise, auditory discrimination, and reading ability in children. *J Exp Soc Psychol* 9:407–422, 1973.

Cohen SA: Cause vs. treatment in reading achievement. *J Learn Disabil* 33:163–166, 1970.

Cokely DR, Gawlik R: A position paper on the relationship between manual English and Sign. *The Deaf American*, May 1973, pp 7–9.

Cole W: Hearing aid gain: a functional approach. *Hear Instrum* 26:22–24, 1975.

Coleman M: An overview of Down's syndrome. *Semin Speech Lang Hear* 1:1, 1980.

Collet L, Gartner M, Moulin A, Kauffman I, Disant F, Morgon A: Evoked otoacoustic emissions and sensorineural hearing loss. *Otolaryngol Head Neck Surg* 115:1060–1062, 1989.

Commission on Education of the Deaf. *Toward Equality: Education of the Deaf. Report to the President and the Congress of the United States.* Washington, DC: Government Printing Office, February 1988.

Condon WS, Sander LW: Neonate movement is synchronized with adult speech: interactional participation and language structure. *Science* 183:99–101, 1974.

Conference on Hearing Screening Services for Preschool Children. Columbus, OH: Maternal & Child Health Bureau, Dept of HEW, Washington, DC, 1977.

Conway A: Mainstreaming from a school for the deaf. *Volta Rev* 81:237, 1979.

Cooper J, Langley L, Meyerhoff W, et al: The significance of negative middle ear pressure. *Laryngoscope* 87:92–97, 1977.

Cooper JC, Gates GA, Owen JH, et al: An abbreviated impedance bridge technique for school screening. *J Speech Hear Disord* 40:260–269, 1975.

Cooper L: Rubella: clinical manifestations and management. *Am J Dis Child* 118:18–29, 1969.

Cooper LF, Jabs EW: Aural atresia associated with multiple congenital anomalies and mental retardation: a new syndrome. *J Pediatr* 110:5, 747–750, 1987.

Cooper LZ, Ziring PR, Ockerse AB, et al: Rubella; clinical manifestations and management. *Am J Dis Child* 118:18–29, 1969.

Cope Y, Lutman ME: Oto-acoustic emissions. In McCormick: *Paediatric Audiology 0–5 Years.* London: Taylor and Francis, 1988, pp 221–245.

Coplan J: Deafness: ever heard of it? Delayed recognition of permanent hearing loss. *Pediatrics* 79(2):206–213, 1987.

Coplan J, Gleason JR: Unclear speech: recognition and significance of unintelligible speech in preschool children. *Pediatrics* 82(2):3, 447–452, 1988.

Coplan J, Gleason JR, Ryan R, Burke MG, Williams ML: Validation of an early language milestone scale in a high-risk population. *Pediatrics* 70:5, 677–683, 1982.

Corliss E: *Facts about Hearing and Hearing Aids. A Consumer's Guide from the National Bureau of Standards, U.S. Dept. of Commerce.* Washington, DC: Government Printing Office, 1971.

Cornett RO: Diagnostic factors bearing on the use of cued speech with hearing-impaired children. *Ear Hear* 6:1, 33–35, 1985.

Costello A: Are mothers stimulating? In Levin R: *Child Alive.* Garden City, NY: Anchor Press/Doubleday, 1975.

Courtois M, Berland M: Ipsilateral no-mold fitting of hearing aids. Oti Congress II, Copenhagen, 3–23, 1972.

Cox LC, Metz DA; ABER in the prescription of hearing aids. *Hear Instrum* 31:12–15, 55, 1980.

Craig W, Craig H: *Verbotonal Instruction for Young Deaf Children: Questions and Replies.* Pamphlet from Western Pennsylvania School for the Deaf, 1972.

Craig WN, Craig H, DiJohnson A: Preschool verbotonal instruction for deaf children. *Volta Rev* 74:236–246, 1972.

Craig WN, Salem JM, Craig HB: Mainstreaming and partial integration of deaf with hearing students. *Am Ann Deaf* 121:63–68, 1976.

Crarioto J: *Pre-School Malnutrition.* Publication No 1282. National Academy of Science: National Research Council, 1966.

Cremers CWRJ, Thijssen HOM, Fischer AJEM: Otological aspects of the earpit—deafness syndrome. *J Otolaryngol* 43:223–239, 1981.

Cremers WRJ, Hoogland GA, Kuypers W: Hearing loss in the cervico-oculo-acoustic (Wildervanck) syndrome. *Arch Otolaryngol* 110:54–57, 1984.

Cross HE, Pfaffenbach DD: Duane's retraction syndrome and associated congenital malformations. *Am J Ophthalmol* 73:442–449, 1972.

Cullen JK, Thompson CL: Release from masking in subjects with temporal lobe resections. Unpublished paper. Kresge Hearing Research Laboratory of the South, New Orleans, 1973.

Cunningham GC: Biochemical screening programs and problems. In Gold EM: *Earlier Recognition of Handicapping Conditions in Childhood: Proceedings of a Bi-Regional Institute.* Berkeley, CA: University of California School of Public Health, 1970, pp 37–41.

Curran J: *Four Basic Factors for Successful Hearing Aid Fittings.* Minneapolis, MN: Maico Hearing Instruments, 1982.

Curran JR: ITE aids for children: survey of attitudes and practices of audiologists. *Hear Instrum* 36(4):20–26, 1985.

Curran JR: Hearing aids. In Lass N, McReynolds L, Northern J, Yoder D (eds): *Handbook of Speech-Language Pathology and Audiology.* Toronto: BC Decker, 1988, pp 1293–1314.

Cyr DG: The vestibular system: pediatric considerations. *Semin Hear* 4:1, 33–46, 1983.

Cyr DG, Brookhouser PE, Valente M, Grossman A: Vestibular evaluation of infants and preschool children. *Otolaryngol Head Neck Surg* 93:4, 463–468, 1985.

Dahl HA: Progressive hearing impairment in children with congenital CMV. *J Speech Hear Disord* 44:220, 1979.

Dahle AJ, McCollister FP: Considerations for evaluating hearing in multiply handicapped children. In *The Multiply Handicapped Child* (Proceedings of a symposium in Edmonton, Alberta). New York: Grune & Stratton, 1983.

Dallos P: *The Auditory Periphery: Biophysics and Physiology*. New York: Academic Press, 1973.

Dallos P: Cochlear neurobiology. *Asha* 30 (issues 6/7): 50–56, 1988.

Dalsgaard S, Dyrlund-Jensen O: Measurement of the insertion gain of hearing aids. *J Audiol Technol* 15:170, 1976.

Danaher EM, Pickett JM: Some masking effects produced by low frequency vowel formants in persons with sensorineural hearing loss. *J Speech Hear Res* 18:261–271, 1975.

Danenberg MA, Loos-Cosgrove M, LoVerde M: Temporary hearing loss and rock music. *Language, Speech and Hearing Services in Schools* 18:267–274, 1987.

Darbyshire JV: A study of the use of high power hearing aids by children with marked degrees of deafness and the possibility of deteriorations in acuity. *Br J Audiol* 10:74–78, 1976.

Darley FI: Identification and audiometry for school-age children; basic procedures. *J Speech Hear Disord* (monogr suppl) 9:26–34, 1961.

Darlington RB: Duration of pre-school effects on later school competence. *Science* 213:1145–1146, 1981.

Davila RR, Brill RG: Guest editorial—P.L. 94–142. *Am Ann Deaf* 121:361, 1976.

Davis GL: CMV and hearing loss: clinical and experimental observations. *Laryngoscope* 89:1681–1688, 1979.

Davis H: Peripheral coding of auditory information. In Rosenblith WA: *Sensory Communication*. Cambridge, MA: MIT Press, 1961.

Davis H: Brainstem and other responses in electric response audiometry. *Ann Otol* 85:3–13, 1976.

Davis H, Hudgins CV, Marquis RJ, et al: The selection of hearing aids. *Laryngoscope* 56:85–115, 1946.

Davis J: Introduction letter to "Developing Your Child's Individualized Educational Program." *Shhh*, November/December 1988, p 26.

Davis JM, Elfenbein J, Schum R, Bentler R: Effects of mild and moderate hearing impairments on language, educational, and psychosocial behavior of children. *J Speech Hear Disord* 51:53–62, 1986.

Davis JM, Shepard NT, Stelmachowicz PG, et al: Characteristics of hearing-impaired children in the public schools. Part II. Psychoeducational data. *J Speech Hear Disord* 46:130–137, 1981.

Davis JW, Mueller HG: Hearing aid selection. Mueller HG, Geoffrey VC (eds): *Communication Disorders in Aging*. Washington, DC: Gallaudet University Press, 1987, ch 14, pp 408–436.

Davis PA: Effects of acoustic stimuli on the waking human brain. *J Neurophysiol* 2:444–499, 1939.

Deatherage BH, Hirsh IJ: Auditory localization of clicks. *J Acoust Soc Am* 31:486–492, 1959.

DeCasper AJ, Fifer WP: Of human bonding: newborns prefer their mothers' voices. *Science* 208:1174–1176, 1980.

Dee A, Rapin I, Ruben RJ: Speech and language development in a parent-infant total communication program. Report to combined otolaryngological spring meetings, Palm Beach, FL, April 30–May 2, 1982.

DeHirsch K, Jansky JJ, Langford WS: *Predicting Reading Failure*. New York: Harper & Row, 1966.

DeHirsh K: Learning disabilities: an overview. *Bull NY Acad Med* 50:459–479, 1974.

Demany I, McKenzie B, Vurpillot E: Rhythm perception in early infancy. *Nature* 266:718–719, 1977.

Dennis JM, Sheldon R, Toubas P, McCaffee A: Identification of hearing loss in the neonatal intensive care unit population. *Am J Otol* 5:201–205, 1984.

Dennis W: *Children of the Creche. Century Psychology Series*. New York: Prentice-Hall, 1973.

Denton DM, Brill RB, Kent MS, et al: Schools for deaf children. In Fine PJ: *Deafness in Infancy and Early Childhood*. New York: Medicom Press, 1974.

Derbyshire AJ, Davis H: The action potential of the auditory nerve. *Am J Physiol* 113:476–504, 1935.

Deutsch CP: Auditory discrimination and learning: social factors. *Merrill-Palmer J Behav Dev* 10:277–296, 1964.

Devens J, Hoyer E, McCroskey R: Dynamic auditory localization by normal and learning disability children. *J Am Audit Soc* 3:172–178, 1978.

Diefendorf AO: Behavioral evaluation of hearing-impaired children. In Bess FH (ed): *Hearing Impairment in Children*. Parkton, MD: York Press, 1988, pp 133–149.

Dirks D: Perception of dichotic and monaural verbal material and cerebral dominance for speech. *Acta Otolaryngol (Stockh)* 58:73–80, 1964.

Dirks D, Carhart R: A survey of reactions from users of binaural and monaural hearing aids. *J Speech Hear Disord* 27:311–321, 1962.

Dobie RA, Berlin CI: Influence of otitis media on hearing and development. *Ann Otol Rhinol Laryngol* 88 (suppl 60):48–53, 1979.

Dodds E, Harford E: Modified earpieces and CROS for high frequency hearing loss. *J Speech Hear Res* 11:204–218, 1968.

Dodge HW Jr, Wood MW, Kennedy RIJ: Craniofacial dysostosis: Crouzon's disease. *Pediatrics* 23:98, 1959.

Dodge PR, Davis H, Feigin RD, et al: Prospective evaluation of hearing impairment as a sequela of acute bacterial meningitis. *N Engl J Med* 311:14, 869–874, 1984.

Doster M: Personal communication. Denver Public Schools Health Department, Denver, CO, 1972.

Douek E, Dodson H, Banister L, et al: Effects of incubator noise on the cochlea of the newborn. *Lancet* 2:1110–1113, 1976.

Downs M: Guest editorial: implanting electrodes? *Asha* 23:567–568, 1981.

Downs M, Gerkin K: Early identification of hearing loss. In Lass N, McReynolds L, Northern J, Yoder D (eds): *Handbook of Speech-Language Pathology and Audiology*. Philadelphia: BC Decker, 1988, pp 1188–1201.

Downs MP: The establishment of hearing aid use: a program for parents. *Maico Audiological Library Series* 4:v, 1966.

Downs MP: The identification of congenital deafness. *Trans Am Acad Ophthalmol Otolaryngol* 74:1208–1214, 1970.

Downs MP: Maintaining children's hearing aids. The role of parents. *Maico Audiological Library Series* 10:1, 1971.

Downs MP: The deafness management quotient. *Hear Speech News*, Jan.-Feb. 1974.

Downs MP (ed): Communication disorders in Down's syndrome. *Semin Speech Lang Hear* 1:1, 1980.

Downs MP: The team approach to congenital deafness. In Mencher G, Gerber S (eds): *Early Management of Hearing Loss*. New York: Grune & Stratton, 1981.

Downs MP: The audiologist and the non-benign conductive hearing loss of otitis media. *Semin Speech Lang Hear* 3:295, 1982a.

Downs MP: Early identification of hearing loss. In Lass NJ, McReynolds LV, Northern JL, et al: *Speech, Language & Hearing*. Philadelphia: WB Saunders, 1982b, ch 41.

Downs MP, Hemenway WG: Report on the hearing screening of 17,000 neonates. *Int Audiol* 8:72–76, 1969.

Downs MP, Jafek B, Wood RP: Comprehensive treatment of children with recurrent serous otitis media. *Otolaryngol Head Neck Surg* 89:658–665, 1981.

Downs MP, Sterritt GM: Identification audiometry for neonates: a preliminary report. *J Audit Res* 4:69–80, 1964.

D'Souza S, McCartney E, Nolan M, et al: Hearing, speech and language in survivors of severe perinatal asphyxia. *Arch Dis Child* 56:245–252, 1981.

Dudich TM, Keiser M, Keith RW: Some relationships between loudness and the acoustic reflex. *Impedance Newsletter* (American Electromedics Corp, Acton, MA) 4:12–15, 1975.

Dupertius SM, Musgrave RH: Experiences with the reconstruction of the congenitally deformed ear. *Plast Reconstr Surg* 23:361–373, 1959.

Durieux-Smith A, Picton T, Edwards C, Goodman JT, MacMurray B: The Crib-O-Gram in the NICU: an evaluation based on brain stem electric response audiometry. *Ear Hear* 6:20–24, 1985.

Dworkin PW: The learning-disabled child. In Gottlieb MI, Williams PE (eds): *Developmental-Behavior Disorders*. New York: Plenum Publishing, 1989.

Dykstra R: Auditory discrimination abilities and beginning reading achievement. *Reading Res O* 1:5–34, 1966.

Eagles EL, Wishik SM, Doerfler LG: Hearing sensitivity and ear disease in children: a prospective study. *Laryngoscope* (monogr):1–274, 1967.

Edwards EP: Kindergarten is too late. *Saturday Rev*:60–79, 1968.

Efron R: Temporal perception, aphasia, and deja vu. *Brain* 86:403–424, 1963.

Eichenwald HF, Fry PC: Nutrition and learning. *Science* 163:644–648, 1969.

Eilers RE, Wilson WR, Moore JM: Developmental changes in speech discrimination in infants. *J Speech Hear Res* 20:4, 766–779, 1977.

Eimas PD: In Cohen LB, Salapatek: *Infant Perception: From Sensation to Cognition*. New York: Academic Press, 1975, vol 2.

Eimas PD, Siqueland ER, Juscyzk P, et al: Speech perception in infants. *Science* 171:303, 1972.

Eimas PD, Tartter VC: On the development of speech perception: mechanisms and analogies. *Adv Child Dev Behav* 13: 1979.

Eisele W, Berry R, Shriner T: Infant sucking response patterns as a conjugate function of change in the sound pressure level of auditory stimuli. *J Speech Hear Res* 18:296–307, 1975.

Eisen NH: Some effects of early sensory deprivation on later behavior: the quondam hard-of-hearing child. *J Abnorm Soc Psychol* 65:338, 1962.

Eisenberg LS, Kirk KI, Thielemeir MA, Luxford WM, Cunningham JK: Cochlear implants in children: speech production and auditory discrimination. *Otolaryngol Clin North Am* 19:409–421, 1986.

Eisenberg RB: Auditory behavior in the human neonate: functional properties of sound and their ontogenetic implications. *Int Audiol* 8:34–45, 1969.

Eisenberg RB: The development of hearing in man: an assessment of current status. *Asha* 12:119–123, 1970.

Eisenberg RB: *Auditory Competence in Early Life*. Baltimore: University Park Press, 1976.

Eldridge R, Berlin CI, Money JW, et al: Cochlear deafness, myopia, and intellectual impairment in an Amish family. *Arch Otolaryngol* 88:49–54, 1968.

Elliot GB, Elliot KA: Some pathological, radiological and clinical implications of the precocious development of the human ear. *Laryngoscope* 74:1160–1171, 1964.

Elliott L: Effects of noise on perception of speech of children and certain handicapped individuals. *Sound Vibration* 16:12, 1982.

Elliott L, Katz D: *Development of a New Children's Test of Speech Discrimination*. St. Louis: Auditec, 1980.

Elliott LL, Hammer MA: Longitudinal changes in auditory discrimination in normal children and children with language-learning problems. *J Speech Hear Disord* 53:467-474, 1988.

Elliott LL, Katz DR: Childrens' pure-tone detection. *J Acoust Soc Am* 67:343–344, 1980.

Elssmann SF, Matkin ND, Sabo MP: Early identification of congenital sensorineural hearing impairment. *Hear J* 40:9, 13–17, 1987.

Ely W: Electroacoustic modifications in hearing aids. In Bess F, Freeman B, Sinclair J (eds): *Amplification in Education*. Washington, DC: AG Bell, 1981, ch 20.

English GM: *Otolaryngology: A Textbook*. New York: Harper & Row, 1976.

English GM, Northern JL, Fria TJ: Chronic otitis media as a cause of sensorineural hearing loss. *Arch Otolaryngol* 98:17–22, 1973.

Erber NP: Use of the auditory numbers test to evaluate speech perception abilities of hearing-impaired children. *J Speech Hear Disord* 45:527, 1980.

Evans EF: The sharpening of cochlear frequency selectivity in the normal and abnormal cochlea. *Audiology* 14:419, 1975.

Evans JR: Auditory and auditory-visual integration skills as they relate to reading. *The Reading Teacher* 22:625–629, 1969.

Everberg G: Further studies on hereditary unilateral deafness. *Acta Otolaryngol (Stockh)* 51:615–635, 1960.

Eviatar L, Eviatar A: The neurovestibular testing of infants and children. In Bluestone CD, Stool SE (eds): *Pediatric Otolaryngology.* Philadelphia: WB Saunders, 1983, pp 199–212, vol I.

Ewing IR, Ewing AWG: The ascertainment of deafness in infancy and early childhood. *J Laryngol Otol* 59:309–338, 1944.

Falk S, Farmer J: Incubator noise and possible deafness. *Arch Otolaryngol* 97:385, 1973.

Falk SA: Combined effects of noise and ototoxic drugs. *Environ Health Perspect* 5–22, 1972.

Falk SA, Woods NF: Hospital noise-levels and potential health hazards. *N Engl J Med* 289:774, 1973.

Fant LJ Jr: *Say It with Hands.* Washington, DC: Gallaudet College, 1964.

Fantz RL: The origin of form perception. *Sci Am* 204:66–72, 1961.

Fay TH: Audiologic and otologic screening of disadvantaged children. In Glorig A, Gerwin K: *Otitis Media.* Springfield, IL: Charles C Thomas, 1972, pp 163–170.

Feagans L: A current view of learning disabilities. *J Pediatr* 102:487–493, 1983.

Fedio P, Van Buren JM: Memory deficits during electrical stimulation of the speech cortex in conscious man. *Brain Lang* 1:29–42, 1974.

Feigin RD, Dodge PR: Bacterial meningitis: newer concepts of pathophysiology and neurologic sequelae. *Pediatr Clin North Am* 23:3, 1976.

Feinmesser M, Tell L: Neonatal screening for detection of deafness. *Arch Otolaryngol* 102(5):297–299, 1976.

Feldman AS, Grimes CT, Grimes LL: Hearing screening in the educational setting. *Semin Speech Lang Hear* 2:101, 1981.

Ferguson DG, Hicks DE, Pfau G: Education of the hearing impaired learner. In Lass NJ, McReynolds LV, Northern JL, et al: *Speech, Language & Hearing.* Toronto: BC Decker, 1988, pp 1265–1277, ch 47.

Fernandez AO, Ronis ML: The Treacher Collins syndrome. *Arch Otolaryngol* 80:505, 1964.

Ferraro JA: Electrocochleography. *Semin Hear* 7:3, 239–337, 1986.

Field TM, Woodson R, Greenberg R, et al: Discrimination and imitation of facial expressions by neonates. *Science* 218:179–181, 1982.

Fifield D, Earnshaw R, Smither M: A new ear impression technique to prevent acoustic feedback with high powered hearing aids. *Volta Rev* 82:33, 1980.

Finitzo-Hieber T: Classroom acoustics. In Roeser RJ, Downs MP (eds): *Auditory Disorders in School Children.* New York: Thieme-Stratton, 1981a, ch 14.

Finitzo-Hieber T: Auditory brainstem response in assessment of infants treated with aminoglycoside antibiotics. In Lerner SA, Matz GJ, Hawkins JE (eds): *Aminoglycoside Ototoxicity.* Boston: Little, Brown, 1981b, ch 18.

Finitzo-Hieber T: Auditory brainstem response: its place in infant audiological evaluations. *Semin Speech Lang Hear* 3:76–87, 1982.

Finitzo-Hieber T, Gerling IJ, Matkin ND, et al: A sound effects recognition test for the pediatric audiologic evaluation. *Ear Hear* 1:271, 1980.

Finitzo-Hieber T, McCracken G, Roeser R, et al: Ototoxicity in neonates treated with gentamicin and kanamycin: results of a four-year controlled follow-up study. *Pediatrics* 63:443, 1979.

Finitzo-Hieber T, Simhadri R, Hieber JP: Auditory brainstem response assessment of postmeningitic infants and children. *Int J Pediatr Otorhinolaryngol* 3:275, 1981.

Fior R: Physiological maturation of auditory function between 3–13 years of age. *Audiology* 11:317–321, 1972.

Fischler RS, Todd WN, Feldman CM: Otitis media and language performance in a cohort of Apache Indian children. *Am J Dis Child* 139:355–360, 1985.

Fisher B: An investigation of binaural hearing aids. *J Laryngol Otol* 73:658–668, 1964.

Fitch JL, Williams TF, Etienne JE: A community based high risk register for hearing loss. *J Speech Hear Disord* 47:373–375, 1982.

Fletcher H: *Speech and Hearing.* New York: Van Nostrand, 1929.

Flexer C: Audiological rehabilitation in the schools. *Asha* 32:4, 44–45, 1990.

Flexer C, Gans D: Comparative evaluation of the auditory responsiveness of normal infants and profoundly multihandicapped children. *J Speech Hear Res* 28:163–168, 1985.

Flexer C, Gans DP: Distribution of auditory response behaviors in normal infants and profoundly multihandicapped children. *J Speech Hear Res* 29:425–429, 1986.

Folsom RC, Widen JE, Wilson WR: Auditory brainstem response in Down's syndrome infants. Paper presented to the American Speech-Language-Hearing Association 1981 Annual Convention, Los Angeles, CA.

Forgus RH: The effect of early perceptual learning on the behavioral organization of adult rats. *J Comp Physiol Psychol* 47:331–336, 1954.

Fosmoe RJ, Holm RS, Hildreth RC: Van Buchem's disease (hyperostosis corticalis generalisata familiaris). *Radiology* 90:771–774, 1968.

Fowler ER: Deafness from mumps. *Arch Pediatr* 77:243–246, 1960.

Fowler FP, Fletcher H: Three million deafened school children: their detection and treatment. *JAMA* 87:1877–1882, 1926.

Frank R, Karlovich R: Ear canal frequency response and speech discrimination performance as a function of hearing aid mold type. *J Audit Res* 13:124–129, 1973.

Frankenburg WK, Camp BW: *Pediatric Screening Tests.* Springfield, IL: Charles C Thomas, 1975.

Frankenburg WK, Dodds JB: The Denver developmental screening test. *J Pediatr* 71:181–189, 1967.

Franklin D: Tactile aids: what are they? *Hearing Journal,* May 1988.

Fraser GR: Our genetical load. *Ann Hum Genet* 25:387–415, 1962.

Fraser GR: Association of congenital deafness with goiter (Pendred's syndrome). A study of 207 families. *Ann Hum Genet* 28:201–249, 1965.

Fraser GR: *The Causes of Profound Deafness in Childhood.* Baltimore: The Johns Hopkins University Press, 1976.

Fraser WI, Cambell BM: A study of six cases of de Lange Amsterdam syndrome, with special attention to voice, speech and language characteristics. *Dev Med Child Neurol* 20:189–198, 1978.

Frazen LE, Elmore J, Nadler HL: Mandibulofacial dysostosis. *Am J Dis Child* 113:405, 1967.

Freedman AM, Kaplan HJ: *Comprehensive Textbook of Psychiatry.* Baltimore: Williams & Wilkins, 1967, pp 1434–1438.

Freeman B, Sinclair J, Riggs D: Electroacoustic performance characteristics of FM auditory trainers. *J Speech Hear Disord* 45:16–26, 1980.

French NR, Steinberg JC: Factors governing the intelligibility of speech sounds. *J Acoust Soc Am* 19:90–119, 1947.

Freyss G, Narcy P, Manac'h Y, et al: Acoustic reflex as a predictor of middle ear effusion. *Ann Otol Rhinol Laryngol* 89 (suppl 68): 196–199, 1980.

Fria T: The auditory brain stem response: background and clinical applications. *Monogr Contemp Audiol* 2(2):1980.

Fria T, LeBlanc J, Kristensen R, et al: Ipsilateral acoustic reflex stimulation in normal and sensorineural impaired ears: a preliminary report. *Can J Otol* 4:695–703, 1975.

Fria TJ, Cantekin EI, Eichler JA: Hearing acuity of children with otitis media with effusion. *Otolaryngol Head Neck Surg* 111:10–16, 1985.

Friedlander BZ: Receptive language development in infancy. *Merrill-Palmer J Behav Dev* 16:7–51, 1970.

Friedman A. Schulman R, Weiss S: Hearing and diabetic neuropathy. *Arch Intern Med* 135:573–576, 1975.

Friedmann I, Fraser GR, Froggatt P: Pathology of the ear in the cardioauditory syndrome of Jervell and Lange-Nielsen. *J Laryngol Otol* 80:451–470, 1966.

Friel-Patti S, Finitzo T: Language learning in a prospective study of otitis media with effusion in the first two years of life. *J Speech Hear Res* 33:188–194, 1990.

Friel-Patti S, Finitzo T, Meyerhoff W, Hieber JP: Speech-language learning and early middle ear disease: a procedural report. In Kavanagh J (ed): *Otitis Media and Child Development.* Parkton, MD: York Press, 129–138, 1986.

Friel-Patti S, Finitzo-Hieber T, Conti G, et al: Language delay in infants associated with middle ear disease and mild, fluctuating hearing impairment. *Pediatr Infect Dis J* 1:104–109, 1982.

Friel-Patti S, Roeser R: Evaluating changes in the communication skills of deaf children using vibrotactile stimulation. *Ear Hear* 4:31–40, 1985.

Froeschels E, Beebe H: Testing hearing of newborn infants. *Arch Otolaryngol* 44:710–714, 1946.

Fromkin V, Krashen S, Curtiss S, et al: The development of language in Genie: a case of language acquisition beyond the "critical period." *Brain Lang* 1:81–107, 1974.

Fryer DG, Winckleman AC, Ways PO, et al: Refsum's disease. *Neurology (Minneap)* 21:162–167, 1971.

Fulton RT, Gorzycki PA, Hull WL: Hearing assessment with young children. *J Speech Hear Disord* 40:397–404, 1975.

Gabbard SA: References for communication disorders related to otitis media. *Semin Speech Lang Hear* 3:351, 1982.

Galambos R, Hecox KE: Clinical applications of the auditory brainstem response. *Otolaryngol Clin North Am* 11:709–721, 1978.

Galambos R, Hicks G, Wilson M: The auditory brainstem response reliably predicts hearing loss in graduates of a tertiary intensive care nursery. *Ear Hear* 5:4, 254–260, 1984.

Galambos R, Hicks G, Wilson MJ: Hearing loss in graduates of a tertiary intensive care nursery. *Ear Hear* 3:87–90, 1982.

Gallagher JC: *Histology of the Human Temporal Bone.* Washington, DC: Armed Forces Institute of Pathology, 1967.

Gans D, Flexer C: Observer bias in the hearing testing of profoundly involved multiply handicapped children. *Ear Hear* 3:309–313, 1982.

Gans DP: Improving behavioral observation audiometry testing and scoring problems. *Ear Hear* 8:92–99, 1987.

Gans DP, Flexer C: Auditory response behavior of severely and profoundly multiply handicapped children. *J Audit Res* 23:137–146, 1983.

Gantz BJ, Tyler RS, Knutson JF, Woodworth G, et al: Evaluation of five different cochlear implant designs: audiological assessment and predictors of performance. *Laryngoscope* 98:1100–1106, 1988.

Gardner H: The forgotten lesson of Monsieur C. *Psychology Today*, August 1973.

Gardner RA, Gardner BT: Teaching sign language to a chimpanzee. *Science* 165:664–672, 1969.

Garretson MD: The need for multiple communication skills in the education process of the deaf. *Rocky Mt Leader* 62:1–8, 1963.

Gauger JS, Clymer EW, Young M, et al: *Hearing Aid Orientation.* Rochester, NY: National Technical Institute for the Deaf, 1980.

Gebhart DE: Tympanostomy tubes in the otitis media prone child. *Laryngoscope* 111:849–865, 1981.

Geers AE, Moog J, Schick B: Acquisition of spoken and signed English by profoundly deaf children. *J Speech Hear Disord* 49:378–388, 1984.

Geers AE, Moog JS: Predicting spoken language acquisition of hearing-impaired children. *J Speech Hear Disord* 52:1, 84–94, 1987.

Geers AE, Schick B: Acquisition of spoken and signed English by hearing-impaired children of hearing-impaired or hearing parents. *J Speech Hear Disord* 53: 136–143, 1988.

Gengel RW, Pascoe D, Shore I: A frequency response procedure for evaluating and selecting hearing aids for severely hearing-impaired children. *J Speech Hear Disord* 36:341–353, 1971.

Gerber SE, Mencher GT: Arousal responses of neonates to wide band and narrow-band noise. Paper presented to the American Speech-Language-Hearing Association, Atlanta, GA, November 1979.

Gerkin KP: Infant hearing screening. *Audiol J Cont Educ* 9:3, 1984.

Gerkin KP: The high risk register for deafness: a tutorial. *Asha* 25:4, 1984.

Gerkin KP, Downs MP: The high risk register for newborn screening programs. *Semin Hear* 5:1, 1984.

Geschwind N: The anatomy of acquired disorders of reading. In Money J (ed): *Reading Disability: Progress and Research Needs for Dyslexia.* Baltimore: Johns Hopkins, 1962.

Geschwind N, Levitsky W: Human brain: left-right asymmetries in temporal speech region. *Science* 161:186–187, 1968.

Gershon A: Infections of fetus and newborn infants. *J Perinat Med* 9:204–206, 1981.

Gesell A: The psychological development of normal and deaf children in their preschool years. *Volta Rev* 58:117–120, 1956.

Gilbert JHV: Babbling and the deaf child: a commentary on Lenneberg et al. (1965) and Lenneberg (1967). *J Child Lang* 9:511–515, 1981.

Gillberg C, Rosenhall U, Johansson E: Auditory brainstem responses in childhood psychosis. *J Autism Dev Disord* 13:2, 181–195, 1983.

Gladney JH, Monteleone PI: Metaphysical dysplasia. Genetic and otolaryngologic aspects. *Arch Otolaryngol* 92:147–153, 1970.

Glorig A, Roberts J: Hearing levels of adults by age and sex. *Vital and Health Statistics*. Washington, DC: Dept of HEW, 1965, series 11.

Goldman R, Sanders JW: Cultural factors and hearing. *Except Child* 35:489–490, 1969.

Goldstein MA: *Problems of the Deaf*. St. Louis: The Laryngoscope Press, 1933.

Goldstein MH, Stark R: Modifications of vocalizations of pre-school deaf children by vibrotactile and visual displays. *J Acoust Soc Am* 59:1477–1481, 1976.

Goldstein MN: Auditory agnosia for speech ("pure word-deafness"). *Brain Lang* 1:195–204, 1974.

Goldstein R: Auditory dysfunction associated with brain impairment. *Postgrad Med* 48:83–85, 1970.

Goldstein R, McRandle CC, Rodman LB: Site of lesion in cases of hearing loss associated with Rh incompatibility: an argument for peripheral impairment. *J Speech Hear Disord* 37:447–450, 1972.

Goldstein R, Rodman LB: Early components of averaged evoked responses to rapidly repeated auditory stimuli. *J Speech Hear Res* 10:697–705, 1967.

Goldstein R, Tait C: Critique of neonatal hearing evaluation. *J Speech Hear Disord* 36:3–18, 1971.

Goodhill V: *Ear Diseases, Deafness and Dizziness*. Hagerstown, MD: Harper and Row, 1979.

Goodman RM, Lackareff S, Gwinup G: Hereditary congenital deafness with onychodystrophy. *Arch Otolaryngol* 90:474–477, 1969.

Gorga MP, Kaminski JR, Beauchaine KA: Auditory brainstem responses from graduates of an intensive care nursery using an insert earphone. *Ear Hear* 9:3, 144–147, 1988.

Gorga MP, Kaminski JR, Beauchaine KL, Jesteadt W, Neely ST: Auditory brainstem responses from children three months to three years of age: normal patterns of response II. *J Speech Hear Res* 32:281–288, 1989.

Gorga MP, Reiland JK, Beauchaine KA, Worthington DW, Jesteadt W: Auditory brainstem responses from graduates of an intensive care nursery: normal patterns of response *J Speech Hear Res* 30:311–318, 1987.

Gorga MP, Worthington DW, Reiland J, Beauchaine KA, Goldgar DE: Some comparisons between auditory brainstem response thresholds, latencies and the pure tone audiogram. *Ear Hear* 6:2, 105–112, 1985.

Gorlin RJ, Anderson RC, Blaw M: Multiple lentigines syndrome. *Am J Dis Child* 117:652–662, 1969.

Gould HJ: Audiologic findings in Pierre Robin. *Ear Hear* 10:211–213, 1989.

Gravel JS: Behavioral assessment of auditory function. *Semin Hear* 10:217–228, 1989.

Green DS: Non-occluding earmolds with CROS and IROS hearing aids. *Arch Otolaryngol* 89:512–522, 1969.

Greenberg D, Wilson W, Moore J, et al: Visual reinforcement audiometry (VRA) with young Down's syndrome children. *J Speech Hear Disord* 43:448–458, 1978.

Greenberg MT: Hearing families with deaf children: stress and functioning as related to communication method. *Am Ann Deaf* 125:1063, 1975.

Greenstein JM, Greenstein BB, McConville K, et al: *Mother-Infant Communication and Language Acquisition in Deaf Infants*. New York: Lexington School for the Deaf, 1976.

Greenway EB: The communication needs of the deaf child. In *Report of the Proceedings of the International Congress on Education of the Deaf*. Washington, DC: Gallaudet College, 1964, pp 433–439.

Gregg JB, Steele JP, Clifford S, Werthman HE: A multidisciplinary study of ear disease in South Dakota. *S Dak J Med* 23:11–20, 1970.

Grier JB, Counter SA, Shearer WM: Prenatal auditory imprinting in chickens. *Science* 155:1692–1693, 1980.

Groothuis JR, Altemeier WA, Wright PF, et al: The evolution and resolution of otitis media in infants: tympanometric findings. In Harford ER, Bess FH, Bluestone CD, et al: *Impedance Screening for Middle Ear Disease in Children*. New York: Grune and Stratton, 1978, pp 105–109.

Groothuis JR, Sell SHW, Wright PF, et al: Otitis media in infancy: tympanometric findings. *Pediatrics* 63:435–442, 1979.

Grundfast K, Carney CJ: *Ear Infections in Your Child*, Hollywood, FL: Compact Books, 1987.

Grundy BL, Heros RC, Tung AS, et al: Intraoperative hypoxia detected by evoked potential monitoring. *Anesth Analg* 60:437–439, 1981.

Grusberg CM, Rudoy R, Nelson JD: Acute mastoiditis in infants and children. *Clin Pediatr* 19:8, 549–553, 1980.

Guberina P, Asp C: *The Verbo-tonal Method for Rehabilitating People with Communication Problems*. International Exchange of Information in Rehabilitation. New York: World Rehabilitation Fund, Inc, 1981, Monograph no 13.

Guiscafre H, Benitex-Diaz L, Martinez MC, Munoz O: Reversible hearing loss after meningitis. *Ann Otol Rhinol Laryngol* 93:229–232, 1984.

Hadeed AJ, Siegel S: Maternal cocaine use during pregnancy: effect on the newborn infant. *Pediatrics* 84:205–210, 1989.

Haggard M, Hughes E: *Objectives, Values and Methods of Screening Children's Hearing—A Review of the Literature*. IHR Internal Reports, series A, no 4. Nottingham, England: Institute of Hearing Research, 1988.

Hall J: Predicting hearing loss from the acoustic reflex. In Jerger J, Northern JL: *Clinical Impedance Audiometry*, ed 2. Acton, MA: American Electromedics Corp., 1980, ch 8.

Hall J, Bleakney M: Hearing loss prediction by the acoustic reflex: comparison of seven methods. *Ear Hear* 2:156, 1981.

Hall J: Contemporary tympanometry. *Semin Hear* 4:319–327, 1987.

Hall JG, Rohrt T: The stapes in osteogenesis imperfecta. *Acta Otolaryngol (Stockh)* 65:345–348, 1968.

Hall JL II: Binaural interaction in the accessory superior olivary nucleus of the cat. *J Acoust Soc Am* 37:814–823, 1965.

Hall JW, Ruth RA: Acoustic reflexes and auditory evoked responses in hearing aid evaluation. *Semin Hear* 6:3, 251–277, 1986.

Hallgren V: Retinitis pigmentosa combined with congenital deafness; with vestibulo-cerebellar ataxia and mental abnormality in a portion of cases. *Acta Psychiatr Scand Suppl* 138:1–101, 1959.

Hanners B, Sitton A: Ears to hear: a daily hearing aid monitoring program. *Volta Rev* 76:530–536, 1974.

Hanshaw J, Scheiner A, Moxley A, et al: School failure and deafness after "silent" congenital cytomegalovirus infection. *N Engl J Med* 295:468, 1976.

Hanson MJ: *Atypical Infant Development*. Baltimore: University Park Press, 1984.

Harboyan G, Mamo J, der Kalonstian V, et al: Congenital corneal dystrophy. Progressive sensorineural deafness in a family. *Arch Ophthalmol* 75:27–32, 1971.

Harford E, Barry J: A rehabilitative approach to the problems of unilateral hearing impairment: the contralateral routing of signals (CROS). *J Speech Hear Disord* 30:121–128, 1965.

Harford ER, Bess FH, Bluestone CD, et al (eds): *Impedance Screening for Middle Ear Disease in Children*. New York: Grune and Stratton, 1978.

Harris D: Action potential suppression, tuning curves and thresholds: comparison with single fiber data. *Hear Res* 1:133, 1979.

Harris JD: Combinations of distortion in speech. The 25% safety factor by multiple-cueing. *Arch Otolaryngol* 72:227–232, 1960.

Harris JD: Pure-tone acuity and the intelligibility of everyday speech. *J Acoust Soc Am* 37:821–830, 1965.

Harris JD: Monaural and binaural speech intelligibility and the stereophonic effect based on temporal cues. *Laryngoscope* 75:428–446, 1965.

Harris S, Ahlfors K, Ivarsson S, Lemmark B, Svanberg L: Congenital cytomegalovirus infection and sensorineural hearing loss. *Ear Hear* 5:352–355, 1984.

Hasenstab MS: *Language Learning and Otitis Media*. Rockville, MD: Aspen Systems Corporation, 1987.

Haskins H: A phonetically balanced test of speech discrimination for children. Unpublished MS degree thesis, 1949. (Cited in O'Neill J and Oyer H: *Applied Audiometry*. New York: Dodd, Mead, 1966.)

Haskins HI, Hardy WG: Clinical studies in stereophonic listening. *Laryngoscope* 70:1427–1433, 1960.

Haug O, Baccaro P, Guilford F: A pure-tone audiogram on the infant: the PIWI technique. *Arch Otolaryngol* 86:101–106, 1967.

Hawkins DB: Comparisons of speech recognition in noise by mildly-to-moderately hearing impaired children using hearing aids and FM systems. *J Speech Hear Disord* 49:409–418, 1984.

Hawkins DB: Clinical ear canal probe tube measurements. *Ear Hear* 85:74–81, 1987.

Hawkins DB, Prosek R, Walden B, Montgomery A: Binaural loudness summation in the hearing impaired. *J Speech Hear Res* 30:37–43, 1987.

Hawkins DB, Schum DJ: Some effects of FM system coupling on hearing aid characteristics. *J Speech Hear Disord*, 50:132–141, 1985.

Hayes E, Babin R, Platz C: The otologic manifestations of mucopolysaccharidoses. *Am J Otol* 2:65, 1980.

Hayman C, Kester F: Eye, ear, nose and throat infection in natives of Alaska. *Northwest Med* 56:423–430, 1957.

Hebb DO: The effects of early experience on problem-solving maturity. *Am Psychol* 2:306–307, 1947.

Hecox K, Galambos R: Brainstem auditory evoked responses in human infants and adults. *Arch Otolaryngol* 99:30–33, 1974.

Hecox K, Squires N, Galambos R: Brainstem auditory evoked responses in man. I. Effect of stimulus rise-fall time and duration. *J Acoust Soc Am* 60:1187–1192, 1976.

Heffernan HP, Simons MR: Temporary increase in sensorineural hearing loss with hearing aid use. *Ann Otol Rhinol Laryngol* 88:86–91, 1979.

Helpern J, Hosford-Dunn H, Malachowski N: Four factors that accurately predict hearing loss in "high risk" neonates. *Ear Hear* 8:1, 21–25, 1987.

Hemenway WG, Berstrom I: Dysplasias of the inner ear. In Bergsma D (ed): *Birth Defects, Atlas and Compendium*. Baltimore: Williams & Wilkins, published for the National Foundation-March of Dimes, 1972.

Hendricks-Munoz KD, Walton JP: Hearing loss in infants with persistent fetal circulation. *Pediatrics* 81:5, 650–656, 1988.

Herbets G: Otological observations on the Treacher Collins Syndrome. *Acta Otolaryngol (Stockh)* 54:457, 1962.

Herrmann C Jr, Aguilar MJ, Sacks OW: Hereditary photomyoclonus associated with diabetes mellitus, deafness, nephropathy and cerebral dysfunction. *Neurology* 14:212–221, 1964.

Hersch B, Amon C: An approach to reporting the diagnosis of hearing loss in parents of a hearing impaired child. Unpublished manuscript. University of Denver, CO, 1973.

Hicks WM, Hicks DE: The Usher's syndrome adolescent: programming implications for school administrators, teachers, and resident advisors. *Am Ann Deaf* 126:422–431, 1981.

Himalstein MR: Phylogeny of the temporal bone and temporomandibular joint. *Ear Nose Throat J* 57:42, 1978.

Hinchcliffe R: Epidemiological aspects of otitis media. In Glorig A, Gerwin K (eds): *Otitis Media*. Springfield, IL: Charles C Thomas, 1972, pp 36–43.

Hitselberger WE, Hughes RL: Bilateral acoustic tumors and neurofibromatosis. *Arch Otolaryngol* 88:700–711, 1968.

Ho M: *Cytomegalovirus, Biology and Infection*. New York: Plenum Medical Book Co, 1982.

Hodges A, Ruth R: Subject related factors influencing the acoustic reflex. *Semin Hear* 8:339–357, 1987.

Hodgson WR: Testing infants and young children. In Katz, J: *Handbook of Clinical Audiology*, ed 3. Baltimore: Williams & Wilkins, 1985, p 650, ch 32.

Hodgson WR: *Hearing Aid Assessment and Use in Audiological Habilitation*, ed 3. Baltimore: Williams & Wilkins, 1986.

Holcomb RK, Corbett EE: *Mainstream—The Delaware Approach.* Newark, DE: Newark School District (Sterk School), 1975.

Holloway G: Auditory-visual integration in language delayed children. *J Learn Disabil* 4:204–208, 1971.

Holm V, Kunze L: Effects of chronic otitis media on language and speech development. *Pediatrics* 43:833, 1969.

Holmes AE, Jones Muir KC, Kemker FJ: Acoustic reflectometry versus tympanometry in pediatric middle ear screenings. *Language, Speech & Hearing Services in Schools*, January 1989, pp 41–49.

Holmes EM: The microtia ear. *Arch Otolaryngol* 49:243–265, 1949.

Holmes LB: Norrie's disease; an X-linked syndrome of retinal malformation, mental retardation, and deafness. *J Pediatr* 70:89–92, 1971.

Holt R, Young W: Acute coalescent mastoiditis. *Otolaryngol Head Neck Surg* 89:317–321, 1981.

Hood DC: Evoked cortical response audiometry. In Bradford L (ed): *Physiological Measures of the Audio-Vestibular System.* New York: Academic Press, 1975, ch 10.

Hood J, Poole J: Tolerable limit of loudness: its clinical and physiological significance. *J Acoust Soc Am* 40:47–53, 1966.

Horn JM: Duration of preschool effects on later school competence. *Science* 213:1145, 1981.

Horton KB: Early intervention through parent training. *Otolaryngol Clin North Am* 8:143–157, 1975.

House WF: Subarachnoid shunt for drainage of hydrops: a report of 63 cases. *Arch Otolaryngol* 79:338–354, 1964.

Hoversten G: A public school audiology program: amplification, maintenance, auditory management, and in-service education. In Bess F, Freeman B, Sinclair J (eds): *Amplification in Education.* Washington, DC: AG Bell, 1981, ch 15.

Hoversten GH, Fornby D: Mainstreaming—the controversy. In Roeser R, Downs M (ed): *Auditory Disorders in School Children.* New York: Thieme-Stratton, 1981, ch 4.

Hoversten G, Fornby D: *Mainstreaming: A Process—Not a Goal.* New York: Thieme Medical Publishers, 1988, ch 4.

Howie VM: Natural history of otitis media. *Ann Otol Rhinol Laryngol Suppl* 19:67–72, 1975.

Howie VM, Ploussard JH: Treatment of serous otitis media with ventilatory tubes. *Clin Pediatr* 13:919, 1974.

Howie VM, Ploussard JH, Sloyer J: The "otitis-prone" condition. *Am J Dis Child* 129:676–678, 1975.

Hull FM, Mielke PW, Timmons RJ, et al: The National Speech and Hearing Survey: preliminary results. *Asha* 13:501–509, 1971.

Humes L, Bess F: Tutorial on the potential deterioration in hearing due to hearing aid usage. *J Speech Hear Res* 46:3–15, 1981.

Humes LE, Kirn EU: The reliability of functional gain. *J Speech Hear Disord* 55:193–197, 1990.

Ide CH, Wollschlaeger PP: Multiple congenital abnormalities associated with cryptophthalmia. *Arch Ophthalmol* 81:640–644, 1969.

Illum P, Kaier HW, Hvidberg-Hansen J, et al: Fifteen cases of Pendred's syndrome. *Arch Otolaryngol* 96:297–304, 1972.

Irwin OC: Infant speech: consonantal sounds according to manner of articulation. *J Speech Hear Disord* 12:402–404, 1947.

Irwin OC: Identification audiometry for school-age children: basic procedures. *J Speech Hear Disord* (monogr) 9:26–34, 1961.

Iwashita H, Inoue N, Araki S, et al: Optic atrophy, neural deafness and distal neurogenic amyotrophy. *Arch Neurol* 22:357–364, 1970.

Jacobson JT (ed): *The Auditory Brainstem Response.* San Diego: College-Hill Press, 1985.

Jacobson JT, Jacobson CA: Application of test performance characteristics in newborn auditory screening. *Semin Hear* 8:2, 133–141, 1987.

Jacobson JT, Morehouse CR: A comparison of auditory brainstem response and behavioral screening in high-risk and normal newborn infants. *Ear Hear* 5:247–253, 1984.

Jacobson JT, Morehouse CR, Johnson MJ: Strategies for infant auditory brain stem response assessment. *Ear Hear* 3:263–270, 1982.

Jaffe B, Hurtado F, Hurtado E: Tympanic membrane mobility in the newborn: with seven months' follow-up. *Laryngoscope* 80:36–48, 1970.

Jaffe BF: Congenital shoulder-neck-auditory anomalies. *Laryngoscope* 58:2119–2139, 1968a.

Jaffe BF: The incidence of ear diseases in the Navajo Indians. *Laryngoscope* 58:2126–2133, 1968b.

Jahn AF, Santos-Sacchi J: *Physiology of the Ear.* New York: Raven Press, 1988.

Jahrsdoerfer RA, Hall JW III: Congenital malformations of the ear. *Am J Otology* 7:267–269, 1986.

Jepsen O: Middle ear muscle reflexes in man. In Jerger J (ed): *Modern Developments in Audiology.* New York: Academic Press, 1963, pp 193–239.

Jerger J: Clinical experience with impedance audiometry. *Arch Otolaryngol* 92:311–324, 1970.

Jerger J: On the evaluation of hearing aid performance. *Asha* 29:9, 49–51, 1987.

Jerger J, Anthony L, Jerger S, et al: Studies in impedance audiometry: III. Middle ear disorders. *Arch Otolaryngol* 99:165–171, 1974a.

Jerger J, Burney P, Mauldin L, et al: Predicting hearing loss from the acoustic reflex. *J Speech Hear Disord* 39:11–22, 1974b.

Jerger J, Chmiel R, Frost J, Coker N: Effect of sleep on the auditory steady state evoked potential. *Ear Hear* 7:4, 240–245, 1986.

Jerger J, Dirks D: Binaural hearing aids: an enigma. *J Acoust Soc Am* 33:537–538, 1961.

Jerger J, Hayes D: The cross-check principle in pediatric audiometry. *Arch Otolaryngol* 102:614–620, 1976.

Jerger J, Hayes D: Diagnostic applications of impedance audiometry: middle ear disorder; sensorineural disorder. In Jerger J, Northern JL (eds): *Clinical Impedance Audiometry*, ed 2. Acton, MA: American Electromedics Corp, 1980, ch 6, pp 109–127.

Jerger J, Hayes D, Anthony L, et al: Factors influencing prediction of hearing level from the acoustic reflex. *Contemp Monogr Audiol* 1:1, 1978.

Jerger J, Hayes D, Jordon C: Clinical experience with auditory brainstem response audiometry in pediatric assessment. *Ear Hear* 1:19–25, 1980.

Jerger J, Hayes D, Smith S, et al: Auditory brainstem response in clinical practice. Course syllabus. Department of Otorhinolaryngology and Communicative Sciences, Baylor College of Medicine, 1981.

Jerger J, Jerger S: Temporary threshold shift in rock-and-roll musicians. *J Speech Hear Res* 13:218–224, 1970.

Jerger J, Jerger S: Auditory findings in brainstem disorders. *Arch Otolaryngol* 99:342–350, 1974.

Jerger J, Jerger S, Mauldin L: Studies in impedance audiometry: I. Normal and sensorineural ears. *Arch Otolaryngol* 96:513–523, 1972.

Jerger J, Lewis N: Binaural hearing aids: are they dangerous for children? *Arch Otolaryngol* 101:480–483, 1975.

Jerger J, Northern JL (eds): *Clinical Impedance Audiometry*, ed 2. Acton, MA: American Electromedics Corp., 1980.

Jerger J, Oliver T, Chmiel R: The auditory middle latency response. *Semin Hear* 9:1, 75–86, 1988.

Jerger J, Oliver T, Stach B: Auditory brainstem response testing strategies. In Jacobson J (ed): *The Auditory Brainstem Response*. San Diego: College-Hill Press, 1985, pp 371–388.

Jerger J, Thelin J: Effects of electroacoustic characteristics of hearing aids on speech understanding. *Bull Prosthet Res* 110:159–197, 1968.

Jerger S: Decision matrix and information theory analyses in the evaluation of neuroaudiologic tests. *Semin Hear* 4:2, 121–132, 1983.

Jerger S: Speech audiometry. In Jerger J (ed): *Pediatric Audiology*. San Diego: College Hill Press, 1984.

Jerger S, Jerger J: Pediatric speech intelligibility test: performance-intensity characteristics. *Ear Hear* 4:138–145, 1983.

Jerger S, Jerger J, Fahad R: Pediatric hearing aid evaluation: case reports. *Ear Hear* 6:5, 240–243, 1985.

Jerger S, Jerger J, Lewis S: Pediatric speech intelligibility test: II. Effect of receptive language age and chronological age. *Int J Pediatr Otorhinolaryngol* 3:101–118, 1981.

Jerger S, Jerger J, Mauldin L, et al: Studies in impedance audiometry: II. Children less than 6 years old. *Arch Otolaryngol* 99:1–9, 1974.

Jerger S, Lewis S, Hawkins J, et al: Pediatric speech intelligibility test: I. Generation of test materials. *Int J Pediatr Otorhinolaryngol* 2:217–230, 1980.

Jervell A, Lange-Nielsen F: Congenital deaf-mutism, functional heart disease with prolongation of the QT interval, and sudden death. *Am Heart J* 54:59–68, 1957.

Jewett D, Williston JS: Auditory evoked far fields averaged from the scalp of humans. *Brain* 94:681–696, 1971.

Jirsa R, Norris TW: Relationship of acoustic gain to aided threshold improvement in children. *J Speech Hear Disord* 43:3, 348–351, 1978.

Johansson B: A new coding amplifier system for the severely hard of hearing. In *Proceedings of the Third International Conference on Acoustics*. Stuttgart, 1959 (published 1961), pp 655–657.

Johansson B: The use of the transposer for the management of the deaf child. *Int Audiol* 5:362–372, 1966.

Johansson B, Wedenberg E, Westin B: Measurement of tone response by the human fetus. *Acta Otolaryngol (Stockh)* 57:188–192, 1964.

Johnson D, Caccamise F: Hearing-impaired populations: optimizing the use of vision for academic, career and communications program planning. *Am Ann Deaf* 126:317, 1981.

Johnson J: Binaural hearing instrument system—the biphasic. *Hear Instrum* 26:20–22, 1975.

Johnson JS, Watrous BS: An acoustic impedance screening program with an American Indian population. In Harford ER, Bess FH, Bluestone CD, et al: *Impedance Screening for Middle Ear Disease in Children*. New York: Grune & Stratton, 1978.

Johnson RL: Chronic otitis media in school age Navajo Indians. *Laryngoscope* 77:1990–1995, 1967.

Johnsson LG, Arenberg K: Cochlear abnormalities in Alport's syndrome. *Otolaryngol Head Neck Surg* 107:340–349, 1981.

Johnston CC, Lawy N, Lord T, et al: Osteopetrosis. A clinical, genetic, metabolic, and morphologic study of the dominantly inherited benign form. *Medicine* 47:149–167, 1968.

Johnston JR: The language delayed child. In Lass NJ, McReynolds LV, Northern JL, Yoder DE (eds): *Speech, Language and Hearing*, vol II. Philadelphia: WB Saunders, 1982, ch 31.

Joint Committee on Infant Hearing: Joint Committee on Infant Hearing 1982 statement. *Asha* 24:1017–1018, 1982.

Joint Committee on Infant Hearing: Joint Committee on Infant Hearing 1991 position statement. *Asha*, in press.

Jones FR, Simmons FB: Early identification of significant hearing loss: the Crib-o-gram. *Hear Instrum* 28:8–10, 1977.

Jones MD, Mulcahy ND: Osteopathia striata, osteopetrosis, and impaired hearing. *Arch Otolaryngol* 87:20–22, 1968.

Jordan I, Gustason G, Rosen R: An update on communication trends in programs for the deaf. *Am Ann Deaf* 125:350–357, 1979.

Jordan IK, Gustason G, Rosen R: Current communication trends in programs for the deaf. *Am Ann Deaf* 121:527–532, 1976.

Jordan O: Mental retardation and hearing defects. *Scand Audiol* 1:29–32, 1972.

Jordan O, Greisen O, Bentzen O: Treatment with binaural hearing aids. *Arch Otolaryngol* 85:319–326, 1967.

Jordan RE, Eagles EL: The relation of air conduction audiometry to otologic abnormalities. *Ann Otol Rhinol Laryngol* 70:819–827, 1961.

Jusczyk PW, Thompson E: Perception of a phonetic contrast in multisyllabic utterances by 2-month-old infants. *Percept Psychophysics* 23:105–109, 1978.

Kaga K, Tanaka Y: Auditory brainstem response and behavioral audiometry. *Otolaryngol Head Neck Surg* 106:564–566, 1980.

Kagan J: Do infants think? *Sci Am* 226:74–82, 1972.

Kahane JC: Pathophysiologic effects of Möbius syndrome on speech and hearing. *Arch Otolaryngol Head Neck Surg* 105:29–34, 1979.

Kamhi AG: Developmental vs. difference theories of mental retardation: a new look. *Am J Ment Defic* 86:1–7, 1982.

Kankkunen B, Thuringer R: Hearing impairment in connection with preauricular tags. *Acta Paediatr Scand* 76:143–146, 1987.

Kannapell BM, Hamilton IB, Bornstein H: *Signs for Instructional Purposes.* Washington, DC: Gallaudet College Press, 1969.

Kaplan S, Goddard J, Van Kleeck M, et al: Ataxia and deafness in children due to bacterial meningitis. *Pediatrics* 52:577–585, 1973.

Kaplan SL, Catlin F, Weaver T, Feigin RD: Onset of hearing loss in children with bacterial meningitis. *Pediatrics* 73:575–579, 1984.

Karchmer M, Trybus R: Who are the deaf children in "mainstream" programs? *Annual Survey of Hearing Impaired Children and Youth*, series R, no 4. Washington, DC: Office of Demographic Studies, Gallaudet College, 1977.

Karmody CS, Schuknecht HF: Deafness in congenital syphilis. *Arch Otolaryngol Head Neck Surg* 83:18–26, 1966.

Kasten R, Braunlin R: Traumatic hearing aid usage: a case study. Presented at the American Speech and Hearing Association Convention, 1970.

Kavanagh JF (ed): *Otitis Media and Child Development.* Parkton, MD: York Press, 1986.

Kavanagh KT, Gould H, McCormick G, Franks R: Comparison of the identifiability of the low intensity ABR and MLR in the mentally handicapped patient. *Ear Hear* 10:2, 124–130, 1989.

Keane WM, Potsic WP, Rowe LD, et al: Meningitis and hearing loss in children. *Arch Otolaryngol* 105:39–44, 1979.

Kearsley R, Snider M, Richie R, et al: Study of relations between psychologic environment and child behavior. *Am J Dis Child* 104:12–20, 1962.

Keith R: Impedance audiometry with neonates. *Arch Otolaryngol* 97:465–467, 1973.

Keith RW: Middle ear functions in neonates. *Arch Otolaryngol* 101:376–379, 1975.

Keith RW (ed): *Central Auditory Dysfunction.* New York: Grune and Stratton, 1977a.

Keith RW: An evaluation of predicting hearing loss from the acoustic reflex. *Arch Otolaryngol Head Neck Surg* 103:419, 1977b.

Keith RW: Commentary. Letter to the editor. *Audiol Hear Educ* 4:28, 1978.

Keith RW (ed): Auditory perceptual problems in children. *Semin Speech Lang Hear* 1:2, 1980a.

Keith RW (ed): *Audiology for the Physician.* Baltimore: Williams & Wilkins, 1980b.

Keith RW (ed): *Central Auditory and Language Disorders in Children.* Houston: College Hill Press, 1981.

Keith RW: Special issue: dichotic listing tests. *Ear Hear* 4:6, 1983.

Keith RW: *SCAN: A Screening Test for Auditory Processing Disorders.* San Antonio, TX: The Psychological Corporation/Harcourt Brace Jovanovich, 1986.

Keith RW: Central auditory tests. In Lass NJ, McReynolds LV, Northern JL, et al (eds): *Handbook of Speech-Language Pathology & Audiology.* Toronto: BC Decker, 1988.

Keith RW: Tests of central auditory function. In Roeser R, Downs M (eds): *Auditory Disorders in School Children.* New York: Thieme Medical Publishers, 1988.

Keith RW, Farrer S: Filtered word testing in the assessment of children with central auditory disorders. *Ear Hear* 12:267–269, 1981.

Keith WJ, Smith RP: Automated pediatric hearing assessment using interactive video images. *Hear Instrum* 38(9):27–28, 1987.

Keleman G: Toxoplasmosis and congenital deafness. *Arch Otolaryngol* 68:547–561, 1958.

Keleman G: Hurler's syndrome and the hearing organ. *J Laryngol* 80:791–803, 1966.

Keleman G, Hooft C, Kluyskens P: The inner ear in autosomal trisomy. *Pract Otorhinolaryngol* (Basel) 30:251–258, 1968.

Kellman N: Noise in the intensive care nursery. *Neonatal Network*, August 1982, pp 8–17.

Kemp DT: Stimulated acoustic emissions from the human auditory system. *J Acoust Soc Am* 64:1386–1391, 1978.

Kemp DT: Towards a model for the origin of cochlear echos. *Hear Res* 2:533–548, 1980.

Kemp DT, Bray P, Alexander L, Brown AM: Acoustic emission cochleography—practical aspects. *Scand Audiol* 25:71–95, 1986.

Kent RD, Osberger MJ, Netsell R, Hustedde CG: Phonetic development in identical twins differing in auditory function. *J Speech Hear Disord* 52:64–75, 1987.

Kenworthy OT, Bess FH, Stahlman MT, Lindstrom DP: Hearing, speech and language outcome in infants with extreme immaturity. *Am J Otol* 5:419–425, 1987.

Kerr G, Smyth GD, Cinnamond M: Congenital syphilitic deafness. *J Laryngol Otol* 87:1–12, 1973.

Kessner DM, Kalk CE: A strategy for evaluating health services. In *Contrasts in Health Status.* Washington, DC: Institute of Medicine, National Academy of Sciences, 1973, vol 2.

Kessner DM, Snow CK, Singer J: Assessment of medical care in children. In *Contrasts in Health Status.* Washington, DC: Institute of Medicine, National Academy of Sciences, 1974, vol 3.

Kiessling J: Hearing aid selection by brainstem audiometry. *Scand Audiol* 11:269–275, 1982.

Killion M: Experimental wideband hearing aid [Abstract]. *J Acoust Soc Am* 59:562, 1976.

Killion M: Transducers, earmolds and sound quality considerations. In Studebaker B, Bess F (eds): *The Vanderbilt Hearing Aid Report: State of the Art—Research Needs.* Nashville, TN: *Monographs Contemporary Audiology*, 1982, pp 104–111.

Kim DO: Cochlear mechanics: implications of electrophysical and acoustic observations. *Hear Res* 2:297–317, 1980.

Kimura D: Cerebral dominance and the perception of verbal stimuli. *Can J Psychol* 15:166–171, 1961.

Kimura D: Left-right differences in the perception of melodies. *Q J Exp Psychol* 16:355–358, 1964.

Kirk SA, McCarthy JP, Kirk WD: *The Illinois Test of Psycholinguistic Abilities*, rev. ed. Urbana: University of Illinois Press, 1968.

Kirkham TH: Duane's syndrome and familial perceptive deafness. *Br J Ophthalmol* 53:335–339, 1969.

Kleffner FR: Hearing losses, hearing aids, and children with language disorders. *J Speech Hear Disord* 38:232–239, 1973.

Klein JO: Epidemiology of otitis media. In Wiet RJ, Coulthard SW: *Otitis Media: Proceedings of the Second National Conference on Otitis Media.* Columbus, OH: Ross Laboratories, 1979, pp 18–20.

Klein JO: Article in *Washington Post*, May 27, 1981.

Klein JO: Epidemiology and natural history of otitis media. *Pediatrics* 71:639–640, 1983.

Klein JO: Feigin RD, McCracken GH: Report of the Task Force on Diagnosis and Management of Meningitis. *Pediatrics* 78:5, 1986.

Kloepfer HW, Laguaite JK, McLaurin JW: The hereditary syndrome of deafness in retinitis pigmentosa. *Laryngoscope* 76:850–862, 1966.

Kodman P: Successful binaural hearing aid users. *Arch Otolaryngol* 74:302–314, 1961.

Koenig W: Subjective effects in binaural hearing. *J Acoust Soc Am* 22:61–62, 1950.

Koenigsberger MR, Chutorian AM, Gold AP, et al: Benign paroxysmal vertigo of childhood. *Neurology* 20:1108–1113, 1970.

Konigsmark BW: Hereditary deafness in man. *N Engl J Med* 281:713–720, 774–778, 827–832, 1969.

Konigsmark BW: Genetic hearing loss with no associated abnormalities: a review. *J Speech Hear Disord* 37:89–99, 1972.

Konigsmark BW, Gorlin RJ: *Genetic and Metabolic Deafness.* Philadelphia: WB Saunders, 1976.

Konigsmark BW, Hollander MB, Berlin CI: Familial neural hearing loss and atopic dermatitis. *JAMA* 204:953–957, 1968.

Konigsmark BW, Mengel MC, Haskins H: Familial congenital moderate neural hearing loss. *J Laryngol* 84:495–506, 1970.

Kos AO, Schuknecht HF, Singer JD: Temporal bone studies in 13–15 and 18 trisomy syndrome. *Arch Otolaryngol* 83:439–445, 1966.

Kossowska E, Goralowna M: Prenatal and neonatal prophylaxis in otorhinolaryngology. *Int J Pediatr Otorhinolaryngol* 2:85–98, 1980.

Kramer SJ, Vertes DR, Condon M: Auditory brainstem responses and clinical follow-up of high-risk infants. *Pediatrics* 83:3, 385–392, 1989.

Kraus N, McGee T, Comperatore C: MLRs in children are consistently present during wakefulness, Stage I, and REM sleep. *Ear Hear* 10:6, 339–345, 1989.

Kruger B: An update on the external ear resonance in infants and young children. *Ear Hear* 8:6, 333–336, 1987.

Kryter K: *The Effects of Noise on Man.* New York: Academic Press, 1970.

Kryter KD: Impairment to hearing from exposure to noise. *J Acoust Soc Am* 53:1211–1234, 1973.

Kryter KD, Ades HW: Studies on the function of the higher acoustic nervous centers in the cat. *Am J Psychol* 56:501–536, 1943.

Kryter KD, Williams C, Green DM: Auditory acuity and the perception of speech. *J Acoust Soc Am* 34:1217–1223, 1962.

Kuczwara LA, Birnholz JC, Klodd DA: Auditory responsiveness in the fetus. *Natl Student Speech Lang Hear Assoc J* 14:12–20, 1984.

Kuhl P: Speech perception in early infancy: perceptual constancy for spectrally dissimilar vowel categories. *J Acoust Soc Am* 66:1668–1679, 1979.

Kuhl P, Miller J: Discrimination of auditory target dimensions in the presence or absence of variation in a second dimension by infants. *Percept Psychophysics* 31:279–292, 1982.

Kuhl PK, Hillenbrand J: Speech perception by young infants: perceptual constancy for categories based on pitch contour. Paper presented at the meeting of the Society for Research in Child Development, San Francisco, March 1979.

Kuzniarz J: Hearing loss and speech intelligibility in noise. In *Proceedings of the International Congress on Noise as a Public Health Problem.* Washington, DC: US Environmental Protection Agency, Office of Noise Abatement Control, 1973, pp 57–71.

Lahey BB, Schaughency EA, Strauss CC, Frame CL: Are attention deficit disorders with and without hyperactivity similar or dissimilar disorders? *J Am Acad Child Adolesc Psychiatry* 23:302–309, 1984.

Lamb I, Norris T: Relative acoustic impedance measurements with mentally retarded children. *Am J Ment Defic* 75:51–56, 1970.

Lamb LE, Norris T: Acoustic impedance measurement. In Fulton, RT, Lloyd LI (eds): *Audiometry for the Retarded.* Baltimore: Williams and Wilkins, 1969, pp 164–209.

Lampe R, Weir M, Spier J, Rhodes M: Acoustic reflectometry in the detection of middle ear effusion. *Pediatrics* 76:75–78, 1985.

Lancioni GE, Coninx F, Smeets PH: A classical conditioning procedure for the hearing assessment of multiply handicapped persons. *J Speech Hear Disord* 54:88–93, 1989.

Lane H: *The Wild Boy of Aveyron.* Cambridge: Harvard University Press, 1977.

Langer LO Jr: Diastrophic dwarfism in early infancy. *Am J Roentgenol* 93:399, 1965.

Langer LO Jr: Achondroplasia; clinical radiologic features with comment on genetic implications. *Clin Pediatr* 7:474–478, 1968.

Langer LO Jr, Baumann PA, Gorlin RJ: *Am J Roentgenol Radium Ther Nucl Med* 100:12–15, 1967.

Langer SK: *Philosophy in a New Key.* Cambridge, MA: Harvard University Press, 1957.

Langford C, Bench J, Wilson I: Some effects of prestimulus activity and length of prestimulus observations on judgments of newborns' responses to sounds. *Audiology* 14:44–52, 1975.

Last JM: *A Dictionary of Epidemiology.* New York: Oxford University Press, 1983.

League R, Parker J, Robertson M, et al: Acoustical environments in incubators and infant oxygen tents. *Prev Med* 1:231, 1972.

Lee L: *The Northwestern Syntax Screening Test.* Evanston, IL: Northwestern University Press, 1971.

Lempert J, Wever EG, Lawrence M: The cochleogram and its clinical application. *Arch Otolaryngol Head Neck Surg* 45:61–67, 1947.

Lenneberg EH: *Biological Foundations of Language.* New York: John Wiley and Sons, 1967.

Leridan Audiscreen: Leridan Associates (USA), 520 Barker Pass Road, Santa Barbara, CA 93108.

Leroy JG, Crocker AC: Clinical definition of Hunter-Hurler phenotypes. A review of 50 patients. *Am J Dis Child* 112:518–530, 1966.

Leshin GJ: Childhood non-organic hearing loss. *J Speech Hear Disord* 25:290–292, 1960.

Leske MC: Prevalence estimates of communicative disorders in the U.S. Language, hearing and vestibular disorders. *Asha* 23:229–236, 1981.

Levine RL: Bilirubin: worked out years ago? *Pediatrics* 64:380–385, 1979.

Levitt H: Recurrent issues underlying the development of tactile sensory aids. *Ear Hear* 9:301–305, 1988.

Levitt H, Nye PW: Sensory training aids for the hearing impaired. In *Proceedings of a Conference, Easton, MD, 1970*. Washington, DC: National Academy of Engineering, Subcommittee on Sensory Aids, 1971.

Lewin R: Starved brains. *Psychology Today*, September 1975, pp 29–33.

Lewis M, Goldberg S: Perceptual-cognitive development in infancy: a generalized expectancy model as a function of the mother-infant interaction. *Merrill-Palmer J Behav Dev* 15:81–100, 1969.

Lewis N: Otitis media and linguistic incompetence. *Arch Otolaryngol* 102:387–390, 1976.

Libby ER (ed): *Binaural Hearing Aid Amplification*. Chicago: Zenetron, Inc, 1980, vols 1 and 2.

Libby ER: Achieving a transparent, smooth, wideband hearing aid response. *Hear Instrum* 32:9–12, 1981.

Libby ER: In search of transparent insertion gain hearing aid responses. In Studebaker G, Bess F (eds): *The Vanderbilt Hearing Aid Report: State of the Art—Research Needs*. Nashville, TN: *Monographs in Contemporary Audiology*, 1982, pp 112–123.

Liberman AM, Cooper FS, Shankweiler DP, et al: Perception of the speech code. *Psychol Rev* 74:431–461, 1967.

Liden G, Kankkonen A: Visual reinforcement audiometry. *Acta Otolaryngol (Stockh)* 67:281–292, 1961.

Liden G, Peterson JL, Bjorkman G: Tympanometry: a method for analysis of middle-ear function. *Acta Otolaryngol (Stockh)* 263:218–224, 1970.

Lieberman P: *On the Origins of Language*. New York: Macmillan, 1975.

Lieberman P, Harris KS, Wolff P, et al: Newborn infant cry and nonhuman primate vocalization. *J Speech Hear Res* 14:718–727, 1971.

Liebman J, Graham JT: Changes in the parameters of the averaged auditory evoked potentials related to the number of data samples analyzed. *J Speech Hear Res* 10:782–785, 1967.

Lim DH: Three dimensional observation of the inner ear with the scanning electron microscope. *Acta Otolaryngol Suppl (Stockh)* 255, 1969.

Lim DJ: Diagnosis and screening. In *Recent Advances in Otitis Media, Report of the Fourth Research Conference. Ann Otol Rhinol Laryngol (Suppl)* 139: 98(4), part 2, 39–41, 1989.

Linden RD, Campbell KB, Hamel G, Picton TW: Human auditory steady state evoked potentials during sleep. *Ear Hear* 6:167–184, 1985.

Lindsay JR: Labyrinthitis of viral origin. In Graham B (ed): *Sensorineural Hearing Process and Disorders*. Boston: Little, Brown, 1967a.

Lindsay JR: Congenital deafness of inflammatory origin. In McConnell F, Ward PH (eds): *Deafness in Childhood*. Nashville, TN: Vanderbilt University Press, 1967b, pp 142–155.

Lindsay JR: Inner ear histopathology in genetically determined congenital deafness. In *Birth Defects, Part IX, Ear*. Baltimore: Williams & Wilkins, for National Foundation-March of Dimes, 1971a.

Lindsay JR: Inner ear pathology in congenital deafness. *Otolaryngol Clin North Am* (Symposium) 4:2, 1971b.

Lindsay JR, Black FO, Donnelly WN: Acrocephalosyndactyly (Apert's syndrome). Temporal bone findings. *Ann Otol Rhinol Laryngol* 84:174–178, 1975.

Lindsay P, Norman D: *Human Information Processing: An Introduction to Psychology*. New York: Academic Press, 1972, fig 7.2, p 95.

Ling D: Implications of hearing aid amplification below 300 cps. *Volta Rev* 66:723–729, 1964.

Ling D: Three experiments on frequency transposition. *Am Ann Deaf* 113:283–294, 1968.

Ling D, Ling AH, Doehring DG: Stimulus response and observer variables in the auditory screening of newborn infants. *J Speech Hear Res* 13:9–18, 1970.

Ling D, Maretic H: Frequency transposition in the teaching of speech to deaf children. *J Speech Hear Res* 14:37–46, 1971.

Ling D: Recent developments affecting the education of hearing-impaired children. *Public Health Rev* 4:117–152, 1975.

Lippe WR: Recent developments in cochlear physiology. *Ear Hear* 7:233–239, 1986.

Lipscomb DM: Noise exposure and its effects. Otocongress II, Copenhagen, 1972.

Lipscomb DM: Mechanisms of the middle ear. In Northern JL (ed): *Hearing Disorders*, ed 2. Boston: Little, Brown, 1984, ch 21.

Lipscomb DM: Anatomy and physiology of the hearing mechanism. In Lass NJ, McReynolds LV, Northern JL, Yoder DE (eds): *Handbook of Speech-Language Pathology & Audiology*. Toronto: BC Decker, 1988, pp 52–76.

Litke RE: Elevated high-frequency hearing in school children. *Arch Otolaryngol* 94:255–257, 1971.

Lloyd LI: Audiological aspects of mental retardation. In Ellis NR (ed): *International Review of Research in Mental Retardation*. New York: Academic Press, 1970, pp 311–374.

Lloyd LI, Spradlin JE, Reid MJ: An operant audiometric procedure for difficult-to-test patients. *J Speech Hear Disord* 33:236–245, 1968.

Loeb G: Single and multichannel cochlear prostheses: rationale, strategies, and potential. In Schindler R and Merzenich M (eds): *Cochlear Implants*. New York: Raven Press, 1985, pp 17–28.

Loeb GE: The functional replacement of the ear. *Sci Am*, Feb 1985, pp 104–111.

Long J, Lucey J, Philip A: Noise and hypoxemia in the intensive care nursery. *Pediatrics* 65:143, 1980.

Lous J, Fiellau-Nikolajsen M: Epidemiology of middle ear effusion and tubal dysfunction. *Int J Pediatr Otorhinolaryngol* 3:303–317, 1981.

Lowe A, Campbell R: Temporal discrimination in aphasoid and normal children. *J Speech Hear Res* 8:313–314, 1965.

Lowe SS, Cullen JK, Thompson CL, et al: Dichotic and monotic simultaneous and time-staggered speech. *J Acoust Soc Am* 47:76, 1970.

Lowenstein B, Preger D Jr: *Diabetes, A New Look at an Old Problem*. New York: Harper & Row, 1976.

Lucker JR: Application of pass-fail criteria to middle ear screening results. *Asha* 22:839, 1980.

Luterman D: *Counseling Parents of Hearing-Impaired Children*. Boston: Little, Brown, 1979.

Luterman D, Chasin J: The deafness management quotient as an indicator of oral success. *Volta Rev* 83:405, 1981.

Luterman DM: A comparison of language skills of hearing impaired children trained in a visual/oral method and an auditory/oral method. *Am Ann Deaf* 121:389–393, 1976.

Lutman M, Mason SM, Sheppard S, Gibbin KP: Differential diagnostic potential of otoacoustic emissions: a case study. *Audiology* 28:205–210, 1989.

Lybarger S: Some comments on CROS. *Natl Hear Aid J* 21:8–33, 1968.

Lybarger S: Earmolds. In Katz J: *Handbook of Clinical Audiology*, ed 2. Baltimore: Williams & Wilkins, 1978.

Lynn GE, Gilroy J: Detection and localization of central auditory disorders. In Northern JL (ed): *Hearing Disorders*, ed 2. Boston: Little, Brown, 1984, ch 16.

Lyon R: Auditory perceptual training: the state of the art. *J Learn Disabil* 10:564–572, 1977.

MacDonald HM: Neonatal asphyxia; I. Relationship of obstetric and neonatal complications to neonatal mortality in consecutive deliveries. *J Pediatr* 96:898–902, 1980.

MacDonald JT, Feinstein S: Hearing loss following *Hemophilus influenzae* meningitis in infancy. *Arch Neurol* 41:1058–1059, 1984.

Mackie K, Dermody P: Use of a monosyllabic adaptive speech test (MAST) with young children. *J Speech Hear Res* 29:275–281, 1986.

Macklin F: Mainstreaming: the cost issue. *Am Ann Deaf* 121:364–365, 1976.

Macrae JH: TTS and recovery from TTS after use of powerful hearing aids. *J Acoust Soc Am* 44:1445–1446, 1968a.

Macrae JH: Recovery from TTS in children with sensorineural deafness. *J Acoust Soc Am* 44:1451, 1968b.

Macrae JH, Farrant RH: The effect of hearing aid use on the residual hearing of children with sensorineural deafness. *Ann Otol Rhinol Laryngol* 74:407–419, 1965.

Madell JR (ed): Mainstreaming the school-aged hearing-impaired child. *Semin Hear* 5:4, 1984.

Mahoney T: High-risk hearing screening of large general newborn populations. *Semin Hear* 5:1, 25–37, 1984.

Mahoney T: Auditory brainstem response hearing aid applications. In Jacobson J (ed): *The Auditory Brainstem Response*. Boston: College-Hill Press, 1985, pp 349–370.

Malkin SF, Freeman RD, Hasting JO: Psychosocial problems of deaf children and their families: a comparative study. *Audiol Hear Educ* Part I—2:3, 21–26; Part II—2:4, 31–38, 1976.

Mandell AJ, Smith CK: Hereditary sensory radicular neuropathy. *Neurology* 10:627–630, 1960.

Mangabeira-Albernaz PL, Fukaka J, Chammas F, et al: The Mondini dysplasia—a clinical study. *ORL* 43:131–152, 1981.

Maniglia JM, Wolff D, Herques AS: Congenital deafness in 13–15 syndrome. *Arch Otolarynol* 92:181–188, 1970.

Marcus RE, Valvasori G: Cochleo-vestibular apparatus; radiologic studies in hereditary and familial hearing loss. *Int Audiol* 9:95–102, 1970.

Mardel M, Hosick E, Windman T, et al: Audiometric comparison of the middle and late components of the adult auditory evoked potential awake and sleep. *Electroencephalogr Clin Neurophysiol* 38:27–33, 1975.

Margolis RH: Tympanometry in infants: state-of-the-art. In Harford ER, Bess FH, Bluestone CD et al (eds): *Impedance Screening for Middle Ear Disease in Children*. New York: Grune & Stratton, 1978, pp 41–56.

Margolis RM: Tympanometry for prediction of middle ear effusion. Letter to the editor. *Arch Otolaryngol* 105:225, 1979.

Markle D, Zaner A: The determination of gain requirements of hearing aids; a new method. *J Audit Res* 6:371–377, 1966.

Marquardt TP, Saxman JH: Language comprehension and auditory discrimination in articulation deficient kindergarten children. *J Speech Hear Res* 15:382–389, 1972.

Marshall L, Brandt JF: Temporary threshold shift from a toy cap gun. *J Speech Hear Disord* 39:163–168, 1974.

Marshall R, Reichtert T, Kerley SM, et al: Auditory function in newborn intensive care unit patients revealed by auditory brain-stem potentials. *J Pediatr* 96:731–735, 1980.

Martensson B: Dominant hereditary nerve deafness. *Arch Otolaryngol* 52:270–274, 1960.

Martin E, Pickett JM: Sensorineural hearing loss and upward spread of masking. *J Speech Hear Res* 13:426–437, 1980.

Martin FN, Clark JG: Audiologic detection of auditory processing disorders in children. *J Am Audiol Soc* 3:140–146, 1977.

Maskarinec AS, Cairns FG, Butterfield EC, et al: Longitudinal observations of individual infants' vocalizations. *J Speech Hear Disord* 46:267–273, 1981.

Masterton RB, Diamond IT: Effects of auditory cortex ablation on discrimination of small binaural time differences. *J Neurophysiol* 27:15–36, 1964.

Matkin A, Matkin N: Benefits of total communication as perceived by parents of hearing-impaired children. *Language, Speech & Hearing Services in Schools* 16:64–74, 1985.

Matkin N: Assessment of hearing sensitivity during the preschool years. In Bess FH (ed): *Childhood Deafness*. New York: Grune and Stratton, 1977.

Matkin N: Amplification for children: current status and future priorities. In Bess F, Freeman B, Sinclair J (eds): *Amplification in Education*. Washington, DC: AG Bell, 1981, ch 12.

Matkin N, Thomas J: The utilization of CROS hearing aids in children. *Maico Audiological Library Series* 10:8, 1972.

Matkin ND: Hearing aids for children. In Hodgson WR (ed): *Hearing Aid Assessment and Use in Audiologic Habilitation*, ed 3. Baltimore: Williams & Wilkins, 1986, pp 170–190.

Matkin ND, Carhart R: Auditory profiles associated with Rh incompatibility. *Arch Otolaryngol* 84:502–513, 1966.

Matkin ND, Carhart R: Hearing acuity and Rh incompatibility: electrodermal thresholds. *Arch Otolaryngol* 87:383–388, 1968.

Matzker J: Two new methods for the assessment of central auditory functions in cases of brain disease. *Ann Otol Rhinol Laryngol* 68:1185–1197, 1959.

Maumenee AE: Congenital hereditary corneal dystrophy. *Am J Ophthalmol* 50:1114–1123, 1960.

May DL, White HH: Familial myoclonus, cerebellar ataxia, and deafness. *Arch Neurol* 19:331–338, 1968.

May J, Brackett D: Adapting the classroom environment. *Semin Hear* 5:4, 405–409, 1984.

McCabe BF: Perilymph fistula: the Iowa experience to date. *Am J Otol* 10:262, 1989.

McCaffrey A: Speech perception in infancy. Personal communication cited in Friedlander (1970).

McCandless G, Keith R: Use of impedance measurements in hearing aid fitting. In Jerger J, Northern JL (eds): *Clinical Impedance Audiometry*, ed 2. Acton, MA: American Electromedics Corp, 1980, pp 203–218, ch 11.

McCandless G, Miller D: Loudness discomfort and hearing aids. *Natl Hear Aid J* 25:7–32, 1972.

McCandless GA: Screening for middle ear disease on the Wind River Indian Reservation. *Hear Instrum* 26:19–20, 1975.

McCandless GA: Hearing aid formulae and their application. In Sandlin RE (ed): *Handbook of Hearing Aid Amplification*, vol 1. Boston: College-Hill Press, 1988, ch 8.

McCandless GA, Allred PL: Tympanometry and emergence of the acoustic reflex in infants. In Harford ER, Bess FH, Bluestone CD, et al (eds): *Impedance Screening for Middle Ear Disease in Children*. New York: Grune & Stratton, 1978, pp 56–67.

McClure WJ: The ostrich syndrome and educators of the deaf. *The Kentucky Standard* (Kentucky School for the Deaf, Danville) 100:5, 1973.

McConnell F, Liff S: The rationale for early identification and intervention. *Otolaryngol Clin North Am* 8:77–87, 1975.

McConnell F, Ward PH (eds): *Deafness in Childhood*. Nashville, TN: Vanderbilt University Press, 1967.

McCroskey R: Wichita Auditory Processing Test. Tulsa, OK: Modern Education Corp, 1984.

McCroskey R, Kidder H: Auditory fusion in learning disabled, reading disabled and normal children. *J Learn Disabil* 13:69–76, 1980.

McDonald F, Studebaker G: Earmold alteration effects as measured in human auditory meatus. *J Acoust Soc Am* 48:1366–1372, 1970.

McDonough ER: Fanconi anemia syndrome. *Arch Otolaryngol* 92:284–285, 1970.

McFarlan D: The voice test of hearing. *Arch Otolaryngol* 5:1–5, 1927.

McFarland WH, Simmons FB, Jones FR: An automated hearing screening technique for newborns. *J Speech Hear Disord* 45:495, 1980.

McIntire MS, Menolascina FJ, Wiley JH: Mongolism—some clinical aspects. *Am J Ment Defic* 69:794, 1965.

McKay H, Sinisterra L, McKay A, et al: Improving cognitive ability in chronically deprived children. *Science* 200:270–278, 1978.

McLaurin JW, Kloepfer HW, Lagnaite JK, et al: Hereditary branchial anomalies and associated hearing impairment. *Laryngoscope* 76:1277–1288, 1966.

McLay K, Maran AGD: Deafness and the Klippel-Feil syndrome. *J Laryngol Otol* 83:175–184, 1969.

McLeod AC, McConnell F, Sweeney A, et al: Clinical variation in Usher's syndrome. *Arch Otolaryngol* 94:321–334, 1971.

McMillan P, Bennett M, Marchant C, Shurin P: Ipsilateral and contralateral acoustic reflexes in neonates. *Ear Hear* 6:6, 320–324, 1985.

McNeill D: Developmental psycholinguistics. In Smith F, Muller GA (eds): *The Genesis of Language: A Psycholinguistic Approach*. Cambridge, MA: MIT Press, 1966.

McReynolds LV: Operant conditioning for investigating speech sound discrimination in aphasic children. *J Speech Hear Res* 9:519–528, 1966.

Meadow KP: The effect of early manual communication and family climate. Doctoral dissertation, University of California, Berkeley, 1968.

Meadow KP, Trybus RJ: Behavioral and emotional problems of deaf children: an overview. In Bradford LJ, Hardy WG (eds): *Hearing and Hearing Impairment*. New York: Grune & Stratton, 1979.

Mecklenburg DJ (ed): Cochlear implants in children. *Semin Hear* 7:4, 1986.

Mecklenburg DJ: The Nucleus children's program. *Am J Otol* 8:436–442, 1987.

Mecklenburg DJ: Cochlear implants and rehabilitative practices. In Sandlin RE (ed): *Handbook of Hearing Aid Amplification*, Vol II. Boston: College-Hill Publishers, 1990, pp 179–202.

Melloni BJ: *Some Pathological Conditions of Eye, Ear, Throat: An Atlas*. Chicago: Abbott Laboratories, 1957.

Melnick M, Bixler D, Nance WE, et al: Familial branchio-oto-renal dysplasia. A new addition to the branchial arch syndrome. *Clin Genet* 9:25–34, 1976.

Melnick W, Eagles EL, Levine HS: Evaluation of a recommended program of identification audiometry with school-age children. *J Hear Disord* 29:3–13, 1964.

Meltzoff AN, Moore MK: Imitation of facial and manual gestures by human neonates. *Science* 198:75–78, 1977.

Mencher G, Gerber S: *Early Management of Hearing Loss*. New York: Grune & Stratton, 1981.

Mencher G, McCulloch B, Derbyshire A, et al: Observer bias as a factor in neonatal hearing screening. *J Speech Hear Res* 20: 27–34, 1977.

Mencher GT: Screening infants for auditory deficits: University of Nebraska Neonatal Hearing Project. *Audiology (Suppl)* 11:69, 1972.

Mencher GT (ed): *Early Identification of Hearing Loss*. Basel: S. Karger, 1976.

Mendel M: Clinical use of primary cortical responses. *Audiology* 19:1–15, 1980.

Mendel M, Goldstein R: The effect of test conditions on the early components of the averaged electroencephalic response. *J Speech Hear Res* 12:344, 1969.

Mendel M, Goldstein R: Stability of the early components of the averaged electroencephalographic response. *J Speech Hear Res* 14:829–840, 1971.

Mendel M, Hosick E, Windman T, et al: Audiometric comparison of the middle and late components of the adult auditory evoked potentials awake and asleep. *Electroencephalogr Clin Neurophysiol* 38:27–33, 1975.

Mendel MI: Middle and late auditory evoked potentials. In Katz J (ed): *Handbook of Clinical Audi-*

ology, ed 3. Baltimore: Williams & Wilkins, 1985, pp 565–581.

Mendelson T, Salamy A, Lenoir M, et al: Brain stem evoked potential findings in children with otitis media. *Arch Otolaryngol* 105:17–20, 1979.

Mengel MC, Konigsmark BW, Berlin CI, et al: Conductive hearing loss and malformed low-set ears as a possible recessive syndrome. *J Med Genet* 6:14–21, 1969.

Menyuk P: *The Development of Speech.* New York: Bobbs-Merrill, 1972.

Menyuk P: Predicting speech and language problems with persistent otitis media. In Kavanagh J (ed): *Otitis Media and Child Development.* Parkton, MD: York Press, 1986, pp 83–96.

Messer SB, Lewis M: Social class and sex differences in the attachment and play behavior of the year-old infant. Paper presented at the meeting of the Eastern Psychiatric Association, Atlantic City, NJ, 1970.

Metz O: The acoustic impedance measured on normal and pathological ears. *Acta Otolaryngol Suppl (Stockh)* 63, 1946.

Metz O: Threshold of reflex contractions of muscles of middle ear and recruitment of loudness. *Arch Otolaryngol* 55:536–543, 1952.

Miller AL, Lehman RH, Geretti R: Unusual audiological findings in cranial-metaphysical dysplasia. *Arch Otolaryngol* 89:861–864, 1969.

Miller GA, Nicely PE: Analysis of perceptual confusions among some English consonants. *J Am Speech Assoc* 27:338–352, 1955.

Miller JD, Rothenberg SJ, Eldredge DH: Preliminary observations on the effects of exposure to noise for seven days on the hearing and inner ear of the chinchilla. *J Acoust Soc Am* 50:1199–1203, 1971.

Mills JH: Noise and children: a review of literature. *J Acoust Soc Am* 58:768–779, 1975.

Mills JH, Gengel RW, Watson CS, et al: Temporary changes for the auditory system due to exposure to noise for one or two days. *J Acoust Soc Am* 48:524–530, 1970.

Milner B, Taylor I, Sperry RW: Lateralized suppression of dichotically presented digits after commissural section in man. *Science* 161:184–186, 1968.

Mindel ED, Vernon M: *They Grow in Silence: The Deaf Child and His Family.* Silver Spring, MD: National Association of the Deaf, 1971, p 23.

Mitchell C: Counseling for the parent. In Roeser R, Downs M (eds): *Auditory Disorders in School Children.* New York: Thieme-Stratton, 1981, ch 19.

Mitchell O, Richards G: Effects of various anesthetic agents on normal and pathological middle ears. *Ear Nose Throat J* 55:36, 1976.

Miyamoto RT, Yune HY, Rosevear WH: Klippel-Feil syndrome and associated ear deformities. *Am J Otol* 5:113–119, 1983.

Mizrahi EM, Dorfman LJ: Sensory evoked potentials: clinical applications in pediatrics. *J Pediatr* 97:1–10, 1980.

Moffat S: *Helping the Child Who Cannot Hear,* Public Affairs Pamphlet 479. The Public Affairs Committee, 381 Park Ave South, New York, NY, 1972.

Molfese DL: Left and right hemisphere involvement in speech perception: electrophysiological correlates. *Percept Psychophysics* 23:237–243, 1978.

Molfese DL: Hemispheric specialization for temporal information: implications for the perception of voicing cues during speech perception. *Brain Lang* 11:285–299, 1980.

Molfese DL, Freeman RB, Palermo DS: The ontogeny of brain lateralization for speech and nonspeech stimuli. *Brain Lang* 2:356–368, 1975.

Molfese DL, Hess TM: Hemispheric specialization for VOT perception in the pre-school child. *J Exp Child Psychol* 26:71–84, 1978.

Molfese DL, Molfese VJ: Hemisphere and stimulus differences are reflected in the cortical responses of newborn infants to speech stimuli. *Dev Psychol* 15:505–511, 1979.

Moller A: The sensitivity of the contraction of the tympanic muscles in man. *Ann Otol Rhinol Laryngol* 71:86–95, 1962.

Moller P: Hearing, middle ear pressure and otopathology in a cleft palate population. *Acta Otolaryngol (Stockh)* 92:521–528, 1981.

Moncur J: Judge reliability in infant testing. *J Speech Hear Res* 11:348–357, 1968.

Mondini C: Anatomica surdi nati sectio. In *DeBononiensi Scientarium et Artium Instituto atque Academia Comentarii,* Vol VII. Bonoia, 1791, pp 419–431.

Montandon PP: Auditory nerve potentials from ear canals of patients with otologic problems. *Ann Otol Rhinol Laryngol* 184:1, 165–168, 1975.

Moog JS, Geers AE: *Grammatical Analysis of Elicited Language—Simple Sentence Level.* St. Louis: Central Institute for the Deaf, 1979.

Moore JM, Thompson G, Thompson M: Auditory localization of infants as a function of reinforcement conditions. *J Speech Hear Disord* 40:29–34, 1975.

Moore JM, Wilson WR, Lillis KE, et al: Earphone auditory threshold of infants utilizing visual reinforcement auditory reinforcement (VR). Poster session, American Speech and Hearing Association meeting, Houston, TX, 1976.

Moore JM, Wilson WR, Thompson G: Visual reinforcement of head-turn responses in infants under twelve months of age. *J Speech Hear Disord* 42:328–334, 1977.

Moore MV: Speech, hearing and language in de Lange syndrome. *J Speech Hear Disord* 35:66–69, 1970.

Morrison JR, Stewart MA: A family study of the hyperactive child syndrome. *Biol Psychiatry* 3:189–195, 1971.

Morse PA: The discrimination of speech and nonspeech stimuli in early infancy. *J Exp Child Psychol* 14:477–492, 1972.

Mueller HG, Hawkins DB: Three important considerations in hearing aid selection. In Sandlin RE (ed): *Handbook of Hearing Aid Amplification,* Vol II. Boston: College-Hill Press, 1990, 31–60.

Mulac A, Gerber SE: Cardiovascular measures. In Gerber S (ed): *Audiometry and Infancy.* New York: Grune & Stratton, 1977.

Murai JI: The sounds of infants. *Studia Phonologica* 3:21–24, 1964.

Murphy KP: Development of hearing in babies. *Child Family* 1, 1962.

Murphy KP: A developmental approach to pediatric audiometry. *Hear Aid J* September 1979, pp 6–32.

Musselman CR, Lindsay PH, Wilson AK: An evaluation of recent trends in preschool programming for hearing-impaired children. *J Speech Hear Disord* 53:71–88, 1988.

Mussen EF: Hearing, listening, and attending: techniques and concepts in auditory training. In Roeser R, Downs M (eds): *Auditory Disorders in School Children.* New York: Thieme-Stratton, 1981, ch 17.

Mussen PH, Conger JJ, Kagan J: *Child Development and Personality.* New York: Harper & Row, 1969.

Myer CM, Farrer SM, Drake AF, Cotton RT: Perilymphatic fistulas in children: rationale for therapy. *Ear Hear* 10:112–116, 1989.

Myers FN, Stool S: The temporal bone in osteoporosis. *Arch Otolaryngol* 89:44–53, 1969.

Myklebust H: *Auditory Disorders in Children.* New York: Grune & Stratton, 1954.

Nagafuchi M: Development of dichotic and monaural hearing abilities in young children. *Acta Otolaryngol (Stockh)* 69:409–414, 1970.

Nager GT: Association of bilateral VIIIth nerve tumors with meningiomas in von Recklinghausen's disease. *Laryngoscope* 74:1220–1265, 1964.

Nager GT: Congenital aural atresia: anatomy and surgical management. In *Birth Defects, Part IX, Ear.* Baltimore: Williams & Wilkins, for National Foundation—March of Dimes, 1971.

Nahmias AJ: The TORCH complex. *Hosp Pract* 9:65–72, 1974.

Nahmias AJ, Norrild B: Herpes simplex virus 1 and 2, basic and clinical aspects. *DM* 25:10, 1979.

Nakazima S: A comparative study of the speech development of Japanese and American English in childhood. *Studia Phonologica* 3:27–39, 1962.

Nance WE: Symposium on Usher's Syndrome, Public Service Programs, Gallaudet College, Washington, DC, 1973.

Nassif R, Harboyan G: Madelung's deformity with conductive hearing loss. *Arch Otolaryngol* 91:175–178, 1970.

National Advisory Committee on Education of the Deaf: *Basic Education Rights for the Hearing Impaired.* Publication No (OE) 73-24001. Washington, DC: Office of Education, Dept of HEW, 1973.

National Center for Health Statistics: *Hearing Sensitivity and Related Findings Among Children,* US DHEW Pub No (HRA) 76–1046.

National Center for Health Statistics: *Hearing Sensitivity and Related Mental Findings Among Youths 12–17 Years,* US DHEW Pub No (HRS) 76–1636. Washington, DC: US Dept of HEW, 1975.

Naulty CM, Weiss IP, Herer G: Progressive sensorineural hearing loss in survivors of persistent fetal circulation. *Ear Hear* 7:74–77, 1986.

Naunton RF: The effect of hearing aid use upon the user's residual hearing. *Laryngoscope* 67:569–576, 1957.

Needleman H: Effects of hearing loss from early recurrent otitis media on speech and language development. In Jaffe B (ed): *Hearing Loss in Children.* Baltimore: University Park Press, 1977, ch 44.

Neff WD: The effects of partial section of the auditory nerve. *J Comp Physiol* 40:203–216, 1947.

Neff WD: Neural mechanisms of auditory discrimination. In Rosenblith WA (ed): *Sensory Communications.* Cambridge, MA: MIT Press, 1961, pp 259–278.

Neisser A: *Cognitive Psychology.* New York: Appleton-Century-Crofts, 1967.

Nelson JM: *Agnosia, Apraxia, Aphasia: Their Value in Cerebral Localization,* ed 2. New York: Hafner Publishing, 1948.

Nelson KB, Ellenberg J: Apgar scores of predictors of chronic neurologic disability. *Pediatrics* 68:36, 1981.

Nelson M, Scott CI: Engelmann's disease (a form of craniodiaphyseal dysplasia). *Birth Defects* 5(4):301, 1969.

Nelson SM, Berry RI: Ear disease and hearing loss among Navajo children—a mass survey. *Laryngoscope* 94:3, 316–323, 1984.

Neuman A, Molinelli P, Hochberg I: Post-meningitic hearing loss: report on three cases. *J Commun Disord* 14:105–111, 1981.

Newby H: *Audiology,* ed 2. New York: Appleton-Century-Crofts, 1964.

Nield T, Ramos AD, Warburton D: Late-onset hearing loss. *Pediatrics* 74:807–808, 1989.

Nield TA, Schrier S, Ramos AD, Platzker ACG, Warburton D: Unexpected hearing loss in high-risk infants. *Pediatrics* 78:3, 417–422, 1986.

Niemeyer W, Sesterhenn G: Calculating the hearing threshold from the stapedius reflex threshold for different sound stimuli. *J Aud Commun* 11:84, 1972.

Niswander P, Ruth R: Prediction of hearing sensitivity from acoustic reflexes in mentally retarded persons. *Am J Ment Defic* 81:474, 1977.

Nober IW: A study of classroom noise as a factor which affects the auditory discrimination performance of primary grade children. EdD thesis, University of Massachusetts, Amherst, MA. *Dissertation Abstracts,* 1973.

Nolte J: *The Human Brain: An Introduction to Its Functional Anatomy,* ed. 2. St. Louis: CV Mosby, 1988.

North FA: Chapter 4. In Frankenburg WK, Camp BW: *Pediatric Screening Tests.* Springfield, IL: Charles C Thomas, 1975.

Northcott W: Freedom through speech: every child's right. *Volta Rev* 83:162–181, 1981.

Northcott WH (ed): The hearing impaired child in a regular classroom: preschool, elementary and secondary years. Washington, DC: AG Bell Association for the Deaf, 1973.

Northcott WH: *Implications of Mainstreaming for the Education of Hearing Impaired Children in the 1980's.* Washington, DC: AG Bell Publications, 1979.

Northern JL, Bergstrom L: Impedance audiometry. *Eye Ear Nose Throat Monogr* 52:404–406, 1973.

Northern JL: Clinical application of acoustic impedance measurements. *Otolaryngol Clin North Am* (Symposium on Congenital Deafness) 4:359–368, 1971a.

Northern JL (ed): *Audiometric Assistant Training Guide.* US Department of HEW, Office of Education, Manpower Development and Training Program. Washington, DC: National Association of Hearing and Speech Agencies, 1971b.

Northern JL, Teter DL, Krug RF: Characteristics of manually communicating deaf adults. *J Speech Hear Disord* 36:71–76, 1971c.

Northern JL: Acoustic impedance in the pediatric population. In Bess F (ed): *Childhood Deafness: Causation, Assessment, and Management.* New York: Grune & Stratton, 1977a.

Northern JL: Impedance audiometry for otologic diagnosis. In Shambaugh C, Shea J (eds): *Proceedings of the Shambaugh Fifth International Workshop on Middle Ear Microsurgery and Fluctuant Hearing Loss*. Huntsville, AL: Strode Publishers, 1977b, p 75.

Northern JL: Hearing aids and acoustic impedance measurements. *Monogr Contemp Audiol* 1:2, 1978a.

Northern JL: Advanced techniques for measuring middle ear function. *Pediatrics* 61:761, 1978b.

Northern JL: Impedance screening in special populations: state of the art. In Harford ER, Bess FH, Bluestone CD, et al (eds): *Impedance Screening for Middle Ear Disease in Children*. New York: Grune & Stratton, 1978c, pp 229–248.

Northern JL: Acoustic impedance measures in the Down's population. *Semin Speech Lang Hear* 1:81, 1980a.

Northern JL: Clinical measurement procedures in impedance audiometry. In Jerger J, Northern JL (eds): *Clinical Impedance Audiometry*, ed 2. Acton, MA: American Electromedics Corp, 1980b, ch 2.

Northern JL: Impedance measurements with distinctive groups. In Jerger J, Northern JL (eds): *Clinical Impedance Audiometry*, ed 2. Acton, MA: American Electromedics Corp, 1980c, ch 10.

Northern JL: Impedance screening: an integral part of hearing screening. *Ann Otol Rhinol Laryngol* 89 (Suppl 68):3, 1980d.

Northern JL: Impedance measurements in infants. In Mencher G, Gerber S (eds): *Early Management of Hearing Loss*. New York: Grune & Stratton, 1981, p 131.

Northern JL: Selection of children for cochlear implantation. *Semin Hear* 7:341–347, 1986.

Northern JL: Recent developments in acoustic immittance measurements in children. In Bess F (ed): *Hearing Impairment in Children*. Parkton, MD: York Press, 1988.

Northern JL, Gabbard SA, Kinder DL: Pediatric considerations in selecting and fitting hearing aids. In Sandlin RE (ed): *Handbook of Hearing Aid Amplification, Vol II*. Boston: College Hill Press, 1990, pp 113–132.

Northern JL, Grimes A: Introduction to acoustic impedance. In Katz J (ed): *Handbook of Clinical Audiology*, ed 2. Baltimore: Williams & Wilkins, 1978.

Northern JL, Lemme M: Hearing and auditory disorders. In Shames GH, Wiig EH (eds): *Human Communication Disorders: An Introduction*, ed 2. Columbus, OH: Charles E Merrill, 1986, pp 416–444.

Northern JL, Walker D, Downs MP, Guggenheim S: Office screening for communicative disorders in young children. In Gottlieb M, Williams J (eds): *Developmental Behavior Disorders*, Vol 2. New York: Plenum Publishing, 1989, pp 213–231.

Nwaesei CG, Van Aerde JV, Boyden M, Perlman M: Changes in auditory brainstem responses in hyperbilirubinemic infants before and after exchange transfusion. *Pediatrics* 74:5, 800-803, 1984.

Oller DK: Infant vocalizations and the development of speech. *Allied Health & Behavioral Sciences* I: 523–549, 1978.

Oller DK: The emergence of the sounds of speech in infants. In Komshian-Yeni G, Kavanagh JF, Ferguson CA (eds): *Child Phonology: Production*, Vol 1. New York: Academic Press, 1980, pp 83–112.

Oller DK, Eilers RE, Vengara KC, LaVoie EC: Tactual vocoders in a multisensory program training speech production and reception. *Volta Rev* 88:21–36, 1986.

Oller DK, Payne SL, Gavin WJ: Tactile speech perception by minimally trained deaf subjects. *J Speech Hear Res* 23:769–778, 1980.

Olsen WO: The effects of noise and reverberation on speech intelligibility. In Bess F, Freeman B, Sinclair J (eds): *Amplification in Education*. Washington, DC: AG Bell, 1981.

Olsen WO, Hawkins DB, Van Tasell DJ: Representations of the long-term spectra of speech. *Ear Hear* (Suppl) 8(5): 100–108, 1987.

Olsen WO, Matkin ND: Speech audiometry. In Rintelmann WF (ed): *Hearing Assessment*. Baltimore: University Park Press, 1979, ch 5.

Olson A, Hipskind N: The relation between levels of pure tones and speech which elicit the acoustic reflex and loudness discomfort. *J Audit Res* 13:71–76, 1973.

Omerod FC: The pathology of congenital deafness. *J Laryngol Otol* 74:919, 1960.

Opheim O: Loss of hearing following the syndrome of Van Der Hoeve-De Kleyn. *Acta Otolaryngol (Stockh)* 65:337, 1968.

Orchik DJ, Dunn JW, McNutt L: Tympanometry as a predictor of middle ear effusion. *Arch Otolaryngol* 104:4–6, 1978a.

Orchik DJ, Morff R, Dunn JW: Impedance audiometry in serous otitis media. *Arch Otolaryngol* 104:409–412, 1978b.

Osberger MJ, Hesketh LJ: Speech and language disorders related to hearing impairment. In Lass et al (eds): *Handbook of Speech-Language Pathology & Audiology*. Toronto: BC Decker, 1988, pp 858–885, ch 29.

Owens E, Kessler DK (eds): *Cochlear Implants in Young Deaf Children*. Boston: College-Hill Press, 1989.

Owens E, Telleen CC: Speech perception with hearing aids and cochlear implants. *Audecibel*, Summer 1981.

Oyler RF, Oyler AL, Matkin ND: Warning: a unilateral hearing loss may be detrimental to a child's academic career. *Hear J* 40(9):18–22, 1987.

Oyler RF, Oyler AL, Matkin ND: Unilateral hearing loss: demographics and educational impact. *Language, Speech & Hearing in Schools* 19:201–210, 1988.

Ozdamar O, Kraus N: Auditory middle-latency response in human. *Audiology* 22:34–49, 1983.

Ozdamar O, Kraus N, Stein L: Auditory brainstem responses in infants recovering from bacterial meningitis: audiological evaluation. *Otolaryngol Head Neck Surg* 109:13–18, 1982.

Ozdamar O, Stein L: Auditory brainstem response (ABR) in unilateral hearing loss. *Laryngoscope* 91:565–574, 1981.

Paden EP, Matthies ML, Novak MA: Recovery from OME-related phonologic delay following tube placement. *J Speech Hear Disord* 54:94–100, 1989.

Paden EP, Novak MA, Beiter AL: Predictors of phonologic inadequacy in young children prone to otitis media. *J Speech Hear Disord* 52:232–242, 1987.

Palfrey JS: Commentary: P.L. 94–142: the Education for all Handicapped Children Act. *J Pediatr* 97:417–419, 1980.

Paluszny MJ: *Autism: A Practical Guide for Parents and Professionals.* Syracuse, NY: Syracuse University Press, 1979.

Palva T, Pulkinen K: Mastoiditis. *J Laryngol Otol* 73:573–577, 1959.

Panjvani ZFK, Henshaw JB: CMV in the perinatal period. *Am J Dis Child* 135:56–60, 1981.

Pannbacker M: Hearing loss and cleft palate. *Cleft Palate J* 6:50–56, 1969.

Pantke OA, Cohen MM Jr: The Waardenburg syndrome. *Birth Defects* 7(7): 147–152, 1971.

Paparella M: Middle ear effusions: definitions and terminology. *Ann Otol Rhinol Laryngol* 85 (suppl 25):8–11, 1976.

Paparella MM: Differential diagnosis of childhood deafness. In Bess F (ed): *Childhood Deafness: Causation, Assessment and Management.* New York: Grune & Stratton, 1977.

Paparella MM, Brady DR: Sensorineural hearing loss in chronic otitis media and mastoiditis. *Arch Otolaryngol* 74:108–115, 1970.

Paparella MM, Suguira S: The pathology of suppurative labyrinthitis. *Ann Otol Rhinol Laryngol* 75:554–586, 1967.

Pappas DG: Hearing impairments and vestibular abnormalities among children with subclinical cytomegalovirus. *Ann Otol Rhinol Laryngol* 92:552–557, 1983.

Pappas DG, Schaibly M: A two-year diagnostic report on bilateral sensorineural hearing loss in infants and children. *Am J Otol* 5:339–343, 1984.

Paradise JL: Pediatrician's view of middle ear effusions: more questions than answers. *Ann Otol Rhinol Laryngol* 85 (suppl 25):20, 1976a.

Paradise JL: Management of middle ear effusions in infants with cleft palate. *Ann Otol Rhinol Laryngol* 85 (suppl 25):285–288, 1976b.

Paradise JL: Otitis media in infants and children. *Pediatrics* 65:917–943, 1980.

Paradise JL: Otitis media during early life: how hazardous to development? A critical review of the evidence. *Pediatrics* 68(6):869–873, 1981.

Paradise JL: Editorial retrospective: tympanometry. *N Engl J Med* 307:1074–1076, 1982.

Paradise JL, Bluestone CD: Diagnosis and management of ear disease in cleft palate infants. *Trans Am Acad Ophthalmol Otolaryngol* 73:709–714, 1969.

Paradise JL, Bluestone CD: Early treatment of the universal otitis media of infants with cleft palate. *Pediatrics* 53:48–54, 1974.

Paradise JL, Rogers KD: On otitis media, child development, and tympanostomy tubes: new answers or old questions? *Pediatrics* 77:1, 88–91, 1986.

Paradise JL, Smith C: Impedance screening for preschool children, state of the art. In Harford E, Bess F, Bluestone C (eds): *Impedance Screening for Middle Ear Disease in Children.* New York: Grune & Stratton, 1978.

Paradise JL, Smith C: Impedance screening for preschool children. *Ann Otol* 88:56, 1979.

Paradise JL, Smith C, Bluestone CD: Tympanometric detection of middle ear effusion in infants and young children. *Pediatrics* 58:198–206, 1976.

Parnes LS, McCabe BF: Perilymph fistula: an important cause of deafness and dizziness in children. *Pediatrics* 80:4, 524–528, 1987.

Pashayan H, Fraser FC, McIntyre J, et al: Bilateral aplasia of the tibia, polydactyly and absent thumbs in a father and daughter. *J Bone Joint Surg* 53B:495–499, 1971.

Pashayan HM, Pruzansky S, Solomon L: The EEC syndrome. *Birth Defects* 10(7):105–127, 1974.

Pass RF, Stasno S: Outcome of symptomatic congenital cytomegalovirus infection results of long-term longitudinal follow-up. *Pediatrics* 66:758–762, 1980.

Passchier-Vermeer W: Noise-induced hearing loss from exposure to intermittent and varying noise. In *Proceedings of the International Congress on Noise as a Public Health Problem, v.s. EPA.* Washington, DC: Office of Noise Abatement Control, 1973, pp 169–200.

Patten BM: *Human Embryology,* ed 3. New York: McGraw-Hill, 1968.

Paul R, Cohen D, Breg W, Watson M, Herman S: Fragile X syndrome: its relations to speech and language disorders. *J Speech Hear Disord* 49:326–336, 1984.

Pauls DL, Shaywitz SE, Kramer PL, Shaywitz BA, Cohen DJ: Demonstration of vertical transmission of attention deficit disorder. *Ann Neurol* 14:363–367, 1983.

Pearson AA, Jacobson AD, VanCalcar R, et al: *The Development of the Ear.* Rochester, NY: Section on Instruction, Home Study Courses, American Academy of Otolaryngology and Ophthalmology, 1970.

Pelton S, Shurin P, Klein J: Persistence of middle ear effusion after otitis media. *Pediatr Res* 11:504, 1977.

Peltzman P, Kitterman JA, Ostwald PF, et al: Effects of incubator noise on human hearing. *J Audit Res* 10:335–339, 1970.

Penfield W, Rasmussen T: *The Cerebral Cortex of Man.* New York: Hafner Publishing, 1968.

Penfield W, Roberts L: *Speech and Brain Mechanisms.* Princeton, NJ: Princeton University Press, 1959.

Perrin JM, Charney E, MacWhinney JB, et al: Sulfioxazole as chemoprophylaxis for recurrent otitis media. *N Engl J Med* 291:664–667, 1974.

Peterson GE, Lehiste I: Revised CNC lists for auditory testing. *J Speech Hear Disord* 27:62, 1962.

Peterson RA: Ophthalmology. In Jaffe B (ed): *Hearing Loss in Children.* Baltimore: University Park Press, 1977.

Petroff MA, Simmons FB, Winzelberg J: Two emerging perilymph fistula "syndromes" in children. *Laryngoscope* 96:498–501, 1986.

Picton RW, Hillyard SA, Krausz H, et al: Human auditory evoked potentials; I. Evaluation of components. *Electroencephalogr Clin Neurophysiol* 36:179–190, 1974.

Pinheiro ML, Musiek FE (eds): *Assessment of Central Auditory Dysfunction: Foundations and Clinical Correlates.* Baltimore: Williams & Wilkins, 1985.

Pollack D: The development of an auditory function. *Otolaryngol Clin North Am* (Symposium on Congenital Deafness) 4:319–335, 1971.

Pollack D: Amplification and auditory/verbal training for the limited hearing infant 0 to 30 months. *Semin Speech Lang Hear* 3:52–67, 1982.

Pollack M: *Amplification for the Hearing-Impaired*, ed 3. New York: Grune & Stratton, 1988.

Pollock KC: The influence of hearing impairment. In Bzoch K (ed): *Communicative Disorders Related to Cleft Lip & Palate*. Boston: Little, Brown, 1979, pp 77–86.

Polvogt LM, Crowe SJ: Anomalies of the cochlea in patients with normal hearing. *Arch Otol Rhinol Laryngol* 46:579–591, 1937.

Popelka GR: *Hearing Assessment with the Acoustic Reflex*. New York: Grune & Stratton, 1981.

Popper A, Fay R (eds): *Comparative Studies of Hearing in Vertebrates* (Proceedings in Life Science Series). Berlin: Springer-Verlag, 1980.

Portmann M, Aran JM: Electro-cochleographic sur le nourrissons et le jeune infant. *Acta Otolaryngol (Stockh)* 71:253–261, 1971.

Potts P, Greenwood J: Hearing aid monitoring. *Lang Speech Hear Serv Sch* 14:163, 1983.

Premack AJ, Premack D: Teaching language to an ape. *Sci Am* 227:92–99, 1972.

Preus M, Fraser FC: The lobster-claw defect with ectodermal defects, cleft lip-palate, tear duct anomaly and renal anomalies. *Clin Genet* 4:369–375, 1973.

Primus MA: Response and reinforcement in operant audiometry. *J Speech Hear Disord* 52:294–299, 1987.

Primus MA, Thompson G: Response strength of young children in operant audiometry. *J Speech Hear Res* 28:539–547, 1985.

Proctor CA, Proctor B: Understanding hereditary nerve deafness. *Arch Otolaryngol* 85:23–40, 1967.

Pumper RW, Yamashiroya HM: *Essentials of Medical Virology*. Philadelphia: WB Saunders, 1975.

Queen S, Moses F, Wood S, et al: The use of immittance screening by the Kansas City, MO public school district. *Semin Speech Lang Hear* 2:119, 1981.

Querleu Q, Renard Z, Crepin G: Perception auditive et reactivite foetale aux stimulations sonores. *J Gynecol Obstet Biol Reprod* 10:307–314, 1981.

Quigley SP: Environment and communication in the language development of deaf children. In Bradford LJ, Hardy WG (eds): *Hearing and Hearing Impairment*. New York: Grune & Stratton, 1979.

Quisling RW, Moore GR, Jahrsdoerfer RA, et al: Osteogenesis imperfecta: a study of 160 family members. *Arch Otolaryngol* 105: 207–211, 1979.

Ramaiya JJ: A study of binaural hearing aid performance. Unpublished MS degree thesis, directed by McConnell F, Vanderbilt University, Nashville, TN, 1971.

Rampp D: *Proceedings of the Memphis State University First Annual Symposium on Auditory Processing and Learning Disabilities*. Memphis State University, TN, 1972.

Rappaport B, Tait C: Acoustic reflex threshold measurement in hearing aid selection. *Arch Otolaryngol* 102:129–132, 1976.

Rawlings BW, Trybus R: Personnel, facilities and services available in schools and classes for hearing impaired children in the United States. *Am Ann Deaf* 123:99–121, 1978.

Redding J, Hargest T, Minsky S: How noisy is intensive care? *Crit Care Med* 5:275, 1977.

Reddy JK, Rao MS: Imitation of facial and manual gestures by human neonates. *Science* 198:75–79, 1977.

Reed D, Dunn W: Epidemiologic studies of otitis media among Eskimo children. *Public Health Rep* 85:699–706, 1970.

Reed D, Struve S, Maynard JE: Otitis media and hearing deficiency among Eskimo children; a cohort study. *Am J Public Health* 57:1657–1662, 1967.

Reed WB, Store VM, Boder E, et al: Pigmentary disorders in association with congenital deafness. *Arch Dermatol* 95:176–186, 1967.

Rees N: The speech pathologist and the reading process. *Asha* 16:225–258, 1974.

Rees NS: Auditory processing factors in language disorders: the view from Procrustes' bed. *J Speech Hear Disord* 38:304–315, 1973.

Rees NS: Saying more than we know: is auditory processing a meaningful concept? In Keith RW (ed): *Central Auditory and Language Disorders in Children*. Houston, TX: College-Hill Press, 1981.

Refetoff A, DeWind LT, DeGroot LJ: Familial syndrome combining deaf-mutism, stippled epiphyses, goiter and abnormally high PBI. *J Clin Endocrinol* 27:279–294, 1967.

Reichert TJ, Cantekin EI, Riding KH, et al: Diagnosis of middle ear effusions in young infants by otoscopy and tympanometry. In Harford ER, Bess FH, Bluestone CD, et al (eds): *Impedance Screening for Middle Ear Disease in Children*. New York: Grune & Stratton, 1978, pp 69–79.

Reid DK, Hresko W: *A Cognitive Approach to Learning Disabilities*. New York: McGraw Hill, 1981.

Reilly K, Owens E, Uken D, et al: Progressive hearing loss in children: hearing aids and other factors. *J Speech Hear Disord* 46:328–334, 1981.

Reisen AH: The development of visual perception in man and chimpanzee. *Science* 106:107–108, 1947.

Reisen AH: Effects of stimulus deprivation on the development and atrophy of the visual sensory system. *Am J Orthopsychiatry* 30:23–36, 1960.

Reynolds BS, Newsom CD, Lovaas OI: Auditory overselectivity in autistic children. *J Abnormal Child Psych* 2(4):253–262, 1974.

Reynolds D, Stagno S, Stubbs G, et al: Inapparent congenital cytomegalovirus infection with elevated cord IgM levels. *N Engl J Med* 290:292, 1974.

Richards BW, Rundle AT: A familial hormonal disorder associated with mental deficiency, deaf mutism and ataxia. *J Ment Defic Res* 3:33–35, 1959.

Richards GB, Mitchell OC, Speight IL: Effects of pentobarbital on intra-aural muscle reflexes in retarded children. *Eye Ear Nose Throat Monogr* 54:69–72, 1975.

Richards IDG, Robert CJ: The at risk infant. *Lancet* 2:711–714, 1967.

Richardson S: A pediatrician's view. In Keith RW (ed): *Central Auditory and Language Disorders in Children*. Houston, TX: College-Hill Press, 1981.

Ridgeway J: Dumb children. *Saturday Review*, August 1969, pp 19–21.

Riedner ED, Levin S, Holliday MJ: Hearing patterns in dominant osteogenesis imperfecta. *Otolaryngol Head Neck Surg* 106:737–740, 1980.

Riggs W Jr, Seibert J: Cockayne's syndrome; roentgen findings. *Am J Roentgenol* 116:623–633, 1972.

Riko K, Hydge ML, Alberti PW: Hearing loss in early infancy: incidence, detection and assessment. *Laryngoscope* 95:137–145, 1985.

Rimoin DL, Edgerton MT: Genetic and clinical heterogeneity in the oral-facial-digital syndrome. *J Pediatr* 71:94–102, 1967.

Rines D, Stelmachowicz P, Gorga M: An alternate method for determining functional gain of hearing aids. *J Speech Hear Res* 27:4, 627–633, 1984.

Rintelmann W, Harford E, Burchfield S: A special case of auditory localization: CROS for blind persons with unilateral hearing loss. *Arch Otolaryngol* 91:284–288, 1970.

Rintelmann WF: Auditory manifestations of Alport's Disease syndrome. *Trans Am Acad Ophthalmol Otolaryngol* 82:375–387, 1976.

Rintelmann WF, Bess FH: High-level amplification and potential hearing loss in children. In Bess FH (ed): *Hearing Impairment in Children*. Parkton, MD: York Press, 1988, pp 278–309.

Rintelmann WF, Borus J: Noise-induced hearing loss and rock and roll music. *Arch Otolaryngol* 88:57–65, 1968.

Rittmanic PA: The mentally retarded and mentally ill. In Rose DE: *Audiological Assessment*. Englewood Cliffs, NJ: Prentice-Hall, 1971, pp 369–401.

Roberts DB: The etiology of bullous myringitis and the role of mycoplasmas in ear disease. A review. *Pediatrics* 65:761–766, 1980.

Roberts JL, Davis H, Phon GL, et al: Auditory brainstem responses in preterm neonates: maturation and follow-up. *J Pediatr* 101:257–263, 1982.

Robertson EO, Peterson JL, Lamb LE: Relative impedance measurements in young children. *Arch Otolaryngol* 88:162–168, 1968.

Robillard TAJ, Gersdorff MCH: Prevention of pre- and perinatal acquired hearing defects: part 1—study of causes. *J Audit Res* 26:207–237, 1986.

Robinette MS, Rhodes DP, Marion MW: Effects of secobarbital on impedance audiometry. *Arch Otolaryngol* 100:351–354, 1974.

Robinson A: Genetic and chromosomal disorders. In Kempe CH, Silver HK, O'Brien D (eds): *Current Pediatric Diagnosis and Treatment*. Los Altos, CA: Lange Medical Publications, 1972.

Robinson DO, Sterling GR: Hearing aids and children in school: a follow-up study. *Volta Rev* 82:229, 1980.

Robinson GC, Wildervanck LS, Chiang TP: Ectrodactyly, ectodermal dysplasia and cleft lip-palate. Its association with conductive hearing loss. *J Pediatr* 82:107–109, 1973.

Roeser R, Downs M: *Auditory Disorders in School Children: The Law, Identification, Remediation*. New York: Thieme-Stratton, 1981.

Roeser RJ: Tactile aids for the profoundly deaf. *Semin Hear* 6:279–298, 1985.

Roeser RJ, Campbell JC, Daly D: Recovery of auditory function following meningitic deafness. *J Speech Hear Disord* 40:405–411, 1975.

Roeser RJ, Glorig A, Gerken GM, et al: A hearing aid malfunction detection unit. *J Speech Hear Disord* 42:351–357, 1977.

Rogers BO: Microtic, lop, cup, and protruding ears. *Plast Reconstr Surg* 41:208–231, 1968.

Rojskjaer C: Presented at the Fifth International Congress of Audiology, Bonn, West Germany, 1960.

Roland P, Finitzo T, Friel-Patti S, Clinton-Brown KC, Stephens KT, Brown O, Coleman JM: Otitis media: incidence, duration and hearing status. *Otolaryngol Head Neck Surg* 115:1049–1053, 1989.

Romer AS: *The Vertebrate Body*, ed 5. Philadelphia: WB Saunders, 1977.

Rood SR, Stool SE: Otologic survey of schools for the deaf. *Am Ann Deaf* 126:113–117, 1981.

Rose DE, Galambos R, Hughes JR: Microelectrode studies of the cochlear nuclei of the cat. *Johns Hopkins Med J* 104:211–251, 1959.

Rosenberg AL, Bergstrom L, Troost BT, et al: Hyperuricemia and neurologic defects. *N Engl J Med* 282:992–997, 1970.

Rosenberg P, Swogger-Rosenberg J: Hearing screening. In Lass NJ, McReynolds LV, Northern JL, et al (eds): *Speech, Language and Hearing*. Philadelphia: WB Saunders, 1982, ch 42.

Rosenblum SM, Arick JR, Krug D, Stubbs E, Young N, Pelson R: Auditory brainstem evoked responses in autistic children. *J Autism Dev Disord* 10:215–225, 1980.

Rosenthal W: Auditory and linguistic interaction in developmental aphasia: evidence from two studies of auditory processing. *Papers and Reports in Child Language Development*, No 4. Stanford University, Committee on Linguistics, 1972.

Rosner J, Simon D: *The Auditory Analysis Test: An Initial Report*. Learning Research & Development Center, University of Pittsburgh, PA, 1970.

Ross M: Changing concepts in hearing aid candidacy. *Eye Ear Nose Throat Monogr* 48:27–34, 1969.

Ross M: Classroom acoustics and speech intelligibility. In Katz J (ed): *Handbook of Clinical Audiology*. Baltimore: Williams & Wilkins, 1972.

Ross M: Hearing aid selection for the preverbal hearing-impaired child. In Pollack M (ed): *Amplification for the Hearing-Impaired*. New York: Grune & Stratton, 1975, ch 6.

Ross M: *Hard of Hearing Children in Regular Schools*. Englewood Cliffs, NJ: Prentice-Hall, 1982.

Ross M, Calvert DR: Guidelines for audiology programs in educational settings. *Volta Rev* 79:153–161, 1977.

Ross M, Lerman J: Hearing aid usage and its effect upon residual hearing: a review of the literature and an investigation. *Arch Otolaryngol Head Neck Surg* 86:57–62, 1967.

Ross M, Lerman J: A picture identification test for hearing-impaired children. *J Speech Hear Res* 13:44–53, 1970.

Ross M, Seewald RC: Hearing aid selection and evaluation with young children. In Bess F (ed): *Hearing Impairment in Children*. Parkton, MD: York Press, 1988, pp 190–213.

Ross M, Tomassetti C: Hearing aid selection for preverbal hearing-impaired children. In Pollack M (ed): *Amplification for the Hearing-Impaired*, ed 2. New York: Grune & Stratton, 1980, ch 6.

Ross N, Giolas T (eds): *Auditory Management of Hearing-Impaired Children*. Baltimore: University Park Press, 1978.

Rossi DF, Sims DG: Acoustic reflex measurement in the severely and profoundly deaf. *Audiol Hear Educ* 3:6–8 1977.

Roswell F, Chall J: *Auditory Blending Test*. New York: Essay Press, 1963.

Roush J, Tait C: Pure-tone and acoustic immittance screening for preschool-aged children: an examination of referral criteria. *Ear Hear* 6:5, 245–250, 1985.

Rozin P, Poritsky S, Sotsky R: American children with reading problems can easily learn to read English represented by Chinese characters. *Science* 171:1264–1267, 1971.

Ruben RJ: Anatomical diagnosis of non-conductive deafness by physiological tests. *Arch Otolaryngol* 78:47–51, 1963.

Ruben RJ: Current treatment of otitis media. *Pediatrics* 77:1, 59–60, 1986.

Ruben RJ, Bordley JE, Nager GT, et al: Human cochlear responses to sound stimuli. *Ann Otol Rhinol Laryngol* 169:459, 1960.

Ruben RJ, Knickerbocker GG, Sekula J, et al: Cochlear microphonics in man. *Laryngoscope* 69:665, 1959.

Ruben RJ, Lieberman AT, Bordley JE: Some observations on cochlear potentials and nerve action potentials in children. *Laryngoscope* 5:545, 1962.

Ruben RJ, Rapin I: Plasticity of the developing auditory system. *Ann Otol Rhinol Laryngol* 89:303–311, 1980.

Ruben RJ, Math R: Serous otitis media associated with sensorineural hearing loss in children. *Laryngoscope* 88:1139–1154, 1978.

Rubin M: Hearing aids for infants and toddlers. In Rubin M (ed): *Hearing Aids: Current Developments and Concepts.* Baltimore: University Park Press, 1976, pp 95–102.

Rubin M: Serous otitis media in severely to profoundly hearing-impaired children, ages 0 to 6. *Volta Rev* 80:81–85, 1978.

Ruckelshaus W: *Report to the President and Congress on Noise.* Rep Admin EPA US Senate Document 92–63, 1972, pp 38–39, ch 1.

Rupp RR: An approach to the communicative needs of the very young hearing impaired child. *J Acad Rehab Audiol* 4:11–22, 1971.

Ruppert ES, Buerk E, Pfordresher MF: Hereditary hearing loss with saddle nose and myopia. *Arch Otolaryngol* 92:95–98, 1970.

Rutter M: Diagnosis and definition. In Rutter M, Schopler E (eds): *Autism: A Reappraisal of Concepts and Treatments.* New York: Plenum Press, 1978, pp 1–26.

Ryan AF, Dallos P: Physiology of the cochlea. In Northern JL (ed): *Hearing Disorders.* Boston: Little, Brown, 1984, ch 22.

Sachs R, Burkhard M: Insert earphone pressure response in real ears and couplers [abstract]. *J Acoust Soc Am* 52 (part 1):183, 1972.

Sachs RM, Miller JD, Grant K: Perceived magnitude of electroacoustic pulses. *Percept Psychophysics* 28:255–262, 1980.

Safer DJ, Allen RD: *Hyperactive Children: Diagnosis and Management.* Baltimore: University Park Press, 1976.

Saito H, Kishimoto S, Furuta M: Temporal bone findings in a patient with Mobius Syndrome. *Ann Otol* 90:80–84, 1981.

Sak RJ, Ruben RJ: Effects of recurrent middle ear effusion in preschool years on language and learning. *J Dev Behav Pediatr* 3:7–11, 1982.

Salamy A, Mendelson T, Tooley W, et al: Contrasts in brainstem function between normal and high-risk infants in early postnatal life. *Early Hum Dev* 4:179–185, 1980.

Salamy A, Eldredge L, Tooley WH: Neonatal status and hearing loss in high-risk infants. *J Pediatr* 114:847–852, 1989.

Salem JM, Fell BP: The impact of P.L. 94-142 on residential schools for the deaf: a follow-up to the 1997 survey. *Am Ann Deaf* 133:68–75, 1988.

Samples JM, Franklin B: Behavioral responses in 7 to 9 month old infants to speech and non-speech stimuli. *J Audit Res* 18:115–123, 1978.

Sanchez-Longo LP, Forster FM: Clinical significance of impairment of sound localization. *Neurology* (Minneap) 8:119–125, 1958.

Sanders D: Noise conditions in normal school classrooms. *Except Child* 31:344–353, 1965.

Sanders DA: *Auditory Perception of Speech. An Introduction to Principles and Problems.* Englewood Cliffs, NJ: Prentice-Hall, 1977.

Sanderson-Leepa M, Rintelmann WF: Articulation functions and test-retest performance of normal-hearing children on three speech discrimination tests: WIPI, PBK-50, and NU Auditory Test No. 6. *J Speech Hear Disord* 41:503, 1976.

Sandlin RE: *Handbook of Hearing Amplification*, vols I and II. Boston: College-Hill Press, 1988, 1990.

Sando I, Baker B, Black PO, et al: Persistence of stapedial artery in trisomy 13–15 syndrome. *Arch Otolaryngol* 96:441–447, 1972.

Sando I, Bergstrom L, Wood RP, et al: Temporal bone findings in trisomy 18 syndrome. *Arch Otolaryngol* 72:913–924, 1968.

Sando I, Hemenway WG, Morgan RW: Histopathology of the temporal bones in mandibulofacial dysostosis. *Trans Am Acad Ophthalmol Otolaryngol* 72:913–924, 1968.

Sando I, Wood RP: Congenital middle ear anomalies. *Otolaryngol Clin North Am* (Symposium) 4:291–318, 1971.

Sarno CN, Clemis JD: A workable approach to the identification of neonatal hearing impairment. *Laryngoscope* 90:1313–1320, 1980.

Sass-Lehrer M, Bodner-Johnson B: Public Law 99-457: a new challenge to early intervention: *Am Ann Deaf* 134:2, 71–77, 1989.

Saunders FA, Hill WA, Simpson CA: Speech perception via the tactile mode. In Levitt H, Pickett JM, Houde RA (eds): *Sensory Aids for the Hearing Impaired.* New York: IEEE Press, 1980.

Savage-Rumbaugh ES, Rumbaugh DM: Chimpanzee problem comprehension: insufficient evidence. *Science* 206:1201–1202, 1979.

Savage-Rumbaugh ES, Rumbaugh DM, Smith ST, et al: Reference: the linguistic essential. *Science* 210:922–925, 1980.

Schafer IA, Scriver CR, Efron ML: Familial hyperprolinemia, cerebral dysfunction, and renal anomalies occurring in a family with hereditary nephropathy and deafness. *N Engl J Med* 267:51–60, 1962.

Scharfenaker SK, Snelling TM, Ferrer-Vinent ST: The otitis media clinic: a multidisciplinary approach to the treatment of otitis media in children. *Rocky Mountain Journal of Communication Disorders*, Fall 1987, pp 3–7.

Schein JD: *The Deaf Community Study of Washington, DC.* Washington, DC: Gallaudet College Press, 1965.

Schein JD, Delk MT: *The Deaf Population of the United States*. Silver Spring, MD: National Association of the Deaf, 1974.

Scheiner AP: Perinatal asphyxia: factors which predict developmental outcome. *Dev Med Child Neurol* 22:102–104, 1980.

Scherz RG, Graga JR, Reichelderfer TE: A typical example of 13–15 trisomy in a Negro boy. *Clin Pediatr* 11:246–248, 1972.

Schildroth A: Recent changes in the educational placement of deaf students. *Am Ann Deaf* 133:2, 61–67, 1988.

Schlesinger HS: The deaf pre-schooler and his many faces. In Lloyd L (ed): *International Seminar of the Vocational Rehabilitation of Deaf Persons*, Washington, DC: US Department of Health, Education and Welfare, 1973.

Schlesinger HS, Meadow KP: Emotional support to parents. In Lillie DL (ed): *Monograph on Parent Programs in Child Development Centers*. Chapel Hill, NC: University of North Carolina, 1972a, pp 13–25.

Schlesinger HS, Meadow KP: *Sound and Sign; Childhood Deafness and Mental Health*. Berkeley: University of California Press, 1972b.

Schneider B, Trehub SE, Bull D: High-frequency sensitivity in infants. *Science* 207:1003–1004, 1980.

Schuchman G: An ear level hearing aid for bilateral atresia. *Arch Otolaryngol* 94:87–88, 1971.

Schuknecht HF: Pathology of sensorineural deafness of genetic origin. In McConnel F, Ward PH (eds): *Deafness in Childhood*. Nashville, TN: Vanderbilt University Press, 1967, pp 69–90.

Schuknecht HF: *Pathology of the Ear*. Cambridge, MA: Harvard University Press, 1974.

Schulman CA: Effects of auditory stimulation on heart rate in premature infants as a function of level of arousal, probability of CNS damage, and conceptional age. *Dev Psychobiol* 2:172–183, 1970a.

Schulman CA: Heart rate response habituation in high-risk premature infants. *Psychophysiology* 6:690–694, 1970b.

Schulman CA, Wade G: The use of heart rate in the audiological evaluation of non-verbal children; II. Clinical trials on an infant population. *Neuropediatrics* 2:197–205, 1970.

Schulman-Galambos C, Galambos R: Brain stem evoked response audiometry in newborn hearing screening. *Arch Otolaryngol* 105:86–90, 1979.

Schuyler V, Rushmer N: *Parent-Infant Habilitation*. Portland, OR: IHR Publications, 1987.

Schwartz D: Current status of techniques for screening and diagnosis of middle ear disease in children. In Bluestone C, Fria TJ, Arjona SK, et al (eds): Controversies in Screening for Middle Ear Disease and Hearing Loss in Children. *Pediatrics* 77:59–74, 1986.

Schwartz D, Schwartz R: Validity of acoustic reflectometry in detecting middle ear effusion. *Pediatrics* 29:739–742, 1987.

Schwartz DM, Larson V: Hearing aid selection and evaluation procedures in children. In Bess F (ed): *Childhood Deafness: Causation, Assessment and Management*. New York: Grune & Stratton, 1977, pp 217–233.

Schwartz DM, Larson VD: A comparison of three hearing aid evaluation procedures for young children. *Arch Otolaryngol* 103:401–406, 1977.

Schwartz DM, Pratt RE, Schwartz JA: Auditory brainstem responses in preterm infants: evidence of peripheral maturity. *Ear Hear* 10:1, 14–22, 1989.

Schwartz DM, Schwartz RH: A comparison of tympanometry and acoustic reflex measurements for detecting middle ear effusion in infants below seven months of age. In Harford ER, Bess FH, Bluestone CD, et al (eds): *Impedance Screening for Middle Ear Disease in Children*. New York: Grune & Stratton, 1978a, pp 91–96.

Schwartz DM, Schwartz RH: Acoustic and otoscopic findings in young children with Down's syndrome. *Arch Otolaryngol* 104:652, 1978b.

Schwartz DM, Schwartz RH: Tympanometric findings in young infants with middle ear effusion: some further observations. *Int J Pediatr Otolaryngol* 2:67–72, 1980.

Schwartz RH, Stool SE, Rodriguez W, et al: Acute otitis media: toward a more precise definition. *Clin Pediatr* 20:549–554, 1981a.

Schwartz RH, Rodriguez W, Khan W: Persistent purulent otitis media. *Clin Pediatr* 20:445–447, 1981b.

Schwartz S: *Choices in Deafness: A Parent's Guide*. Montgomery, MD: Woodbine House, 1987.

Seewald R, Ross M: Amplification for young hearing-impaired children. In Pollack MC (ed): *Amplification for the Hearing-Impaired*, ed 3. New York: Grune & Stratton, 1988, pp 213–267.

Seewald RC, Ross M, Spiro MK: Selecting amplification characteristics for young hearing-impairing children. *Ear Hear* 6:1, 48–53, 1985.

Seitz MR, Kisiel DL: Hearing aid assessment and the auditory brainstem response. In Sandlin RE (ed): *Handbook of Hearing Aid Amplification*, vol II. Boston: College Hill Press, 1990, pp 203–224.

Sell EJ, Gaines JA, Gluckman C, Williams E: Persistent fetal circulation, neurodevelopmental outcome. *Am J Dis Child* 139:25–28, 1985.

Semel E, Wiig E: Comprehension of syntactic structures and critical verbal elements by children with learning disabilities. *J Learn Disabil* 8:46–53, 1975.

Senturia BH: Classification of middle ear effusions: definitions and terminology. *Ann Otol Rhinol Laryngol* 85 (suppl 25):15–17, 1976.

Senturia BH, Bluestone CD, Klein JO, et al: Report of the Ad Hoc Committee on Definition and Classification of Otitis Media and Otitis Media with Effusion. *Ann Otol Rhinol Laryngol* 89 (suppl 68):3–4, 1980.

Sever JL, Ellenberg JH, Ley AC, Madden DL, Fuccillo DA, Tzan NR, Edmonds DM: Toxoplasmosis: maternal and pediatric findings in 23,000 pregnancies. *Pediatrics* 82:2, 1988.

Shah CP, Chandler D, Dale R: Delay in referral of children with impaired hearing. *Volta Rev* 80:207, 1978.

Shallop JK, Mecklenburg DJ: Technical aspects of cochlear implants. In Sandlin RE (ed): *Handbook of Hearing Aid Amplification*, vol I. Boston: College-Hill Press, 1988, pp 265–280.

Shankweiler D, Studdert-Kennedy M: Hemispheric specialization for speech perception. *J Acoust Soc Am* 48:579–594, 1970.

Shanon E, Himelfarb M, Gold S: Auditory function in Friedreich's ataxia. *Otolaryngol Head Neck Surg* 107:254–256, 1981.

Shapiro I, et al: Ossicular discontinuity with intact acoustic reflex. *Otolaryngol Head Neck Surg* 107:576–578, 1981.

Shaywitz SE: Early recognition of educational vulnerability: technical report. State Department of Education, Hartford, CT, 1986.

Shaywitz SE, Shaywitz BA: Attention deficit disorder: current perspectives. *Pediatr Neurol* 3:129–135, 1987.

Shemen LJ, Mitchell DP, Farkashidy J: Cockayne syndrome—an audiologic and temporal bone analysis. *Am J Otol* 5:300–307, 1984.

Shimizu H: Editorial: clinical use of auditory brain stem response; issues and answers. *Ear Hear* 2:3–4, 1981.

Shinefield HR: Cytomegalovirus in utero. In Bergsma D (ed): *Birth Defects: Atlas and Compendium*. Baltimore: Williams & Wilkins, 1973, p 324.

Shulman K: Hydrocephaly. In Bergsma D (ed): *Birth Defects: Atlas and Compendium*. Baltimore: Williams & Wilkins, 1973.

Shurin PA, Pelton SI, Donner A, et al: Persistence of middle ear effusion after acute otitis media in children. *N Engl J Med* 300:1121–1123, 1979.

Shurin PA, Pelton SI, Klein JO: Otitis media in the newborn infant. *Ann Otol Rhinol Laryngol* 85 (suppl 25):216–222, 1976.

Siegel J, McCracken G: Aminoglycoside ototoxicity in children. In Lerner SA, Matz GJ, Hawkins JE (eds): *Aminoglycoside Ototoxicity*. Boston: Little, Brown, 1981, ch 24.

Siegel-Sadewitz V, Shprintzen R: The relationship of communication disorders to syndrome identification. *J Speech Hear Disord* 47:338–354, 1982.

Siegenthaler B, Haspiel G: *Development of Two Standardized Measures of Hearing for Speech by Children*. Washington, DC: Cooperative Research Program, Project 2372, United States Office of Education, 1966.

Siervogel RM, Roche AF, Johnson DL, et al: Longitudinal study of hearing in children; II. Cross-sectional studies of noise exposure as measured by dosimetry. *J Acoust Soc Am* 71:372–377, 1982.

Silman S (ed): *The Acoustic Reflex: Basic Principles and Clinical Applications*. New York: Academic Press, 1984.

Silman S, Gelfand S, Emmer M: Acoustic reflex in hearing loss identification and prediction. *Semin Hear* 8:379–390, 1987.

Silman S, Gelfand S, Silverman C: Late-onset auditory deprivation: effects of monaural versus bilateral hearing aids. *J Acoust Soc Am* 76(5): 1357–1362, 1984.

Silver HK: The de Lange syndrome. *Am J Med Dis Child* 108:523–529, 1964.

Silverman SR, Lane HS: Deaf children. In David H, Silverman SR (eds): *Hearing and Deafness*, ed 3. New York: Holt, Rinehart & Winston, 1970.

Simmons D: Developing your child's individualized educational program. *Shhh*, November/December 1988, pp 26–30.

Simmons FB: Automated hearing screening test for newborns: the Crib-o-gram. In Mencher G (ed): *Early Identification of Hearing Loss*. Basel: Karger, 1976, pp 171–180.

Simmons FB: Patterns of deafness in newborns. *Laryngoscope* 90:448, 1980a.

Simmons FB: Diagnosis and rehabilitation of deaf newborns, part II. *Asha* 22:475, 1980b.

Simmons FB: Comment on hearing loss in graduates of a tertiary intensive care nursery. *Ear Hear* 3:188, 1982.

Simmons FB, Glattke TJ: Electrocochleography. In Bradford L (ed): *Physiological Measures of the Audio-Vestibular System*. New York: Academic Press, 1975, ch 5.

Simmons FB, Russ FN: Automated newborn hearing screening, the Crib-o-gram. *Arch Otolaryngol* 100:1–7, 1974.

Singh S, Bresman MJ: Menkes' "kinky hair syndrome" (trichopolio dystrophy). *Am J Dis Child* 125:572–578, 1973.

Singh SP, Rock EH, Shulman A: Klippel-Feil syndrome with unexplained conductive hearing loss. *Laryngoscope* 79:113–117, 1969.

Siqueland E, Hoenigmann N: Infant responsivity to pure tone stimulation. *J Audit Res* 13:321–327, 1973.

Siqueland ER, DeLucia CA: Visual reinforcement of nonnutritive sucking in human infants. *Science* 165:1144–1146, 1969.

Sitnick V, Rushmer N, Arpan R: *Parent-Infant Communication: A Program of Clinical and Home Training for Parents and Hearing-Impaired Infants*. Portland, OR: Good Samaritan Hospital and Medical Center, 1978.

Skinner MW: The hearing of speech during language acquisition. *Otolaryngol Clin North Am* 11:631–650, 1978.

Skinner MW: *Hearing Aid Evaluation*. Englewood Cliffs, NJ: Prentice Hall, 1988.

Skinner P, Glattke TJ: Electrophysiologic response audiometry: state-of-the-art. *J Speech Hear Disord* 42:170–198, 1977.

Sly RM, Sambie MF, Fernandes DA, et al: Tympanometry in kindergarten children. *Ann Allergy* 44:1–7, 1980.

Smith D, Wilson A: *The Child With Down's Syndrome (Mongolism): Causes, Characteristics and Acceptance*. Philadelphia: WB Saunders, 1973.

Smith DW: The number 18 trisomy syndrome. *J Pediatr* 60:513, 1962.

Smith K, Hodgson W: The effects of systematic reinforcement on the speech discrimination responses of normal and hearing-impaired children. *J Audit Res* 10:110–117, 1970.

Smith MWF: Beyond "COR": new technology in pediatric behavioral testing. *Hear Instrum* 38(9):19–21, 1987.

Smith RD: The use of developmental screening tests by primary-care pediatricians. *J Pediatr* 93:524–527, 1978.

Snell RS: *Clinical Embryology for Medical Students*, ed 2. Boston: Little, Brown, 1975.

Snyder L: Have we prepared the language-disordered child for school? *Topics in Language Disorders & Learning Disabilities* 1:29–49, 1980.

Sohmer H, Feinmesser M: Cochlear action potentials recorded from the external ear in man. *Ann Otolaryngol* 76:427–435, 1967.

Sparkes RS, Graham CB: Camurati-Englemann disease. Genetics and clinical manifestations with a review of the literature. *J Med Genet* 9:73–85, 1972.

Sparks D, Kuhl P, Edmonds A, Gray G: Investigating the MESA (Multipoint Electrotactile Speech Aid): the transmission of segmental features of speech. *J Acoust Soc Am* 63:246–257, 1978.

Sparks S: Speech and language in fetal alcohol syndrome. *Asha* 26:27–31, 1984.

Sparling J, Lewis I: *Learning Games for the First Three Years.* New York: Berkley Books, 1979.

1968, Special Education for Handicapped Children. First Annual Report. Washington, DC: US Department of Health, Education and Welfare, 1968.

Sperry R: Some effects of disconnecting the cerebral hemispheres. *Science* 217:1223–1226, 1982.

Spitz RA: *A Genetic Field Theory of Ego Formation: Its Implications for Pathology.* New York: International Universities Press, 1959.

Spoendlin H: The innervation of the organ of Corti. *J Laryngol Otol* 81:717–738, 1967.

Spoendlin H: Innervation patterns in the organ of Corti of the cat. *Acta Otolaryngol (Stockh)* 67:239–254, 1969.

Spoendlin H: Congenital stapes ankylosis and fusion of carpal and tarsal bones as a dominant hereditary syndrome. *Acta Otol Rhinol Laryngol* 206:173–179, 1974.

Spoor A, Eggermont JJ: Electrocochleography as a method of objective audiogram determination. In Hirsh SK, Eldredge DH, Hirsh IJ, et al (eds): *Hearing and Davis.* St. Louis, MO: Washington University Press, 1976, pp 411–418.

Sprague B, Wiley T, Goldstein R: Tympanometric and acoustic-reflex studies in neonates. *J Speech Hear Res* 28:265–272, 1985.

Spreng M, Keidal WG: Separierung von Cerebroaudiogramm (CAG), Neuroaudiogramm (NAG), und Otoaudiogramm (OAG) in der Objecktiven Audiometrie. *Arch Klin Exp Ohren Nasen Kehlkopfheilk* 189:225, 1967.

Spring DR, Dale PA: Discrimination of linguistic stress in early infancy. *J Speech Hear Res* 20:224–232, 1977.

Stach BA, Jerger JF: Immittance measures in auditory disorders. In Jacobson J, Northern J (eds): *Diagnostic Audiology.* Boston: College-Hill Press, 1990, ch 6.

Stagno S: Auditory and visual defects resulting from symptomatic and sub-clinical congenital CMV and toxoplasma infections. *Pediatrics* 59:669–678, 1977.

Stagno, S, Pass RF, Dworsky ME, Henderson RE, Moore EG, Walton P, Alford CA: Congenital cytomegalovirus infection: the relative importance of primary and recurrent maternal infection. *N Engl J Med* 306:945–949, 1982.

Staller SJ, Beiter AL, Brimacombe JA, Mecklenburg DJ: Pediatric performance with the Nucleus 22-Channel Cochlear Implant System. *Am J Otol,* in press.

Staller SJ, Lunde LKM: Auditory brainstem response and electrocochleography. In Lass N, McReynolds LV, Northern JL, Yoder DE (eds): *Handbook of Speech-Language Pathology and Audiology.* Toronto: BC Decker, 1166–1187, 1988.

Standards and Recommendations for Hospital Care for Newborn Infants, ed 6. Evanston, IL: American Academy of Pediatrics, Committee of Fetus and Newborn, 1977.

Stanley RJ, Puritz EM, Birggaman RA, et al: Sensory radicular neuropathy. *Arch Dermatol* 111:760–762, 1975.

Stark EW, Borton TE: Klippel-Feil syndrome and associated hearing loss. *Arch Otolaryngol* 97:415–419, 1973.

Stark R: Stages of speech development in the first year of life. In Yeni-Komshiow G, Kavanagh J, Ferguson C (eds): *Child Phonology: Volume 1—Production.* New York: Academic Press, 1980.

Stark RE, Tallal P: Selection of children with specific language deficits. *J Speech Hear Disord* 46:114–122, 1981.

Starr A, Amlie RN, Martin WH, et al: Development of auditory function in newborn infants revealed by auditory brainstem potentials. *Pediatrics* 60:831–839, 1977.

Stein L, Ozdamar O, Kraus N, et al: Follow-up of infants screened by auditory brainstem response (ABR) in the NICU. *J Pediatr* 103: 447–453, 1983a.

Stein L, Clark S, Kraus N: The hearing-impaired infant: patterns of identification and habilitation. *Ear Hear* 4:5, 232–236, 1983b.

Stein L, Ozdamar O, Schnabel M: Auditory brainstem responses (ABR) with suspected deaf-blind children. *Ear Hear* 1(2):30–40, 1981.

Stein LK, Jabaley T: Early identification and parent counseling. In Stein L, Mendel E, Jabaley T (eds): *Deafness and Mental Health.* New York: Grune & Stratton, 1981.

Stein LK, Jabaley T, Spitz R, Stoakley D, McGee T: The hearing-impaired infants: patterns of identification and habilitation revisited. *Ear Hear* 11:3, 201–205, 1990.

Stein LK, Kraus N: Auditory evoked potentials with special populations. *Semin Hear* 9:1, 35–46, 1988.

Stein LK, Kraus N, Ozdamar O, Cartee C, Jabaley T, Jeantet C, Reed N: Hearing loss in an institutionalized mentally retarded population. *Otolaryngol Head Neck Surg* 113:32–35, 1987.

Stevens PR, Macfayden WAL: Familial incidence of juvenile diabetes mellitus progressive optic atrophy, and neurogenic deafness. *Br J Ophthalmol* 56:496–500, 1972.

Stevens S, House A (1972): Cited in Eimas P: Speech perceptions in early infancy. In *From Sensation to Cognition.* New York: Academic Press, 1975, vol 2.

Stewart JM, Bergstrom L: Familial hand abnormality and sensori-neural deafness, a new syndrome. *J Pediatr* 78:102–110, 1971.

Stewart TC: *Counseling Parents of Exceptional Children.* Columbus, OH: CE Merrill, 1978.

Stockard JE, Stockard JJ, Westmoreland B, et al: Brainstem auditory evoked responses: normal variation as a function of stimulus and subject characteristics. *Arch Neurol* 36:823–831, 1979.

Stockard JE, Westmoreland BF: Technical considerations in the recording and interpretation of the brainstem auditory evoked potential for neonatal neurologic diagnosis. *Am J EEG Technol* 21:31–54, 1981.

Stoel-Gammon C, Otomo K: Babbling development of hearing impaired and normally hearing subjects. *J Speech Hear Disord* 51:33–41, 1986.

Stokoe WC, Casterline DC, Croneberg CG: *A Dictionary of American Sign Language on Linguistic Prin-*

ciples. Washington, DC: Gallaudet College Press, 1965.

Stool S, Anticaglia J: Electric otoscopy—a basic pediatric skill. *Clin Pediatr* 12:420, 1973.

Stool SE: Diagnosis and treatment of ear disease in cleft palate children. In Bzoch K: *Communicative Disorders Related to Cleft Lip and Palate.* Boston: Little, Brown, 1971, pp 264–273.

Stool SE, Marshak G, Stanievich J, et al: *Otitis Media: Current Concepts, Incidence, Pathogenesis, Diagnosis and Management.* Pamphlet companion to an exhibit, Department of Otolaryngology, Children's Hospital, Pittsburgh, PA, 1982.

Storer T: *General Zoology,* ed 6. New York: McGraw-Hill, 1979.

Stratton HJM: Gonadal dysgenesis and the ears. *J Laryngol Otol* 79:343–346, 1965.

Strauss M: A clinical pathologic study of the hearing loss in congenital cytomegalovirus infection. *Laryngoscope* 95:951–962, 1985.

Strauss M, Davis GL: Viral disease of the labyrinth: review of the literature and discussion of the role of cytomegalovirus in congenital deafness. *Ann Otol Rhinol Laryngol* 82:577–583, 1973.

Stream RW, Stream KS: Counseling the parents of the hearing impaired child. In Martin F (ed): *Pediatric Audiology.* Englewood Cliffs, NJ: Prentice-Hall, 1978, ch 9.

Stubblefield HH, Young CE: Central auditory dysfunction in learning disabled children. *J Learn Disabil* 8:89–94, 1975.

Stuckless ER (ed): Deafness and rubella: infants in the 60's, adults in the 80's. *Am Ann Deaf* 125:959, 1980.

Studdert-Kennedy M: Speech perception. In Lass N (ed): *Contemporary Issues in Experimental Phonetics.* New York: Academic Press, 1976.

Studdert-Kennedy M, Shankweiler D: Hemispheric specialization for speech perception. *J Acoust Soc Am* 48:579–594, 1970.

Studebaker GA, Hochberg I (eds): *Acoustical Factors Affecting Hearing Aid Performance.* Baltimore: University Park Press, 1980.

Sugar HS: The oculoauriculovertebral dysplasia syndrome of Goldenhar. *Am J Ophthalmol* 62:678, 1966.

Sullivan RF: An acoustic coupling-based classification system for hearing aid fittings. *Hearing Instruments,* Part I, 36:9, 25, 1985; Parts II and III, 36:12, 17, and 36:12, 20, 1985.

Survey of Hearing Impaired Children and Youth: Washington, DC: Gallaudet College Office of Demographic Studies, series D, vol 9, 1971.

Suzuki T, Ogiba Y: Conditioned orientation audiometry. *Arch Otolaryngol* 74:192–198, 1961.

Sylvester PE: Some unusual findings in a family with Friedreich's ataxia. *Arch Dis Child* 33:217–221, 1958.

Sylvester PE: Spino-cerebellar degeneration, hormonal disorder, hypogonadism, deaf-mutism, and mental deficiency. *J Ment Defic Res* 16:203–214, 1972.

Szatmari P, Offord DR, Boyle MH: Ontario Child Health Study: prevalence of attention deficit disorder with hyperactivity. *J Child Psychol Psychiat* 30:219–230, 1989.

Tallal P: Rapid auditory processing in normal and disordered language development. *J Speech Hear Res* 19:561–571, 1976.

Tallal P: Auditory perceptual factors in language and learning disabilities. In Knights R, Bakker D (eds): *The Neuropsychology of Learning Disabilities.* Baltimore: University Park Press, 1976.

Tallal P: Neuropsychological research approaches to the study of central auditory processing. *Hum Commun Canada* 9:17–22, 1985.

Tallal P, Piercy M: Defects of non-verbal auditory perception in children with developmental aphasia. *Nature* 241:468–469, 1973a.

Tallal P, Piercy M: Developmental aphasia: impaired rate of nonverbal processing as a function of sensory modality. *Neuropsychologia* 11:389–398, 1973b.

Tallal P, Piercy M: Developmental aphasia: rate of auditory processing and selective impairment of consonant perception. *Neuropsychologia* 12:83–93, 1974.

Tallal P, Piercy M: Developmental aphasia: the perception of brief vowels and extended stop consonants. *Neuropsychologia* 13:69–74, 1975.

Tanguay PE, Edwards RM: Electrophysiological studies of autism: the whisper of the bang. *J Autism Dev Disord* 12:2, 177–184, 1982a.

Tanguay PE, Edwards RM, Buchwald J, Schwafel J, Allen V: Auditory brainstem responses in autistic children. *Arch Gen Psychiatry* 39:174–180, 1982b.

Taylor AI: Autosomal trisomy syndromes: a detailed study of twenty-seven cases of Edward's syndrome and twenty-seven cases of Patan's syndrome. *J Med Genet* 5:227, 1968.

Taylor D, Mencher GT: Neonatal responses, the effect of infant state and auditory stimuli. *Arch Otolaryngol* 95:120–124, 1972.

Teele D, Teele J: Detection of middle ear effusion by acoustic reflectometry. *J Pediatrics* 104:832–838, 1984.

Teele DW, Klein JO, Rosner BA: Epidemiology of otitis media in children. *Ann Otol Rhinol Laryngol* 89 (suppl 68):5–6, 1980a.

Teele DW, Klein JO, Rosner B: Epidemiology of otitis media in children. Proceedings of 2nd International Symposium: Recurrent Advances in Otitis Media with Effusion. *Ann Otol Rhinol Laryngol* (suppl 68) 89(3): (part 2):5–6, 1980b.

Teele DW, Klein JO, Rosner BA, Greater Boston Otitis Media Study Group: Otitis media with effusion during the first three years of life and development of speech and language. *Pediatrics* 74:2, 282–287, 1984.

Templin M: Vocabulary problems of the deaf child. *Int Audiol* 5:349, 1966.

Terrace HS, Pettito LA, Sanders RJ, et al: Can an ape create a sentence? *Science* 206:891–902, 1979.

Tervoort B: Development of languages and the critical period. The young deaf child: identification and management. *Acta Otolaryngol Suppl (Stockh)* 206:247–251, 1964.

Thompson CI, Stafford MR, Cullen JK, et al: Interaural intensity differences in dichotic speech perception. Paper presented at the 83rd meeting of the Acoustical Society of America, Buffalo, NY, 1972.

Thompson G: Structure and function of the central auditory system. *Semin Hear* 4:81–95, 1983.

Thompson G, Folsom R: Hearing assessment of at-risk infants. *Clin Pediatr* 20:257–267, 1981.

Thompson G, Folsom RC: A comparison of two conditioning procedures in the use of visual reinforcement audiometry (VRA). *J Speech Hear Disord* 49:241–245, 1984.

Thompson G, Wilson W, Moore J: Application of visual reinforcement audiometry (VRA) to low-functioning children. *J Speech Hear Disord* 44:80–90, 1979.

Thompson M, Thompson G: Responses of infants and young children as a function of auditory stimuli and test month. *J Speech Hear Res* 15:699–707, 1972.

Thompson M, Thompson G: Mainstreaming: a closer look. *Am Ann Deaf* 126:395–401, 1981.

Thompson M, Thompson G, Vethivelu S: A comparison of audiometric test methods for 2-year-old children. *J Speech Hear Disord* 54:174–179, 1989.

Thompson P, Northern J: Audiometric monitoring of patients treated with ototoxic drugs. In Lerner SA, Matz GJ, Hawkins JE (eds): *Aminoglycoside Ototoxicity*. Boston: Little, Brown, 1981, ch 15.

Thompson RC Jr, Gaull GE, Horwitz SJ, et al: Hereditary hyperphosphatasia. Studies of three siblings. *Am J Med* 47:209–219, 1969.

Thomsen J, Tos M: Spontaneous improvement of secretory otitis—a long-term study. *Acta Otolaryngol* 92:493–499, 1981.

Thomsen KA, Terkildsen K, Arnfred J: Middle ear pressure during anesthesia. *Arch Otolaryngol Head Neck Surg* 82:609, 1965.

Thorner M, Remein OR: *Principles and Procedures in the Evaluation of Screening for Disease*, Public Health Service Publication #846. Washington, DC: Public Health Monograph N., 1967.

Tibbling L: The rotatory nystagmus response in children. *Acta Otolaryngol (Stockh)* 68:459–467, 1969.

Tietz W: A syndrome of deaf-mutism associated with albinism showing dominant autosomal inheritance. *Am J Hum Genet* 15:259–264, 1963.

Titche LL, Windrem EO, Searmel WL: Hearing aids and hearing deterioration. *Ann Otol Rhinol Laryngol* 86:357, 1977.

Torgersen AM, Kringlen E: Genetic aspects of temperamental differences in infants: a study of same-sexed twins. *J Am Acad Child Psychol* 17:433–444, 1978.

Tos M: Spontaneous improvement of secretory otitis and impedance screening. *Otolaryngol Head Neck Surg* 106:345–349, 1980a.

Tos M: Treatment of cholesteatoma in children. *Am J Otol* 4:189, 1983.

Townsend T, Olsen C: Performance of new hearing aids using the ANSI S3.22-1976 standard. *J Speech Hear Disord* 47:376, 1982.

Townsend T, Wavrek D: Clinical use of ANSI hearing aid measurements. *Asha* 25:25–30, 1983.

Trehub SE, Bull D, Schneider BA: Infants' detection of speech in noise. *J Speech Hear Res* 24:202–206, 1981.

Trehub SE, Schneider BA, Endman M: Developmental changes in infants' sensitivity to octave-band noises. *J Exp Child Psychol* 29: 282–293, 1980.

Trevarthen C: Early attempts at speech. In Levin R: *Child Alive*. Garden City, NY: Anchor Press/Doubleday, 1975.

Turner G: A second family with renal, vaginal and middle ear anomalies. *J Pediatr* 76:641, 1970.

Turner RG: Recommended guidelines for infant screening: analysis, *Asha* 32:9, 57–61, 1990.

Turnure C: Response to voice of mother and stranger by babies in the first year. Paper presented at meeting of the Society for Research in Child Development, Santa Monica, CA, March 1969.

Ueda K, Hisanaga S, Nishida Y, et al: Low birthweight and congenital rubella syndrome. *Clin Pediatr* 20:730–733, 1981.

US Dept of HEW, Nat'l Center for Health Statistics: *Hearing Levels of Children by Demographic and Socioeconomic Characteristics*, pub no (HSM) 72-1025. Washington, DC: Government Printing Office, 1972.

US Dept of HEW, Office of Education: Education of Handicapped Children: Assistance to States. *Federal Register*, November 29, 1976, vol 41, no 230.

Uzgiris IC: Socio-cultural factors in cognitive development. In Haywood HC (ed): *Social-Cultural Aspects of Mental Retardation*. New York: Appleton-Century, 1970.

Uzgiris IC, Hunt, JMcV: An instrument for assessing infant psychological development. Mimeographed paper, Psychological Development Laboratory, University of Illinois, Urbana-Champaign, IL, 1966.

Vaughan V, McKay RJ, Behrman R: *Nelson Textbook of Pediatrics*, ed 11. Philadelphia: WB Saunders, 1979.

Ventry IM: Research design issues in studies of effects of middle ear effusion. *Pediatrics* 71:644, 1983.

Vernon J: Meningitis and deafness: the problem, its physical, audiological, and educational manifestations in deaf children. *Laryngoscope* 77:1856–1874, 1967.

Vernon M: Meningitis and deafness: the problem, its physical, audiological, and educational manifestations in deaf children. *Laryngoscope* 77:1856–1874, 1967.

Vernon M: *Multiply Handicapped Deaf Children*. Research Monograph, Council for Exceptional Children, 1–112, 1969.

Vernon M, Hicks D: Relationship of rubella, *Herpes simplex*, cytomegalovirus and certain other viral disabilities. *Am Ann Deaf* 125:529–534, 1980.

Vernon M. Klein N: Hearing impairment in the 1980's. *Hear Aid J* 35:17, 1982.

Vernon M, Prickett H: Mainstreaming: issues and a model plan. *Audiol Hear Educ* 2:5–11, 1976.

Vienny H, Despland PA, Lutschg J, Deonna T, Dutoit-Marco ML, Gander C: Early diagnosis and evolution of deafness in childhood bacterial meningitis: a study using brainstem auditory evoked potentials. *Pediatrics* 73:579–586, 1984.

Vogel S: Syntactic abilities in normal and dyslexic children. *J Learn Disabil* 7:103–110, 1974.

Volkmar FR, Cohen DJ: Infantile autism and the pervasive developmental disorders. *Developmental & Behavioral Pediatrics* 7(5):324–329, 1986.

Voron DA, Hatfield HH, Kalkhoff RK: Multiple lentigines syndrome. *Am J Med* 60:447–456, 1976.

Vulliamy DG, Normandale PA: Craniofacial dysostosis in a Dorset family. *Arch Dis Child* 41:375, 1966.

Vuorenkoski V, Wasz-Hockert O, Lind J, et al: Training the auditory perception of some specific types of abnormal pain cry in newborn and young infants. Quarterly Program Statistical Report; Speech Transcription Laboratory, Royal Institute of Technology, Stockholm, No. 4, 1971, pp 37–48.

Vuori M, Lahikainen EA, Peltonen T: Perceptive deafness in connection with mumps. *Acta Otolaryngol (Stockh)* 55:231–236, 1962.

Wachs TD, Uzgiris IC, Hunt JMcV: Cognitive development in infants to different age levels and from different environmental backgrounds: an exploratory investigation. *Merrill-Palmer J Behav Dev* 17:283–317, 1971.

Wahl RA, Dick M: Congenital deafness with cardiac arrhythmia: the Jervell and Lange-Nielsen syndrome. *Am Ann Deaf* 125:34, 1980.

Walden BE, Demorest ME, Hepler EL: Self-report approach to assessing benefit derived from amplification. *J Speech Hear Res* 27:49–56, 1984.

Waldon EF: Audio-reflexometry in testing hearing of very young children. *Audiology* 12:14–20, 1973.

Walker D, Downs MP, Gugenheim S, Northern JL: Early language milestone scale and language screening of young children. *Pediatrics* 83(2):284–288, 1989.

Walker ML, Cervette MJ, Newberg N, Moss SD, Storrs BB: Auditory brainstem responses in neonatal hydrocephalus. *Concepts Pediatr Neurosurg* 7:142–152, 1987.

Walker WG: Renal tubular acidosis and deafness. *Birth Defects* 7(4):126, 1971.

Wallace IF, Gravel JS, McCarton CM, Stapells DR, Bernstein RS, Ruben RJ: Otitis media, auditory sensitivity, and language outcomes at one year. *Laryngoscope* 98:64–70, 1988.

Ward PH, Lindsay JR, Warner NE: Cytomegalic inclusion disease affecting the temporal bone. *Laryngoscope* 75:628–636, 1965.

Warren WS, Stool SE: Otitis media in low birth weight infants. *J Pediatr* 79:740–743, 1971.

Watson DO: *Talk with Your Hands.* Winneconne, WI, 1964.

Weatherby L, Bennett M: The neonatal acoustic reflex. *Scand Audiol* 9:103–110, 1980.

Weber B: Validation of observer judgments in behavioral observation audiometry. *J Speech Hear Disord* 34:350–355, 1969.

Weber B: Comparison of two approaches to behavioral observation audiometry. *J Speech Hear Res* 13:823–825, 1970.

Weber H: Colorado's statewide hearing screening program utilizing visual reinforcement audiometry. *Hear Instrum* 38(9):22–24, 1987.

Weber HJ, McGovern FJ, Zink D: An evaluation of 1000 children with hearing loss. *J Speech Hear Disord* 32:343–354, 1967.

Webster DB, Webster M: Neonatal sound deprivation affects brainstem auditory nuclei. *Arch Otolaryngol* 103:392–396, 1977.

Webster DB, Webster M: Effects of neonatal conductive loss on brainstem auditory nuclei. *Ann Otol Rhinol Laryngol* 88:684–688, 1979.

Webster DB, Webster M: Mouse brainstem auditory nuclei development. *Ann Otol Rhinol Laryngol* 89 (suppl 68):254–256, 1980.

Wegman M: Annual summary of vital statistics—1986. *Pediatrics* 80(6):817–827, 1987.

Weiner R, Koppelman J: From birth to five: serving the youngest handicapped children. Alexandria, VA: Capitol Publications, 1987.

Weinstein RL, Kliman B, Scully RE: Familial syndrome of primary testicular insufficiency with normal virilization, blindness, deafness, and metabolic abnormalities. *N Engl J Med* 281:969–977, 1969.

Weir RH: Some questions on the child's learning of phonology. In Smith F, Miller G (eds): *The Genesis of Language.* Cambridge, MA: MIT Press, 1966, pp 153–169.

Weiss KL, Goodwin MW, Moores DF: Characteristics of young deaf children and early intervention programs. Research Report 91, Department of HEW, Bureau of Education for the Handicapped, 1975.

Wender EH: Learning disabilities in children. *Pediatr Rev* 3:91–98, 1981.

Wepman Test of Auditory Discrimination: Language Research Associates, 1958.

Wetherby AM, Koegal R, Mendel M: Central auditory nervous system dysfunction in autistic individuals. *J Speech Hear Res* 24:420–429, 1981.

Wever EG, Bray CW: Auditory nerve impulses. *Science* 71:215, 1930.

Wever EG, Lawrence M: *Physiological Acoustics.* Princeton, NJ: Princeton University Press, 1954.

Wever EG, Neff WD: A further study of the effects of partial section of the auditory nerve. *J Comp Physiol Psychol* 40:217–226, 1947.

Whitely RJ: The natural history of H.S.V. infection of mother and newborn. *Pediatrics* 66:489–494, 1980.

Wiig E, Semel E: *Language Disabilities in Children and Adolescents.* Columbus, OH: Merrill, 1976.

Wiig E, Semel E: *Language Assessment and Intervention for the Learning Disabled.* Columbus, OH: Merrill, 1980.

Willeford JA: Central auditory function in children with learning disabilities. *Audiol Hear Educ* 2:12–20, 1976.

Willeford JA, Burleigh JM: *Handbook of Central Auditory Processing Disorders in Children.* New York: Grune & Stratton, 1985.

Williams A, Williams M, Walker C, et al: The Robin anomalad (Pierre Robin syndrome)—follow-up study. *Arch Dis Child* 56:663–668, 1981.

Wilson L, Doehring D, Hirsh I: Auditory discrimination learning by aphasic and non-aphasic children. *J Speech Hear Res* 3:130–137, 1960.

Wilson MD, Evans MB, Dawson RL, et al: Disturbed children in special schools. *Spec Educ Forward Trends* 4:8–10, 1977.

Wilson WR, Folson RC, Widen JE: Hearing impairment in Down's syndrome children. Paper presented at the Elks 1982 International Symposium, The Multiply Handicapped Hearing Impaired Child, Edmonton, Canada, 1982.

Wilson WR, Moore JM, Thompson G: Sound-field auditory thresholds of infants utilizing visual reinforcement audiometry (VRA). Paper read at the American Speech and Hearing Association Annual Convention, Houston, TX, 1976.

Wilson WR, Thompson G: Behavioral audiometry. In Jerger J (ed): *Pediatric Audiology,* San Diego: College-Hill Press, 1984, pp 1–44.

Windle-Taylor P, Emery PJ, Phelps PD: Ear deformities associated with the Klippel-Feil syndrome. *Ann Otol* 90:210–216, 1981.

Winter JSD, Kohn G, Mellman WJ, et al: A familial syndrome of renal, genital and middle ear anomalies. *J Pediatr* 72:88–93, 1968.

Withrow MS: The federal role in services to hearing-impaired people. In Roeser R, Downs MP (eds): *Auditory Disorders in School Children.* New York: Thieme-Stratton, 1981.

Wolf-Schein E, Sudhalter V, Cohen I, et al: Speech-language and the fragile X syndrome: initial findings. *Asha* 29:35–38, 1987.

Woodford CM: Speech-language pathologists' knowledge and skills regarding hearing aids. *Language, Speech & Hearing Services in Schools* 18:312–322, 1987.

Woolf CM, Dolowitz DA, Aldous HE: Congenital deafness associated with piebaldness. *Arch Otolaryngol* 82:244-250, 1965.

Worthington DW, Peters JF: Quantifiable hearing and no ABR: paradox or error? *Ear Hear* 1:281–285, 1980.

Wright LB, Rybak LP: Crib-o-gram (COG) and ABR: effect of variables on test results. *J Acoust Soc Am* (suppl 1) 74:540–544, 1983.

Wright P, McConnell K, Thompson J, Vaughn W, Sells S: A longitudinal study of the detection of otitis media in the first two years of life. *Int J Pediatr Otorhinolaryngol* 10:245–252, 1985.

Yarrow LJ, Rubinstein JL, Pedersen FA, et al: Dimensions of early stimulation and their differential effects on infant development. *Merrill-Palmer J Behav Dev* 18:205–218, 1971.

Yoneshige Y, Elliott LL: Pure-tone sensitivity and ear canal pressure at threshold in children and adults. *J Acoust Soc Am* 70:1272–1276, 1981.

Yost WA, Nielsen DW: *Fundamentals of Hearing.* New York: Holt, Rinehart & Winston, 1977.

Yost WA, Nielsen DW: *Fundamentals of Hearing: An Introduction,* (ed 2). New York: Holt, Rinehart and Winston, 1985.

Young DF, Eldridge R, Gardner WJ: Bilateral acoustic neuroma in a large kindred. *JAMA* 214:347–353, 1970.

Yules RB: Hearing in cleft patients. *Arch Otolaryngol* 91:319–323, 1970.

Zack L, Kaufman J: How adequate is the concept of perceptual deficit for education. *J Learn Disabil* 5:351–356, 1972.

Zellweger H, Smith JK, Grutzner P: The Marshall syndrome; report of a new family. *J Pediatr* 84:868–871, 1974.

Zemlin WR: *Speech and Hearing Science,* ed 3. Englewood Cliffs, NJ: Prentice-Hall, 1988.

Zigler E: Developmental versus different theories in mental retardation and the problem of motivation. *Am J Ment Defic* 73:536–556, 1969.

Zigmund N: Intrasensory and intersensory processes in normal and dyslexic children. Unpublished doctoral dissertation, Northwestern University, Evanston, IL, 1966.

Zigmund N: Maturation of auditory processes in children with learning disabilities. In Tampol L (ed): *Introduction to Learning Disabilities.* Springfield, IL: Charles C Thomas, 1973.

Zink GD: Hearing aids children wear: a longitudinal study of performance. *Volta Rev* 74:41–51, 1972.

Zizz CA, Glattke TJ: Reliability of spontaneous otoacoustic emission suppression tuning curve measures. *J Speech Hear Res* 31:616–619, 1988.

Zoller MK, Ruhe DJ, Dunster JR: Tympanometry screening in developmentally delayed individuals. *J Audit Res* 25:15–25, 1985.

Zonis RD: Chronic otitis media in the Southwestern American Indian. *Arch Otolaryngol* 88:40–45, 1968.

Zurif EB, Sait PE: The laterality effect in lingual-auditory tracking. *J Acoust Soc Am* 49:1874–1880, 1970.

Zwislocki J: An acoustic method for clinical examination of the ear. *J Speech Hear Res* 6:303–314, 1963.

INDEX

411